ATLAS *of*

ENDOVASCULAR VENOUS SURGERY

SECOND EDITION

ATLAS *of* ENDOVASCULAR VENOUS SURGERY

Jose I. Almeida, MD, FACS

Founder, Miami Vein
Voluntary Professor of Surgery
Division of Vascular and Endovascular Surgery
University of Miami Miller School of Medicine
Miami, Florida

ELSEVIER

ELSEVIER

1600 John F. Kennedy Blvd.
Ste 1600
Philadelphia, PA 19103-2899

ATLAS OF ENDOVASCULAR VENOUS SURGERY, SECOND EDITION   ISBN: 978-0-323-51139-1

Previous edition copyrighted 2012.

Library of Congress Control Number: 2018949538

Content Strategist: Russell Gabbedy
Senior Content Development Specialist: Joan Ryan
Publishing Services Manager: Catherine Jackson
Senior Project Manager: Daniel Fitzgerald
Designer: Patrick Ferguson

Printed in China.

Last digit is the print number: 9 8 7 6 5 4 3 2 1

Working together
to grow libraries in
developing countries

www.elsevier.com • www.bookaid.org

To my loving wife of 25 years, Yvette Angela Almeida, who has raised our four children and managed the complex affairs of our family and my surgical practice. Without her, I would be a mess.

To my mother, Estrella Almeida, who instilled the traditional values of faith, family, and education, which I strive to maintain every day.

To my father, Jose Almeida, MD, who died on April 16, 2009. He served as the chief medical officer for the CIA-trained force of Cuban exiles whose unsuccessful attempt to overthrow the Cuban government of Fidel Castro is now known as the Bay of Pigs Invasion. After release from his 2-year incarceration as a political prisoner of Cuba, my father went on to train at the renowned Menninger School of Psychiatry in Topeka, Kansas. He practiced psychiatry in West Palm Beach, Florida, until he died at home from multiple sclerosis at the age of 75.

To the memory of Robert Zeppa, MD, Chairman of Surgery at the University of Miami–Jackson Memorial Hospital, under whom I received my general surgery residency training.

CONTRIBUTORS

Andrew M. Abi-Chaker, MD
Vascular Surgery Resident
Division of Vascular and Endovascular Surgery
University of Miami
Jackson Memorial Hospital
Miami, Florida
  Venous Diagnostic Tools
  Iliocaval and Femoral Venous Occlusive Disease

Ashley Nicole Adamovich, MD
Department of Radiology
University of South Florida
Tampa, Florida
  Endovenous Management of Central and Upper Extremity Veins

Rima Ahmad, MD
Clinical Instructor
University of Vermont College of Medicine
Burlington, Vermont
  Radiofrequency Thermal Ablation: Current Data

Jose I. Almeida, MD, FACS
Founder, Miami Vein
Voluntary Professor of Surgery
Division of Vascular and Endovascular Surgery
University of Miami Miller School of Medicine
Miami, Florida
  Venous Anatomy
  Venous Diagnostic Tools
  Endovenous Thermal Ablation of Saphenous Reflux
  Treatment of Perforating Veins
  Treatment of Varicosed Tributary Veins
  Endovenous Approach to Recurrent Varicose Veins
  Thromboembolic Disease
  Endothermal Heat-Induced Thrombosis
  Iliocaval and Femoral Venous Occlusive Disease

Guilherme Dabus, MD, FAHA
Director, Fellowship
Neuroendovascular Surgery
Miami Cardiac & Vascular Institute
Miami, Florida
  Venous Malformations

Michael C. Dalsing, MD
Professor Emeritus
Division of Vascular Surgery
Indiana University
Indianapolis, Indiana
  Deep Venous Incompetence and Valve Repair

Alan M. Dietzek, MD, RPVI, FACS
Network Chief
Vascular & Endovascular Surgery
Western Connecticut Health Network
Linda and Stephen R. Cohen Chair in Vascular Surgery
Danbury Hospital
Clinical Professor of Surgery
University of Vermont College of Medicine
Burlington, Vermont
  Radiofrequency Thermal Ablation: Current Data

Steve Elias, MD, FACS, FACPh
Director
Center for Vein Disease
Englewood Hospital and Medical Center
Englewood, New Jersey
  Nonthermal Ablation of Saphenous Reflux

Mark J. Garcia, MD, MS, FSIR, FACR
Founder and Medical Director
EndoVascular Consultants
Wilmington, Delaware
  Pharmacomechanical Thrombolysis

Monika Lecomte Gloviczki, MD, PhD
Research Fellow, Emeritus
Department of Internal Medicine and the Gonda Vascular
Center
Mayo Clinic
Rochester, Minnesota
  Evidence-Based Summary of Guidelines From the Society for
  Vascular Surgery and the American Venous Forum

Peter Gloviczki, MD, FACS
Joe M. and Ruth Roberts Professor and Chair, Emeritus
Division of Vascular and Endovascular Surgery
Mayo Clinic
Rochester, Minnesota
  Pelvic Venous Disorders
  Nutcracker Syndrome
  Evidence-Based Summary of Guidelines From the Society for
  Vascular Surgery and the American Venous Forum

Issam Kably, MD
Assistant Professor
Vascular and Interventional Radiology
University of Miami Miller School of Medicine
Miami, Florida
  New Concepts in the Management of Pulmonary Embolus

Lowell S. Kabnick, MD
Associate Professor
Department of Surgery
Director of NYU Vein Center
New York University Langone Health
New York, New York
Laser Thermal Ablation: Current Data
Endothermal Heat-Induced Thrombosis

Manju Kalra, MBBS
Professor
Vascular and Endovascular Surgery
Mayo Clinic
Rochester, Minnesota
Nutcracker Syndrome

Robert L. Kistner, MD
Clinical Professor of Surgery
University of Hawaii
Honolulu, Hawaii
Deep Venous Incompetence and Valve Repair

Nicos Labropoulos, PhD, DIC, RVT
Professor of Surgery
Department of Surgery
Division of Vascular Surgery
Stony Brook University Medical Center
Stony Brook, New York
Venous Pathophysiology
Postthrombotic Syndrome

Timothy K. Liem, MD, MBA
Professor of Surgery
Knight Cardiovascular Institute
Oregon Health & Science University
Portland, Oregon
Thromboembolic Disease
Endovenous Placement of Inferior Vena Caval Filters

Edward G. Mackay, MD
Private Practice
Palm Harbor, Florida
Treatment of Spider Telangiectasias

Rafael D. Malgor, MD, FACS
Assistant Professor of Surgery
Eastern Virginia Medical School
Norfolk, Virginia
Venous Pathophysiology
Postthrombotic Syndrome

William Marston, MD
Chief
Division of Vascular Surgery
Professor
Department of Surgery
University of North Carolina School of Medicine
Chapel Hill, North Carolina
Venous Ulcers

Mark H. Meissner, MD, FACS
Professor of Venous and Lymphatic Disorders
Division of Vascular and Endovascular Surgery
University of Washington
Seattle, Washington
Pelvic Venous Disorders
Evidence-Based Summary of Guidelines From the Society for Vascular Surgery and the American Venous Forum

Marc A. Passman, MD
Professor
Division of Vascular Surgery and Endovascular Therapy
Department of Surgery
University of Alabama at Birmingham
Birmingham, Alabama
Severity Scoring and Outcomes Measurement

Constantino S. Peña, MD
Assistant Professor
Department of Radiology
University of South Florida
Tampa, Florida
Medical Director of Vascular Imaging
Baptist Cardiac and Vascular Institute
Miami, Florida
Endovenous Management of Central and Upper Extremity Veins
Venous Malformations

Seshadri Raju, MD, FACS
Vascular Surgeon
The Rane Center
Jackson, Mississippi
Venous Hemodynamics

Michele N. Richard, MD
Clinical Instructor
University of Vermont College of Medicine
Burlington, Vermont
Radiofrequency Thermal Ablation: Current Data

Mikel Sadek, MD
Assistant Professor
Department of Surgery
Chief
Vascular Surgery
Bellevue Hospital
New York University Langone Health
New York, New York
Laser Thermal Ablation: Current Data
Endothermal Heat-Induced Thrombosis

Jason Thomas Salsamendi, MD
Associate Professor
Vascular and Interventional Radiology
University of Miami Miller School of Medicine
Miami, Florida
New Concepts in the Management of Pulmonary Embolus

Priscila Gisselle Sanchez Aguirre, MD
Division of Vascular and Endovascular Surgery
Leonard M. Miller School of Medicine
University of Miami
Miami, Florida
Venous Diagnostic Tools
Iliocaval and Femoral Venous Occlusive Disease

Jan M. Sloves, RVT, RCS, FASE
Technical Director of Vascular Imaging
Mount Sinai Beth Israel-Mount Sinai Health System
New York, New York
Venous Diagnostic Tools

FOREWORD

Advances in the field of endovascular venous surgery created the stimulus for a second edition of this material under the editorship of Jose Almeida following the enthusiastic reception of the first edition in 2011. This field is undergoing rapid development in breadth and depth for both diagnosis and treatment of venous disease. These changes include new techniques and refinements of established procedures that are best expressed by the visual display afforded in the atlas format. The presentations allow the practitioner to grasp subtleties that are often poorly appreciated through descriptive formats limited to the written word.

The need for this atlas presentation is dictated by the requirement for accuracy in transmitting critical details of technique that are best understood by a visual presentation to supplement the written word. Just as we understand that the training of the surgeon requires clinical experience in addition to academic understanding, so there is the need for visual understanding of the technical steps that are the key to performing successful procedures in open and minimally invasive endovascular surgery. The strength of the atlas is that it displays technical procedures in visual steps, and in many instances there are videos with audio to link the key steps into a full presentation of the procedure. The picture supplemented by the written explanation provides the nearest thing to the real-time experience of watching or participating in a technical operation.

Dr. Almeida has chosen recognized experts to join him in detailing the intricacies of successful technique in the various fields of endovascular procedures. The range of subjects covers the active endovascular field at this time, making it safe to predict this atlas will address a basic need for those who are working in the endovascular field.

Robert L. Kistner, MD

PREFACE

This book was conceived as a well-illustrated technical guide for the endovascular surgical management of venous diseases. This second edition of the *Atlas of Endovascular Venous Surgery* builds on the first edition; it remains a text atlas, but I hope that it will eventually grow into an authoritative reference for venous disease. Currently, the best evidence-based reference of venous disorders is the *Handbook of Venous Disorders: Guidelines of the American Venous Forum,* edited by Peter Gloviczki, MD. This second edition of the *Atlas of Endovascular Venous Surgery* should serve as a nice companion to the *Handbook of Venous Disorders* because it beautifully illustrates the technical aspects of endovenous vascular surgery through full-color illustrations, photographs, and radiologic (ultrasound, fluoroscopy, contrast venography, and cross-sectional) images. We are pleased that the current book is bundled as a print and Web version. It also contains video presentations.

This second edition includes five brand new chapters covering venous hemodynamics, new concepts in the management of pulmonary embolus, endothermal heat-induced thrombosis, deep venous incompetence and valve repair, and nutcracker syndrome. It features significant updates throughout, including new devices in the management of thromboembolic disease, aggressive techniques for recanalizing iliofemoral venous occlusions, new nomenclature and endovascular approach to the treatment of pelvic venous disorders, new nonthermal devices for saphenous vein ablation, new stents for treatment of iliac vein obstruction, new devices for clot management, and endovascular and open repair of deep vein obstruction and reflux.

All this work would not have been possible without the excellent contributions of the coauthors—all world-renowned experts—who prepared many of the chapters that make up this book.

A special recognition goes to the beautiful artistic renderings prepared by Tiffany Davanzo. Her illustrations really make the technical details of the procedures self-explanatory.

Finally, we appreciate the assistance of many individuals at Elsevier, especially Joan Ryan the Senior Content Development Specialist. Their efforts, combined with those of many other copyeditors, artists, and printers, helped to assemble this final product.

Jose I. Almeida, MD, FACS

CONTENTS

VIDEO CONTENTS

ATLAS *of*

ENDOVASCULAR VENOUS SURGERY

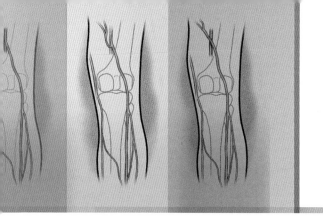

Venous Anatomy

Jose I. Almeida

HISTORICAL BACKGROUND

Chronic venous diseases include a spectrum of clinical findings ranging from spider telangiectasias and varicose veins to debilitating venous ulceration. Varicose veins without skin changes are present in about 20% of the general population, and they are slightly more frequent in women.

References to varicose veins are found in early Egyptian and Greek writings and confirm that venous disease was recognized in ancient times. A votive tablet in the National Museum in Athens showing a man holding an enlarged leg with a varicose vein is frequently featured in many historical writings regarding venous disease.

The venous system originates at the capillary level and progressively increases in size as the conduits move proximally toward the heart. The venules are the smallest structures, and the vena cava is the largest. It is critical that all endovascular venous surgeons understand the anatomic relationships between the thoracic, abdominal, and extremity venous systems, especially from the anatomic standpoint (Fig. 1.1). Veins of the lower extremities are the most germane to this book and are divided into three systems: deep, superficial, and perforating. Lower extremity veins are located in two compartments: deep and superficial. The deep compartment is bounded by the muscular fascia. The superficial compartment is bounded below by the muscular fascia and above by the dermis. The term *perforating veins* is reserved for veins that perforate the muscular fascia and connect superficial veins with deep veins. The term *communicating veins* is used to describe veins that connect with other veins of the same compartment.

The vein wall is composed of three layers: intima, media, and adventitia. Notably, the muscular tunica media is much thinner in a vein than in a pressurized artery. Venous valves are an extension of the intimal layer, have a bicuspid structure, and support unidirectional flow (Fig. 1.2).

VENOUS SYSTEM OVERVIEW

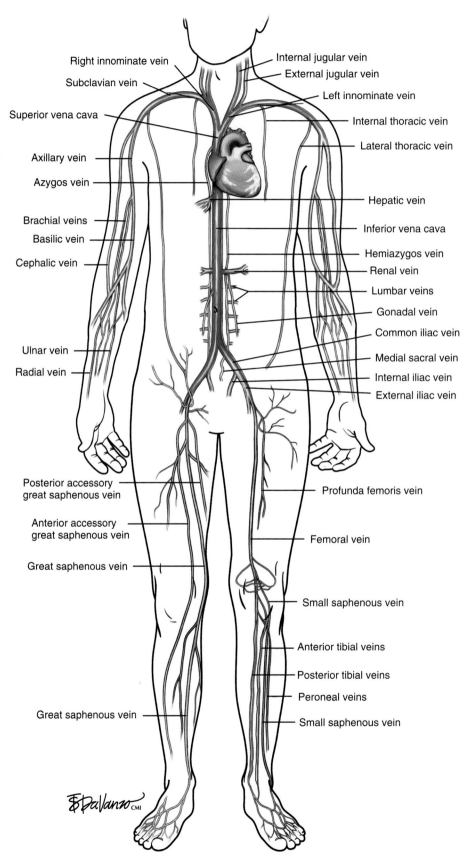

Right innominate vein

Subclavian vein

Superior vena cava

Axillary vein

Azygos vein

Brachial veins

Basilic vein

Cephalic vein

Ulnar vein

Radial vein

Posterior accessory
great saphenous vein

Anterior accessory
great saphenous vein

Great saphenous vein

Great saphenous vein

Internal jugular vein

External jugular vein

Left innominate vein

Internal thoracic vein

Lateral thoracic vein

Hepatic vein

Inferior vena cava

Hemiazygos vein

Renal vein

Lumbar veins

Gonadal vein

Common iliac vein

Medial sacral vein

Internal iliac vein

External iliac vein

Profunda femoris vein

Femoral vein

Small saphenous vein

Anterior tibial veins

Posterior tibial veins

Peroneal veins

Small saphenous vein

■ Fig. 1.1

VENOUS STRUCTURE

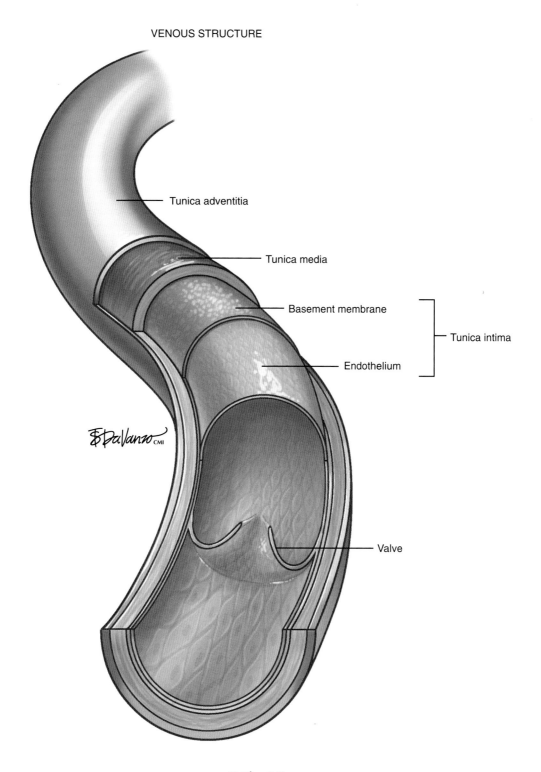

■ **Fig. 1.2**

Surgeons who perform thermal or chemical ablation therapy of the great saphenous vein (GSV) and its related structures must have a good understanding of the saphenous canal. The importance of the saphenous canal in relation to B-mode ultrasound anatomy is detailed in Chapter 4. A cross section of the saphenous canal (Fig. 1.3) depicts many of the critical relationships referable to GSV treatment; the most important is how it courses atop the muscular fascia in a quasi-envelope called the *saphenous fascia*. The saphenous fascia is the portion of the membranous layer of the subcutaneous tissue that overlies the saphenous veins. Veins coursing parallel to the saphenous canal are termed *accessory veins*; those coursing oblique to the canal are called *circumflex veins*. Compressible structures superficial to the muscular fascia are potential targets for treatment, but treating those structures deep to the muscular fascia may lead to a disastrous outcome. Noncompressible structures generally represent major arteries. Perforating veins must pierce the muscular fascia as they drain blood from the superficial to deep systems.

As diagnostic and therapeutic options for venous disorders expanded, the nomenclature proposed in 2002 by the International Interdisciplinary Committee[1] required revision. The nomenclature was extended and further refined,[2] taking into account recent improvements in ultrasound and clinical surgical anatomy. The term *great saphenous vein* should be used instead of terms such as *long saphenous vein, greater saphenous vein,* or *internal saphenous vein*. The LSV abbreviation, used to describe both the *long saphenous vein* and *lesser saphenous vein*, was clearly problematic. For this reason, these terms have been eliminated. Similarly, the term *small saphenous vein*, abbreviated as SSV, should be used instead of the terms *short, external,* or *lesser saphenous vein.*

The GSV originates at the medial foot and receives deep pedal tributaries as it courses to the medial malleolus. From the medial ankle, the GSV ascends anteromedially within the calf and continues a medial course to the knee and into the thigh. The termination point of the GSV into the common femoral vein is a confluence called the *saphenofemoral junction* (SFJ) (Fig. 1.4).

SAPHENOUS CANAL CROSS SECTION

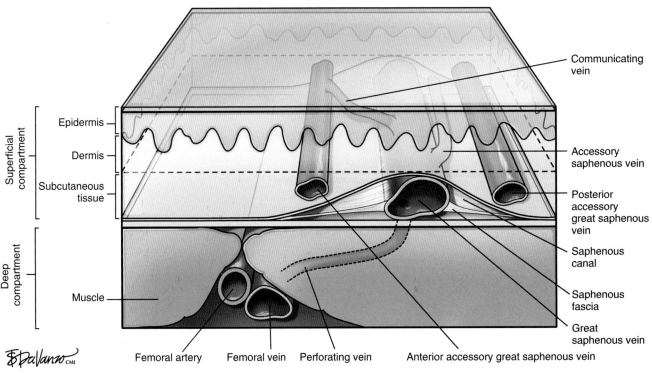

■ Fig. 1.3

SUPERFICIAL VENOUS ANATOMY (ANTERIOR)

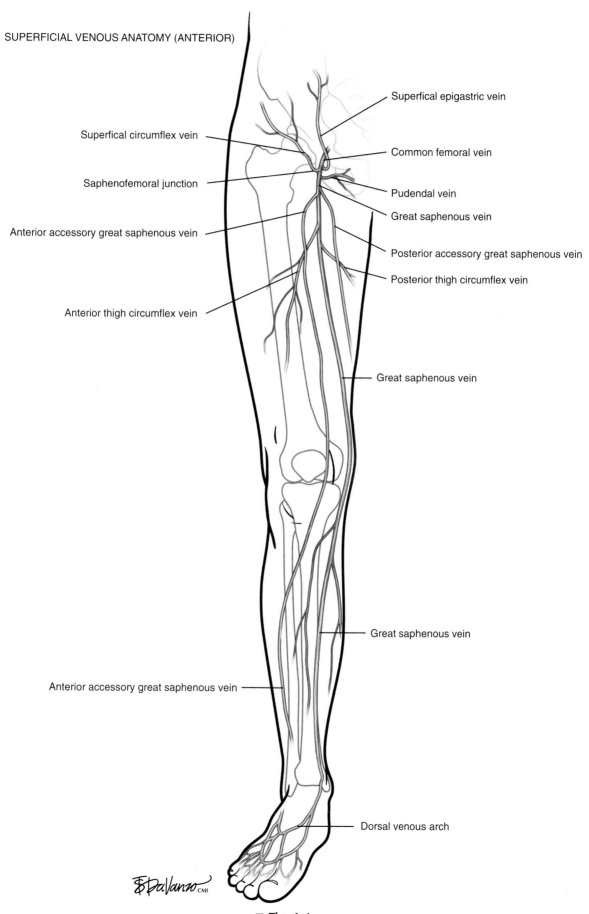

Superfical epigastric vein

Superfical circumflex vein

Common femoral vein

Saphenofemoral junction

Pudendal vein

Great saphenous vein

Anterior accessory great saphenous vein

Posterior accessory great saphenous vein

Posterior thigh circumflex vein

Anterior thigh circumflex vein

Great saphenous vein

Great saphenous vein

Anterior accessory great saphenous vein

Dorsal venous arch

■ **Fig. 1.4**

The terminal valve of the GSV is located within the junction itself. A subterminal valve can often be identified approximately 1 cm distal to the terminal valve. From the upper calf to the groin, the GSV is usually contained within the saphenous compartment. Visualization of this fascial envelope is an important landmark in identifying the GSV with duplex ultrasound. The saphenous compartment is bounded superficially by a hyperechoic saphenous fascia and deeply by the muscular fascia of the limb.

At the groin, the GSV drains blood from the external pudendal, superficial epigastric, and external circumflex iliac veins just before it enters the common femoral vein confluence. As in all human anatomy, variations are crucial to recognize, to guide the correct diagnosis and treatment. Historically, the GSV has been reported to be duplicated in the thigh in as many as 20% of subjects. However, recent examinations have demonstrated that true duplication, with two veins within one saphenous compartment, occurs in less than 1% of cases. Large extrafascial veins, which are termed *accessory saphenous veins*, can run parallel to the GSV and take on the characteristics of duplicated veins.

The accessory saphenous veins are venous segments that ascend in a plane parallel to the saphenous veins. They may be anterior, posterior, or superficial to the main trunk. (A A G S V) The term *anterior accessory great saphenous vein* describes any venous segment ascending parallel to the GSV and located anteriorly, both in the leg and in the thigh. The term *posterior accessory great saphenous vein* (PAGSV) is consistent with any venous segment ascending parallel to the GSV and located posteriorly, both in the leg and in the thigh. The leg segment corresponds to the popular terms *Leonardo's vein* or *posterior arch vein*. The term *superficial accessory great saphenous vein* is considered to be any venous segment ascending parallel to the GSV and located just superficial to the saphenous fascia, both in the leg and in the thigh.

Circumflex veins, by definition, drain into the GSV from an oblique direction. The posterior thigh circumflex vein is present in virtually every case; however, the anterior thigh circumflex vein is less common.

The SSV originates in the lateral foot and passes posterolaterally in the lower calf. The SSV lies above the deep fascia in the midline as it reaches the upper calf, where it pierces the two heads of the gastrocnemius muscle and courses cephalad until it enters the popliteal space. In approximately two-thirds of patients, the SSV drains entirely into the popliteal vein just above the knee at the saphenopopliteal junction (SPJ). In as many as one-third of patients, the cranial extension of the SSV drains into a posterior medial tributary of the GSV or directly into the GSV (vein of Giacomini) or into the femoral vein via a thigh perforating vein.

In variant drainage, a standard SPJ may or may not be present. The SSV is truly duplicated in 4% of cases; most often, this is segmental and primarily involves the midportion of the vein (Fig. 1.5).

SUPERFICIAL VENOUS ANATOMY (POSTERIOR)

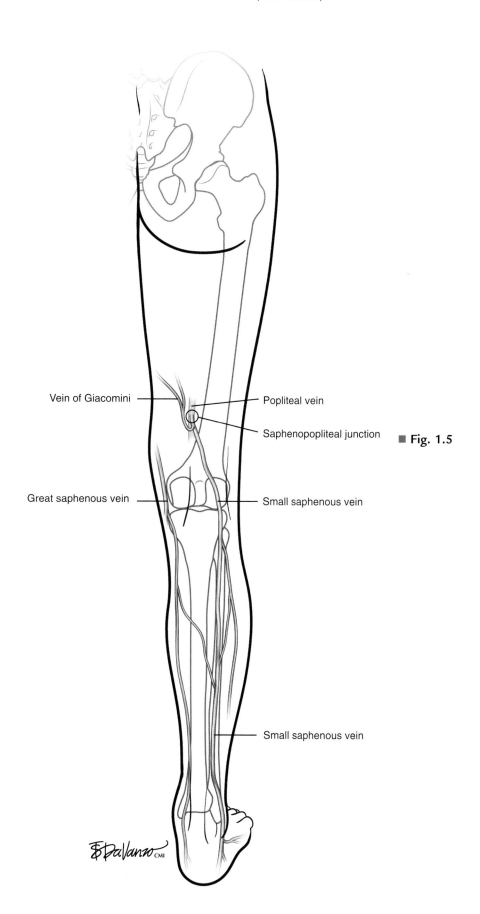

Vein of Giacomini

Popliteal vein

Saphenopopliteal junction

■ **Fig. 1.5**

Great saphenous vein

Small saphenous vein

Small saphenous vein

PERFORATING VEINS

Identifying perforating veins based on the original descriptions of investigators (i.e., Cockett, Sherman, Dodd) is falling into disfavor. Descriptive terms based on topography, which designate the anatomic location, have become the contemporary approach. Perforating veins pass through defects in the deep fascia to connect deep and superficial veins of the calf or thigh. Venous valves prevent reflux of blood from the deep veins into the superficial system. Perforating veins may connect the GSV to the deep system at the femoral, posterior tibial, gastrocnemius, and soleal vein levels. Located between the ankle and the knee are perforating veins, formerly known as Cockett perforators, that connect the posterior tibial venous system with the PAGSV of the calf (also known as the posterior arch vein) (Fig. 1.6).

PERFORATING VEINS

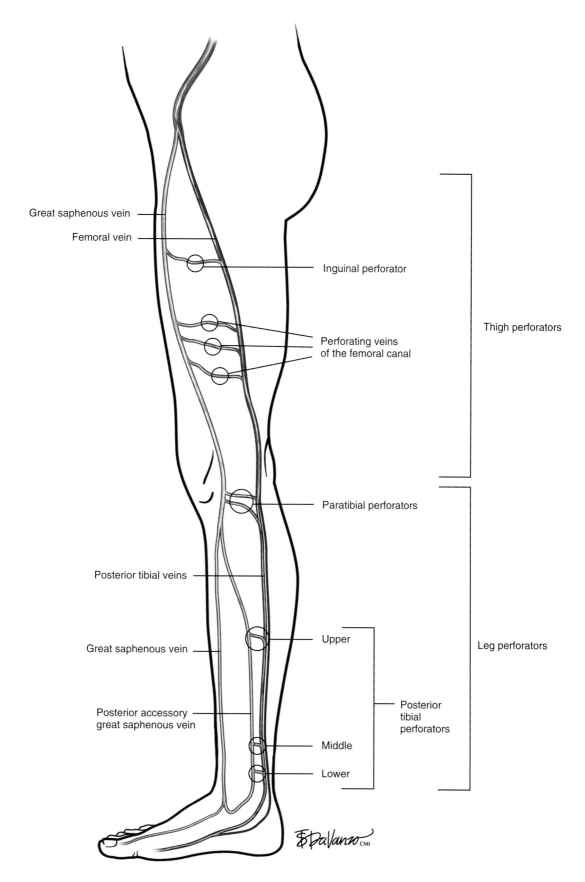

Great saphenous vein

Femoral vein

Inguinal perforator

Perforating veins
of the femoral canal

Thigh perforators

Paratibial perforators

Posterior tibial veins

Great saphenous vein

Upper

Posterior accessory
great saphenous vein

Posterior
tibial
perforators

Leg perforators

Middle

Lower

■ Fig. 1.6

Deep Veins

Below the knee, there are six named axial veins that are generally paired and are located on either side of a corresponding named artery. The names of the three pairs of deep veins in the leg are the anterior tibial, posterior tibial, and peroneal veins. In addition, venous sinusoids within the deep calf muscle coalesce to form the nonaxial soleal and gastrocnemius venous plexi, which ultimately drain into the peroneal veins at the level of the midcalf. In the lower popliteal space, the anterior and posterior tibial veins join with the peroneal veins to become the popliteal vein.

At the upper margin of the popliteal fossa, above the adductor canal, the femoral vein originates from the popliteal vein. The "superficial femoral vein" terminology was clearly problematic and has been abandoned because the femoral vein is a deep structure. The deep femoral vein (profunda femoris) drains the deep muscles of the lateral thigh, communicates with the popliteal vein, and serves as a critical collateral vessel in cases where the femoral vein occludes with thrombus. The common femoral vein runs from the confluence of the femoral vein and the deep femoral vein to the external iliac vein at the level of the inguinal ligament (Figs. 1.7 and 1.8).

Above the inguinal ligament, the external iliac vein represents the final common pathway of lower extremity venous drainage. The external iliac vein is joined by the internal iliac vein (hypogastric), which drains pelvic blood to form the common iliac vein. The union of the right and left common iliac veins forms the inferior vena cava (IVC) at about the level of the fourth lumbar vertebrae.

The IVC continues the journey in a cephalad direction as it leaves the pelvis, enters the abdomen, and terminates in the thoracic cavity. In the abdomen, the IVC picks up paired lumbar veins, the right gonadal vein, the right and left renal veins, and the entire hepatic venous drainage (right, middle, and left hepatics). The IVC is joined by the superior vena cava (SVC), the azygos vein, and the coronary sinus as all four structures empty into the right atrium of the heart.

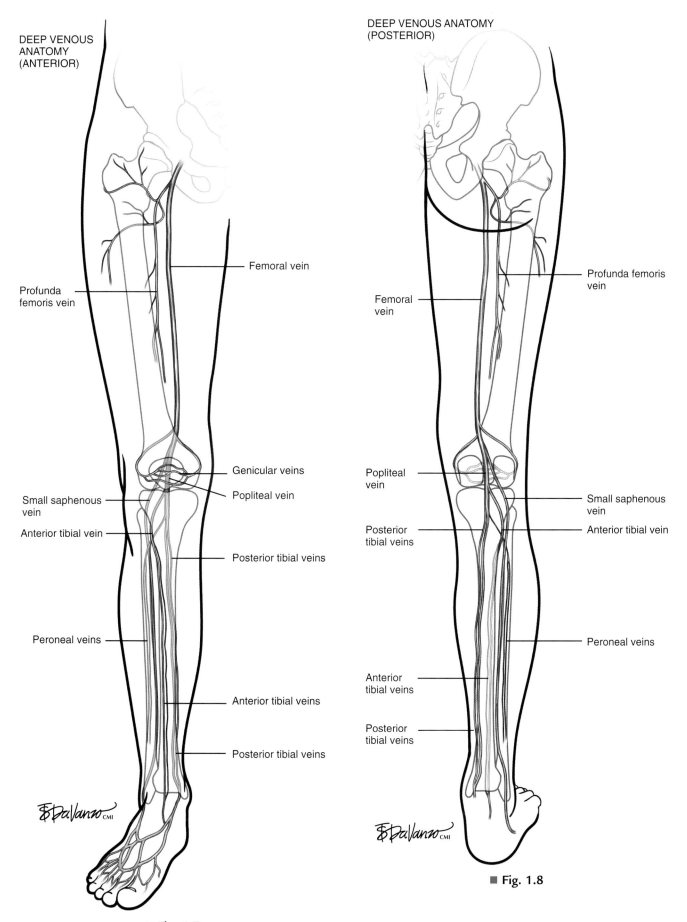

DEEP VENOUS
ANATOMY
(ANTERIOR)

Profunda
femoris vein

Femoral vein

Genicular veins

Popliteal vein

Small saphenous
vein

Anterior tibial vein

Posterior tibial veins

Peroneal veins

Anterior tibial veins

Posterior tibial veins

■ Fig. 1.7

DEEP VENOUS ANATOMY
(POSTERIOR)

Femoral
vein

Profunda femoris
vein

Popliteal
vein

Small saphenous
vein

Posterior
tibial veins

Anterior tibial vein

Anterior
tibial veins

Peroneal veins

Posterior
tibial veins

■ Fig. 1.8

Upper Extremity Veins

Venous blood from the hand drains into the forearm via the deep radial and ulnar veins and the superficial cephalic and basilic veins. In the upper arm, deep drainage from the paired brachial veins enters the axillary vein at the shoulder. The axillary vein also drains the superficial tissues via the cephalic vein (which enters the deltopectoral groove) and the basilic veins of the medial arm. The subclavian vein is protected by the clavicle as it carries upper extremity blood from the axillary vein. The subclavian vein then picks up drainage from the head and neck via the jugular veins and ultimately empties into the innominate veins of the thoracic cavity. Right and left innominate veins drain into the SVC and enter the right atrium of the heart. The SVC also receives venous blood from the azygos system, which drains the thoracic cage via intercostal veins and ultimately enters the SVC (Fig. 1.9).

UPPER EXTREMITY VENOUS ANATOMY

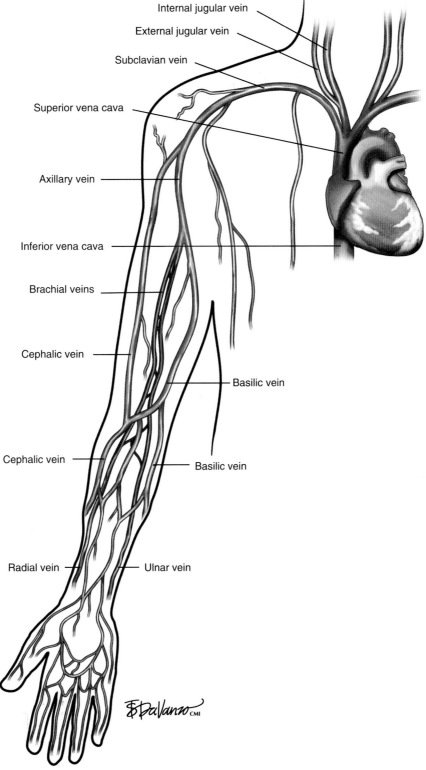

■ **Fig. 1.9**

Lower Extremity Nerves

The posterior division of the femoral nerve provides sensory fibers to the inner surface of the leg (saphenous nerve), to the quadriceps muscles (muscular branches), and to the hip and knee joints. The saphenous nerve descends beneath the sartorius muscle, winding around its posterior edge and exiting at the adductor canal. The infrapatellar branch pierces the sartorius muscle and courses anteriorly to the infrapatellar region. The descending branch passes down the medial aspect of the leg juxtaposed to the great saphenous vein and here is at highest risk for injury from thermal ablation procedures. At the lower third of the leg, it divides into two branches: one of the branches of the descending portion of the saphenous nerve courses along the medial border of the tibia and ends at the ankle, whereas the other branch passes anterior to the ankle and is distributed to the medial aspect of the foot, sometimes reaching as far as the metatarsophalangeal joint of the great toe (Fig. 1.10).

NERVES OF THE LEG (ANTERIOR)

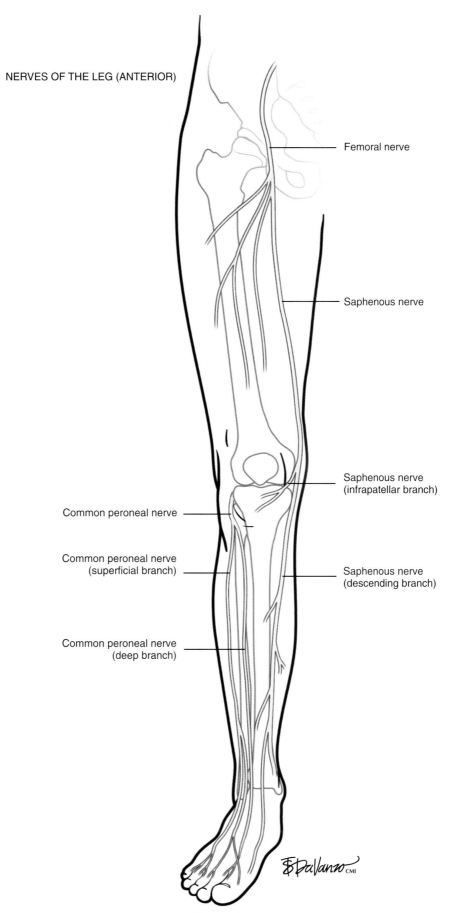

Femoral nerve

Saphenous nerve

Saphenous nerve
(infrapatellar branch)

Common peroneal nerve

Common peroneal nerve
(superficial branch)

Saphenous nerve
(descending branch)

Common peroneal nerve
(deep branch)

■ Fig. 1.10

The most interesting issue referable to surgical work in the popliteal space is clearly the neuroanatomy. The sciatic nerve descends the posterior thigh and divides into the tibial and common peroneal nerves in the popliteal area (Fig. 1.11). The exact location of this division can range several centimeters proximally or several centimeters distally. The tibial nerve continues its descent to the ankle, and its innervation mostly affects motor function. The common peroneal nerve, however, divides near the zone of the head of the fibula, into deep and superficial branches. The common peroneal nerve courses anteriorly around the fibula, taking a sharp turn as it rounds the fibular neck to enter the anterior compartment. Because of the sharp turn, the nerve is more tethered than the superficial branch; immediately below the fibular head, the deep peroneal nerve lies on the anterior cortex of the fibula for a distance of 3 to 4 cm. The deep peroneal nerve innervates the dorsiflexors of the leg and, when injured, results in the dramatic foot drop. The tissues innervated by the superficial peroneal nerve provide only sensory information for interpretation in the brain.

There is a natural flare at the midcalf level where the inferior border of the medial and lateral heads of the gastrocnemius muscles is located. The sural nerve is a sensory nerve, which innervates the skin of the posterolateral aspect of the distal third of leg, the lateral malleolus, along the lateral side of the foot and little toe.

The sural nerve is formed by the union of the medial sural cutaneous nerve (MSCN) and the lateral sural cutaneous nerve (LSCN). When viewed from the posterior position, the sural nerve is arranged like the letter "Y" in most persons. The MSCN is a branch of the tibial nerve, and the LSCN originates from the common peroneal nerve. The site of union is usually in the lower third of the leg or just below the ankle.[3] The SSV travels in proximity to the sural nerve in the lower leg, where the nerve is joined at the midline. Where the gastrocnemius muscle bellies become prominent in the upper calf, the sural nerve is separated into the MSCN and LSCN. Therefore the SSV in the upper calf is distanced from the sural nerve, making this segment safer for thermal ablation.

NERVES OF THE LEG (POSTERIOR)

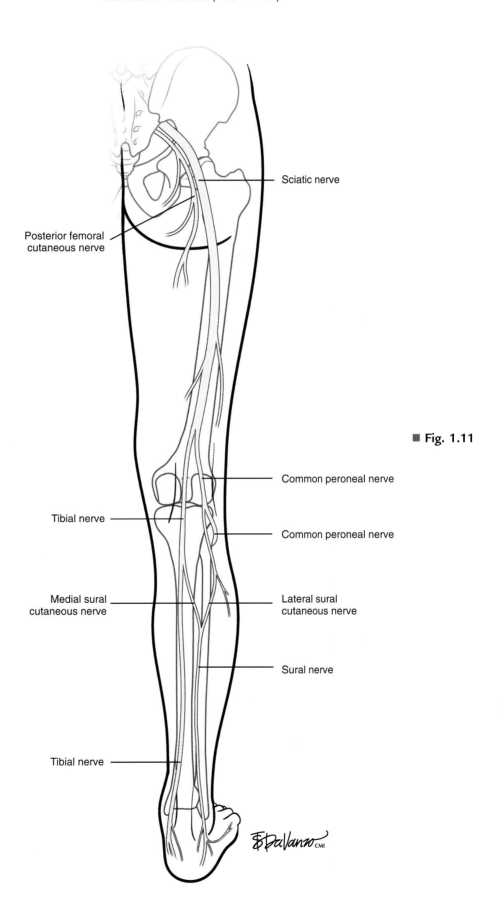

■ **Fig. 1.11**

Sciatic nerve

Posterior femoral
cutaneous nerve

Common peroneal nerve

Tibial nerve

Common peroneal nerve

Medial sural
cutaneous nerve

Lateral sural
cutaneous nerve

Sural nerve

Tibial nerve

As stated earlier, B-mode ultrasound has made it possible to develop an accurate diagnosis and treatment plan for patients with venous disease. The main reference point of the ultrasound examination is at the inguinal crease where the GSV empties into the common femoral vein. In the first cross section of Fig. 1.12, one can study the saphenofemoral junction as it looks using B-mode (gray scale) ultrasound.

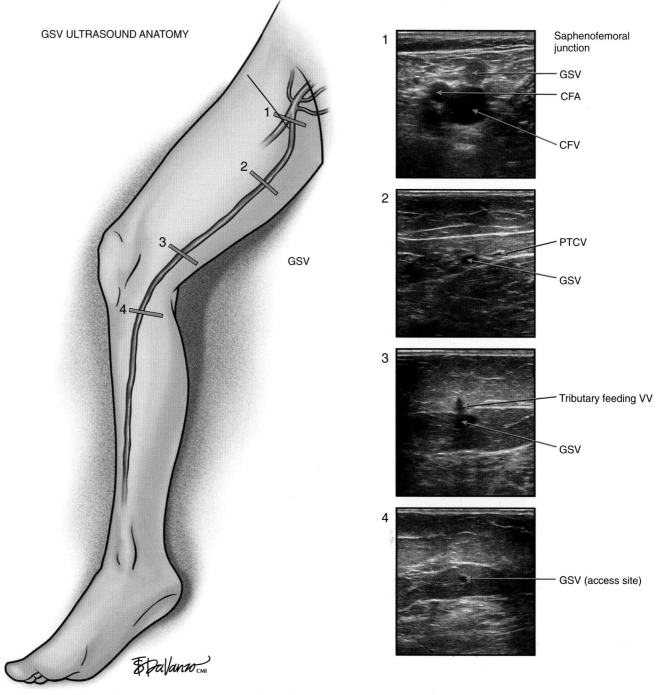

■ **Fig. 1.12** *CFA,* Common femoral artery; *CFV,* common femoral vein; *GSV,* great saphenous vein; *PTCV,* posterior thigh circumflex vein; *VV,* veins.

ETIOLOGY AND NATURAL HISTORY OF DISEASE

Early theories were based on the belief that varicose veins resulted from the effects of venous hypertension secondary to valvular incompetence at the saphenofemoral or saphenopopliteal junction, resulting in retrograde flow of blood down a hydrostatic pressure gradient. Unfortunately, there is little evidence of a constitutive valvular abnormality in primary venous disease. The theories do not explain why truncal varicosities are often found below competent valves, why normal valves are often seen between variceal segments, or why venous dilation often precedes valvular incompetence.[4,5] Rather than being initiated at the saphenofemoral junction, both detailed studies of surgical specimens and ultrasound observation suggest that primary valvular incompetence is a multicentric process that develops simultaneously in discontinuous venous segments.[6]

Histologic and ultrastructural studies of varicose saphenous veins have found hypertrophy of the vein wall with increased collagen content,[7] together with disruption of the orderly arrangements of smooth muscle cells and elastin fibers.[8,9] Cultures of smooth muscle cells from varicose saphenous veins have demonstrated disturbed collagen synthesis, overproduction of collagen type I, and reduced synthesis of collagen type III.[10] Because collagen type I is thought to confer rigidity and collagen type III to confer distensibility to tissues, such changes could contribute to the weakness and reduced elasticity of varicose veins. A complicating factor is the heterogeneity of the varicose vein wall; hypertrophic segments can alternate with thinner atrophic segments with fewer smooth muscle cells and reduced extracellular matrix.

Despite advances in our understanding of varicose veins, the underlying etiology remains elusive. Varicose veins demonstrate diverse histologic abnormalities, including irregular thickening of the intima, fibrosis between the intima and adventitia, atrophy and disruption of elastic fibers, thickening of individual collagen fibers, and disorganization of the muscular layers in varicosed tributaries.[11–15] Varicose veins have increased collagen with a decrease in smooth muscle and elastin content.[16,17] Most recent evidence suggests that such changes in the vein wall precede the development of reflux.[18,19] The exact cause of primary valvular incompetence in superficial veins remains unknown. However, valvular incompetence is thought to result as a phenomenon secondary to dilatation of weakened vein walls, with enlargement of the valve ring preventing adaptation of the leaflets.[17] Interestingly, studies suggest the strength of the valves is far greater than the strength of the venous wall.[19]

PEARLS AND PITFALLS

Successful treatment is predicated on an accurate diagnosis. In the field of endovascular venous surgery, the key to diagnostic accuracy is a thorough understanding of venous anatomy.

REFERENCES

1. Caggiati A, Bergan JJ, Gloviczki P, et al. International Interdisciplinary Consensus Committee on Venous Anatomical Terminology. Nomenclature of the veins of the lower limbs: an international interdisciplinary consensus statement. *J Vasc Surg.* 2002;36:416–422.

2. Caggiati A, Bergan JJ, Gloviczki P, et al. Nomenclature of the veins of the lower limb: extensions, refinements, and clinical application. *J Vasc Surg.* 2005;41:719–724.

3. Mahakkanukrauh P, Chomsung R. Anatomical variations of the sural nerve. *Clin Anat.* 2002;15:263–266.

4. Alexander CJ. The theoretical basis of varicose vein formation. *Med J Aust.* 1972;1:258–261.

5. Cotton LT. Varicose veins. Gross anatomy and development. *Br J Surg.* 1961;48:589–597.

6. Labropoulos N, Giannoukas AD, Delis K, et al. Where does venous reflux start? *J Vasc Surg.* 1997;26:736–742.

7. Travers JP, Brookes CE, Evans J, et al. Assessment of wall structure and composition of varicose veins with reference to collagen, elastin and smooth muscle content. *Eur J Vasc Endovasc Surg.* 1996;11:230–237.

8. Porto LC, Ferreira MA, Costa AM, et al. Immunolabeling of type IV collagen, laminin, and alpha-smooth muscle actin cells in the intima of normal and varicose saphenous veins. *Angiology.* 1998;49:391–398.

9. Wali MA, Eid RA. Changes of elastic and collagen fibers in varicose veins. *Int Angiol.* 2002;21:337–343.

10. Sansilvestri-Morel P, Rupin A, Badier-Commander C, et al. Imbalance in the synthesis of collagen type I and collagen type III in smooth muscle cells derived from human varicose veins. *J Vasc Res.* 2001;38:560–568.

11. Ascher E, Jacob T, Hingorani A, et al. Expression of molecular mediators of apoptosis and their role in the pathogenesis of lower-extremity varicose veins. *J Vasc Surg.* 2001;33:1080–1086.

12. Bouissou H, Julian M, Pieraggi MT, et al. Vein morphology. *Phlebology.* 1988;3(suppl 1):1–11.

13. Jones GT, Solomon C, Moaveni A, et al. Venous morphology predicts class of chronic venous insufficiency. *Eur J Vasc Endovasc Surg.* 1999;18:349–354.

14. Lowell RC, Gloviczki P, Miller VM. In vitro evaluation of endothelial and smooth muscle function of primary varicose veins. *J Vasc Surg.* 1992;16:679–686.

15. Porto LC, Azizi MA, Pelajo-Machado M, et al. Elastic fibers in saphenous varicose veins. *Angiology.* 2002;53:131–140.

16. Travers JP, Brookes CE, Evans J, et al. Assessment of wall structure and composition of varicose veins with reference to collagen, elastin and smooth muscle content. *Eur J Vasc Endovasc Surg.* 1996;11:230–237.

17. Gandhi RH, Irizarry E, Nackman GB, et al. Analysis of the connective tissue matrix and proteolytic activity of primary varicose veins. *J Vasc Surg.* 1993;18:814–820.

18. Rose SS, Ahmed A. Some thoughts on the aetiology of varicose veins. *J Cardiovasc Surg (Torino).* 1986;27:534–543.

19. Cotton LT. Varicose veins. Gross anatomy and development. *Br J Surg.* 1961;48:589–597.

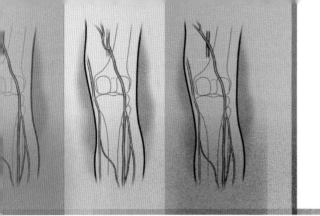

CHAPTER 2

Venous Hemodynamics

Seshadri Raju

VOLUME-PRESSURE CURVE

The volume-pressure (V-P) curve is central to venous hemodynamics. Its effect is manifest in many aspects of venous function. Because veins are thin-walled collapsible tubes, the V-P curve is governed by the *Tube law,* which is displayed in Fig. 2.1.[1] The curve is sigmoid. The functionally relevant parts are the horizontal and terminal vertical limbs in the physiologic pressure range of 5 to 15 mm Hg. The curve is remarkable for its asynchronous nature. The horizontal portion is called the *"bending"* regimen during which a large volume (≈ 80% of total) accumulates with little increase in transmural pressure. During this phase, the vein simply "uncollapses" with movement of the wall (bending) without a perimeter increase. Beyond this point, there is stretching of the vein wall ("stretching" regimen), which increases the perimeter of the venous tube. A sharp increase in the transmural pressure is noted during this regimen, yielding the terminal vertical component of the curve. This portion represents most of the pressure, but only around 20% of the venous volume. This remarkable property permits the storage function of the veins where 70% of the total blood volume resides. Large volumes can be accommodated with considerable flux with little expenditure of energy (pressure). Another example of the utility of this property is shown in Fig. 2.2. A valve station is shown with a valve refluxing into the segment below. The pressure in the infravalvular segment will remain low until 70% to 80% of its capacity is filled by reflux. Only then will there be a pressure rise, a central cause of chronic venous disease (CVD). Without this pressure buffering "shocks," pressure rise will occur sooner and steeper, causing reverberating fluid waves (water hammer) that will be more damaging. Decreased compliance of the infravalvular segment results in the dramatic shortening of pressure recovery times, more so than reflux itself in experimental set-ups.[2,3]

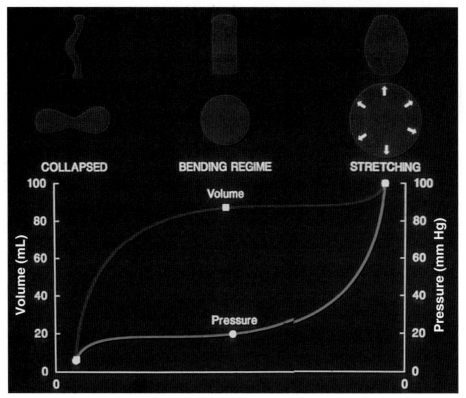

■ **Fig. 2.1** Tube law: asynchronous volume pressure relationship.

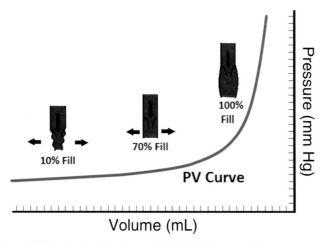

■ **Fig. 2.2** Natural shocks in the lower limb. Volume and accompanying pressure changes in the segment below a refluxing valve are shown.

Venous drainage from the various microvascular beds will be the best during the bending regimen when the venous pressure is the lowest, maximizing the drainage gradient. Nature has provided the abdominal and calf pumps to periodically collapse the major collecting veins into the bending regimen. Venous drainage in the upper body is increased during phases of increased negative pressure with inspiration.

Effect of Poor Compliance

Fig. 2.3 shows the effect of a worsening compliance. The curves were derived from 1-ply and 5-ply Penrose tubing to mimic normal and post-thrombotic veins.[4] The volume ratio of the bending versus stretching regimen dramatically shrinks from the normal 8:1 ratio *(blue curve)* to nearly 1:1 in the poorly compliant vein *(green curve)*. The effect of this on a centimeter-long cylindric conduit is depicted beside the respective curves. The caliber of a poorly compliant vein is about half of normal at a comparable physiologic pressure range; the prevailing pressure is unable to open the conduit to its normal caliber because of decreased compliance. Caliber reduction exponentially increases flow resistance (14–20 times here, shown as units in square boxes), resulting in the elevation of peripheral venous pressure, which is at the root of many of the clinical manifestations of CVD. Note that the bending regimen (counter-intuitively) bears the brunt of this volume reduction; the venous tube is no longer able to uncollapse so easily at prevailing pressures to achieve normal caliber although wall stretch is also affected.

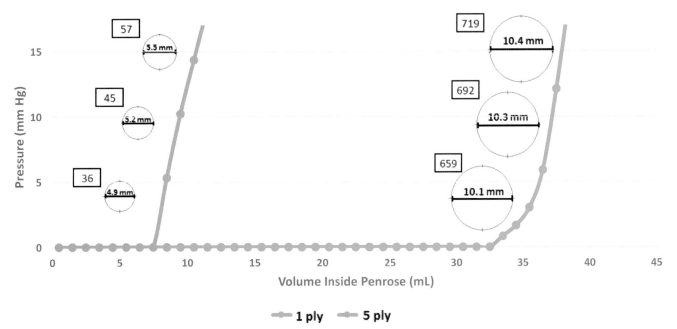

■ **Fig. 2.3** Volume-pressure curves in 1-ply and 5-ply Penrose tubing. *(From Raju S, Crim W, Buck W. Factors influencing peripheral venous pressure in an experimental model.* J Vasc Surg Venous Lymphat Disord. *2017;5:864–874.)*

The Geometric Factor in Venous Flow

The importance of conduit caliber in flow resistance/conductance is well known in the arterial system. The relationship is exponential because the geometric term πr^4 enters the Poiseuille equation in the fourth power. The surprising power of this relationship in the venous system is illustrated in Fig. 2.4. Tributary confluence is an important function of the venous drainage system. Consider two tributaries, each 1 cm in diameter, joining to form a parent trunk (left). The parent needs to be only 20% larger than each of the daughter vessels to accommodate the flow from both without elevating the peripheral pressure. In the center panel is shown an iliac vein 16 mm in diameter. If it is occluded, 256 4-mm sized collaterals will be required to carry the flow without raising the peripheral pressure. The right panel shows a "minor" iliac vein stenosis; the caliber is reduced a mere 2 mm from 16 mm for a 13% diameter stenosis. However, the conductance will be nearly cut in half from 4100 to 2400 units, meaning the peripheral venous pressure will almost double.

Venous Pressure and Flow

Peripheral venous pressure in the supine position has two components: (1) a passive or static component that occurs from venous fill and (2) a dynamic component generated by the pumping action of the heart. The static component, officially termed *mean circulatory pressure* or MCP for short, is also referred to as *dead man's pressure* because it reflects the volume contained in the circulatory tube if the heart were to stop pumping. It is remarkably constant at about 8 mm Hg, regardless of body size. It reflects the V-P curve point prevailing in the normal circulatory system. With cardiac action, the capillary

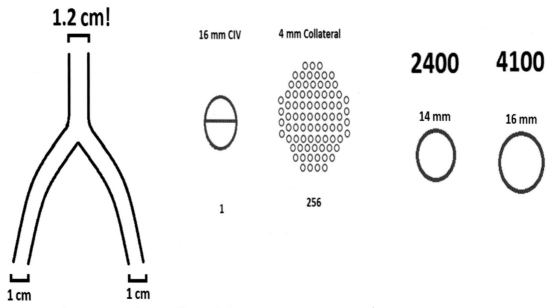

■ **Fig. 2.4** Surprising effects of the "geometric factor" (πr^4) in the Poiseuille equation. *CIV*, Common iliac vein. *(From Raju S, Crim W, Buck W. Factors influencing peripheral venous pressure in an experimental model. J Vasc Surg Venous Lymphat Disord. 2017;5:864–874.)*

venous pressure at the venous end is around 24 mm Hg and the right atrial pressure is near 0 mm Hg. The resulting gradient provides the force for venous circulation and underlies Guyton's theory of venous return control of cardiac function.[5]

The venous bed of the lower limb is a rich network even as the sponge-like multitude of smaller vessels in the calf coalesce to form larger conduits in the thigh and beyond. The flow resistance offered by the large venous trunks is very low, and the pressure gradient is only 0.1 mm Hg or less per cm length. This low resistance combined with rich collateral potential in the calf and thigh (not so rich in the pelvis) means that it is virtually impossible to cut off arterial perfusion of the lower limb unless there is substantial sacrifice or acute extensive thrombosis of the network, such as in phlegmasia cerulae dolens. The compromise of even major trunks, such as the femoral vein (harvest for bypass) or the inferior vena cava interruption, are attended with only a transient increase in the peripheral pressure and edema before the rapid development of collateral pathways restore homeostasis.

Postural Changes

Dramatic adverse changes in the peripheral venous pressure take place when the posture changes from supine to erect.[6] The gravity component increases the peripheral venous pressure from less than 11 mm Hg to 90 to 100 mm Hg, depending upon the height of the individual. The arterial-venous (A-V) gradient itself remains unchanged because an equal amount of gravity pressure is added to the arterial side as well. However, the peripheral bed is enormously dilated, and pressures are increased at both ends of the capillary. Fluid turnover and net fluid outflow increase severalfold. The net negative fluid balance increases, imperiling homeostasis without compensatory mechanisms. This comes in the form of arteriolar vasoconstriction (venoarteriolar reflux), which reduces the arterial capillary pressure by about 10 to 15 mm Hg. Lymph clearance increases 5-fold from supine levels. These mechanisms are not quite enough because even healthy individuals experience ankle edema after some hours of erect posture. A major protective mechanism is calf pump action, which intermittently lowers venous pressure, facilitating increased fluid absorption at the venous capillary. Royal guards drawn from the young and fit in London were famously noted to faint from fluid loss into the tissues when forced to stand motionless at attention, inadvertently "decommissioning" their calf pump in the process. It has been stated that the development from quadruped to bipedal posture is an evolutionary-as-yet-incomplete work in progress.

About 500 mL of blood translocate from veins in the chest to occupy the dilated venous space in the limbs. Stroke volume decreases by about 30%, and limb perfusion falls by about 50% because of increased arteriolar tone. The source of this vasoconstriction is somewhat of a mystery.[7] Bayliss, who highlighted the phenomenon, attributed it to vascular smooth muscle reaction to increased transmural pressure. If so, this would be a positive feedback mechanism that would perpetuate, and not correct, a noxious event. There is tentative experimental evidence that the vasoconstriction is perpetuated through a venoarteriolar axonal reflux emanating from distended veins.[8]

The venous blood volume is adequate to fill the entire venous tree in the supine position. In the erect position, venous blood pools into the distended lower limb veins, leaving inadequate volume to fill the entire venous space. The upper end of the erect venous blood column falls to a level slightly above the clavicle, with the cervical veins collapsing shut above this level. Curiously, the venous pressure measured at the foot level is about 5 to 10 mm Hg less than the pressure represented by the standing venous column. The traditional explanation that the negative pleural pressure negates part of the column pressure is probably incorrect. A more likely explanation is that the erect venous pressure represents only the venous column extending from the foot to the zero-pressure level at the right atrium.[9] The column segment in the superior vena cava of around 8 to 10 mm Hg pressure is not represented. This is because the two columns are not stationary but are fluids moving in opposite directions toward the zero-pressure point. This can be readily demonstrated in an experimental model simulation (Fig. 2.5).

Calf Pump Mechanics

Calf volume changes with calf exercise are monitored through air plethysmography (APG). Pressure changes with calf pump contraction are monitored through a needle in the dorsal foot vein, as it reflects deep venous pressure (ambulatory venous pressure). In a typical curve, the resting pressure of around 90 mm Hg declines to about 30 to 40 mm Hg with ten tip-toe stands. The percentage pressure drop from resting is considered abnormal if it is less than 50%. A complementary index is the time for the pressure to recover back to resting level from arterial inflow. A venous refilling time (VTF) of less than 20 seconds is considered abnormal (Fig. 2.6, *bottom curve*). It is noteworthy that simultaneous calf volume monitored by APG recovers (recovery time [RT]) in about one-third of the time (see Fig. 2.6, *top curve*), a manifestation of the asynchronous pressure volume relationship. The underlying mechanics can be better appreciated by reviewing the sequence of events that occur with calf pump action (Fig. 2.7).[10] After calf pump ejection, the popliteal valve closes, collapsing the emptied venous segments below.

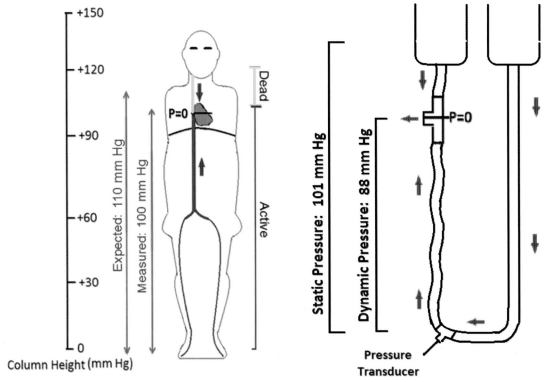

■ **Fig. 2.5** Discrepancy between standing column height and foot venous pressure explained in an experimental model. *P = 0*, P (pressure) = 0 (pressure units = mm Hg). *(From Raju S, Varney E, Flowers W, et al. Effect of external positive and negative pressure on venous flow in an experimental model. Eur J Vasc Endovasc Surg. 2016;51:275–284.)*

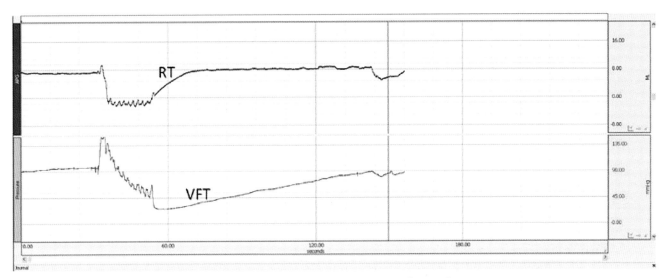

■ **Fig. 2.6** Simultaneous volume *(top)* and pressure *(bottom)* recovery curves after calf exercise. *RT,* Refill time (seconds); *VFT,* venous filling time (seconds). *(From Raju S, Ward Jr M, Jones TL. Quantifying saphenous reflux.* J Vasc Surg Venous Lymphat Disord. *2015;3:8–17.)*

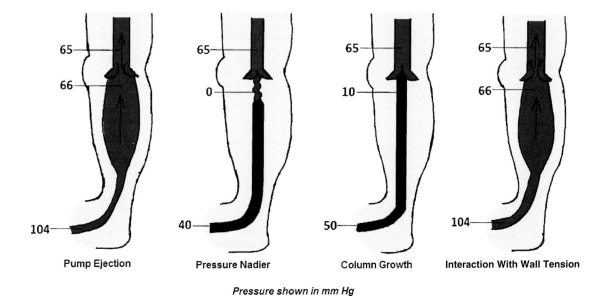

Pressure shown in mm Hg

■ **Fig. 2.7** Sequence of pressure changes after calf pump ejection. *(From Raju S, Ward Jr M, Jones TL. Quantifying saphenous reflux.* J Vasc Surg Venous Lymphat Disord. *2015;3:8–17.)*

There is column segmentation, one each above and below the popliteal valve, respectively. Pressure measurements have shown that a pressure of 50 to 65 mm Hg prevails above the popliteal valve whereas the short column below registers a pressure of around 30 mm Hg at the foot level. The pressure below the valve in the collapsed segment is 0 mm Hg at this stage because of the column segmentation by the valve. The refill of the calf pump occurs from inflow from the venular capillaries. This is typically around 2.2 mL/s as measured by a venous filling index (VFI) parameter of APG. One can envision the blood column in the calf pump gradually growing in height from the inflow touching the popliteal valve. The pressure in the upper part of the calf pump may register 10 mm Hg in the example shown, from a combination of column height and fill pressure. The popliteal valve can pop open only when continuing inflow into the calf pump distends the pump, generating enough pressure (>50 mm Hg) to overcome this level of pressure above the valve. It is clear that wall stretching (compliance) of the calf venous pump is intimately involved in pressure recovery and VFT. Growth in column height alone is not enough to achieve column restitution after calf pump action. A shortened VFT and increased VFI are often interpreted as indicating the presence of reflux, which hastens the refill of the calf. A short VFT can occur from a number of other calf pump abnormalities: poor ejection (stiff pump), small capacitance, or poor compliance (stiff conduit), as shown in Fig. 2.8.[3] In the experimental model shown, poor compliance resulted in more severe shortening of VFT than either reflux or poor ejection alone. Post-thrombotic limbs with a combination of poor compliance and reflux have the most severe shortening of VFT in clinical experience. Venous ulcers in such limbs with a VFT of less than 4 seconds are nearly impossible to heal by any mode of treatment. Many of the calf pump abnormalities can be sorted out by using a combination of ambulatory pressure measurement and APG. Reflux is an extrinsic and major cause of calf pump dysfunction. Reflux can be buffered if pump capacitance, compliance, and ejection fraction are increased (Fig. 2.9). In post-thrombotic limbs, the effects of reflux are worsened by intrinsic abnormalities of the calf pump.

Increased inflow from the microcirculation (e.g., A-V fistula) can also result in a short VFT.

The assumption that dorsal foot venous pressure reflects deep venous pressure is true only at the pressure nadir. Because of the presence of multiple valves and different rates of segmental inflow, different segments can transiently refill to different pressures during recovery with different recovery times.[11] Once equilibrium is achieved and flow resumes, the deep veins (posterior tibial) register a pressure 1 to 2 mm Hg higher than the saphenous vein.[6] Many of the perforators will remain closed because of this flow pressure differential.

Perforators

Functional aspects and the role of perforators in CVD is a source of continuing controversy. Perforator valves are oriented to drain the superficial system into the deep during calf pump diastole, preventing reverse flow during calf systole. However, a bidirectional flow appears to be normal in some perforators near the ankle.[12] A significant perforator reflux is defined as more than 500 ms in a perforator greater than 3.5 mm in caliber. This is, however, a qualitative definition. Perforator reflux has no measurable effect on ambulatory venous pressure. However, there is a local pathologic effect (probably related to shear rather than pressure) as demonstrated by the healing of ulcers when perforators immediately below the ulcer bed are ablated.

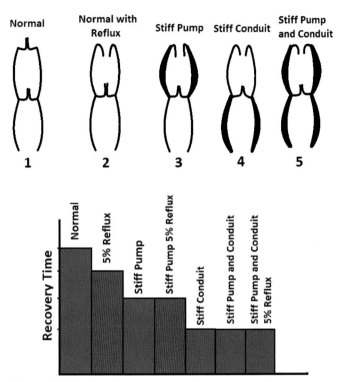

■ **Fig. 2.8** Effect of reflux, poor ejection and poor compliance in an experimental model of calf pump.

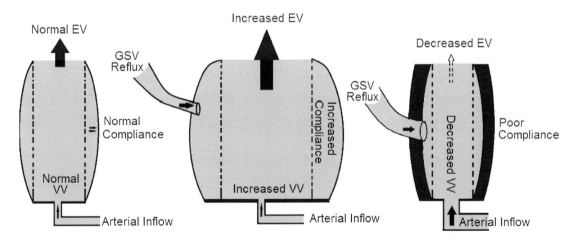

Normal   Abnormal

■ **Fig. 2.9** Effect of reflux on calf pump. Reflux may be buffered or made worse by calf pump mechanics. *EV,* Ejection volume (mL); *GSV,* great saphenous vein; *VV,* venous volume (mL). *(From Raju S, Ward Jr M, Jones TL. Quantifying saphenous reflux.* J Vasc Surg Venous Lymphat Disord. *2015;3:8–17.)*

Reflux

The pathophysiologic basis of CVD is microvascular injury.[13] There is strong experimental evidence that reflux shear initiates the injury. Reflux also causes ambulatory venous hypertension, which sustains the injury in a vicious cycle. The importance of shear in the pathogenesis of varicosities is highlighted by the observation that varices become less distended after the ablation of refluxive saphenous veins even though erect pressures in the varices do not change. The probable explanation is the elimination of vasodilatory nitrous oxide and cytokines induced by reflux shear.

A reverse pressure gradient must be present for reflux to occur. Reflux will readily occur after calf pump action if the valves are incompetent. This is because calf pump contractions and ambulation results in a reverse gradient of 50+ mm Hg between the common femoral vein and tibial veins. Reflux will occur until the gradient vanishes because of the calf pump refill from venular inflow and reflux, commonly 10 to 15 seconds. Current guidelines define significant reflux as greater than a 1-second duration. This definition is qualitative as reflux quantity is not part of it. What is the quantity of reflux necessary to impact the calf pump function? The powerful calf muscles eject about 30 to 60 mL per contraction. A reflux quantity of more than 30 mL is probably a threshold beyond that which the overload and compromise of calf muscle function can occur. In a clinical analysis, only saphenous veins larger than 5 mm in caliber were found to deliver this amount of reflux in 10 to 15 seconds after a calf pump contraction (Fig. 2.10).[14] The reverse case is not true; a refluxive saphenous vein larger than 5 mm in size may or may not deliver this quantity of reflux to shorten VFT; only about one-half the number of saphenous veins larger than 5 mm refluxed more than 30 mL in Fig. 2.10. The blue curve represents the reflux potential of various saphenous calibers calculated from the Poiseuille law. None in this series reached their maximum reflux volume potential. This is probably because reentry perforators may not be large in number and size to deliver the entirety of reflux volume that can potentially pass through a large saphenous vein. It can be shown from the Poiseuille law (conductance is related to πr^4) that about 4000 perforators, each 2 mm in caliber, will be required to unload into the calf all of the reflux volume that a 6-mm saphenous vein can physically transmit. Large caliber saphenous veins restricted by the bottleneck of reentry perforators to deliver reflux into the calf have low reflux velocity, short reflux duration, or both (Fig. 2.11).

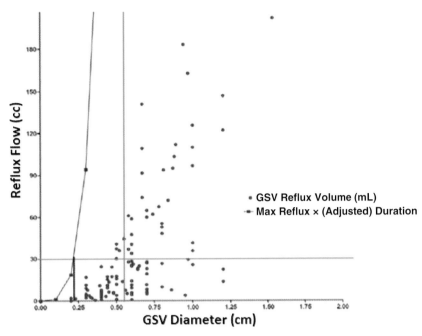

■ Fig. 2.10 An analysis of saphenous size and quantity of measured reflux *(red dots)*. The *horizontal green line* represents 30 cc reflux line. The *vertical green line* represents a saphenous caliber of 5.5 mm. Saphenous veins smaller than this caliber refluxed less than 30 cc with only three exceptions. About half the larger saphenous veins refluxed more than the 30-cc threshold and others less. *GSV,* Great saphenous vein. *(From Raju S, Ward Jr M, Jones TL. Quantifying saphenous reflux.* J Vasc Surg Venous Lymphat Disord. *2015;3:8–17.)*

GSV Reflux: Diameter: 0.62 cm; Area: 0.30 cm²; Velocity: 3 cm/s; Duration: 4.9 s
Reflux Volume: 4.5 mL

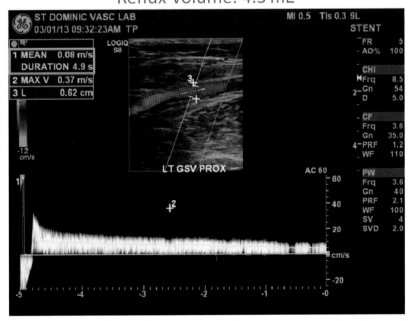

■ Fig. 2.11 A large caliber saphenous vein refluxing only a small volume of reflux. Reflux velocity and duration were low. *GSV,* Great saphenous vein.

Obstruction

Peripheral venous hypertension can result from a variety of central and peripheral factors listed in Table 2.1.[4] Obstruction is a major cause. Silent iliac vein obstruction occurs in about two-thirds of the general population.[15] Secondary insults, such as trauma (e.g., joint replacement), cellulitis, deep venous thrombosis, or onset of reflux, can precipitate symptoms.[16] The effect of peripheral venous hypertension is insidious and constant, working "24/7" both in the supine and erect positions, unlike reflux, which is limited to the hours spent in mobility.

The caliber of the iliac femoral outflow is a critical factor in obstructive peripheral venous hypertension in the lower limb. This is because the arterial inflow into each lower limb at rest is more or less fixed at around 12% of cardiac index.[17] Unless outflow matches inflow, pressure homeostasis cannot be maintained. This means that there is an optimum caliber of the terminal iliac venous outflow necessary to keep the peripheral venous pressure in the normal range (<11 mm Hg). This is best illustrated by the analogy of a dam across a river (Fig. 2.12). The water depth in the reservoir is an analogue of the pressure in conduit flows.[1]

TABLE 2.1 Central and Peripheral Mechanisms Causing Peripheral Venous Hypertension

Central Mechanisms	Clinical Analogue/Comment
• Increased arterial inflow into the limb	• AV fistula
• Elevated right atrial pressure	• Congestive heart failure
• Increased intraabdominal pressure	• Morbid obesity
• Iliac vein stenosis	• May-Thurner syndrome
Peripheral Mechanisms	
• Decreased native unstretched caliber	• Maldevelopment; insufficient upscaling at venous confluence
• Decreased compliance	• Decreased compliance reduces functional caliber, organized thrombus can reduce luminal caliber
• Focal stenosis	• Nearly 2/3 of the general population will have silent iliac vein stenosis
• Venous tone	• Quantitative caliber effect of venous tone is unknown
• Postcapillary inflow	• Rate of arterial inflow into the calf is increased in CVD limbs

AV, Arteriovenous; *CVD*, chronic venous disease.

The water level will be stable (normal) if the outflow conduit caliber is optimum, that is, if it matches inflow; if the outflow is smaller (stenosis), the water level/pressure will rise and collateral overflow may occur. It is common practice to temporarily lower the reservoir level by increasing outflow for energy generation during high-demand season. Note: the river flow will remain unchanged if the dam were to be removed.

The optimal caliber of common iliac vein outflow calculates to be around 18 mm from the Poiseuille equation and intravascular ultrasound observations.[18] The optimum caliber values for the entire iliac-femoral segments are shown in Table 2.2.

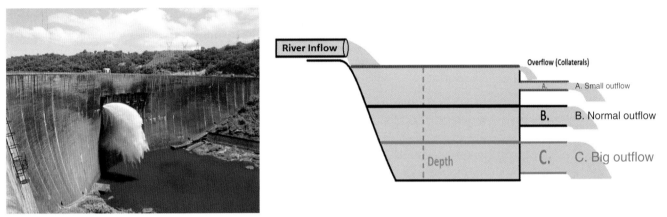

■ **Fig. 2.12** The Kariba Dam across the Zambezi River *(left).* The storage schematics is shown on the *right. (From Raju S, Crim W, Buck W. Factors influencing peripheral venous pressure in an experimental model. J Vasc Surg Venous Lymphat Disord. 2017;5:864–874.)*

TABLE 2.2 Optimal Caliber of the Iliac-Femoral Vein Segments

Vessel Segment	Diameter	Area
CIV	16 mm	200 mm^2
EIV	14 mm	150 mm^2
CFV	12 mm	110 mm^2

CIV, Common iliac vein; *CFV,* common femoral vein; *EIV,* external iliac vein.

The optimal caliber should be used as a reference in calculating common iliac vein stenosis. Long diffuse stenosis of the iliac veins (Rokitanski stenosis) is not uncommon (Fig. 2.13).[19] These are long diffuse lesions without focal cues. A venogram may appear normal because of the internal scale. Intravascular ultrasound (IVUS) shows a diffuse area stenosis of about 65%. If the adjacent segment is used as a reference in stenosis calculation, an underestimation will result in such cases. As with the river dam analogy, stent correction of iliac vein flow has been shown to lower the peripheral venous pressure but the arterial inflow remains unchanged.[20]

Venous Flow Through the Abdomen

Venous flow through thin-walled collapsible tubes has many counterintuitive flow properties, and even more when they are surrounded by a pressurized chamber.[1] This occurs in lower limb flow as the iliac-caval veins transit through the abdomen with a positive pressure that varies 2 to 5 mm Hg with respiration. In obese patients, intra-abdominal pressure can be as high as 15 mm Hg.[21] When external pressure is applied, the flow inside the collapsible tube slows, raising the peripheral venous pressure.[9] This may be the basis of CVD manifestations in a subset of obese patients in whom an iliac vein stenosis cannot be found on IVUS examination.[21]

There are even more unexpected flow features associated with this set-up, known as a *Starling resister,* named after the English physiologist Ernest Starling, who first devised the experimental model (Fig. 2.14).[20] Flow in an externally compressed collapsible tube is no longer controlled by pressure gradient between the inflow and outflow ends per the Poiseuille equation. The external pressure (e.g., abdominal pressure) becomes the sole driving force of flow in the enclosed collapsible tube. Lowering the pressure at the outflow end has no effect on the flow. A similar phenomenon occurs in gas dynamics (choking) and open channel flows (waterfall).[1] There is some evidence that these flow features are present in the inferior vena cava but remain to be fully elucidated.[22]

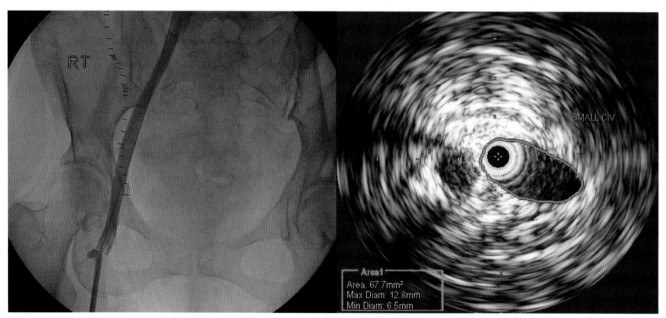

◾ **Fig. 2.13** Right iliac venogram showing diffuse narrow lesion characteristic of Rokitanski stenosis *(left panel).* Corresponding intravascular ultrasound image depicting intraluminal area reduction of right common iliac vein *(right panel).* *(From Raju S, Davis M. Anomalous features of iliac vein stenosis that affect diagnosis and treatment.* J Vasc Surg Venous Lymphat Disord. *2014;2:260–267.)*

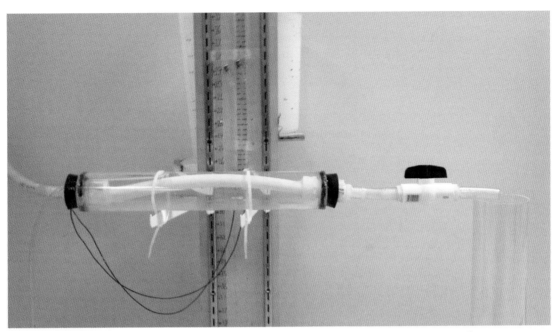

■ **Fig. 2.14** An experimental model of Starling resistor. *(From Raju S, Kirk O, Davis, M, Olivier J. Hemodynamics of "critical" venous stenosis and stent treatment.* J Vasc Surg Venous Lymphat Disord. *2014;2:52–59.)*

REFERENCES

1. Shapiro AH. Steady flow in collapsible tubes. *J Biomech Eng.* 1977;99:126–147.
2. Raju S, Green AB, Fredericks RK, et al. Tube collapse and valve closure in ambulatory venous pressure regulation: studies with a mechanical model. *J Endovasc Surg.* 1998;5(1):42–51.
3. Raju S, Hudson CA, Fredericks R, et al. Studies in calf venous pump function utilizing a two-valve experimental model. *Eur J Vasc Endovasc Surg.* 1999;17(6):521–532.
4. Raju S, Crim W, Buck W. Factors influencing peripheral venous pressure in an experimental model. *J Vasc Surg Venous Lymphat Disord.* 2017;In press.
5. Guyton AC, Lindsey AW, Abernathy B, et al. Venous return at various right atrial pressures and the normal venous return curve. *Am J Physiol.* 1957;189(3):609–615.
6. Strandness DE, Sumner DS. *Hemodynamics for Surgeons.* New York: Grune & Stratton; 1975:xi.
7. Gauer OH, Thorn HL. Postural changes in the circulation. In: Hamilton WF, ed. *Handbook of Physiology. Circulation. 3.* Baltimore. MD: Am Physiol Soc Williams & Wilkins; 1965:2409–2439.
8. Burton AC. *Physiology and Biophysics of the Circulation; an Introductory Text.* 2nd ed. Chicago: Year Book Medical Publishers; 1972.
9. Raju S, Varney E, Flowers W, et al. Effect of external positive and negative pressure on venous flow in an experimental model. *Eur J Vasc Endovasc Surg.* 2016;51(2):275–284.
10. Raju S, Fredericks R, Lishman P, et al. Observations on the calf venous pump mechanism: determinants of postexercise pressure. *J Vasc Surg.* 1993;17(3):459–469.
11. Neglen P, Raju S. Differences in pressures of the popliteal, long saphenous, and dorsal foot veins. *J Vasc Surg.* 2000;32(5):894–901.
12. Sarin S, Scurr JH, Smith PD. Medial calf perforators in venous disease: the significance of outward flow. *J Vasc Surg.* 1992;16(1):40–46.

13. Pascarella L, Schonbein GW, Bergan JJ. Microcirculation and venous ulcers: a review. *Ann Vasc Surg.* 2005;19(6):921–927.

14. Raju S, Ward M Jr, Jones T. Quantifying saphenous reflux. *J Vasc Surg Venous Lymphat Disord.* 2015;3:8–17.

15. Kibbe MR, Ujiki M, Goodwin AL, et al. Iliac vein compression in an asymptomatic patient population. *J Vasc Surg.* 2004;39(5):937–943.

16. Raju S, Neglen P. High prevalence of nonthrombotic iliac vein lesions in chronic venous disease: a permissive role in pathogenicity. *J Vasc Surg.* 2006;44(1):136–143, discussion 44.

17. Nichols W, O'Rourke M, Vlachopoulos C. *McDonald's Blood Flow in Arteries: Theoretical, Experimental and Clinical Principles.* 6th ed. Boca Raton. FL: CRC Press; 2011.

18. Raju S, Buck W, Crim W, et al. Optimal sizing of iliac vein stents. *Phlebology.* 2017;In Press.

19. Raju S, Davis M. Anomalous features of iliac vein stenosis that affect diagnosis and treatment. *J Vasc Surg Venous Lymphat Disord.* 2014;2(3):260–267.

20. Raju S, Kirk O, Davis M, et al. Hemodynamics of 'critical' venous stenosis and stent treatment. *J Vasc Surg Venous Lymphat Disord.* 2014;2:52–59.

21. Raju S, Darcey R, Neglen P. Iliac-caval stenting in the obese. *J Vasc Surg.* 2009;50(5):1114–1120.

22. Guyton AC, Adkins LH. Quantitative aspects of the collapse factor in relation to venous return. *Am J Physiol.* 1954;177(3):523–527.

Venous Pathophysiology

Rafael D. Malgor and Nicos Labropoulos

ETIOLOGY AND NATURAL HISTORY OF DISEASE

Primary Venous Disease

Primary venous disease affects two-thirds of patients with chronic venous disease (CVD). The most accepted theory is based on increased venous hydrostatic pressure transmitted to the vein wall, causing smooth muscle relaxation, endothelial damage, and extracellular matrix degradation with subsequent vein wall weakening and wall dilatation.[1] It has also been suggested that valve damage may occur because of local inflammation.[2] Leukocyte migration, plasma-granulocyte activation, and increased activity of metalloproteinases causing degradation of the valve leaflets support that theory.[2,3] Fig. 3.1 summarizes the pathophysiologic pathways of CVD.

Superficial veins are most commonly involved in primary CVD, followed by perforators and deep veins.[4] It has been shown that reflux starts in superficial veins in more than 80% of patients. In the early stages of CVD, reflux is found in the great saphenous vein (GSV) and its tributaries without almost any junctional involvement (Fig. 3.2). This is followed by reflux in the small saphenous vein (SSV) system (Fig. 3.3) and nonsaphenous veins (Fig. 3.4). Patients with competent saphenous, perforators, and deep veins may also present with tributary reflux in 10% of cases, with the GSV tributaries being affected in 65% of cases.

Text continued on p. 42

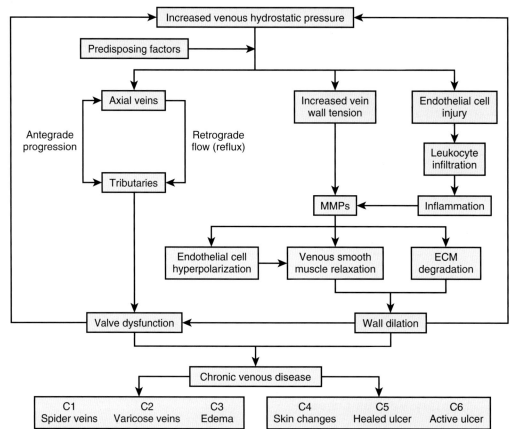

■ **Fig. 3.1** Mechanisms of varicose vein formation. Increased hydrostatic pressure and wall tension in individuals with predisposing risk factors cause matrix metalloproteinase (MMP) activation and changes in the endothelium and vascular smooth-muscle function. In addition, leukocyte wall infiltration and inflammation activate MMPs and lead to extracellular matrix (ECM) degradation, venous wall weakening, and wall/valve fibrosis. Although a possible mechanism may involve primary valve insufficiency in both the axial and tributary veins, this likely represents a secondary event from primary venous wall changes and dilation. Persistent venous wall dilation and valvular dysfunction lead to increased hydrostatic pressure. MMP-mediated vein wall dilation with secondary valve dysfunction leads to chronic venous disease (CVD) and varicose vein formation. The early stages of CVD are maintained within the vasculature, leading to clinical signs of varicose veins, whereas more advanced CVD causes progression of chronic venous insufficiency affecting surrounding tissues and leading to skin changes and ulcer formation. *(From Raffetto JD, Khalil RA. Mechanisms of varicose vein formation: valve dysfunction and wall dilation.* Phlebology. *2008;23:85–98.)*

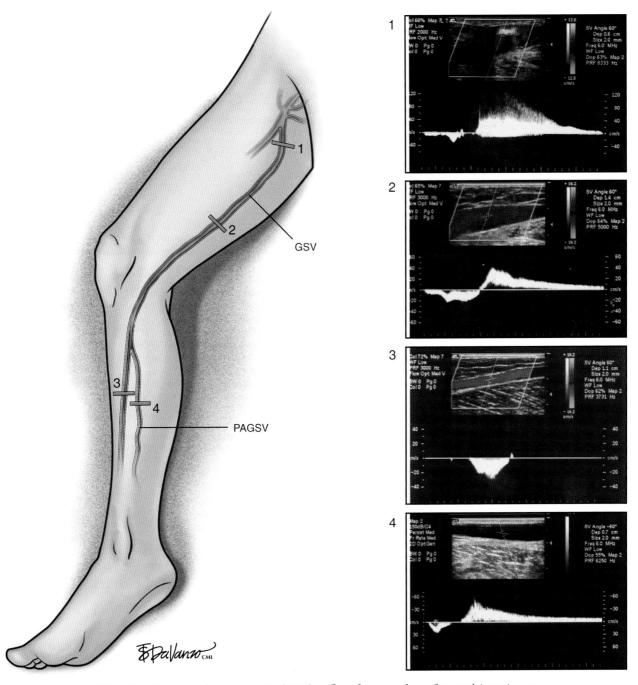

■ **Fig. 3.2** Great saphenous vein (GSV) reflux from saphenofemoral junction to upper calf and the posterior accessory calf vein. The below-knee segment of GSV is normal. *PAGSV*, Posterior accessory great saphenous vein.

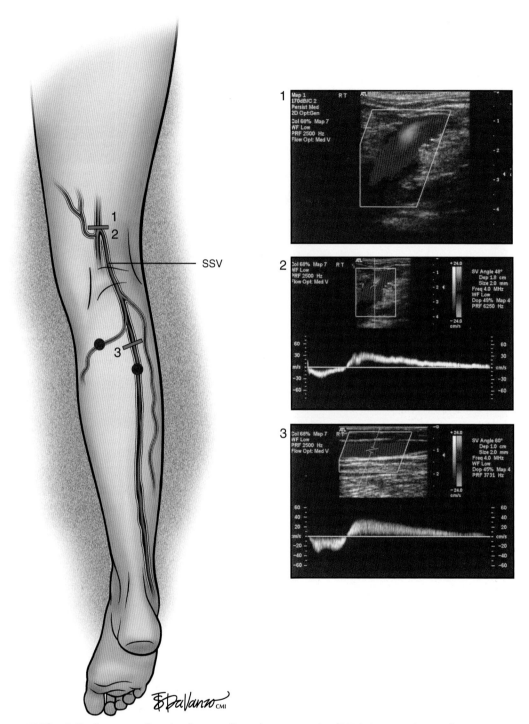

■ **Fig. 3.3** Severe reflux in the small saphenous vein (SSV) in a patient who presented with CEAP (clinical, etiologic, anatomic, pathophysiologic) classes 1 through 4, itching, and pain during prolonged standing. Reflux was also found in two tributaries and two perforator veins *(red dots)*.

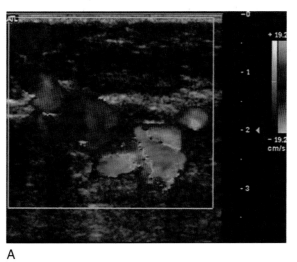

A

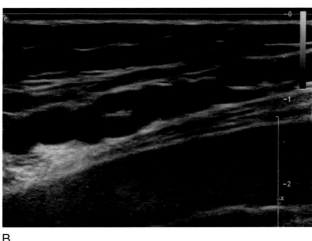

B

■ **Fig. 3.4** Nonsaphenous vein reflux. (A) Vulvar vein reflux in a female patient with a history of three pregnancies. The veins from this region are very tortuous and extend in a nonpredicted manner in the extremity. (B) Sciatic nerve vein reflux giving rise to popliteal fossa varicosities emerging in the posterolateral calf.

Isolated primary deep-vein reflux is rare. It may present as either segmental or axial reflux extending from the femoral vein in the thigh to the below-knee popliteal vein. The most frequent location of primary deep-vein reflux is the common femoral vein, followed by the femoral and popliteal veins[5] (Fig. 3.5). Because most deep venous reflux is deemed to be caused by superficial venous reflux propagation, both common femoral and femoral vein reflux are associated with GSV incompetence and popliteal vein reflux is associated with SSV and/or gastrocnemial vein incompetence[5] (Fig. 3.6). In addition, deep-vein reflux has a shorter duration compared with superficial venous reflux. Association between deep and superficial venous reflux ranges from 5% to 38%.[5–8]

Perforator vein (PV) reflux in primary CVD always occurs in association with superficial vein reflux.[9] Essentially, PVs become incompetent secondary to either ascending extension of superficial vein reflux or descending propagation of the reflux in a reentry fashion (Fig. 3.7). Most often, PV reflux originates from the GSV system and renders the deep veins incompetent in 13% of cases.[9] Deep-vein reflux secondary to PV reflux is usually segmental and has a short duration.[9]

Text continued on p. 50

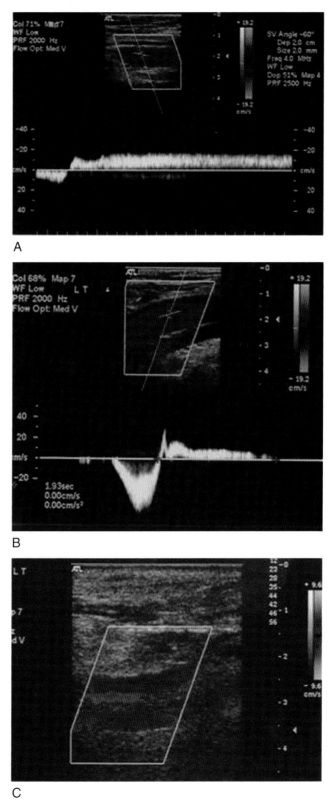

■ **Fig. 3.5** Examples of postthrombotic reflux from three patients. (A) Severe reflux in the femoral vein in a patient who had previous extensive deep venous thrombosis from the common femoral to calf veins. (B) Popliteal vein reflux in a patient who presented with swelling and pain. (C) Reflux in both posterior tibial veins, which have the same color as the artery in the middle.

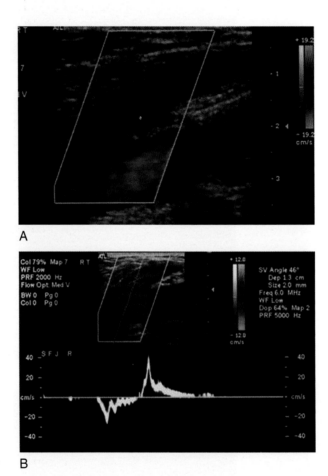

■ **Fig. 3.6** Imaging of the saphenofemoral junction (SFJ). (A) Cephalad flow is seen in the SFJ during distal compression. The saphenous vein has a normal diameter and is competent. (B) SFJ reflux renders the common femoral vein incompetent. In such cases, in patients with primary chronic venous disease, correction of the saphenous reflux abolishes the common femoral vein reflux.

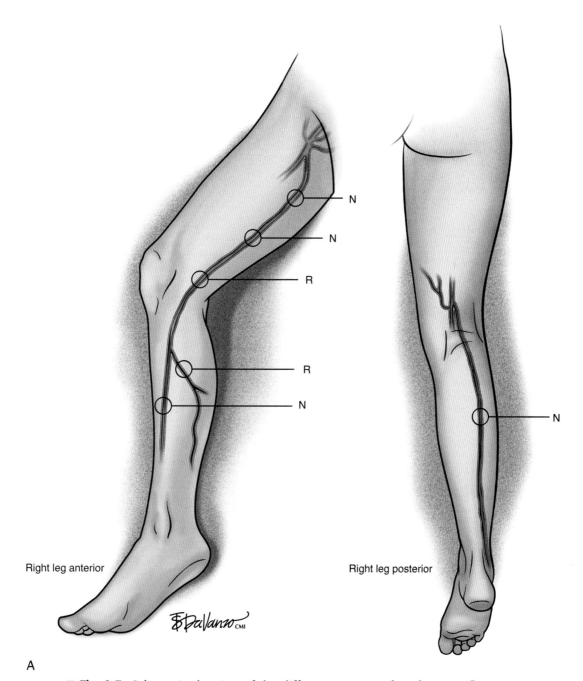

Right leg anterior

Right leg posterior

A

■ **Fig. 3.7** Schematic drawing of the different patterns of perforator reflux development. (A and B) Reflux developed in descending manner in a reentry perforator at the lower medial calf. *N,* Normal; *R,* reflux.

Continued

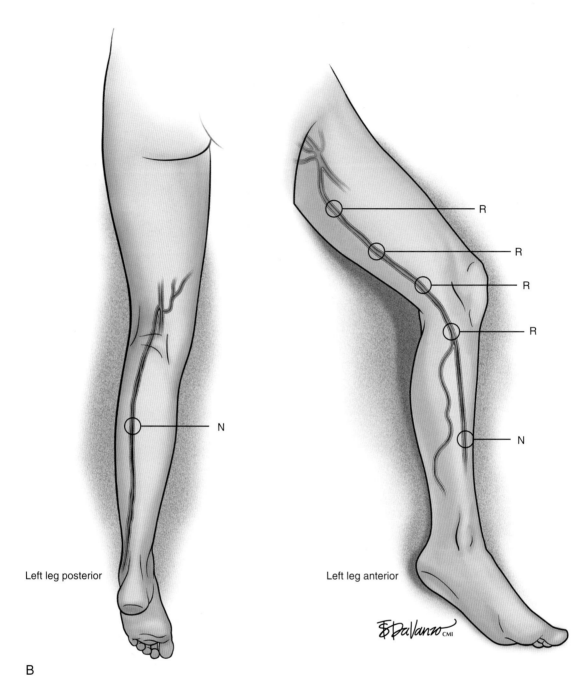

Left leg posterior

Left leg anterior

B

■ **Fig. 3.7** Schematic drawing of the different patterns of perforator reflux development. (A and B) Reflux developed in descending manner in a reentry perforator at the lower medial calf. *N,* Normal; *R,* reflux.

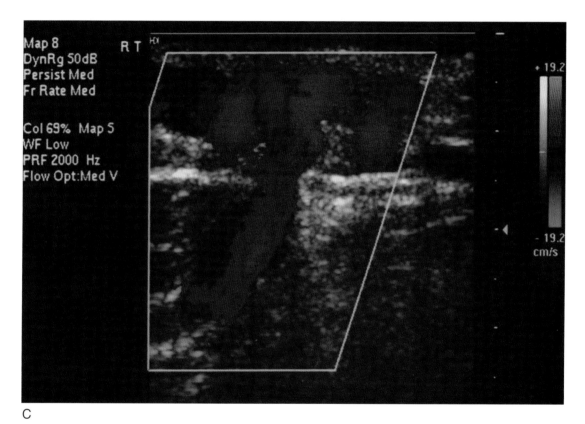

C

■ **Fig. 3.7, cont'd** (C) Baseline ultrasound examination in a 53-year-old female patient with a long-standing history of chronic venous disease. On the right limb, she had great saphenous vein (GSV) reflux from the lower thigh to the upper calf and in the posterior calf accessory vein. On the left limb, she had reflux in the GSV from the saphenofemoral junction to the upper calf and the posterior accessory calf vein. There was no perforator vein reflux at this time.

Continued

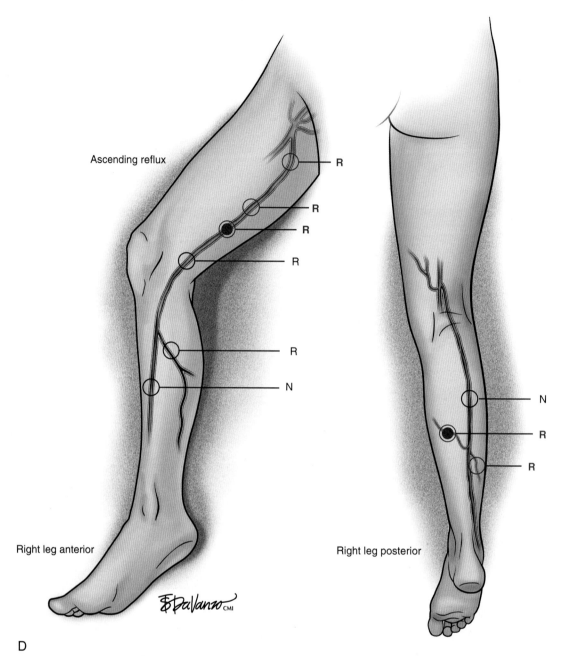

Ascending reflux

R
R
R
R

R

N

Right leg anterior

S DaVanzo CMI

N

R

R

Right leg posterior

D

■ **Fig. 3.7, cont'd** (D and E) During the second examination at 38 months on the right limb, the patient developed ascending reflux in the GSV, a perforator vein at the thigh, a new reflux site in a posterior calf tributary, and a midcalf perforator. On the left limb, she developed a reentry type of reflux in a medial perforator vein from the posterior calf accessory vein. She had worsening of her disease from CEAP (clinical, etiologic, anatomic, pathophysiologic) class 2 to 3 in the right limb and from class 3 to 4A in the left limb. She also became symptomatic in the left limb, with aching and itching along the varicosities of medial calf. The *red dot* indicates reflux in a perforator vein. The *red letters* and *lines* indicate the new sites of reflux in the second examination.

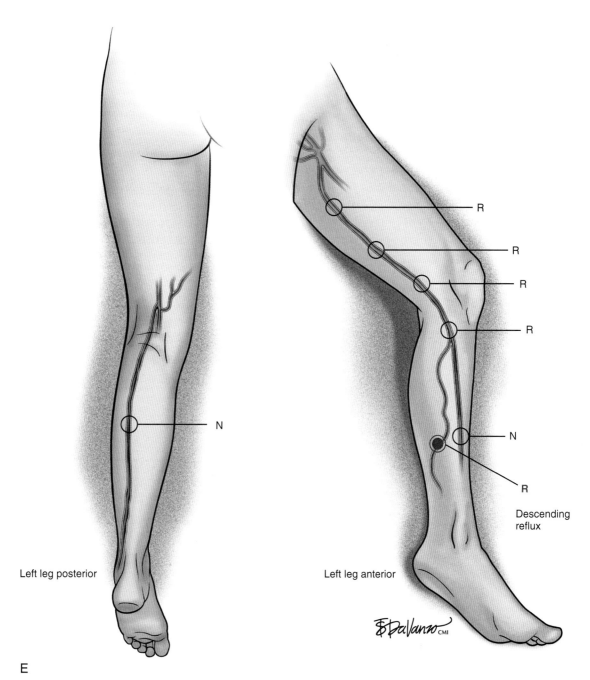

Left leg posterior

Left leg anterior

R

R

R

R

N

N

R

Descending
reflux

E

■ **Fig. 3.7, cont'd** For legend see opposite page.

Secondary Venous Disease

Secondary venous disease is caused by a thrombotic event or is secondary to trauma. The incidence of arteriovenous fistula (AVF) as the cause of secondary CVD is reduced compared with postthrombotic CVD (Fig. 3.8).

Most frequently, AVFs are created when both common femoral vessels are inadvertently punctured during endovascular procedures or secondary to penetrating or blunt traumatic injuries. Animal models based on AVF creation have been used to explain the findings of CVD.[10] Initially, lower resistance in the distal portion of the artery and pulsatile flow in the vein are noted. Venous hypertension supervenes, distending the veins and causing some degree of edema in the limb but no reflux. Subsequently, the valves are unable to appose what portends the reflux. Continuous venous hypertension and reflux entail

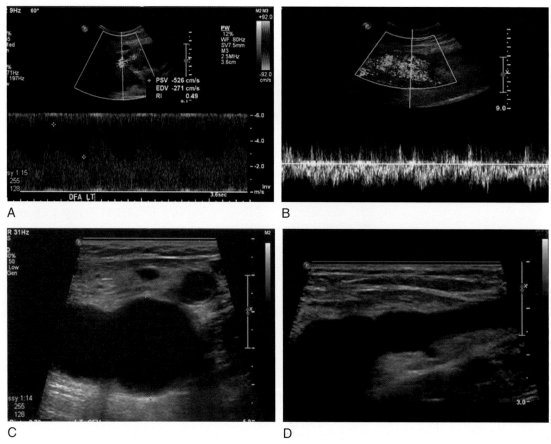

■ **Fig. 3.8** Arteriovenous fistula causing significant venous hypertension (swelling of the entire limb, pain, and discoloration) in a male patient after a gunshot wound in the left groin. (A) Fistula between the deep femoral artery and the common femoral vein. There are high velocities with a low resistance pattern. (B) Waveform with turbulent flow in the common femoral vein proximal to the fistula. (C) The common femoral vein is dilated (2.8 cm) because of the local high pressure. (D) Dilatation of the saphenofemoral junction and the great saphenous vein with continuous reflux (not shown).

valve atrophy and arterialization of the venous wall in the long term. In humans, the occurrence of CVD secondary to AVFs is rare and requires a long course to generate clinical impairment that is frequently devastating.

Deep venous thrombosis (DVT) is a result of stasis, endothelial damage, and/or hypercoagulable state. The predisposing factors for DVT, and therefore secondary CVD, are well established, including pregnancy, operations, immobilization, malignancy, trauma, and obesity. Patients who sustain inherited disorders (i.e., active protein C resistance, protein S, and antithrombin III deficiency) are also prone to develop thromboembolic events.

Regardless of the initial thrombi formation, the majority of the limbs evolve with thrombus resolution. Notably, only one-third of the patients with secondary CVD develop postthrombotic syndrome (PTS), which consists of signs and symptoms such as pain, edema, heaviness, and intolerance to efforts that may progress to skin changes and ulcers (Fig. 3.9). Often, patients with PTS have a combination of reflux and obstruction (Fig. 3.10). PTS represents the most severe manifestation of secondary CVD, carrying significant socioeconomic impact, and is discussed in Chapter 17.

At the other extreme of secondary CVD are patients who develop DVT with no symptoms. This specific group of patients may have a total silent course of the disease for decades, being diagnosed with DVT during postoperative screening ultrasound or for nonrelated diagnostic purposes. The incidence of PTS in this subset of patients is low.

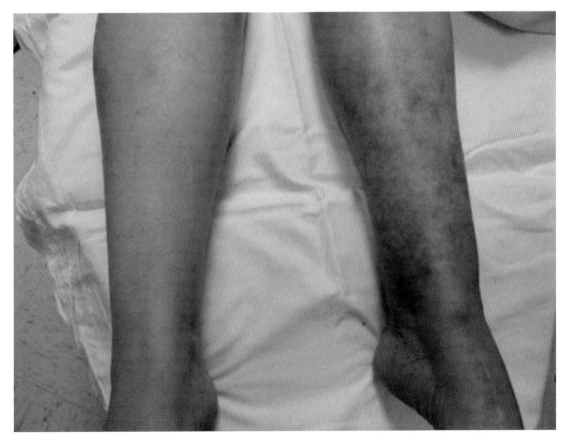

■ **Fig. 3.9** Skin discoloration and swelling in patient with postthrombotic deep venous disease.

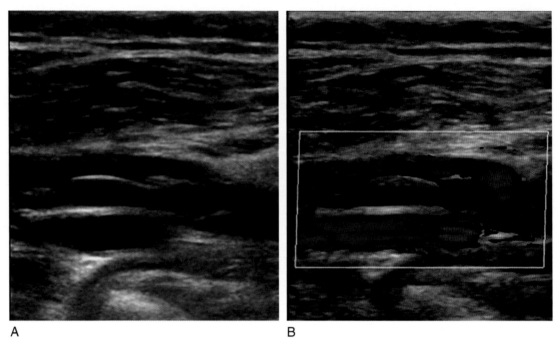

A   B

■ **Fig. 3.10** Patient with leg edema and skin changes with partial recanalization of the popliteal vein. (A) Synechiae are clearly seen in the lumen of the vein. (B) Multiple flow channels are seen through the synechiae. Patients with reflux and obstruction are more likely to develop postthrombotic signs and symptoms.

The location of the DVT and its extent have been investigated. Involvement of at least one proximal deep-vein segment was proposed as a mandatory condition for the development of CVD. Three anatomic and hemodynamic patterns are found following an episode of DVT: reflux, obstruction, or a combination of reflux and obstruction. In that scenario, reflux is caused by destruction of the valves secondary to inflammation. It has been hypothesized that leukocyte infiltration in the venous wall causes amplification and activation of metalloproteinases, leading to venous wall and valve damage.[1]

Failure to resolve an obstruction by either partial or complete recanalization of the thrombosed segment is found in less than 10% of cases.[11,12] Partial recanalization is known to have higher incidence of reflux than complete recanalized segments, and calf veins are more prone to undergo recanalization than proximal segments.[11,12] The role of location of the occlusion has been investigated. In a 1-year prospective study of 70 limbs, recanalization rate was lower in femoral veins, whereas all calf veins had complete recanalization. Finally, patients with reflux or obstruction present with milder changes and symptoms than those with both abnormalities. The presence of reflux and outflow obstruction in the same limb leads to higher rates of skin damage.[13,14]

Congenital

Congenital vascular malformations contribute to between 1% and 3% of CVD. Pure venous malformations are rare and present as an isolated cluster of veins that abuts surrounding tissues, including soft tissue and bone. The most common congenital malformation involving veins is Klippel-Trenaunay syndrome, which is characterized by varicose veins, limb hypertrophy, and port-wine stains[15] (Fig. 3.11). Agenesis of valves and segments of the deep veins is rare but is known to cause CVD.[16]

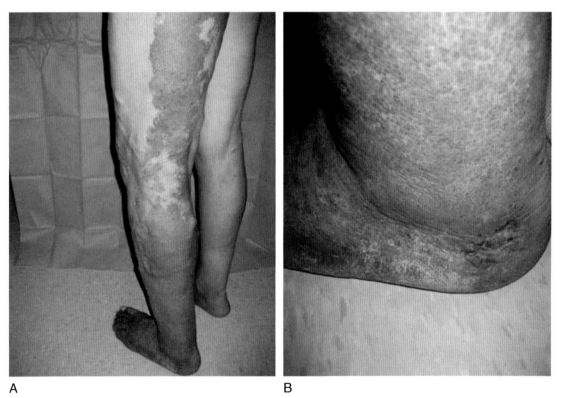

A   B

■ **Fig. 3.11** Klippel-Trenaunay syndrome in a young, female patient who presented with pain and ulceration. The left limb has the typical discoloration and enlargement seen in patients with this syndrome. There were no anomalies seen in the deep axial veins. Reflux was found in multiple superficial, perforator, and muscular veins.

Natural History

CVD slowly evolves over time and is classified based on its clinical (telangiectasias to skin damage), etiologic (primary, secondary, or congenital), anatomic (superficial, deep, or perforators), and pathophysiologic (reflux, obstruction, or both) patterns (CEAP).[17] The clinical portion of the score is extensively used because of its simplicity, being cited as initial stages of CVD, including telangiectasias and varicose veins (C1–C2), and chronic venous insufficiency, including edema, skin changes, and ulcers (C3–C6).

Because the venous pressure increases in the lower-extremity veins for hydrostatic reasons during standing, it has been believed that reflux develops in a retrograde fashion. However, multiple studies have demonstrated that this is not true.[18–21] Predominantly, reflux starts from the saphenous veins and their tributaries and progresses proximally, distally, or in both directions.[22] In a longitudinal study of 116 limbs, progression of reflux occurred in 31 limbs. GSV and tributaries were the most common anatomic sites affected by reflux progression, followed by perforator veins. Some 17 limbs had extension of preexisting reflux in a proximal or distal direction, or both, and 14 limbs had reflux in a new segment that was independent of the preexisting site. Among patients with new signs or symptoms, documented reflux progression by duplex ultrasound was found in 53.8%, which was significantly higher than the 23.3% of patients without new symptoms ($P = .04$). Bernardini et al.[23] corroborated the findings that the reflux most frequently starts in the GSV and its tributaries, reporting progression of venous disease in 94% of the patients in a mean period of 4 years. Further evidence is provided by interventional studies in which reflux in the saphenous vein was corrected after eliminating reflux in the saphenous tributaries.[24–26]

Recent research on microenvironment changes on the lower-extremity veins, such as wall thickness and microvalves damage, have shown to be linked to disease progression.[27,28] Findings of a human in vivo study by Labropoulos et al. demonstrated that venous wall thickness increases with age and patients with venous reflux have thicker vein walls compared with same-age patients without vein reflux (Fig. 3.12).[27] The authors hypothesize that vein wall thickness is likely an early finding even before venous reflux is present.[27] Vincent et al., using scanning electron microscopy, studied limbs injected with resin to study micro valve insufficiency.[28] Their findings showed that valvular incompetence can occur independently in small superficial veins can happen before saphenous vein trunk reflux occurs.[28] On clinical grounds, high progression rate of CVD from varicose veins with no other signs and symptoms (CEAP C2) to higher chronic venous insufficiency (CVI) classes was demonstrated to be about 20% involving nonsaphenous veins and up to 32% involving saphenous veins based on the last findings of the Bonn vein study, which included 3072 participants.[29]

Secondary CVD was found to progress faster than primary CVD,[12] for reasons that are likely to be multivariate. The presence of reflux and obstruction aggravates the clinical status of patients, as shown in a study by Johnson et al.[13] In a cohort of 64 patients, overall progression of the CEAP clinical class occurred in 31.5%. Notably, secondary CVD CEAP class 4 to 6 was observed in 4% of the limbs at a 1-year period, increasing to 25% at 5-year follow-up.[14] Inflammation was also found to be worse in patients with more advanced venous disease (skin damage, ulcerations), which is noted by using duplex ultrasound that is positive for abnormal flow patterns within both the venous and arterial system.

Prandoni et al. analyzed the data of 1626 consecutive patients and found that residual thrombosis, unknown origin, and thrombophilia are risk factors for recurrent DVT over a period of 10 years.[30] Long-term follow-up with duplex ultrasound in a prospective cohort of 153 patients with recurrent DVT showed increased risk of skin damage (C4–C6) in patients with previous recurrent ipsilateral DVT.[31]

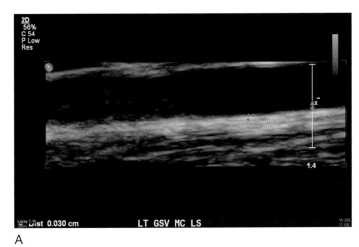

A

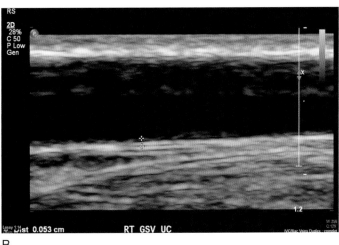

B

■ **Fig. 3.12** (A) A 48-year-old female patient with asymptomatic venous disease (no venous signs and symptoms). A lower-extremity, duplex ultrasound demonstrated no saphenous vein reflux, but showed normal great saphenous vein (GSV) wall thickness (patient: 0.3 mm; normal range 0.3 ± 0.03 mm). (B) 38-year-old female with history of four pregnancies, three live children, presents 3 years after her last pregnancy with bilateral, lower-extremity edema, heaviness, itching, and pain on standing. She has undergone bilateral GSV ablation in the past. Reflux on both below-knee GSV and accessory saphenous vein were demonstrated with duplex ultrasound. Note the wall thickness of the remaining right, below-knee GSV (0.5 mm).

An overview of clinical distribution (reflux, obstruction, or both), classification, and pathophysiology of CVD in consecutive patients attending a vascular clinic is shown in Fig. 3.13. Most patients have primary vein reflux, which is most often found in the superficial veins and varicose veins. Skin damage is present in about one-third of the patients, whereas isolated deep-vein reflux and obstruction are uncommon.[32]

PEARLS AND PITFALLS

A complete understanding of venous pathophysiology is essential to offer an adequate treatment for patients with CVD. The relationship between deep and superficial venous reflux, obesity, and dilated veins with no reflux deserves attention.

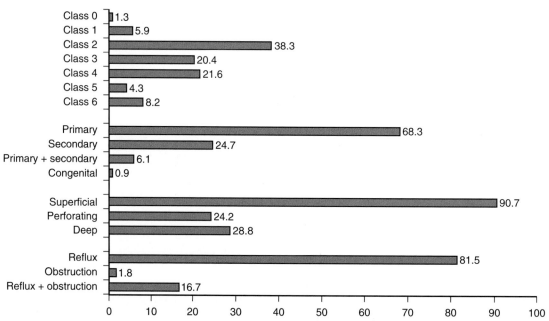

■ **Fig. 3.13** Presentation of 1000 consecutive limbs with chronic venous disease (CVD) according to CEAP (clinical, etiologic, anatomic, pathophysiologic) classification. In the anatomic classification, for simplicity, only the overall contribution of each system is shown. This classification has allowed better communication and comparisons in the medical literature because CVD terminology is more specific and has been adopted worldwide.

Obesity

An association between obesity and CVD has been identified. The role of obesity as a causative versus an aggravating factor remains debatable. It is known that obese patients have higher intraabdominal pressure compared with nonobese patients and have reduced distensibility of the veins that could explain the higher incidence of CVD. Van Rij et al.[33] reported an increased incidence of more severe CVD (CEAP 4–6) in obese patients compared with nonobese patients. Interestingly, the authors concluded that obese patients have better venous calf muscle pump than nonobese patients. Sedentary behavior may explain the reduced effect of the pump to compensate reflux (Fig. 3.14).

Padberg et al. also reported a correlation between higher body mass index (BMI) and severity of CVD[34] in a cohort of morbidly obese patients (BMI > 40). Obese patients had longer mean ulcer healing time, up to 7 months. Notably, 62% of those patients had no anatomic evidence of reflux despite severe CVD changes.[34] Perhaps the disease in that subset of patients may be secondary to microcirculatory changes or even segmental venous hypertension associated with lymphatic drainage impairment. Therefore a high level of suspicion should be raised when evaluating such patients because venous reflux may not be the cause of skin damage.

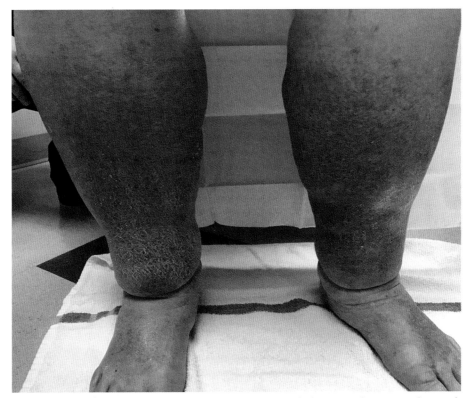

■ **Fig. 3.14** A 65-year-old morbidly obese male with longstanding complaint of bilateral lower-extremity edema, heaviness, and skin discoloration along with lipodermatosclerosis. Bilateral lower-extremity venous duplex showed no deep, superficial, or perforator vein reflux or obstruction.

Effects of Superficial Vein Reflux on the Deep Veins

The role of superficial venous reflux as a causative factor for deep venous reflux has been investigated. Over the past three decades, selected patients with CVD who presented with deep venous reflux, advanced venous stasis, and skin damage have been subject to multiple techniques to improve venous return, including valve transposition, repair, or even axillary vein transfer.[35]

Because isolated deep venous reflux is rare, the current concept of flow overload in the superficial venous system causing venous hypertension and valve dysfunction has been stated. Transmission of the reflux through perforators and saphenofemoral junctions is likely to explain deep venous reflux in association with superficial venous reflux.

Several authors have advocated treatment of superficial venous reflux, instead of direct procedures, to correct deep venous reflux. Walsh et al.[6] performed GSV stripping in 29 limbs with primary CVD, including only CEAP classes 1 through 3, and achieved success abolishing femoral vein reflux in 93% of the cases. In a similar subset of patients including only CEAP classes 1 through 3, Sales et al.[8] achieved hemodynamic normalization of the deep veins in 94% of the patients. However, at the other extreme of the disease presentation, Padberg et al.[34] treated 11 limbs with active ulcers and obtained hemodynamic success in only 27%. All perforators were ligated, and GSV stripping was performed. Nonetheless, the patients did improve, and the ulcers healed with no recurrence at mean 16-month follow-up. Ciostek et al. analyzed photoplethysmography and duplex ultrasound reflux parameters following GSV ablation in 11 patients with secondary CVI and found no statistically significant improvement in deep venous reflux.[36]

The rationale for treating superficial venous reflux before any deep venous intervention is based on clinical and hemodynamic findings. Patients with superficial reflux associated with deep venous reflux present with milder, deep-vein impairment than patients with isolated axial deep venous reflux, suggesting propagation and therefore response to a secondary mechanism as seen in study of 152 limbs.[5] In addition, deep-vein reflux is abolished in patients with initial disease after saphenous vein interruption, corroborating the former mechanism of superficial venous reflux propagation.[6,8] Hemodynamic results may be compromised in patients with skin damage or secondary CVD caused by prolonged inflammatory changes and more severe dilation of the deep veins (Fig. 3.15).

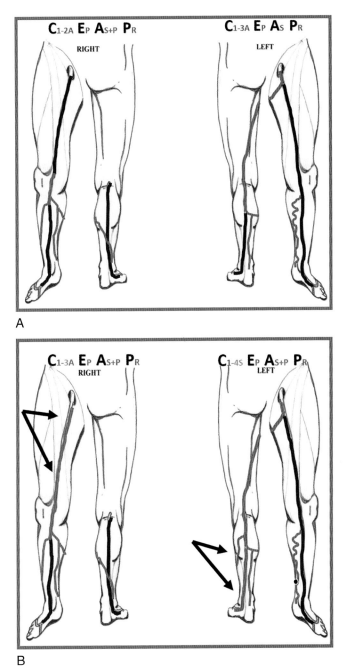

■ Fig. 3.15 A 52-year-old female patient with two previous pregnancies has left lower-extremity varicose veins and right lower-extremity varicose veins, along with edema. Her family history was positive for symptomatic venous disease. (A) Initial presentation at her first physical examination and duplex ultrasound. (B) Progression of venous disease recorded 26 months following initial clinical assessment. Note the clinical progression to lower-extremity edema on the right and skin damage on the left. New segments of saphenous vein reflux have developed *(black arrows).*

FIVE SALIENT REFERENCES

Labropoulos N, Gasparis AP, Tassiopoulos AK. Prospective evaluation of the clinical deterioration in post-thrombotic limbs. *J Vasc Surg.* 2009;50:826–830.

Labropoulos N, Jen J, Jen H, et al. Recurrent deep vein thrombosis: long-term incidence and natural history. *Ann Surg.* 2010;251:749–753.

Labropoulos N, Leon L, Kwon S, et al. Study of the venous reflux progression. *J Vasc Surg.* 2005;41:291–295.

Prandoni P, Noventa F, Ghirarduzzi A, et al. The risk of recurrent venous thromboembolism after discontinuing anticoagulation in patients with acute proximal deep vein thrombosis or pulmonary embolism. A prospective cohort study in 1,626 patients. *Haematologica.* 2007;92:199–205.

Raffetto JD, Khalil RA. Mechanisms of varicose vein formation: valve dysfunction and wall dilation. *Phlebology.* 2008;23:85–98.

REFERENCES

1. Raffetto JD, Khalil RA. Mechanisms of varicose vein formation: valve dysfunction and wall dilation. *Phlebology.* 2008;23(2):85–98.
2. Coleridge Smith PD, Thomas P, Scurr JH, et al. Causes of venous ulceration: a new hypothesis. *Br Med J (Clin Res Ed).* 1988;296(6638):1726–1727.
3. Raffetto JD, Qiao X, Koledova VV, et al. Prolonged increases in vein wall tension increase matrix metalloproteinases and decrease constriction in rat vena cava: potential implications in varicose veins. *J Vasc Surg.* 2008;48(2):447–456.
4. Labropoulos N, Leon L, Kwon S, et al. Study of the venous reflux progression. *J Vasc Surg.* 2005;41(2):291–295.
5. Labropoulos N, Tassiopoulos AK, Kang SS, et al. Prevalence of deep venous reflux in patients with primary superficial vein incompetence. *J Vasc Surg.* 2000;32(4):663–668.
6. Walsh JC, Bergan JJ, Beeman S, et al. Femoral venous reflux abolished by greater saphenous vein stripping. *Ann Vasc Surg.* 1994;8(6):566–570.
7. Puggioni A, Lurie F, Kistner RL, et al. How often is deep venous reflux eliminated after saphenous vein ablation? *J Vasc Surg.* 2003;38(3):517–521.
8. Sales CM, Bilof ML, Petrillo KA, et al. Correction of lower extremity deep venous incompetence by ablation of superficial venous reflux. *Ann Vasc Surg.* 1996;10(2):186–189.
9. Labropoulos N, Tassiopoulos AK, Bhatti AF, et al. Development of reflux in the perforator veins in limbs with primary venous disease. *J Vasc Surg.* 2006;43(3):558–562.
10. Bergan JJ, Pascarella L, Schmid-Schonbein GW. Pathogenesis of primary chronic venous disease: insights from animal models of venous hypertension. *J Vasc Surg.* 2008;47(1):183–192.
11. Yamaki T, Nozaki M. Patterns of venous insufficiency after an acute deep vein thrombosis. *J Am Coll Surg.* 2005;201(2):231–238.
12. Labropoulos N, Gasparis AP, Pefanis D, et al. Secondary chronic venous disease progresses faster than primary. *J Vasc Surg.* 2009;49(3):704–710.
13. Johnson BF, Manzo RA, Bergelin RO, et al. Relationship between changes in the deep venous system and the development of the postthrombotic syndrome after an acute episode of lower limb deep vein thrombosis: a one- to six-year follow-up. *J Vasc Surg.* 1995;21(2):307–312, discussion 313.
14. Labropoulos N, Gasparis AP, Tassiopoulos AK. Prospective evaluation of the clinical deterioration in post-thrombotic limbs. *J Vasc Surg.* 2009;50(4):826–830.
15. Lee BB, Bergan J, Gloviczki P, et al. Diagnosis and treatment of venous malformations Consensus Document of the International Union of Phlebology (IUP)-2009. *Int Angiol.* 2009;28(6):434–451.
16. Gloviczki P, Duncan A, Kalra M, et al. Vascular malformations: an update. *Perspect Vasc Surg Endovasc Ther.* 2009;21(2):133–148.

17. Eklof B, Rutherford RB, Bergan JJ, et al. Revision of the CEAP classification for chronic venous disorders: consensus statement. *J Vasc Surg.* 2004;40(6):1248–1252.

18. Labropoulos N, Delis K, Nicolaides AN, et al. The role of the distribution and anatomic extent of reflux in the development of signs and symptoms in chronic venous insufficiency. *J Vasc Surg.* 1996;23(3):504–510.

19. Caggiati A, Rosi C, Heyn R, et al. Age-related variations of varicose veins anatomy. *J Vasc Surg.* 2006;44(6):1291–1295.

20. Pittaluga P, Chastane S, Rea B, et al. Classification of saphenous refluxes: implications for treatment. *Phlebology.* 2008;23(1):2–9.

21. Garcia-Gimeno M, Rodriguez-Camarero S, Tagarro-Villalba S, et al. Duplex mapping of 2036 primary varicose veins. *J Vasc Surg.* 2009;49(3):681–689.

22. Labropoulos N, Giannoukas AD, Delis K, et al. Where does venous reflux start? *J Vasc Surg.* 1997;26(5):736–742.

23. Bernardini E, De Rango P, Piccioli R, et al. Development of primary superficial venous insufficiency: the ascending theory. Observational and hemodynamic data from a 9-year experience. *Ann Vasc Surg.* 2010;24(6):709–720.

24. Labropoulos N, Leon L, Engelhorn CA, et al. Sapheno-femoral junction reflux in patients with a normal saphenous trunk. *Eur J Vasc Endovasc Surg.* 2004;28(6):595–599.

25. Pittaluga P, Chastanet S, Rea B, et al. Midterm results of the surgical treatment of varices by phlebectomy with conservation of a refluxing saphenous vein. *J Vasc Surg.* 2009;50(1):107–118.

26. Pittaluga P, Chastanet S, Locret T, et al. The effect of isolated phlebectomy on reflux and diameter of the great saphenous vein: a prospective study. *Eur J Vasc Endovasc Surg.* 2010;40(1):122–128.

27. Labropoulos N, Summers K, Sanchez I, et al. Saphenous vein wall thickness in age and venous reflux-associated remodeling in adults. *J Vasc Surg Venous Lymphat Disord.* 2017;5(2):216–223.

28. Vincent JR, Jones GT, Hill GB, et al. Failure of microvenous valves in small superficial veins is a key to the skin changes of venous insufficiency. *J Vasc Surg.* 2011;54(suppl 6):62S–69S. e61-63.

29. Pannier F, Rabe E. Progression in venous pathology. *Phlebology.* 2015;30(suppl 1):95–97.

30. Prandoni P, Noventa F, Ghirarduzzi A, et al. The risk of recurrent venous thromboembolism after discontinuing anticoagulation in patients with acute proximal deep vein thrombosis or pulmonary embolism. A prospective cohort study in 1,626 patients. *Haematologica.* 2007;92(2):199–205.

31. Labropoulos N, Jen J, Jen H, et al. Recurrent deep vein thrombosis long-term incidence and natural history. *Ann Surg.* 2010;251(4):749–753.

32. Labropoulos N. Hemodynamic changes according to the CEAP classification. *Phlebolymphology.* 2003;40:125–129.

33. van Rij AM, De Alwis CS, Jiang P, et al. Obesity and impaired venous function. *Eur J Vasc Endovasc Surg.* 2008;35(6):739–744.

34. Padberg F Jr, Cerveira JJ, Lal BK, et al. Does severe venous insufficiency have a different etiology in the morbidly obese? Is it venous? *J Vasc Surg.* 2003;37(1):79–85.

35. Raju S. Venous insufficiency of the lower limb and stasis ulceration. Changing concepts and management. *Ann Surg.* 1983;197(6):688–697.

36. Ciostek P, Michalak J, Noszczyk W. Improvement in deep vein haemodynamics following surgery for varicose veins. *Eur J Vasc Endovasc Surg.* 2004;28(5):473–478.

CHAPTER 4

Venous Diagnostic Tools

Jan M. Sloves, Jose I. Almeida,
Priscila Gisselle Sanchez Aguirre, and
Andrew M. Abi-Chaker

HISTORICAL BACKGROUND

Of the 25 million Americans with venous disease, approximately 7 million exhibit serious symptoms such as edema, skin changes, and venous ulcers. One million seek formal medical advice annually. Diagnostic testing is used to identify, grade, and follow venous insufficiency and to define deep venous thrombosis (DVT). Because more patients will be presenting for therapy as a result of improved outcomes with endovenous techniques over traditional surgery, diagnostic testing will take on increasing importance. For the purpose of this chapter, diagnostic testing includes the various plethysmography devices, color flow duplex imaging, intravascular ultrasound, and cross-sectional imaging. The goal of these studies is to provide accurate information describing the hemodynamic or anatomic characteristics of the patient with chronic venous insufficiency (Fig. 4.1).[1]

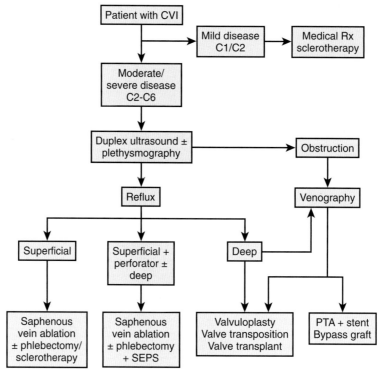

■ **Fig. 4.1** Algorithm for determining treatment of chronic venous insufficiency. *CVI*, Chronic venous insufficiency; *PTA*, percutaneous transluminal angioplasty; *Rx*, treatment; *SEPS*, subfascial endoscopic perforator vein surgery.

ETIOLOGY AND NATURAL HISTORY OF DISEASE

The venous system in the lower extremities is composed of three interconnected parts: the deep system, the perforating system, and the superficial system. In healthy veins, blood flows toward the right side of the heart (i.e., upward) and from the superficial system to the deep system (i.e., inward), driven by the venous muscular pump and unidirectional valves. Lower-extremity muscle compartments contract during ambulation; this contraction compresses the deep veins, producing a pumping action, which propels blood upward toward the right side of the heart. Transient pressures in the deep system have been recorded as high as 5 atmospheres (atm) during strenuous lower-extremity exertion. This pumping action secondary to ambulation has the effect of reducing pressure within the superficial system (Figs. 4.2 and 4.3).

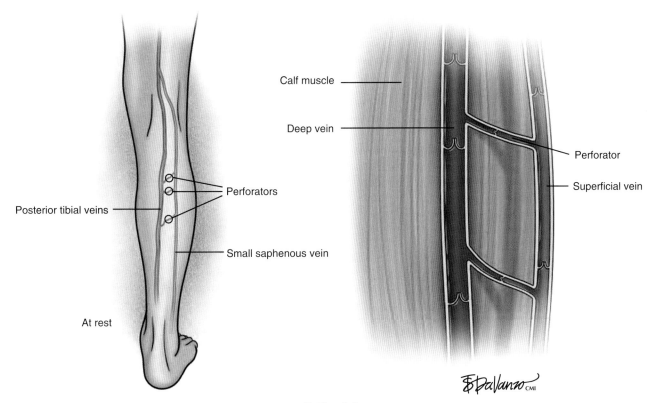

Calf muscle

Deep vein

Perforator

Superficial vein

Perforators

Posterior tibial veins

Small saphenous vein

At rest

■ **Fig. 4.2**

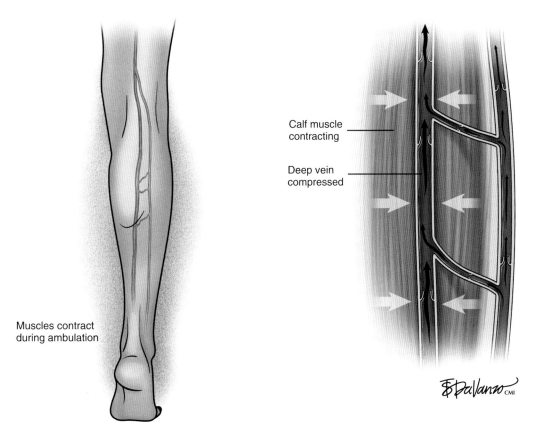

Calf muscle
contracting

Deep vein
compressed

Muscles contract
during ambulation

■ **Fig. 4.3**

All three venous systems of the lower extremity are subjected to hydrostatic pressure. A fluid column has weight and can produce a pressure gradient. In an individual who has a height of 6 feet (183 cm), the distance from the level of the right atrium to the ankle is 120 cm, and this produces a hydrostatic pressure of approximately 90 mm Hg (Fig. 4.4). Deep veins can withstand elevated pressure because the fascia in which they exist limits dilation. In contrast, the superficial system, surrounded by fat and elastic skin, is constructed for low pressure. Therefore elevated pressure in the superficial system can produce dilation, elongation, and valve failure. Dilation increases the diameter of the veins and elongation causes them to be more tortuous.

Because of valve failure, supraphysiologic pressure develops in the superficial venous system and venous dilation ensues (other theories suggest that it is the vein wall that fails with subsequent loss of valvular coaptation). With dilation and multiple valve failure, venous blood will flow in the direction of the pressure gradient, which is downward and outward. This flow direction is directly opposite physiologic flow (i.e., upward and inward). The early result is varicose veins and telangiectasia, which are visible on the skin surface. Symptoms of early or mild superficial venous incompetence produce low-level pain, edema, burning, throbbing, and leg cramping. As the disease progresses, patients can develop venous stasis changes that can lead to debilitating severe soft-tissue ulceration. Based on hemodynamics and clinical experience, symptoms can improve dramatically on elimination of high pressure or flow in diseased, superficial, venous channels.

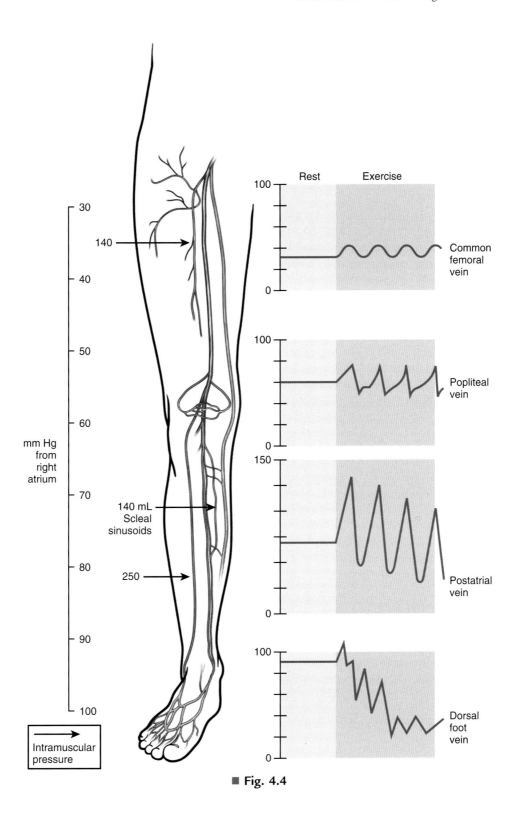

■ Fig. 4.4

INSTRUMENTATION

Plethysmography

To understand lower-extremity venous hemodynamics, venous pressure measurements by dorsal foot vein cannulation can be instructive. The cannula tubing is connected to a fluid column. With the subject standing erect, the fluid column will rise to the level of the right atrium. This is caused by the fact that right atrial pressure is near zero and, therefore the dorsal foot vein pressure at the cannulation site is almost entirely based on the subject's hydrostatic blood column (the subject's blood and the fluid in the column have nearly the same specific weight). When the subject is asked to perform repeated ankle flexion, the fluid column drops to between 50% and 60% of its resting height. This simulates walking and the reduction in superficial venous pressure secondary to the ambulatory venous pump. In subjects with venous insufficiency, the fluid column will not drop to normal levels. If a subject's fluid column falls to normal levels during occlusion of the superficial system, the observer knows the deep system is intact and the superficial system is incompetent. If the fluid column remains elevated with exclusion of the superficial system, the observer knows the deep system is incompetent. Physiologic venous testing is based on these principles (Figs. 4.4 and 4.5).

Plethysmographs are devices that measure volume change. During the past 50 years, plethysmographs have been developed and used clinically with completely different principles. Descriptions of four plethysmographs are given next.

Impedance Plethysmograph

The impedance plethysmograph (IPG) is based on a fundamental principle of electronics, which states that voltage (V) across a segment is equal to the impedance (Z) of the segment multiplied by the current (I) flowing through the segment ($V = Z \times I$). It is possible to isolate a portion of a limb (e.g., thigh, calf) and subject the limb segment to a standard and known current while measuring the voltage across the segment (blood, subcutaneous tissue, and even bone versus impedance). In practice, the operator places circular electrodes around the segment of interest, generally the proximal calf, and connects the electrodes to the electrical console. The subject is asked to perform a series of maneuvers, and outputs from the device are recorded. This method has been used with success by some investigators in the assessment of DVT and venous insufficiency.

Straingauge Plethysmograph

A straingauge plethysmograph (SGP) measures the circumference of a limb segment, which is related to the segment cross-sectional area. The cross-sectional area multiplied by length equals the volume. The device is constructed using a small, hollow, elastic tube filled with mercury and an electrical circuit capable of measuring voltage across the tubing length. The tube containing the mercury is carefully placed around the limb segment of interest and connected to the electrical circuit. The subject is asked to perform a series of maneuvers, and outputs from the device are recorded. As the limb segment circumference is changed secondary to venous blood volume, the length of the elastic tube changes. By measuring circumference as a function of time, venous blood volume as a function of time may be measured.

Photoplethysmograph

Photoplethysmographs (PPGs) are not true plethysmographs because they measure cutaneous microvasculature. PPG instrumentation includes a surface transducer, which is taped to the lower leg just above the medial malleolus and connected to an electrical circuit. The electrical circuit excites the transducer and records and interprets the returning signal. The PPG transducer is designed with an infrared light–emitting diode and a photosensor. The transducer transmits light to the skin, which is both scattered and absorbed by the tissue in the illuminated field. Blood is more opaque than surrounding tissue and therefore attenuates the reflected signal more than other tissue in the field. The intensity of reflected light is reduced with more blood in the field. If the electrical circuit filters the higher-frequency, arterial pulsations, it is possible to register a signal, which qualitatively corresponds to venous volume in the segment of interest.

Air Plethysmograph

An air bladder (cuff) is connected to a console via a single rubber tube, and any change in limb volume is measured by a pressure change within the bladder. If limb volume increases, the bladder volume will decrease, but the bladder pressure will increase. An air plethysmograph (APG) can detect changes in venous limb volume secondary to various patient maneuvers. The APG is used in the clinical assessment of venous insufficiency and DVT. The use of the APG is based on the use of air bladders, which are devices similar to standard blood-pressure cuffs. Physiologic parameters related to chronic

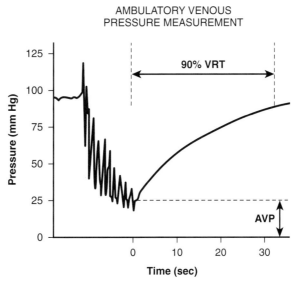

■ **Fig. 4.5** *AVP,* Ambulatory venous pressure; *VRT,* venous refilling time.

venous disease such as chronic obstruction, valvular reflux, calf muscle pump function, and venous hypertension can be measured (Figs. 4.6 and 4.7).

Plethysmography for Venous Insufficiency

Venous insufficiency is characterized by misdirected flow between the three venous systems of the lower extremity. When the patient is supine, the venous pressure in the lower extremities is slightly above right atrial pressure (about 0 mm Hg). In the erect position, the lower-extremity venous pressure increases due to the hydrostatic column of blood extending from the right atrium to the segment of interest. Because veins are compliant, venous blood volume in the segment of interest increases. This volume increase is displayed on a graph from which measurements may be taken.

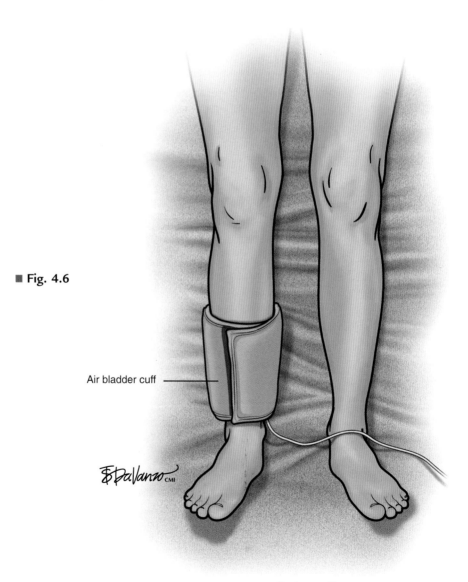

■ Fig. 4.6

Air bladder cuff

Supine position

First, the patient is supine, and outflow testing identifies obstruction and the degree of superficial collateralization. Next, the patient is asked to stand, and the filling rate of the veins by reflux through incompetent valves is measured. The patient is then asked to perform a toe-up exercise, and the calf muscle pump function is measured as an ejection fraction (EF). Finally, the patient performs 10 toe-ups quickly, and a noninvasive measure of ambulatory venous pressure is completed.

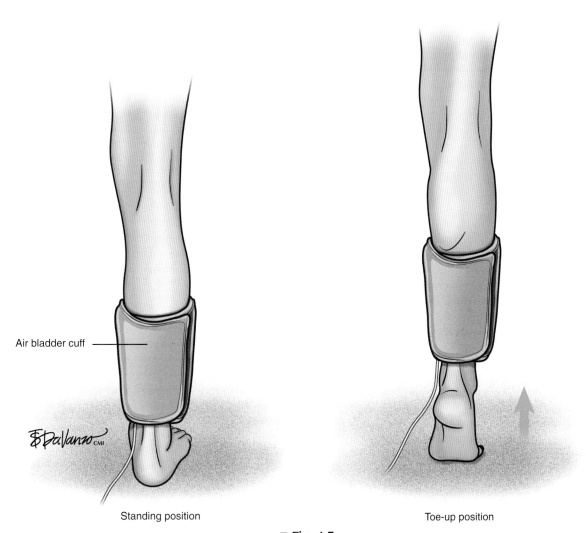

Air bladder cuff

Standing position

Toe-up position

■ **Fig. 4.7**

Venous Filling Index

Briefly, venous filling index (VFI) represents the average filling rate of the veins to 90% of the total venous volume (VV) after first being emptied by gravity. The VFI does not rely on the calf muscle pump for complete vein emptying. EF represents the efficiency of the calf muscle pump and is analogous to left ventricular EF used in cardiology. Residual volume fraction (RVF) is proportional to the invasively measured ambulatory venous pressure, which is a global measurement related to severity of disease. It is important to recognize that VFI measures thigh-to-calf reflux only. Perforator reflux has no effect on VFI, nor does reflux isolated to either the calf or the thigh.

The patient must help in obtaining a clean VFI trace by standing up smoothly and without bumping the cuff. Remind the patient to relax the leg muscles and keep the knee slightly bent to prevent popliteal entrapment.

Ejection Fraction

The EF test consists of three steps. First, the patient applies equal weight on both legs. Next, the patient does their best toe-up effort using both legs equally and without supporting their weight on the support frame, which is used only for balance. The patient remains in the toe-up position for several seconds until the ejection volume is stable (plateau). Finally, the patient returns to the resting position by removing their weight from the test leg with the toe just touching the floor. The veins will quickly refill.

Patients with poor outflow (deep vein obstruction) will take longer to expel calf blood with the single toe-up movement. If the patient were to perform the toe-up exercise quickly, less blood would be ejected past the obstructed vein and the calf pump would appear less effective.

The possible causes of poor calf muscle pump are (1) nonvenous-related problems, including arthritis, ankylosis, and neurologic deficit (whatever prevents the patient from performing a good toe-up movement); (2) proximal obstruction that prevents blood from quickly exiting the calf veins; (3) incompetent calf perforator veins that shunt blood from the deep to the superficial system within the calf; and (4) calf varicosities that retain a large venous volume not expelled with calf muscle contraction.

Residual Volume Fraction

Before beginning the RVF test, one should be certain that VFI testing is completed. The exercise hyperemia resulting from the 10 toe-ups will almost certainly increase VFI and may be mistaken as reflux. The 10 toe-ups are performed similarly to the single toe-up in the EF test, but they are done quickly, approximately one per second. After that, the veins are allowed to refill while the patient stands in the resting position (all weight on the nontested leg). Finally, the patient is returned to the supine position with the operator holding the heel/ankle of the test leg up at 45 degrees with the knee slightly bent. This position is held until an ending baseline is reached. The ending baseline (after the RVF test) may be higher or lower than the baseline value at the beginning of the VFI test.

Recently, the RVF test has been modified by having the patient walk on a treadmill. Walking is no longer simulated by the 10 toe-up movements and the effect of the calf pump is a more accurate reflection of ambulating. Treadmill testing better shows the subtle differences in calf pump function found with the use of compression stockings. The toe-up movement may be such an overpowering use of the calf pump that the effect of compression stockings is overwhelmed and unnoticed.

DEEP VENOUS THROMBOSIS BY PLETHYSMOGRAPHY

The deep venous system is not only a conduit for returning blood to the right side of the heart but is also a storage or capacitant system. This means its volume changes rapidly relative to pressure. If one examines a vein at low pressure, the walls are nearly fully collapsed and only a small flow channel is present. It takes very little increase in internal fluid pressure to expand the flow channel of a vein. Finally, if there is obstruction in a segment of deep vein, despite rich venous collateral channels, venous pressure distal to the obstruction will increase. Examination by plethysmography makes use of these two principles (i.e., volume change with increased pressure and resistance).

Typically, a plethysmograph transducer is placed at the calf or distal thigh with the patient lying supine on a table. In the case of APG, the transducer is an air bladder inflated to 5 mm Hg; in the case of PPG, the transducer is a light-emitting diode. Proximal to the transducer, a method of rapidly occluding the deep system must be used. For all transducers, this can be a thigh cuff inflated rapidly by a hand bulb or automatic inflator.

With the transducer recording a stable venous signal at 5 mm per second chart speed, the pressure in the proximal occluding cuff is rapidly elevated to 50 mm Hg. The transducer is measuring absolute levels of volume. With the increased pressure in the proximal cuff, venous blood in the deep system cannot pass under the cuff until the venous pressure reaches approximately occluding cuff pressure. This increase in venous pressure (i.e., pooling) develops because the proximal cuff does not obstruct the arterial inflow. After about 20 to 40 seconds, pressure in the distal venous system reaches the pressure in the occluding cuff and venous volume reaches a plateau. Once the plateau has been reached, the operator rapidly releases the pressure in the occluding cuff. The pooled venous blood can then return to the right side of the heart via the larger veins upstream. Two measures of venous hemodynamics are taken during this test. First, there is the volume increase from the baseline to the plateau. This is known as *segmental venous capacitance* and represents the blood storage capacity of the segment vein. This is generally quoted in millimeters of deflection or milliliters if the system is calibrated to volume. The second measurement is the slope of the volume-time curve immediately after the pressure in the occluding cuff is released. This is known as *maximum venous outflow*, which represents resistance to blood flow in the deep system and may be quoted in millimeters of deflection per second or milliliters per second if the system is calibrated to volume.

This technique has been largely replaced by duplex ultrasound, which is much more sensitive and specific for the detection of DVT.

DUPLEX ULTRASOUND

Duplex ultrasound has become the gold standard in the diagnosis of both DVTs and venous insufficiency and has replaced the use of venous plethysmographs, continuous wave Doppler signals, and contrast venography. Power Doppler, color flow, pulsed-wave Doppler signals with high-resolution B-mode imaging provide exquisite images and characterize state-of-the-art duplex ultrasound (Figs. 4.8–4.12).

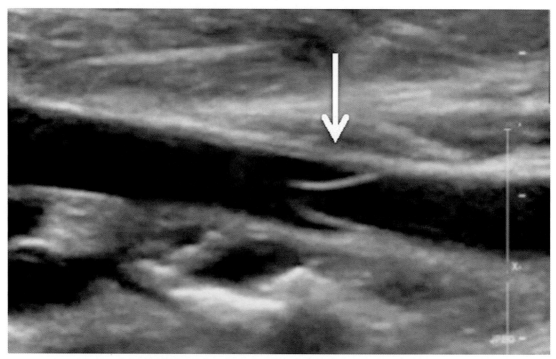

■ **Fig. 4.8** Bicuspid valve femoral vein *(arrow)*.

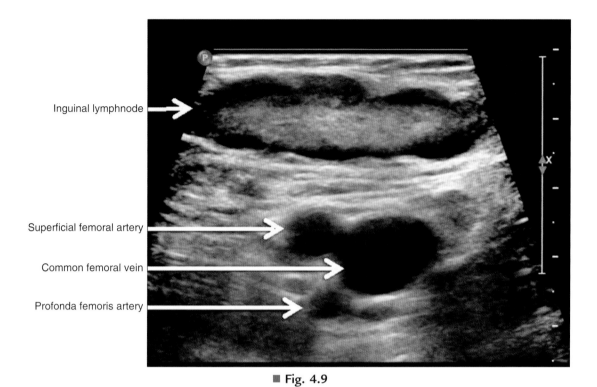

Inguinal lymphnode

Superficial femoral artery

Common femoral vein

Profonda femoris artery

■ Fig. 4.9

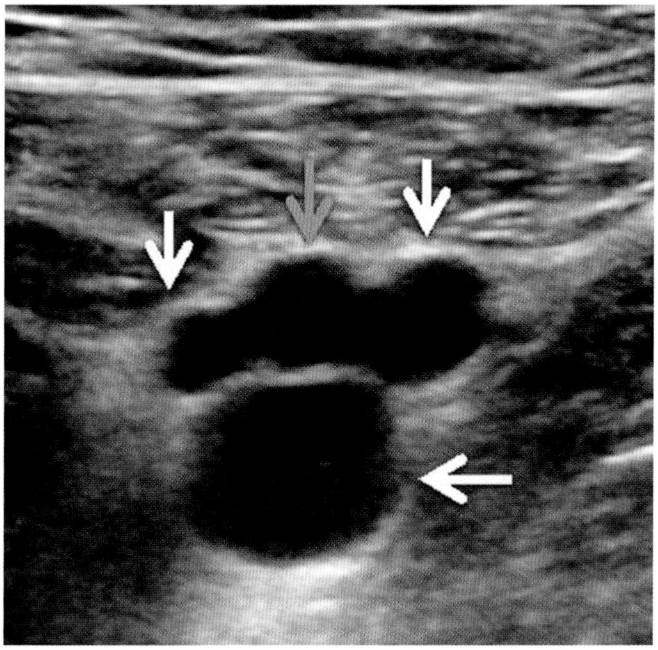

■ **Fig. 4.10** Triplicate femoral vein *(white arrows)* and superficial femoral artery *(blue arrow).*

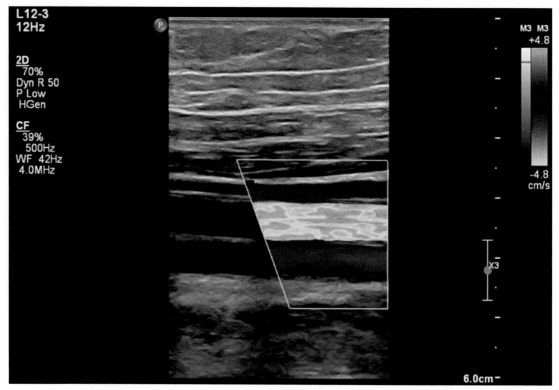

■ **Fig. 4.11** Color flow image of duplicated femoral vein.

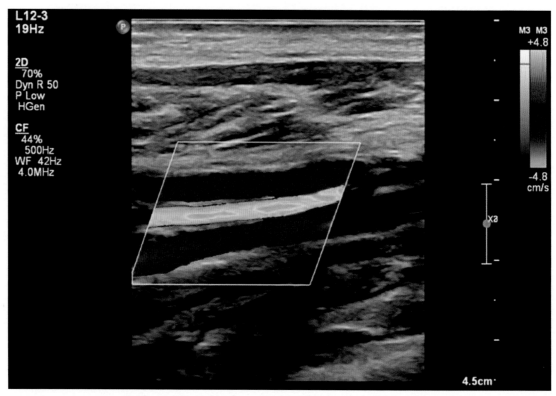

■ **Fig. 4.12** Color flow image of posterior tibial veins.

Panoramic Imaging

Panoramic imaging has emerged as a clinical tool that can be widely used in the diagnosis of venous disease. The benefits of using a longitudinal extended field of view or panoramic imaging is its ability to demonstrate the disease state as well as having the capability to measure vessel lengths beyond 30 cm. As we know, one of the pitfalls associated with a linear transducer is that it only has an approximate footprint of 4 cm in length.

Panoramic image views can be acquired with the use of a curved or linear array transducer. The first step is to optimize the image by adjusting the depth of view, overall gain, and time-gain compensation (TGC). Once the panoramic mode is activated, the operator then advances the transducer over the area of interest. The real-time portion of the image is then replaced by a static section, thus creating an extended field of view. Panoramic imaging uses an image-registration algorithm that identifies image signatures within each frame to provide a sense of the direction and magnitude for each of the transducer movements. Compound-imaging techniques and smoothing functions will automatically reduce noise, clutter, and artifacts, such as vessel pulsations, to provide a superlative image quality. After image acquisition, the operator can trim, zoom, rotate, and measure distance by adding a ruler to the extended field-of-view image. In addition, chroma tint can be used to further enhance the image that, in some clinical settings, may be beneficial when differentiating between plaque, thrombus, or wall stent abnormalities.

In the clinical setting, panoramic imaging can be helpful for both preprocedural and postprocedural planning. Incorporating panoramic-imaging views is useful for guiding the endovascular specialist with a navigational planning tool or a "direct road map" of the peripheral vasculature and the surrounding soft tissue (Fig. 4.13). It will provide an image in an angiographic format, which is anatomically familiar to most interventionalists and used to demonstrate anatomic pathologies. This can include thrombotic, occlusive, or aneurysmal disease states, as well as other pathologies such as masses, cystic structures, or muscular skeletal abnormalities.

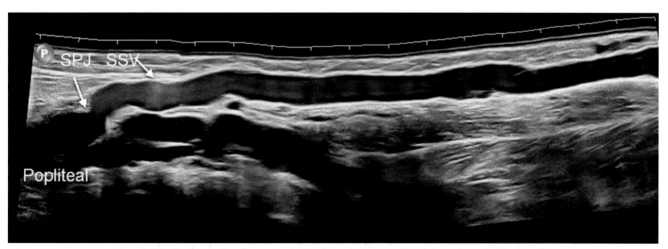

■ **Fig. 4.13** Panoramic chroma view of saphenopopliteal junction (SPJ). Small saphenous vein (SSV) is 16 mm long.

Chroma Imaging

Greyscale imaging is an essential component in the venous duplex examination. In some clinical instances, color-coding the image with a chroma tint is an important first step in optimizing and improving the visual quality. In patients who have a challenging body habitus, this feature can help define and accentuate difficult anatomic structures commonly found within the vessel walls such as thrombi, catheters, filters, or stents. The rationale for coloring the greyscale images is that the human eye has an increased sensitivity to differentiate more color variations than shades of grey. Traditionally, greyscale imaging has become the standard hue for use in ultrasound examinations. Current ultrasound systems have a multitude of chroma tints available with different color schemes that would benefit both greyscale and spectral Doppler waveforms (Fig. 4.14).

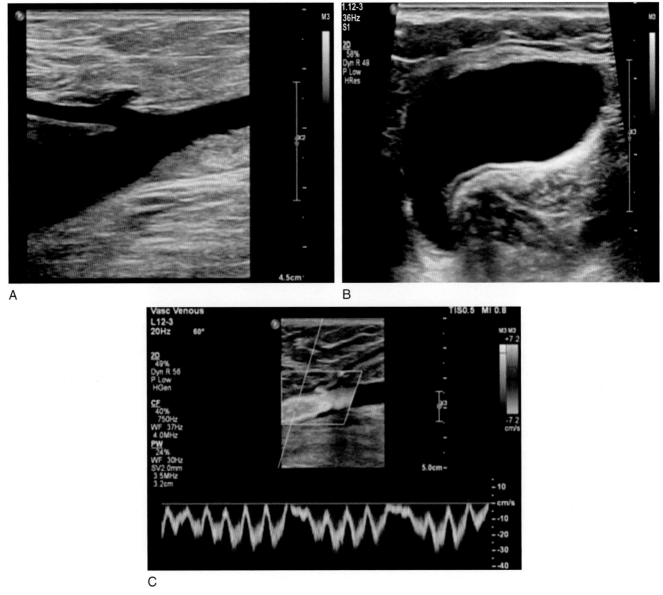

■ **Fig. 4.14** Chroma. (A) Saphenofemoral junction, (B) popliteal fossa cyst, and (C) pulsed Doppler waveform with chroma.

Color Power Angio

Color power angio (CPA) is a modality used in the evaluation of blood flow determination. It can provide the amplitude of the returning Doppler shifted signals demonstrated from the motion of the red blood cells; however, this method does not display absolute velocity information or the direction of blood flow. An important feature is that it can enable the evaluation of slow blood flow because it is less angle dependent and not subject to aliasing, thus an important reason why this mode is superior to conventional color flow imaging. A challenge that we come across when using CPA is its tendency to be prone to motion artifact.

Because of its high sensitivity to slow blood flow, CPA can also be useful when documenting perfusion within the abdominal organs and vasculature, lesions/masses, and blood vessels. The CPA mode has a multitude of uses within the iliocaval region and lower extremity venous circulation. It can be helpful when confirming acute occlusion, as well as determining flow within chronically diseased vein segments, examining areas of stenosis, and demonstrating flow within serpiginous collateral vein networks. In addition, CPA can be beneficial with post ablation surveillance where recanalization of flow is suspected and helpful in demonstrating vein/mass compression or in-stent restenosis.

Depending on the clinical scenario, the operator must be familiar with making the necessary adjustments to the CPA presets concerning the scale, gain, wall filter, and persistence settings. These maneuvers are essential to defining the precise pathology, and failure to do so can lead to a misdiagnosis. Bidirectional color power Doppler is a newer CPA mode feature that uses multiple sound beams and the autocorrelation technique. This allows for simultaneous color mapping of red and blue, indicating the direction of blood flow (Fig. 4.15).

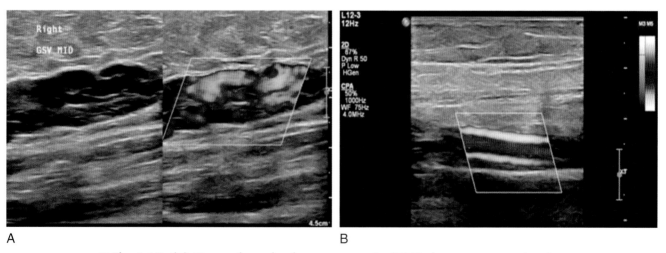

A   B

■ **Fig. 4.15** (A) Greyscale and color power angio (CPA) demonstrate previously ablated great saphenous vein with recanalization of flow. (B) Bidirectional CPA demonstrates flow in the posterior tibial veins in a patient with postthrombotic syndrome.

Three-Dimensional Imaging

Over the last decade, three-dimensional (3D) ultrasound has revolutionized the way clinicians diagnose, provide treatment, and manage patients with a variety of anomalies. 3D ultrasound is a valuable tool used in various fields, including applications in cardiac, obstetric, abdominal, and vascular studies. At present, it is possible for 3D ultrasound to construct high-resolution volume images that are comparable with those produced by computed tomography (CT) and magnetic resonance imaging (MRI) modalities at a lower cost and within a shorter time interval.

In some clinical scenarios, 3D imaging is the modality of choice used for direct visualization in defining precise anatomic locations and pathologies, as well as becoming indispensable in guiding surgical and percutaneous procedures. These advancements are, in part, because of the transducer design, ease of workflow, and computer software algorithms. The examinations are performed with a single transducer made up of a matrix array technology constructed of thousands of active elements providing performance in two-dimensional (2D), 3D, and four-dimensional image planes. It is important to recognize that a 2D transducer will only show one image plane at a time. However, an advantage to using a 3D transducer is its ability to simultaneously capture multiple image planes.

Moreover, the 3D transducer can be used in the biplane mode that displays two separate 2D planes. Biplane imaging allows for the operator to target the reference plane, view the region of interest, and move onto the second plane to observe an additional planar image (Fig. 4.16). Once this region has been identified, the operator can acquire a single image or cineloop.

The two most commonly used 3D techniques are multiplanar reformatting (MPR) and volume rendering (VR). When initiating the MPR dataset, the screen will be divided into four quadrants, three of which represent the X, Y, Z axes or orthogonal planes (i.e., longitudinal, transverse, and coronal) with the fourth representing the rendered image or cineloop. Once the dataset has been acquired, it can then be manipulated on the

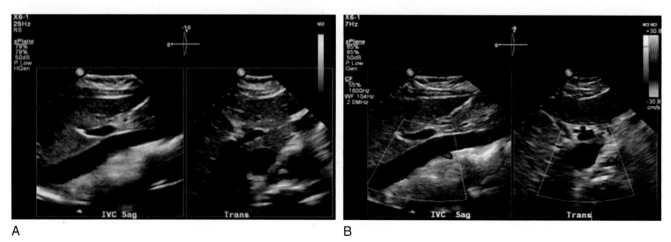

A   B

■ **Fig. 4.16** Biplane greyscale (A) and color flow (B) images of the inferior vena cava.

ultrasound system or off line on a picture-archiving and communication system with quantification software the same way CT and MRI images are viewed. During the postprocessing phase, the acquired images captured in the X, Y, Z, and slice MPR planes, as with cineloops, can be cropped in different axis planes to define the anatomic structures and pathology in question (Fig. 4.17). In addition, images acquired with color flow or power Doppler can be cropped, rotated, and further optimized with various postprocessing features such as gain, steering options, zoom, and chroma tint; use of these features will allow for the acquisition of precise images.

Although 2D duplex ultrasound is a reliable imaging modality, there are clinical scenarios when more information is required. For example, when obtaining 2D measurements for organs, the data gathered can vary and be inaccurate at times because of anatomic boundaries. With 3D imaging, the operator has the ability to acquire datasets via simplified volume acquisition, hence having more options and flexibility to manipulate the transducer, view the desired anatomic image planes, and define the potential segments. As a result, the operator captures a complete examination with better qualitative and quantitative information, reducing the overall study time and allowing for more accuracy in making the clinical diagnosis.

In the clinical setting, 3D ultrasound can be used during a variety of clinical scenarios as follows: when evaluating the severity of vessel obstruction, filter patency and position, wall stent abnormalities, stenotic lesions and aneurysmal segments. Furthermore, 3D ultrasound aids in confirming potential tumor invasion of adjacent vascular structures, defining areas of tortuosity and kinking, determining characteristics of vascular lesions, evaluating for suspected venous compression, and defining vascular organ perfusion.

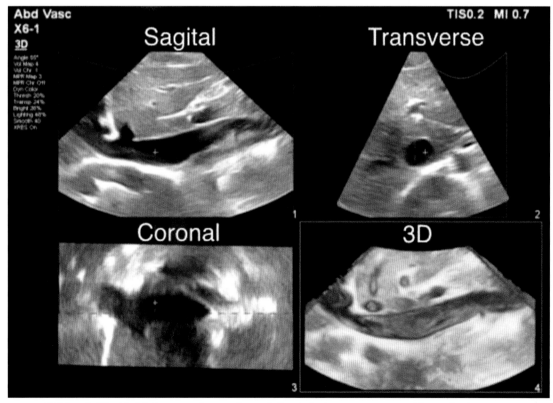

■ **Fig. 4.17** Multiplanar reformatting of the inferior vena cava with sagittal, transverse, coronal, and 3D-rendered images.

In conclusion, it is evident that 3D imaging modality offers a multitude of advantages. It plays a role in assessing for different types of deep and superficial venous pathology, and because of its affordability compared with cross-sectional imaging, could allow for mainstream use in clinical practice setting. A particular benefit for the endovascular specialist is its usefulness in planning a course of action before an invasive procedure. As this technology continues to be developed, we should expect that 3D ultrasound imaging would eventually become part of the mainstay in the clinical setting.

Deep Venous System

Choosing the right transducer for a certain patient, illness, or vein is important. Axial resolution and tissue penetration are inversely related. A 4-MHz to 7-MHz linear-array transducer is optimal for assessing most veins, which normally lie between 1 and 3 cm below the skin. Very shallow veins can be examined with higher-frequency transducers to achieve better resolution. Deep veins such as those in the abdomen or pelvis, or veins in obese or edematous patients are better assessed by using lower frequency curvilinear transducers for deeper penetration.

Low blood flow settings are used most often. The pulse repetition frequency (PRF, or the number of pulses transmitted per second) is set at 1500 Hz or lower. When vein stenosis or arteriovenous fistulae are suspected, PRF should be increased because blood flow velocity is considerably elevated. The imaging focus should be set at the far wall (in relation to the skin) to achieve better lateral resolution. The lumen of the vein should be set to appear dark in the absence of stasis and thrombosis. TGC (or increasing amplification of ultrasound echoes with depth to compensate for their progressive attenuation) is set according to the echogenicity and location of the examined tissues to improve imaging. The weaker the signal seen with increasing depth, the higher the gain that will be required. When velocity waveforms are obtained, gain should be set so that the background is dark to avoid overestimation. The insonation angle is often set at 0 degrees. However, because most veins run parallel to the skin, this angle has to be set to parallel the vein flow channel. An angle of insonation of 45 to 60 degrees between the transducer and the vein should be used to achieve the optimum Doppler waveform.

The examination should be performed on a flat examining table in which the patient's lower extremities are placed in the dependent position at approximately 15 degrees. This slight angle dilates the deep system, which makes the identification of veins easier and improves the velocity signals. Deep vein interrogation from the level of the inguinal ligament to the ankle should include the common femoral, femoral, popliteal, and tibial veins. The deep femoral vein should also be included, especially in cases where femoral vein thrombosis has been identified.

The evaluation begins at the groin using greyscale imaging. Usually seen are the common femoral vein, common femoral artery, and great saphenous vein (GSV), forming a "Mickey Mouse" image (Fig. 4.18). As the probe continues distally, the technologist should focus on keeping the superficial femoral artery and the femoral vein in clear view. The popliteal artery and the popliteal vein are difficult to visualize in the adductor canal, therefore these structures are identified from behind by placing the probe in the popliteal crease. In the calf, the duplicated posterior tibial and peroneal veins, with their associated single arteries, can be viewed from a medial approach as they travel between the muscle bellies. Similarly, the gastrocnemius and soleus veins are identified; however, they are located within the muscular bellies. In general, the anterior tibial veins are not interrogated because they are rarely pathologic.

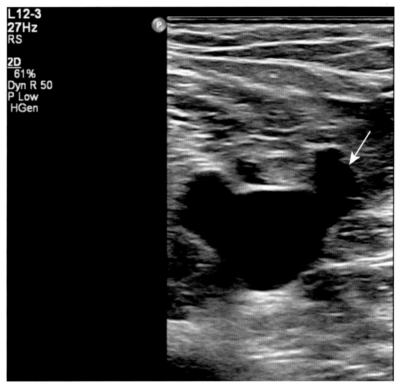

■ **Fig. 4.18** "Mickey Mouse" sign *(arrow)* at saphenofemoral junction (short-axis view).

With the probe, the operator can compress the vein in the short-axis view. The ability to fully compress the vein walls and obliterate the venous lumen momentarily confirms vein patency and absence of thrombus formation (Fig. 4.19). If the technologist identifies the thrombus, the next step is to determine its age. Acute thrombi are characterized by vein dilatation and noncompressible echolucent material, whereas chronic thrombi take on a speckled, hyperechoic, ultrasonic appearance.

If the evaluated system from the common femoral vein through the tibial veins is compressible and no evidence of thrombus formation is seen, the study is considered negative for DVT. The technologist may use the Doppler portion of the duplex system in the long-axis view to verify artery versus vein and determine flow direction. Color Doppler signals, power Doppler signals, compression maneuvers, and respiratory maneuvers can be used to supplement this procedure if necessary. Normal veins have spontaneous flow, which is phasic with respiration (Fig. 4.20).

It is crucial to assess the iliac veins and the inferior vena cava (IVC) when disease is suspected at that level. In this case, however, flow is evaluated chiefly because compression can be difficult and uncomfortable. Asymmetry of flow velocity, waveform, and pattern at rest and during flow augmentation in the common femoral vein (CFV) indicates proximal obstruction. However, the absence of asymmetry cannot exclude obstruction. Accordingly, when iliocaval obstruction is suspected, the full extent of these veins must be imaged. The presence of stenosis, usually from extrinsic compression, is recognized by the mosaic color, which denotes poststenotic turbulence, an abnormal Doppler waveform at the stenotic area, slow flow, spontaneous contrast, and vein dilatation

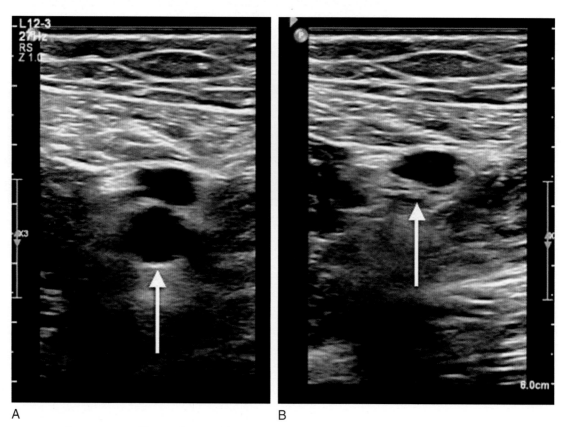

A   B

■ **Fig. 4.19** Midfemoral vein (short-axis view). *Arrows* show vein before compression (A) and after (B).

before the stenosis (Fig. 4.21). The reduction in vein diameter can be measured by planimetry to compare the smallest lumen with the normal lumen and by the peak vein velocity ratio (poststenotic/prestenotic). The four components that should be examined are visualization, compressibility, flow, and augmentation.[2]

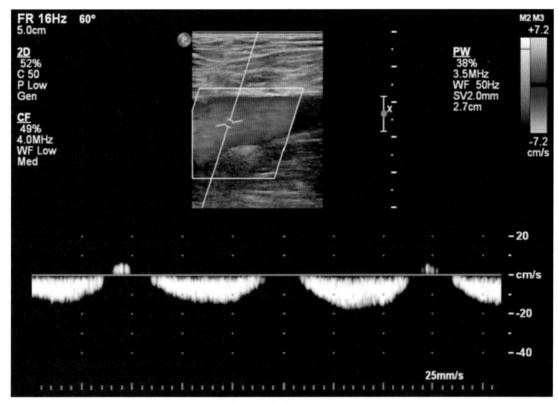

■ **Fig. 4.20** Phasic flow.

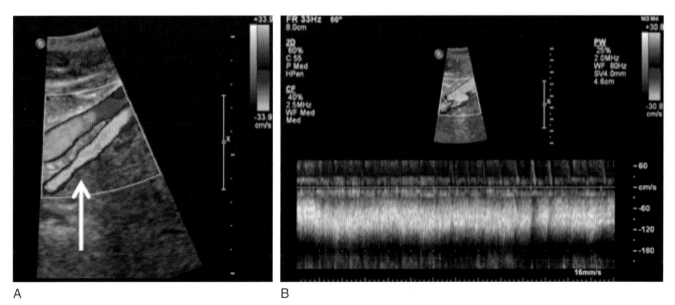

■ **Fig. 4.21** (A) Color flow image of external iliac venous stenosis *(white arrow)*. (B) Pulsed wave Doppler demonstrates continuous flow at site of stenosis.

Acute Thrombosis

A fresh thrombus is mostly hypoechoic, homogeneous, partially compressible, seen in a dilated vein, and sometimes floating.[2] Veins with acute thrombosis are echolucent and distended with smooth walls. Acute thrombus is spongy on compression but will obviate the vein walls from coapting. There is a poorly defined transition from an acute to subacute thrombosis. This is mostly characterized by the mixed hypohyperechoic heterogeneous thrombus seen on imaging (Figs. 4.22–4.25). Other findings such as lower extremity edema can corroborate the clinical presentation (Fig. 4.26).

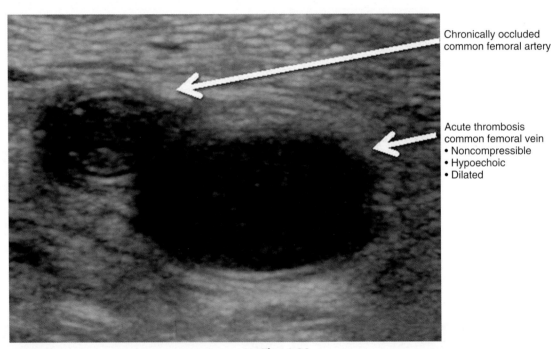

Chronically occluded
common femoral artery

Acute thrombosis
common femoral vein
• Noncompressible
• Hypoechoic
• Dilated

■ Fig. 4.22

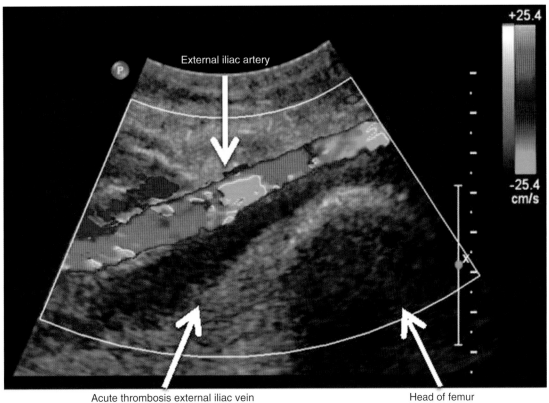

■ **Fig. 4.23**

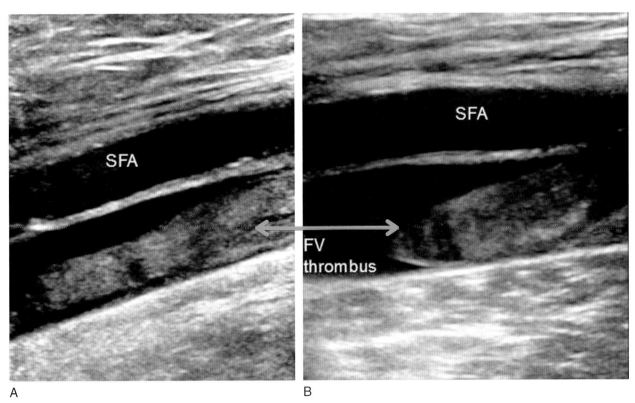

■ **Fig. 4.24** Partially occlusive subacute deep vein thrombosis in femoral vein (FV). Note that the vein is noncompressible, mixed hypoechoic and hyperechoic, and less dilated than acute. *SFA*, Superficial femoral artery.

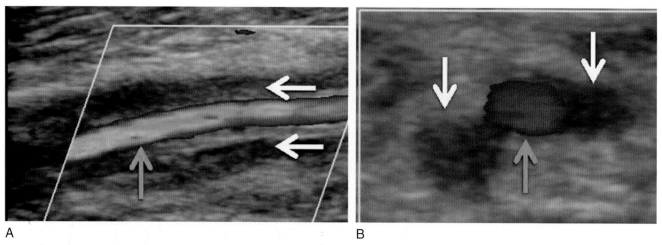

A   B

■ **Fig. 4.25** Long-axis (A) and short-axis (B) views of subacute thrombosis in posterior tibial veins *(white arrows)* and artery *(blue arrows)*. Note that the veins are noncompressible, mixed hypoechoic and hyperechoic, and less dilated than acute.

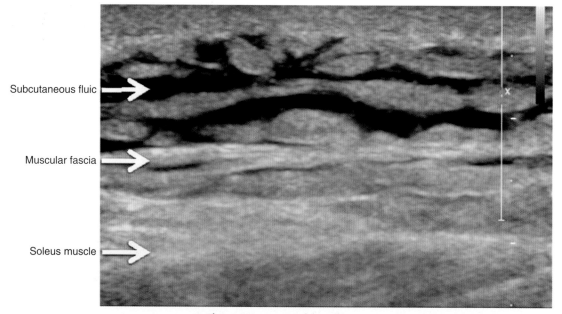

Subcutaneous fluic

Muscular fascia

Soleus muscle

■ **Fig. 4.26** Lower leg edema.

Chronic Thrombosis

Chronic thrombosis is characterized by the presence of an organized hyperechoic heterogeneous noncompressible thrombus firmly adherent to the vein wall on duplex ultrasound.[2] Chronic thrombus is firm. Chronic thrombi are echogenic, contracted with thick and irregular walls, and usually demonstrate multiple channels or collateralization. Intraluminal webs and wall thickening, with or without reflux, indicate previous thrombosis and can cause functional obstruction. The presence of dilated collateral veins is more indicative of obstruction, but their absence cannot exclude it. Veins can also fully recanalize without any anatomic obstruction (Figs. 4.27 and 4.28).

There also exists a poorly defined transition from subacute to chronic thrombosis (Fig. 4.29).

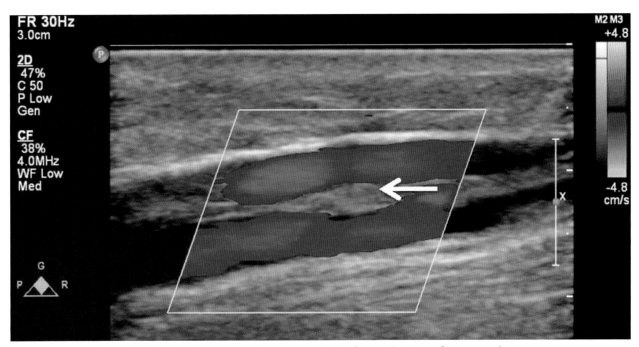

■ **Fig. 4.27** Chronic deep vein thrombosis in femoral vein. After recanalization, color flow *(blue)* and fibrous strand *(arrow)*.

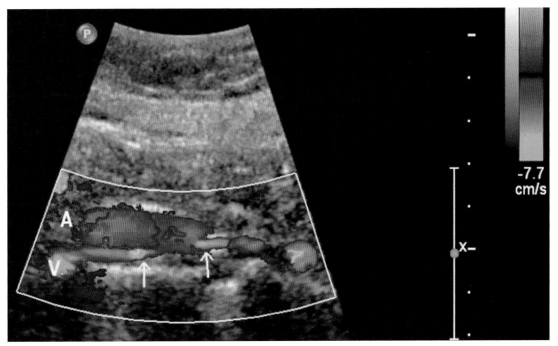

■ **Fig. 4.28** Chronic postthrombotic disease in common iliac vein *(arrows)*. *A,* Artery; *V,* vein.

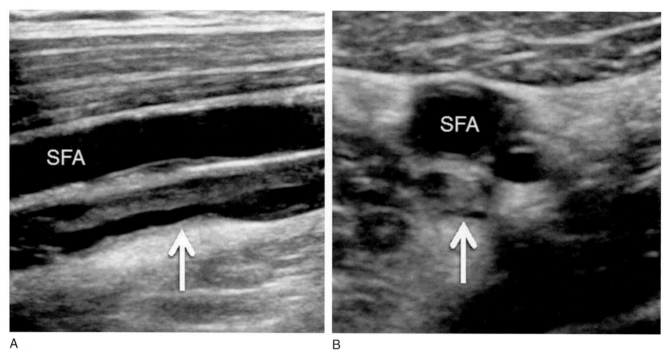

A   B

■ **Fig. 4.29** Long-axis (A) and short-axis (B) views of subacute/chronic deep vein thrombosis in femoral vein. Recanalization of thrombosis indicated by *arrows. SFA,* Superficial femoral artery.

Superficial Venous System

For superficial venous studies, patients are examined in the standing position. The patient rotates the leg of interest to expose the medial surface of the lower extremity from the groin to the ankle. To the extent possible, weight should be shifted from the leg of interest to relax the musculature. A standing stool with arm support may be necessary.

Once positioned, the operator begins at the groin and produces the Mickey Mouse landmark described earlier. Starting from the three-vessel image in the transverse view, the probe moves down the leg following the course of the GSV. The normal GSV extends from the saphenofemoral junction to the ankle and is enveloped by superficial fascia above and muscular fascia below. Diameter measurements are recorded in millimeters, and the presence of reflux (positive or negative) is documented at the saphenofemoral junction, midthigh, and below knee. If reflux is present, the duration of retrograde flow in seconds is also documented.

Reflux is determined at locations of interest using the following technique.[3] The operator adjusts the color box of the duplex system in the measurement location. The velocity scale is adjusted (maximum 25 cm/s). While a signal is being obtained, the technologist compresses the calf (below the probe) in a brisk manner. The vein highlighted in the color box should demonstrate an increase in velocity toward the heart with compression. On release, the vein should demonstrate no velocity or minimal velocity away from the heart. We have found that reflux (venous flow away from the heart after release) lasting between 0.5 and 2 seconds is mild. Reflux is severe if present for longer than 2 seconds.

The same evaluation is repeated posteriorly for the small saphenous vein (SSV). This vein originates in the distal calf and can terminate in the upper thigh. We access this vessel with ultrasound by rotating the subject to expose the back of the legs. We identify the SSV at the distal calf and advance over its course (Fig. 4.30). Multiple levels may be assessed; however, we generally record a characteristic SSV diameter (in millimeters) and assess reflux in the most diseased location.

It is important to note that there are variations in superficial venous anatomy. For example, the GSV may be quite small and complemented by an anterior accessory saphenous vein, which may be competent or incompetent. Further, the GSV may be tortuous or exit the saphenous canal in portions of its course (Fig. 4.31). In addition,

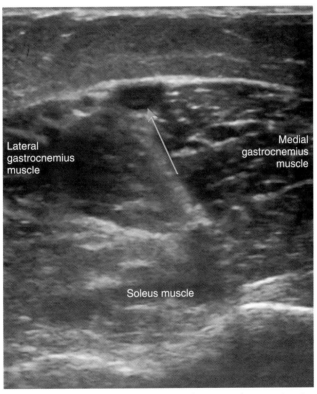

■ **Fig. 4.30** Small saphenous vein (*arrow;* short axis view).

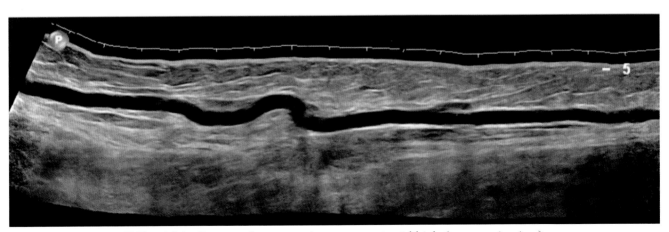

■ **Fig. 4.31** Great saphenous vein tortuous at midthigh (panoramic view).

the GSV may exhibit postthrombotic changes in cases of prior superficial thrombophlebitis (Fig. 4.32).

The lower extremity has some common perforators that play significant roles in venous insufficiency. In clinical practice, perforating veins previously associated frequently with names of authorities (e.g., Hunter, Dodd) have been replaced by descriptive terms designating location. Perforating veins with clinical relevance are usually found in the midthigh, upper calf, or ankle (Fig. 4.33). If present, perforators should be assessed regarding diameter, degree of reflux, and extension to other superficial structures.

Duplex ultrasound is not only diagnostic but also plays a crucial role in endovenous ablation for catheter positioning, monitoring the success of vein closure procedures (Fig. 4.34), and placement of tumescent anesthesia (Fig. 4.35). In addition, it is mandatory for intraluminal placement of foam sclerosants (Fig. 4.36).

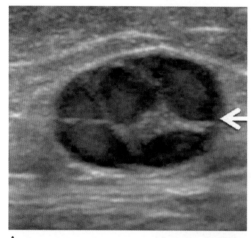

A

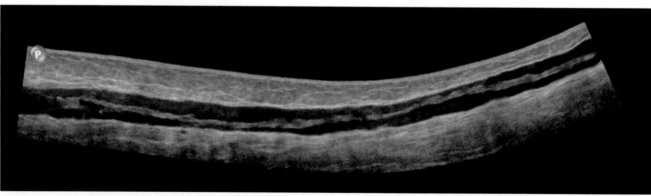

B

■ **Fig. 4.32** (A) Great saphenous vein (GVS) webs *(arrow)* indicate previous thrombosis (short-axis view, greyscale). (B) GVS recanalization and intraluminal fibrosis (panoramic view, greyscale).

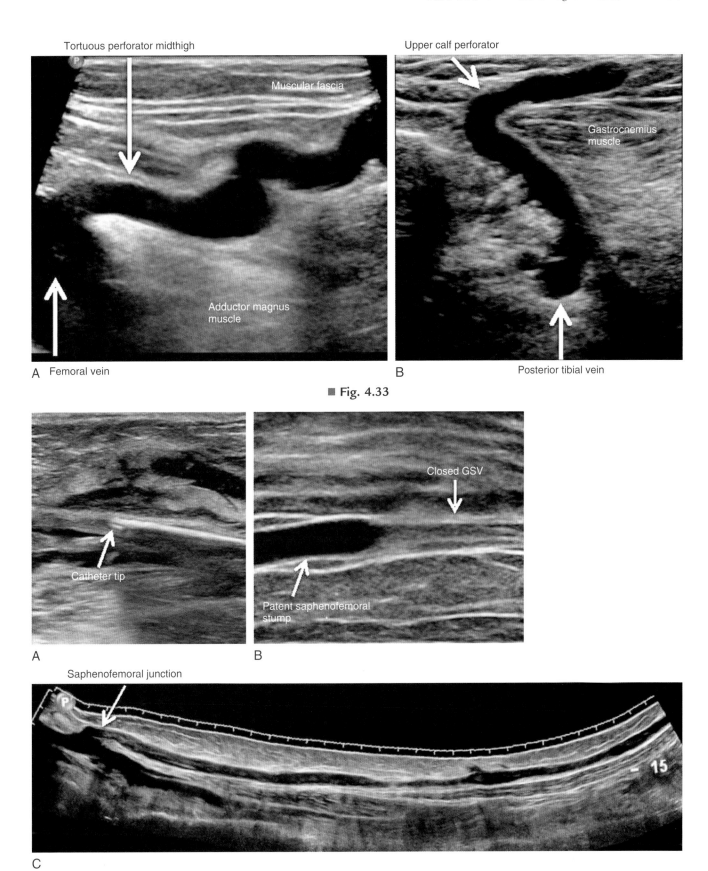

Tortuous perforator midthigh

Muscular fascia

Adductor magnus
muscle

A Femoral vein

Upper calf perforator

Gastrocnemius
muscle

B Posterior tibial vein

■ Fig. 4.33

Catheter tip

A

Closed GSV

Patent saphenofemoral
stump

B

Saphenofemoral junction

C

■ **Fig. 4.34** (A) Radiofrequency ablation (RFA) catheter with tumescent.
(B) Great saphenous vein after stab phlebectomy RFA. (C) Stab phlebectomy
RFA with occlusion (panoramic view).

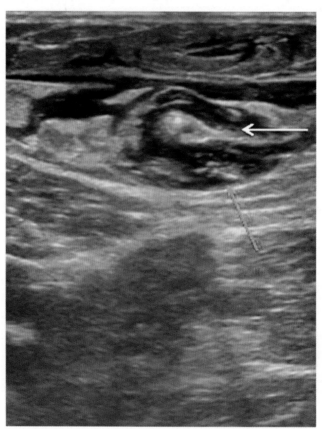

■ **Fig. 4.35** Compressed great saphenous vein with intraluminal laser fiber *(white arrow)*. Perivenous tumescent anesthesia *(blue arrow)* (short-axis view, greyscale).

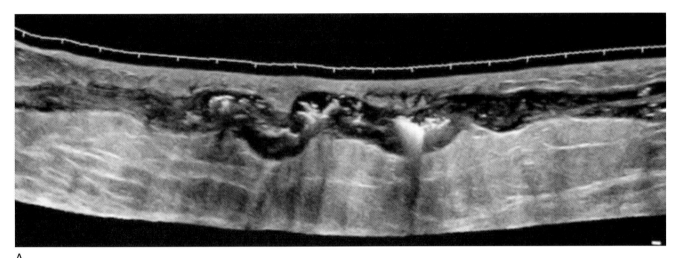

A

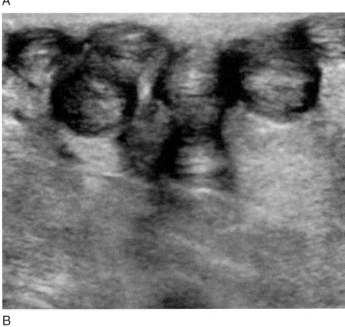

B

■ **Fig. 4.36** (A) Great saphenous vein after ultrasound-guided foam sclerotherapy (UGFS; panoramic view). (B) Surface varicose veins after UGFS (short-axis view).

Image Optimization

Image optimization plays a central role in the quality of our venous duplex examinations. The goal is to use each respective transducer in such a way that the images produced are of the highest quality and contain enough diagnostic information to assist the clinician in making an accurate diagnosis. Thus the images acquired will drive the interpretation.

Current ultrasound technology demonstrates improvement in the processing power, penetration, transducer frequencies, image quality, and workflow. Typically, systems are configured with linear and curved array transducers equipped with standard manufacturer tissue specific presets for each vascular bed. From an engineering perspective, there have been advancements made that relate to improved optimization. For example, there is a control button that can automatically optimize the gain and TGC that will directly improve the greyscale image found on most systems.

Having automated functions and presets are usually just a starting point with which to begin the examination. It is imperative that the operator acquires the technical skills and an understanding with which to properly use the controls as they relate to greyscale, color flow, and pulsed Doppler. Adequate skills coupled with making the necessary adjustments to the settings will aid in defining the anatomy and pathology, regardless of the patient's body habitus (which at times can make the acquisition of images challenging).

There are two components of image optimization. The first underscores proper scanning techniques and modalities used to demonstrate venous hemodynamics. This is achieved by correctly using color flow and pulsed Doppler. The second concerns the constant improvement of image resolution throughout the course of the examination with all three duplex modalities, greyscale, color flow, and pulse wave Doppler.

Understanding the sonographic echo texture within the lower extremities is important in optimizing the greyscale image contour. When the transducer receives a returning echo signal, its amplitude is represented by the overall degree of brightness, which is referred to as the *echogenicity*. It is a fusion of the acquired reflected signals that finalizes the image. The stronger reflections tend to provide brighter signals known as *hyperechoic*, whereas the weaker and more diffuse reflections produce grey signals known as *hypoechoic*. When there is no reflection, it produces dark signals that are known as *anechoic*. This happens because the beam passes directly through these structures without significant reflection.

Deeper structures will often appear as hypoechoic. This is because the attenuation limits the beam's transmissibility to reach certain structures, resulting in an echo signal that is much weaker on return.

The sonographic presentation of arteries and veins are described as *anechoic* (Fig. 4.37) Tendons are mostly described as *hyperechoic* in their appearance. Muscles are noted to be heterogeneous in their echotexture, with a mixture of hyperechoic lines within a hypoechoic tissue background. Fat tends to appear as hypoechoic with irregular hyperechoic lines. The presentation of nerves can range from hyperechoic to hypoechoic, depending on the frequency of the transducer used. The contour of bone demonstrates hyperechoic lines with hypoechoic shadowing.

From a technical perspective, the echogenicity of various structures is a function of the underlying tissue characteristics. For example, ultrasound waves scatter a great deal when going through fat tissue, thus resulting in the haze we see in fatty areas. Another example is when the ultrasound waves attenuate as they travel through muscle, resulting in an image that appears darker. With scarcely any ultrasound reflection travelling through the vessel lumen, the resulting appearance will be black.

When performing venous duplex examinations, choose a transducer with the highest frequency that will achieve the best resolution possible with sufficient penetration for that specific tissue type. It is not unusual for the operator to use more than one transducer during the course of a study. Typically, transducer frequencies used in venous imaging ranges from 3 to 14 MHz, depending on the specific area of interest. The frequency of the transducer determines the axial image resolution and allowable image depth. As the frequency increases, so will the resolution; however, the depth of penetration will

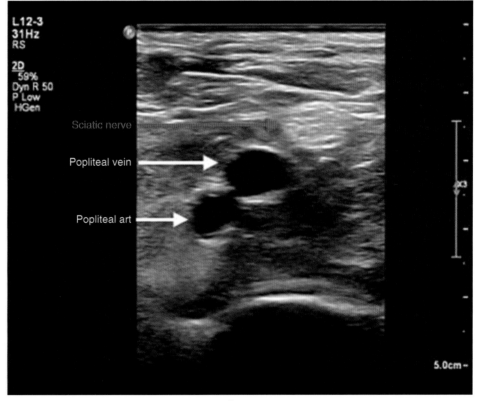

■ Fig. 4.37

decrease. This is because tissue penetration is inversely related to the transducer frequency. In general, for any given transducer, the operator can select the frequency range within which to operate the probe. By switching between a higher and lower frequency in the same transducer, the operator can trade-off between resolution and penetration. Below are some examples that demonstrate the trade-offs made when switching between high-frequency and low-frequency modes using the same transducer (Fig. 4.38).

Harmonic imaging is a technique that provides improved image quality when compared with fundamental ultrasound imaging. Greyscale imaging is used for defining the vessel lumen, detecting various degrees of obstruction, and depicting structures within surrounding soft tissues. A key factor when using harmonics is its ability to provide better greyscale contrast resolution. When needed, the operator can select between different harmonic frequency settings established by the system's respective manufacturer presets. Using harmonic imaging will allow for improved penetration at lower frequencies; this can be particularly helpful when examining technically difficult patients. As an example, Fig. 4.39 demonstrates the difference in vessel clarity between harmonic and fundamental imaging.

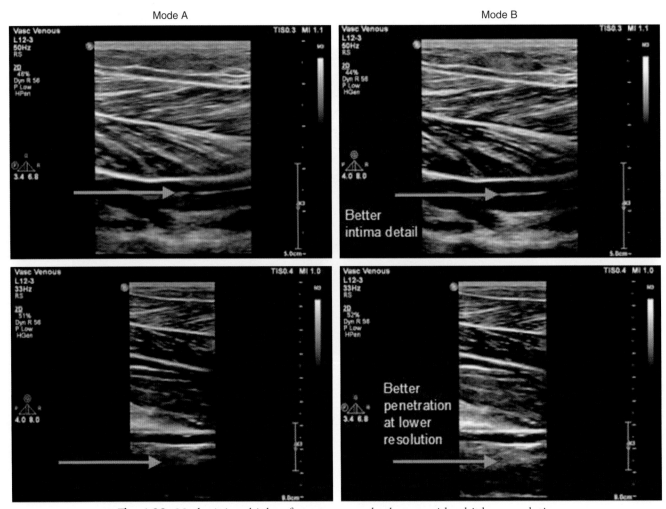

■ **Fig. 4.38** Mode A is a higher frequency mode that provides higher resolution with less penetration. Mode B is a lower frequency mode that provides more penetration with slightly lower resolution.

For more technically difficult patients, when there is not enough penetration with all harmonic modes, the operator can switch to the fundamental imaging modality. When using the fundamental mode, there will be some haze noted within the vessel lumen; however, this will not limit the operator's ability to achieve the desired depth of penetration. This is an important point to consider when the operator cannot reach the level of penetration when using harmonic imaging.

Another option to consider when examining a technically difficult or obese patient is to switch from a linear-array transducer to a curved-array transducer. Examination of these patients typically poses a challenge with penetration across the thigh, especially at the Hunter canal and the calf. The presence of increased adiposity will certainly increase the risk of potentially missing any disease. Using a curved-array transducer with harmonics below the inguinal ligament will provide the operator with an imaging depth up to 30 cm and an extended field of view of 11 cm. Once the depth of penetration is achieved, further adjustments made to the controls regarding the sector width, gain, focal zone, and TGC will be necessary to better define the vessel in question. In this scenario, with the use of color flow the operator should decrease the scale, increase the gain, and increase the persistence to achieve adequate color filling. Furthermore, the curved-array transducer will provide another benefit because it can measure structures greater

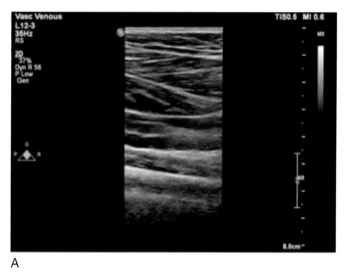

A

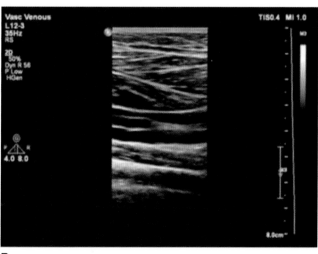

B

■ **Fig. 4.39** Fundamental (A) and harmonic (B) imaging (sagittal view).

than 4 cm in length, whereas the linear-array transducer cannot (Fig. 4.40). This is usually helpful when the operator comes across an incidental finding during the examination.

At the onset of the examination and before image acquisition, it is important to recognize that the optimal greyscale gain contains a mixed range of signals that are low and high in their overall amplitude. If the gain is set too high, the echo signal will be obliterated, and this will result in loss of image resolution. Conversely, if the gain settings are too low and the image produced is dark, abnormalities can be masked, thus resulting in decreased sensitivity. Altering the depth, harmonic frequencies, focal zone, and TGC are essential in attaining superlative resolution. Ideally, the focal zone should be set at or just below the target area of significance. The TGC settings provide exact corrections to the gain at specific depths throughout the image and can have a profound influence on the overall image quality. Examples are shown in Figs. 4.41 through 4.46, while Fig. 4.47 summarizes steps for image optimization.

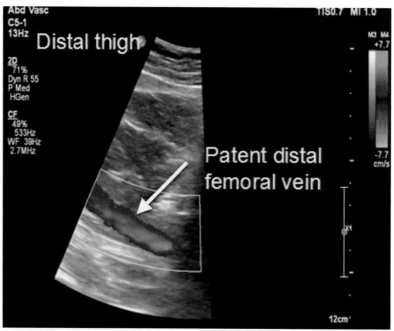

■ **Fig. 4.40** Ultrasound image from a curved arrary transducer used on a technically difficult patient (sagittal view, color flow).

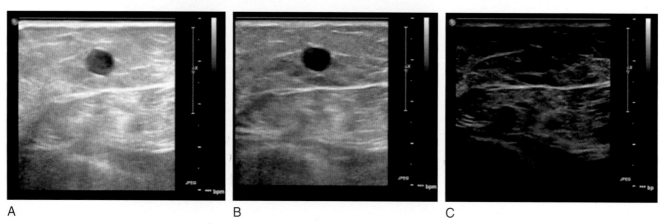

A   B   C

■ **Fig. 4.41** Great saphenous vein (short-axis view, greyscale). (A) Over-gain, (B) optimal gain, and (C) under gained.

Overall gain set too low

Optimal gain

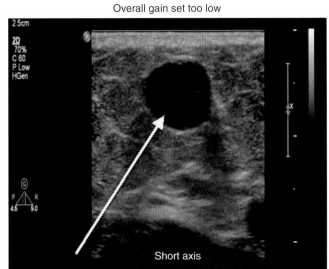

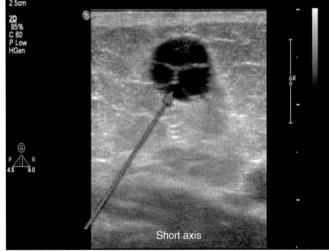

Chronic GSV disease is masked *(white arrow).*

Overall gain is adjusted brighter to depict the chronic GSV disease *(red arrow).*

■ **Fig. 4.42**

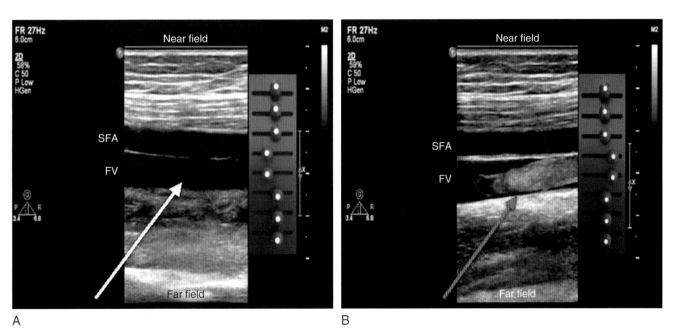

A   B

■ **Fig. 4.43** Time gain compensation (TCG) provides precise gain adjustments at the depth of interest. (A) TCGs are set too dark across the mid portion of the image, masking the disease *(white arrow).* (B) TCGs are adjusted to depict the vessel walls and acute disease *(red arrow). FV,* Femoral vein; *SFA,* superficial femoral artery.

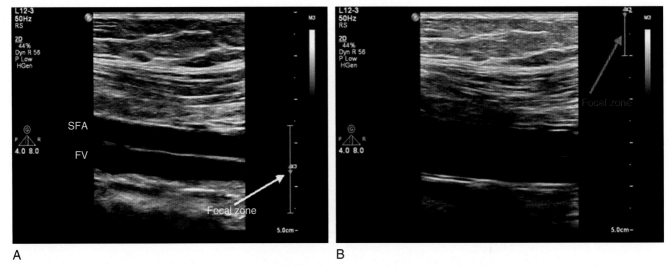

■ **Fig. 4.44** Mid femoral vein (saggital view). (A) Focal zone is placed at the area of interest and displays excellent vessel image detail. (B) Focal zone is placed away from the area of interest, resulting in a loss of vessel image detail. *FV*, Femoral vein; *SFA*, superficial femoral artery.

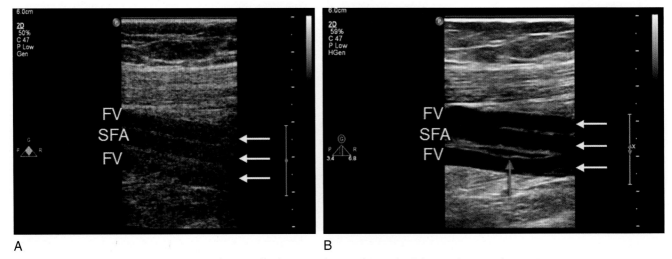

■ **Fig. 4.45** Femoral vein duplication (sagittal view). (A) Fundamental imaging reveals poorly defined vessel walls and artifact within all three vessels *(white arrows)*. (B) Harmonic imaging defines the integrity of the vessel walls and depicts the chronic disease within the FV *(red arrow)*. *FV*, Femoral vein; *SFA*, superficial femoral artery.

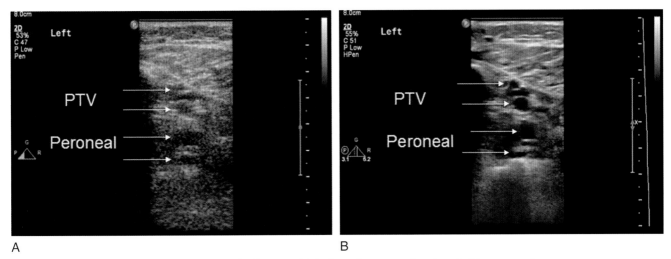

■ **Fig. 4.46** Posterior tibial veins (PTVs) and peroneal veins *(white arrows)* at midcalf level (short axis view). (A) Fundamental imaging. Postthrombotic syndrome patient with poorly visualized PTVs and peroneal veins. (B) Harmonic imaging. Switching to a penetration harmonic setting provides better presentation and improved detail of the vessel walls.

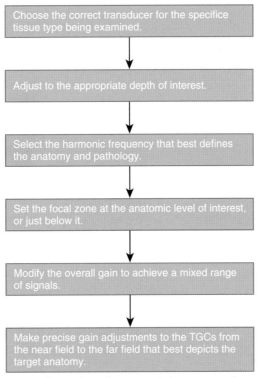

■ **Fig. 4.47** Flow chart for optimizing greyscale settings.

Ultrasound Artifacts

The presence of artifacts is an inherent limitation to all ultrasound imaging modalities and can obscure disease states, thus negatively impacting the reliability of the examination. A full discussion of ultrasound artifacts is beyond the scope of this text, however, the operator should be familiar with, and be able to identify, those typically encountered during the venous duplex examination. If a particular image does not seem to fit with the clinical context or other ultrasound findings, the operator should consider imaging artifact as a potential cause. The most common artifacts encountered are aliasing, misuse of color gain and scale, and improper steering/angle techniques. Examples are shown in Fig. 4.48.

Color Flow Imaging

The color flow settings must be appropriately optimized during the scan to ensure the correct diagnosis is determined. The color flow Doppler mode reveals various hues of red and blue that are ascribed to demonstrate flow. The operator will be in control of which colors will indicate a positive or negative shift. Typically, arteries are color-coded in red and veins are color-coded in blue. The operator should remain cognizant that the presentation can change based on the orientation of the transducer and direction of flow within the vessel. Color flow can demonstrate the presence, absence, and direction of blood flow. During the performance of the scan and later during its interpretation, careful attention to the color settings related to the gain, scale, wall filter, and persistence are implemented during the examination. Here are some points to consider when using the color flow. If the gain is set too low, flow can be missed even though adequate flow may be present. The color gain should be set as high as possible without demonstrating any random color artifacts. Ultimately, when the gain is appropriately set, there will be complete color or "wall-to-wall" filling of the vessel. It is important to recognize that excessive gain can potentially mask disease within the vessel lumen (Fig. 4.49). Avoidance of the color gain spilling into the surrounding tissue is essential.

In conjunction with the color gain, the color velocity scale will need to be adjusted during the course of the examination, thus allowing the operator to compensate for any unexpected range of velocities encountered. When making adjustments, the operator must keep in mind that the color velocity scale has a broad range of velocities and flow aliasing may occur. Aliasing can occur if the scale is set too low, even under normal conditions, as well as when there is an area with elevated velocities, as seen in conditions like venous stenosis or in mass compression. Furthermore, recognizing when to adjust the color flow settings is paramount to demonstrating the clinical findings (Fig. 4.50).

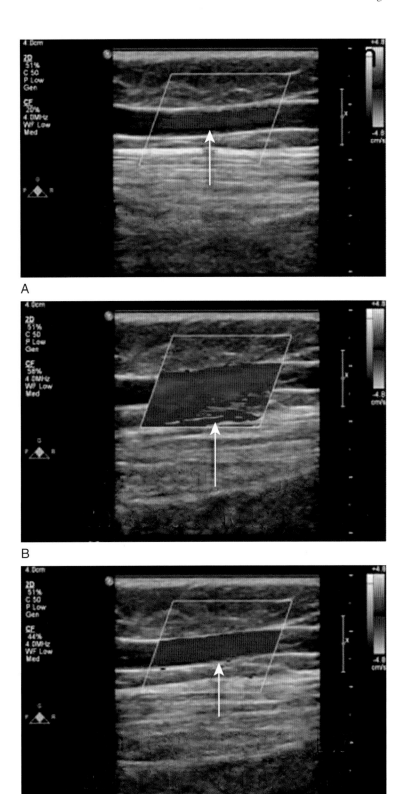

■ **Fig. 4.48** Great saphenous vein (sagittal view). (A) Color flow is undergained, thus the vein lacks color filling. (B) Color flow is overgained, resulting in color spilling into the surrounding tissue. (C) Optimal color gain is achieved, with wall-to-wall color filling within the vein lumen.

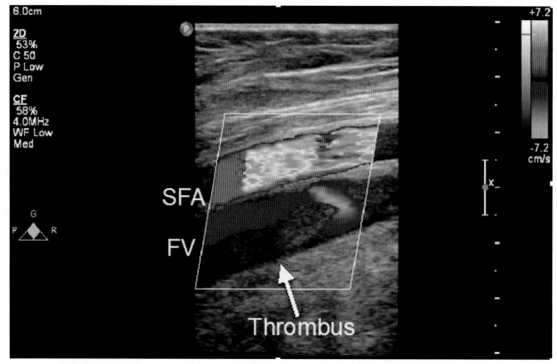

■ **Fig. 4.49** Femoral vein (FV; sagittal view). In this color flow image, the settings were optimized to reflect flow around the partially occlusive thrombus. The color scale, color gain, and wall filter were decreased. *SFA*, Superficial femoral artery.

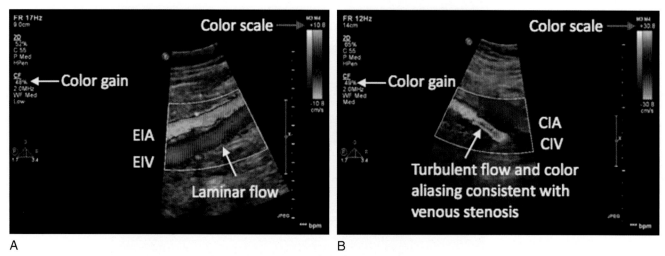

■ **Fig. 4.50** (A) *EIA*, External iliac artery; *EIV*, external iliac vein. (B) *CIA*, Common iliac artery; *CIV*, common iliac vein.

When performing an examination without evidence of a color Doppler shift within the vessel, the operator must consider that the color velocity scale is set too high. To correct this and to obtain a color Doppler shift, the velocity scale must be decreased to produce the desired flow within the vessel. Observably, when decreasing the color scale, the color gain will also need to be decreased to avoid excessive color bleeding out into the surrounding tissue. This is caused by an increased sensitivity when the scale is decreased, and demonstrates why precise adjustments of the color velocity scale are essential to avoid any inaccurate interpretations. As we should expect, the goal is to demonstrate accurate venous flow hemodynamics (Fig. 4.51).

The operator typically makes adjustments to the size, shape, and location of the color box during the examination. When the box size is increased, the frame rate will decrease and so will the image resolution. The objective is to use a small color box over the area of interest that will in turn produce fast frame rates and increase the image resolution (Fig. 4.52).

To achieve the goal of a color Doppler shift when using a linear array transducer, the operator must make adjustments to the color box. When the angle is nearer to the 90-degree mark, the resulting image will lack color flow within the vessel lumen and there will be no identifiable color Doppler shift. Therefore the goal is to make adjustments with an angle nearer to the 0-degree or 180-degree mark to achieve the color Doppler shift (Fig. 4.53).

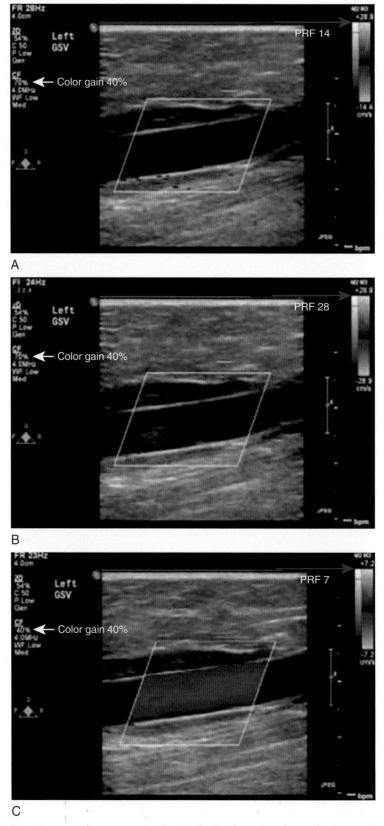

■ **Fig. 4.51** Great saphenous vein (sagittal view) and color velocity scale *(white arrows)*. (A) Color scale is preset at default setting with no color Doppler shift. (B) Color scale is increased with no color Doppler shift. (C) The color scale is decreased to produce a color Doppler shift. The color gain was decreased to avoid bleeding into the surrounding tissue. *PRF*, Pulse repetition frequency.

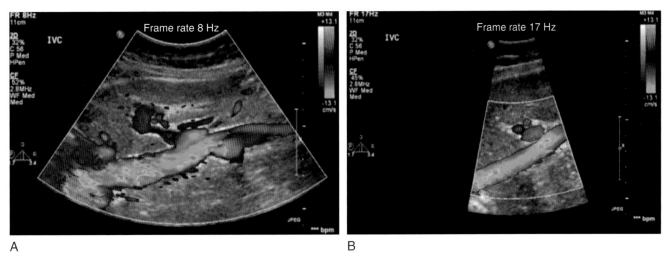

A   B

■ **Fig. 4.52** Inferior vena cava (sagittal view) and color box. (A) Oversized color box will decrease the frame rate and image resolution. (B) Reducing the color box size will increase frame rate and improve resolution.

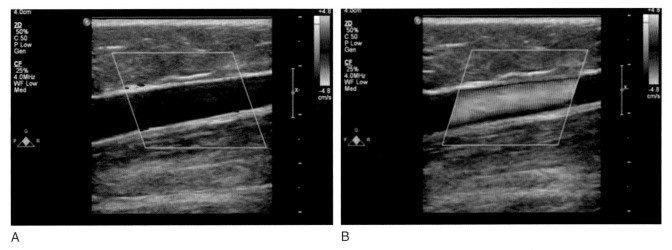

A   B

■ **Fig. 4.53** Great saphenous vein and color box steering. (A) Incorrect color box steering produces no color Doppler shift. (B) With optimal color box steering, color Doppler shift is achieved.

Pulsed Wave Doppler

The pulsed wave Doppler mode is used to evaluate venous flow and to provide quantifiable information about patency, incompetence, and obstruction. The significance of this mode cannot be underrated. The deep venous system demonstrates inconsistencies in the normal appearance of pulsed wave Doppler waveforms. This is caused in part by changes with respiration, volume, right-sided heart pressures, vessel depth, and body habitus. Furthermore, the amplitude of the pulsed Doppler waveforms will decrease the further away from the heart the waveforms are acquired.

Thus optimizing these settings to obtain waveforms depicting phasic, nonphasic, or bidirectional flows are required for obtaining a quality examination. An accurate depiction of these waveforms is central to making the diagnosis. The operator will be required to make adjustments to the manufacturer presets that will include the scale, gain, wall filter, baseline, sweep speed, and flow direction. When performing a pulsed Doppler examination, the angle of incidence should be kept between 45 and 60 degrees, parallel to the vessel walls.

Here are some points to consider when optimizing the pulsed wave Doppler mode. When obtaining pulsed Doppler waveforms, the gain should be kept below 50%; otherwise this will distort the integrity and the characteristics of the waveform (Fig. 4.54). While performing the pulsed Doppler portion of the examination, the waveforms gathered should be indicative of the hemodynamic changes found within the vessel lumen. Increasing the gain should coincide with the severity of disease—that is, a situation where there is the presence of compression or stenosis (Fig. 4.55). During image acquisition, pay careful attention to the direction of flow. The color flow portion of the image and the pulsed Doppler waveform must be in the same direction (Fig. 4.56).

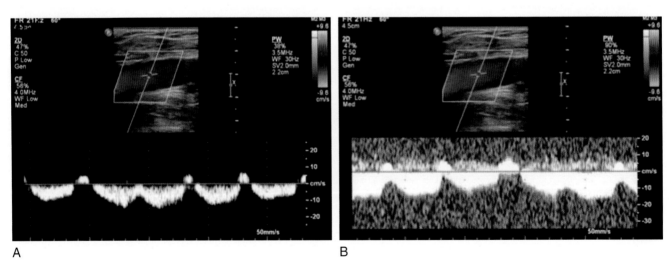

A   B

■ **Fig. 4.54** Common femoral vein, phasic flow, and pulsed wave Doppler. (A) Optimal gain. Pulsed Doppler gain is set at 38%. (B) Over-gain. Pulsed Doppler gain is set at 90%.

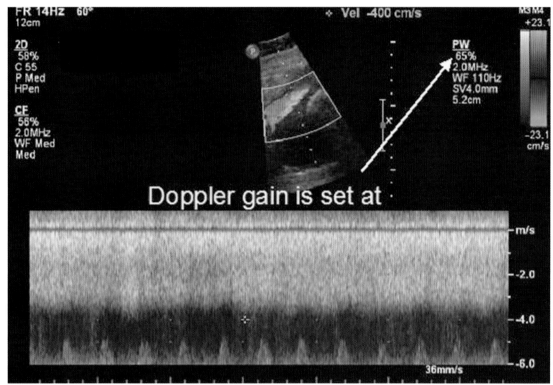

■ **Fig. 4.55** External iliac vein. A high-velocity continuous flow waveform from a postthrombotic patient is shown here (Doppler gain is set at 65%).

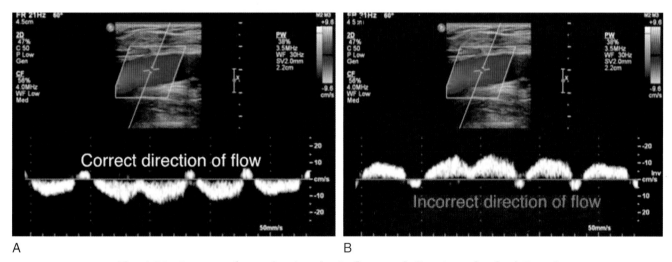

A   B

■ **Fig. 4.56** Common femoral vein, phasic flow, and direction of pulsed Doppler waveform. (A) Color flow and pulsed Doppler wave form shown below the baseline (correct). (B) Pulsed Doppler waveform inverted above the baseline (incorrect).

When examining the bilateral common femoral and iliac veins, the patient should be free of any restrictive undergarments, so as to avoid any unnecessary compression, as well as excessive probe pressure, which could lead to false-positive results. When obtaining bilateral CFV waveforms, it is imperative to set the Doppler scale the same on both sides and use a slow, sweep speed. Recognizing obvious and subtle changes in the waveform contour of the common femoral veins is essential to diagnosing an outflow obstruction. Venous flow is typically 10 to 20 cm per second. If the spectral velocity scale is inadvertently changed and significantly increased, the waveforms will be difficult to interpret (Figs. 4.57–4.60).

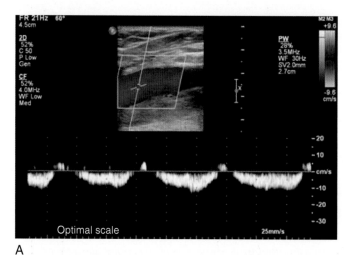

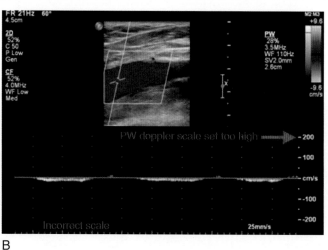

■ **Fig. 4.57** Common femoral vein and pulsed Doppler waveforms. (A) Spectral scale: ± 10-15 cm/s. Phasic flow acquired with a slow sweep speed. (B) Spectral scale; ± 200 cm/s. Same waveform acquired with a slow sweep speed and an increased pulsed wave Doppler scale. The increased scale makes this waveform uninterpretable.

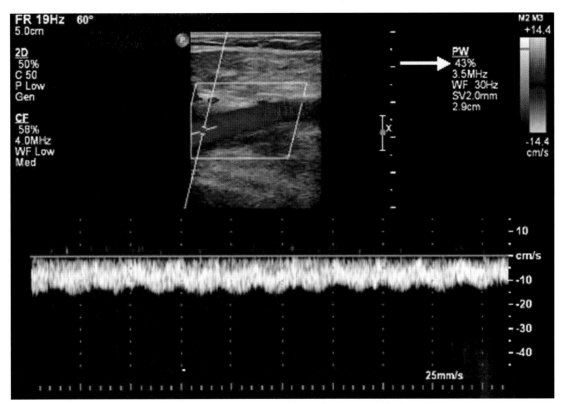

■ **Fig. 4.58** Common femoral vein, nonphasic flow. Pulsed Doppler waveform was acquired with a slow sweep speed and a gain *(arrow)* set at 43%. This waveform is consistent with proximal obstruction.

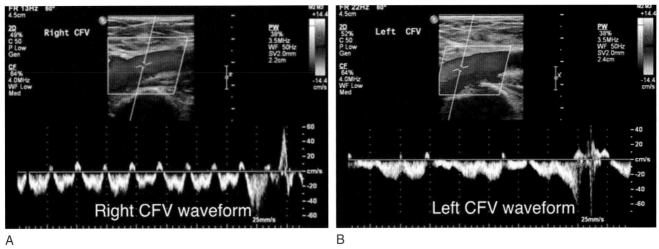

A

B

C

■ **Fig. 4.59** Bilateral common femoral veins (CFVs) and pulsed Doppler waveforms. The right (A) and left (B) pulsed Doppler waveforms from a 48-year-old woman with a nonhealing ulcer are shown. Both CFV waveforms depict phasic flow; however, waveform B is significantly different in its contour than waveform A. This example demonstrates that phasic flow can be maintained in the presence of May-Thurner syndrome. (C) The transverse greyscale image depicts the right CIA crossing over the left CIV against the spine. *CIA,* Common iliac artery *CIV,* common iliac vein.

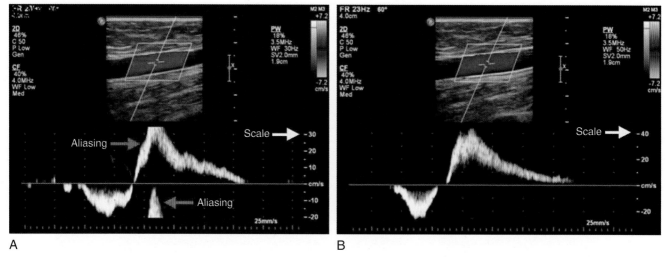

■ **Fig. 4.60** Great saphenous vein reflux acquired with a slow sweep. (A) Pulsed Doppler waveform demonstrates aliasing artifact that is wrapping around the baseline. (B) The same waveform has been optimized by increasing the pulsed wave Doppler scale and baseline shift.

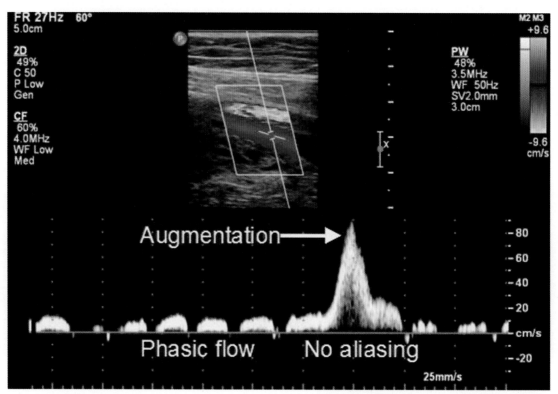

■ **Fig. 4.61** Femoral vein (sagittal view). Pulsed Doppler waveform acquired with a slow sweep speed and manual augmentation without aliasing.

During the duplex examination, the distal augmentation maneuver can be performed manually or automatically. When obtaining a pulsed Doppler waveform, artifacts related to aliasing must be eliminated. They occur when the velocity exceeds the Nyquist limit. Aliasing can be eliminated by increasing the Doppler velocity scale and by adjusting the baseline shift. Optimally, the use of a slow, sweep speed is desired to allow for the appreciation of venous flow and to measure the entire length of reflux (Figs. 4.61 and 4.62).

In conclusion, the accuracy of the venous duplex examination is directly related to the quality of the images acquired. The operator must be well trained with a thorough understanding of image acquisition, including the pitfalls and techniques used to optimize image resolution. The end result should always be a high-quality examination for all patients to assist in making an accurate diagnosis.

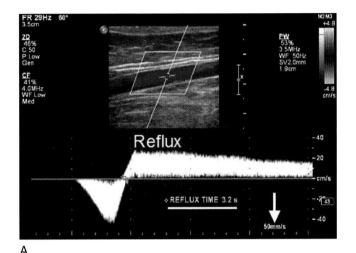

A

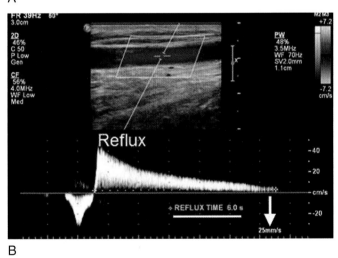

B

■ **Fig. 4.62** Great saphenous vein reflux and sweep speeds *(arrows)*. (A) Pulsed Doppler waveform acquired with manual augmentation and a fast sweep speed. Measured reflux time was 3.2 s. Using a fast sweep speed does not allow for the entire length of the reflux to be measured. (B) Pulsed Doppler waveform acquired with manual augmentation and a slow sweep speed. This allows for the entire length to be measured. Reflux time was 6 s.

Venography

Contrast venography has been widely used to establish the diagnosis of acute and/or chronic thrombotic disease, anatomic variants, and hemodynamic malfunctions of the venous system, iliac vein compression syndrome, and postthrombotic syndrome. Venography used to be the gold standard diagnostic modality for these lesions. However, several studies have shown that venography is not sensitive for quantifying nonocclusive iliac vein lesions and verifying resolution of thrombus following lytic therapy. Venography is best used in conjunction with intravascular ultrasound (IVUS, providing imaging for blood-thrombus-lumen wall interfaces) for proper diagnosis and treatment of the aforementioned lesions (Fig. 4.63).

When compared with IVUS, venography has several limitations. First, it is generally used in a single plane, failing to demonstrate 3D anatomy of the vessel, which limits the diagnosis of external venous compression. Multiple views improve the diagnostic sensitivity of venography at the expense of additional toxic radiation and contrast. Other limitations of venography are contrast stasis which can obscure underlying lesions and limited visualization in obese patients. Discrete stenosis can be missed from contrast flowing through and around the defects within the vein.

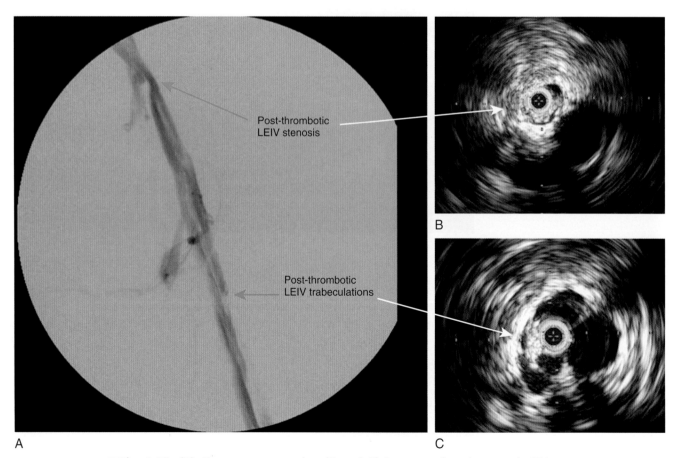

■ **Fig. 4.63** (A) Contrast venography. (B and C) Intravascular ultrasound. *EIA,* External iliac artery; *LEIV,* left external iliac vein.

Intravascular Ultrasound

IVUS of the deep axial veins can provide a 360-degree, 2D, greyscale image of lumen and vessel wall structures. IVUS has become a necessary adjunct to venography when performing catheter-based femoroiliocaval interventions because landmarks, venous branches, external compression, acute and chronic thrombus, fibrosis, mural thickening, spurs, and trabeculations may all be visualized. IVUS can provide real-time, cross-sectional imaging during thromboembolic procedures by imaging the blood-thrombus-lumen wall interfaces not easily seen with venography, and IVUS planimetry aids in vein measurement. Magnetic resonance venography (MRV) and CT venography can provide preprocedural and postprocedural imaging assessments but do not provide imaging during the case. Traditional duplex ultrasound can provide adequate imaging of some axial veins of the extremities, but generally long-penetration depths in the abdomen and pelvis, and single-plane limitations cannot provide the same real-time luminal imaging that is often necessary for these endovascular procedures. IVUS may have other potential advantages such as imaging of the landing zone for the distal part of the stent and assessing the extent of lumen restoration.

Cross-Sectional Imaging

Computed Tomography Venography

The first diagnoses of caval and iliofemoral thrombi on CT were made in the 1980s. CT has some advantages over MRI for venous imaging: (1) less dependence on the technologist, (2) extended anatomic coverage (lower extremities, abdomen, and pelvis) in a single continuous data set, and (3) generally very high spatial resolution. 3D reconstructions can be performed more easily than with MRI, and they often include osseous structures for easy anatomic reference. Disadvantages of CT with respect to MRI include exposure of the patient to ionizing radiation, higher incidence of allergic reaction to iodinated contrast than to gadolinium, lower vessel-to-background contrast, and low intravascular concentration of iodine leading to a high incidence of nondiagnostic studies. In addition, CT does not afford the ability to adequately image veins without contrast or to quantify magnitude or direction of venous flow (Fig. 4.64).

Magnetic Resonance Venography

Advantages of MRV include the lack of ionizing radiation, an extremely low incidence of allergic reactions to gadolinium contrast, higher vessel-to-background image contrast, the ability to obtain dynamic time-resolved imaging, the ability to quantify direction and magnitude of flow, the ability to perform noncontrast venous imaging, and the availability of a blood pool–bound contrast agent, which maintains a very high intravascular contrast concentration, allowing high-resolution imaging up to an hour after contrast administration. MRV can also quantify direction and volume of flow using phase-contrast techniques. Such techniques may be useful, for example, in documenting reversal of flow in gonadal or hypogastric vessels, indicating hemodynamic significance of a proximal stenosis in the iliac or renal vessels (Fig. 4.65). Disadvantages of MRV include more dependence on the skill of the operator, longer scan time, more time-consuming 3D postprocessing, and a risk of nephrogenic systemic fibrosis when administering gadolinium contrast

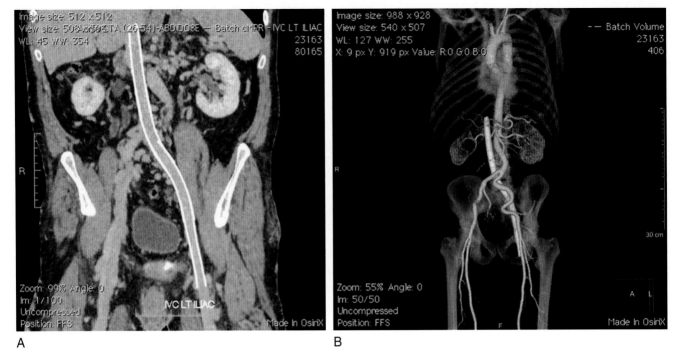

A   B

■ **Fig. 4.64** Noncontrast (A) and volume-rendered (B) computed tomography scans for a patient with left iliocaval stent in place. Note the right iliac vein occlusion with drainage via the azygous system.

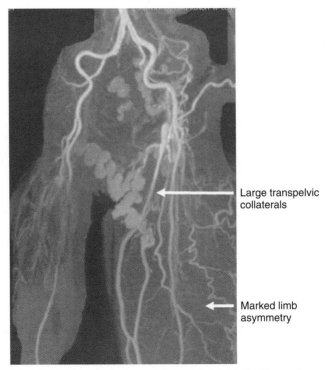

Large transpelvic collaterals

Marked limb asymmetry

■ **Fig. 4.65** Magnetic resonance venography of left iliac vein occlusion.

agents to patients with advanced renal insufficiency. The spatial resolution of MRV is often lower than that of CT venography. Many patients have implanted devices that are not compatible with MRI, including pacemakers, implanted defibrillators, spinal stimulators, and medication pumps.

REFERENCES

1. Marston WA. PPG, APG, duplex: which noninvasive tests are most appropriate for the management of patients with chronic venous insufficiency? *Semin Vasc Surg.* 2002;15:13–20.
2. Labropoulos N, Borge M, Pierce K, et al. Criteria for defining significant central vein stenosis with duplex ultrasound. *J Vasc Surg.* 2007;46:101–107.
3. Raines JK, Almeida JI. Role of physiologic testing in venous disorders. In: Bergan JJ, ed. *The Vein Book.* San Diego: Elsevier; 2007:47–55.

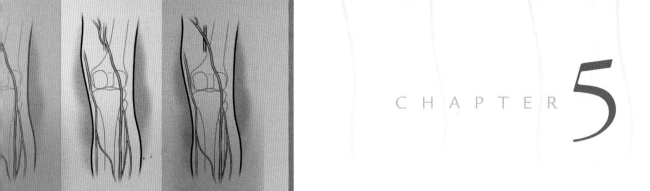

CHAPTER 5

Endovenous Thermal Ablation of Saphenous Reflux

Jose I. Almeida

HISTORICAL BACKGROUND

Treatment of this disorder has evolved from sclerotherapy to open radical surgery and then to the use of sophisticated technology, such as thermal and nonthermal catheter-based ablation.

The exact historical point in time when saphenous vein incompetence was recognized as a source of venous hypertension is unclear; however, Trendelenburg promulgated saphenofemoral ligation in 1891.[1] In the early 20th century, stripping of the saphenous veins was added to proximal ligation. Keller[2] described an internal stripper in 1905. Hence high ligation of the great saphenous vein (GSV) at the saphenofemoral junction (SFJ) followed by GSV stripping from groin to knee or ankle was the standard of care and was performed in the hospital setting for about 100 years.

The two methods of thermal ablation in comprehensive vein centers at present are the VNUS ClosureFAST procedure, which uses a catheter to direct radiofrequency (RF) energy from a dedicated generator (VNUS Medical Technologies, Inc., Sunnyvale, CA), and endovenous laser ablation (EVLA), which uses a laser fiber and generator to produce focused heat (multiple manufacturers). Both RF and EVLA are catheter-based endovascular interventions that use electromagnetic energy to destroy the refluxing saphenous system. Nonthermal techniques are discussed in Chapter 8.

RF catheters were the first devices to become available to venous surgeons for endovenous thermal ablation of the GSV after garnering US Food and Drug Administration approval in 1999. In 2002, endovascular ablation of the GSV using laser energy became available in the United States.

ETIOLOGY AND NATURAL HISTORY OF DISEASE

The majority of patients (60%–70%) with varicose veins have an incompetent SFJ and GSV reflux.[3] It is critical to recognize that bulging varicose veins are usually associated with an underlying source of venous hypertension, and treatment of the source is as important as treatment of the actual varicose vein.

Chronic venous disorders generally result from primary venous insufficiency or secondary processes, such as acute deep venous thrombosis (DVT) or trauma. An analysis of chronic venous disease (CVD) indicated that primary valvular incompetence was present in 70% to 80% of cases; secondary valvular incompetence was caused by trauma or DVT in 18% to 25%, and congenital anomaly was present in 1% to 3% of cases.[4]

PATIENT SELECTION

Patients with CVD will usually present to a physician with concerns referable to both medical symptoms and cosmetic appearance of their disease. Patient satisfaction results from identifying and properly treating the patient's primary concerns, which may include medical and/or cosmetic issues. Not all symptomatic patients are aware of their symptoms because the onset may be insidious. Symptoms may include leg heaviness, pain or tenderness along the course of a vein, pruritus, burning, restlessness, night cramps, edema, skin changes, and paresthesias. After treatment, patients are often surprised to realize how much discomfort they had accepted as normal. Pain caused by CVD is often improved by walking or by elevating the legs. The pain of arterial insufficiency, conversely, is worsened by ambulation and elevation. Pain and other symptoms of venous disease may intensify with the menstrual cycle, pregnancy, and in response to exogenous hormonal therapy (i.e., oral contraceptives).

As is customary for any medical condition, the physician must begin with a careful history and physical examination. The primary purpose of the clinical examination of the patient presenting with CVD is to classify the subject using the popular CEAP system[5,6] (clinical [telangiectasias to skin damage], etiologic [primary, secondary, or congenital], anatomic [superficial, deep, or perforators], and pathophysiologic [reflux, obstruction, or both] patterns). For each of these major classifications, there are subgroups. For the work described in this chapter, clinical signs emerge as the most important and are grouped as follows: C1, spider telangiectasias; C2, varicose veins (Fig. 5.1); C3, edema; C4, lipodermatosclerosis; C5, healed ulcer; and C6, active ulcer. Regarding treatment, the class (C) is the most important parameter to establish during the initial encounter. Treatment algorithms for chronic venous insufficiency ([CVI]; i.e., patients with more severe disease [C4, C5, C6]) are discussed in other sections of this book. This chapter focuses on the treatment of C2 disease.

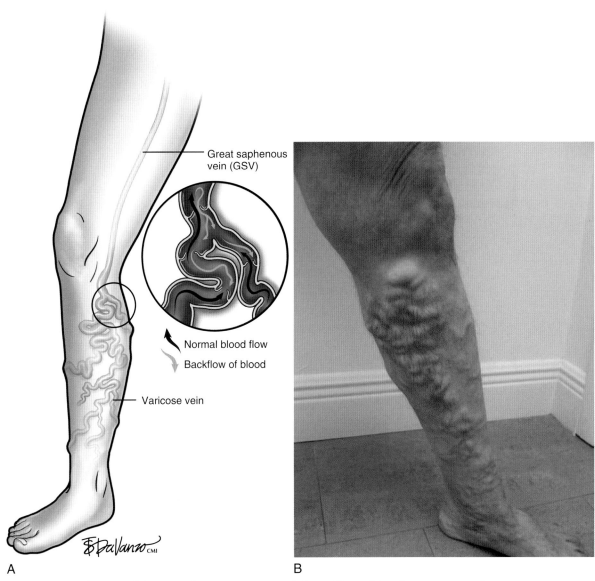

Great saphenous
vein (GSV)

Normal blood flow

Backflow of blood

Varicose vein

A

B

■ **Fig. 5.1** (B) Typical varicose veins of the calf resulting from great saphenous
vein incompetence.

ENDOVASCULAR INSTRUMENTATION

Device choice is a matter of physician preference. Our center and other investigators have compared the efficacy of RF and EVLA. The ablation data are slightly better for EVLA.[7,8] A few years ago, we published our 3-year data showing 94% success with RF and 98% success with laser.[9] However, in current practice, the results are closer to 95% success with either technology. Current RF and EVLA data are presented in Chapters 6 and 7.

Fig. 5.2 depicts the general layout of an office-based venous surgery suite. An operating table with a back table is prepared in the usual sterile manner. The laptop ultrasound system is mounted on a movable cart, and the thermal ablation equipment is in close proximity to allow easy viewing of the display panels by the operator. Hemodynamic monitoring equipment (heart rate, blood pressure, oxygen saturation) is available and is used during cases offering conscious sedation. If local anesthesia without sedation is used, hemodynamic monitoring is not required in most states.

Endovascular Laser

- Diode laser: 810-nm, 940-nm, 980-nm, and 1470-nm wavelengths are available
- Nd:YAG laser: 1319-nm and 1320-nm wavelengths are commercially available
- Standard microintroducer sheaths are used for ultrasound-guided percutaneous access
- Sheaths of differing lengths are available to accommodate a 600-μm-diameter laser fiber (bare tip or covered tip)
- Occasionally, for ablation of short veins, the laser fiber can be placed directly through a microsheath under ultrasound control; recently, smaller, 400-μm-diameter fibers have become available for perforator vein ablation
- For GSV ablation, the fiber tip is positioned 2 to 3 cm distal to the common femoral vein (CFV)

Radiofrequency

- RF generator
  - A 7-Fr coaxial introducer sheath, 7-cm or 11-cm lengths
- For GSV ablation, the RF heating elements are positioned 2 to 3 cm distal to the CFV; occasionally, the RF catheters require coaxial navigation through tortuous vessels by tracking over a 0.025-inch (0.0635-cm) guidewire

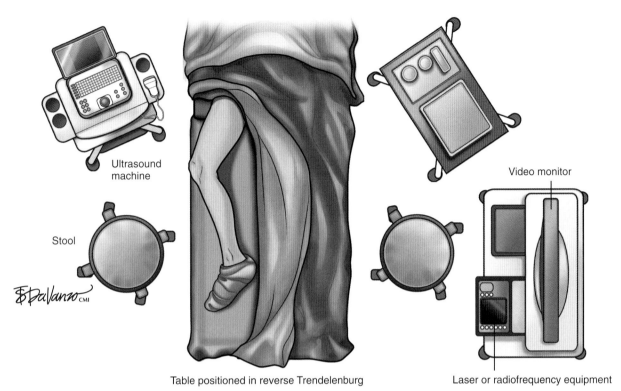

Table positioned in reverse Trendelenburg

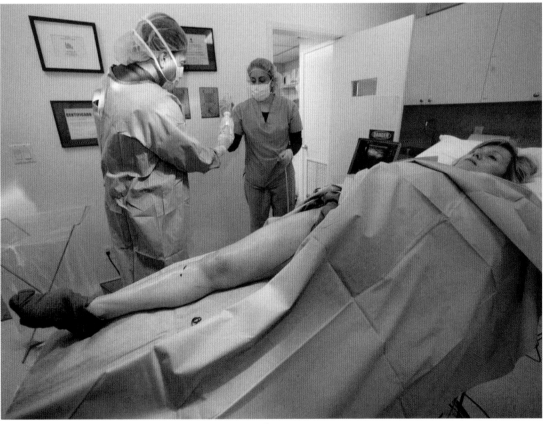

■ Fig. 5.2

TUMESCENT ANESTHESIA DELIVERY

A 30-mL syringe with a 25-gauge needle is preferred if anesthesia is delivered by the operator. Extension sets with three-way stopcocks are useful if an assistant is available to push the anesthetic solution. Alternatively, tumescent anesthesia infusion pumps are commercially available.

IMAGING

- Diagnostic workup with color flow duplex ultrasound imaging is adequate in the majority of patients presenting with lower extremity venous disease
- One should be familiar with the anatomy of the GSV, anterior accessory saphenous vein, posterior accessory saphenous vein, thigh circumflex veins, small saphenous vein (SSV), Giacomini vein, perforating veins of the thigh and calf, and the deep venous system
- The GSV and SSV are identified sonographically in their respective saphenous canals (Fig. 5.3); if they are determined to be incompetent on duplex imaging, they may be sources of venous hypertension and are considered for endovenous ablation
- Vein diameters, obtained via duplex ultrasound imaging, with the patient in the standing position, must be documented to guide energy delivery
- The ideal imaging system incorporates color flow duplex ultrasound with a 5-MHz to 7-MHz linear array transducer; the newer laptop-style platforms are adequate for superficial vein work
- A sterile bag is required to isolate the ultrasound transducer from the prepped lower extremity (see Fig. 5.2)

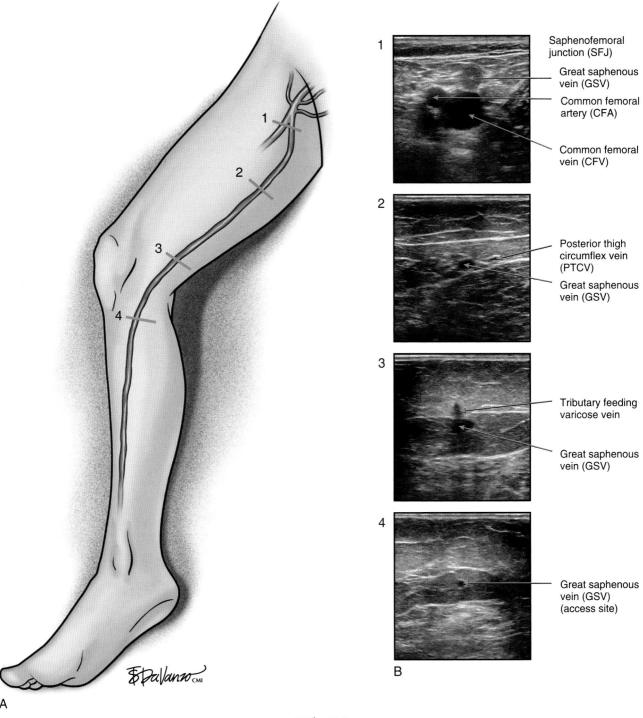

■ Fig. 5.3

Continued

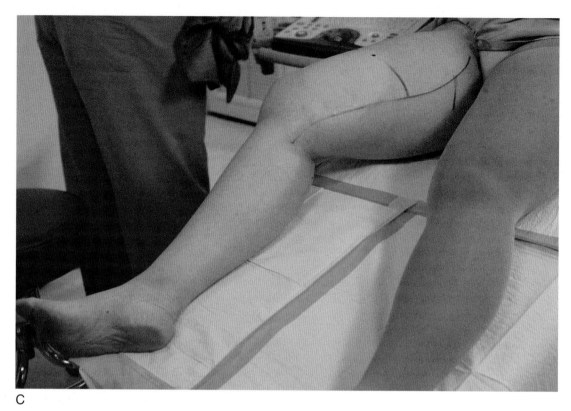

C

■ **Fig. 5.3, cont'd** (C) Preparing for preprocedure ultrasound scan. This is referred to as "reading" the vein. The surgeon will create an image in their "mind's eye" before beginning the procedure.

ACCESS AND CLOSURE

The surgeon begins by placing a wheal of local anesthesia on the skin access site with a syringe and small (25-gauge to 30-gauge) needle (Fig. 5.4). The access needle is then held at an approximately 45-degree angle, 1 inch (2.54 cm) from the ultrasound probe, and the target vein will be located at the tip of an imaginary triangle where the ultrasound beam and the tip of the access needle meet under the skin. For large veins (> 5-mm diameter), an 18-gauge needle is used. For smaller diameter veins (< 5-mm diameter), a 21-gauge needle and micropuncture assembly are preferred (Fig. 5.5).

The needle tip is guided to the roof of the vein using ultrasound to visualize where the puncture will take place. Usually one will tent the roof of the vein with a gentle push, easily seen with ultrasound imaging, before a more forceful motion for entry. Aspiration of dark nonpulsatile blood into a connected syringe confirms venous entry (Fig. 5.6).

- A 4-Fr or 5-Fr microintroducer kit contains a 21-gauge needle, 0.018-inch-diameter (0.045-cm diameter) × 40-cm-length guidewire, and a microintroducer/sheath set
- Percutaneous access is obtained with a 21-gauge needle under ultrasound control for both EVLA and RF procedures
- A 0.035-inch-diameter (0.088-cm-diameter), 150-cm-length, J-tipped guidewire is placed through the microintroducer sheath and navigated to the target site
- If the surgeon is unable to traverse tortuous segments, a second entry site above the tortuosity is created, and the vein is treated as two separate segments; to minimize procedure costs, the use of expensive, interventional glide wires is discouraged

- For the GSV, access is obtained percutaneously at the most distal segment of axial vein reflux; this is usually below the knee at the level of Boyd perforating vein
- For SSV treatment, access is obtained at the midcalf posteriorly, where the gastrocnemius muscle becomes prominent
- One should not introduce wires, sheaths, fibers, and/or catheters into the common femoral vein; they should be parked at the SFJ, 1 cm distal to the CFV before treatment

Text continued on p. 134

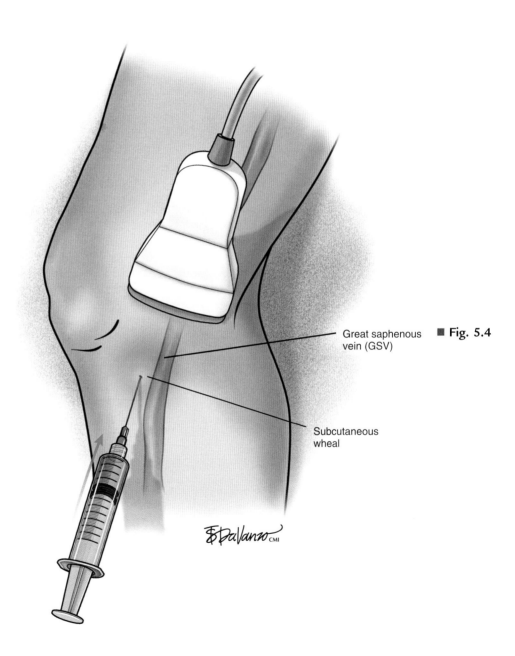

Great saphenous vein (GSV)

Subcutaneous wheal

■ **Fig. 5.4**

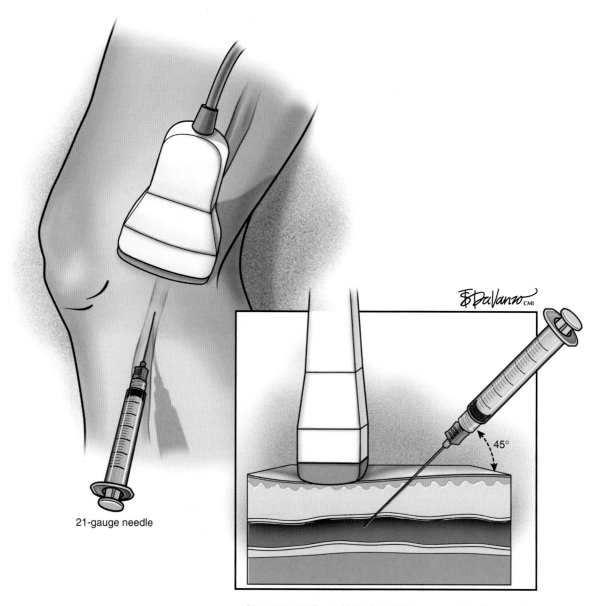

21-gauge needle

21-gauge needle positioned at 45-degree angle to ultrasound

A

■ Fig. 5.5

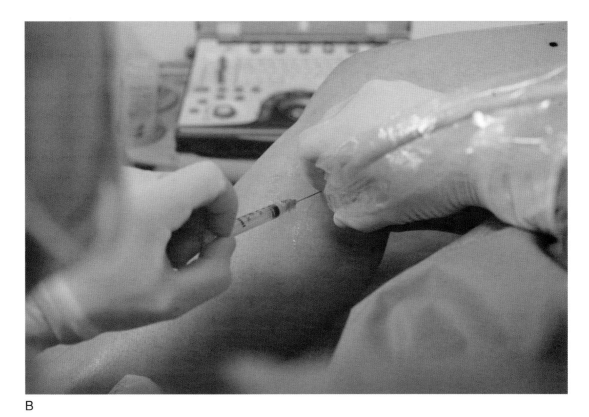

B

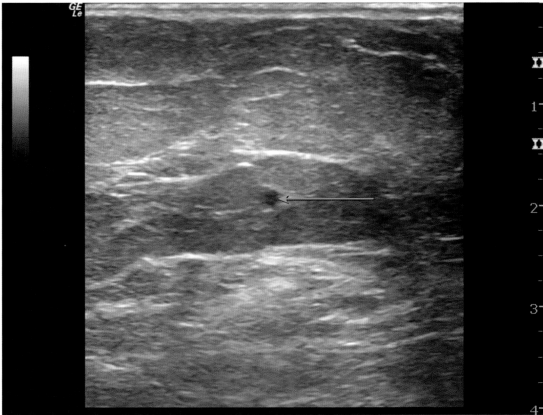

C

■ **Fig. 5.5, cont'd** (C) Cross-sectional ultrasound image of great saphenous vein (the target vein) *(arrow).*

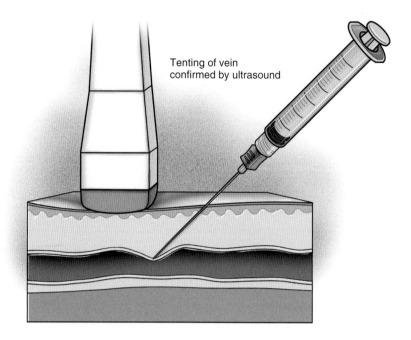

Tenting of vein
confirmed by ultrasound

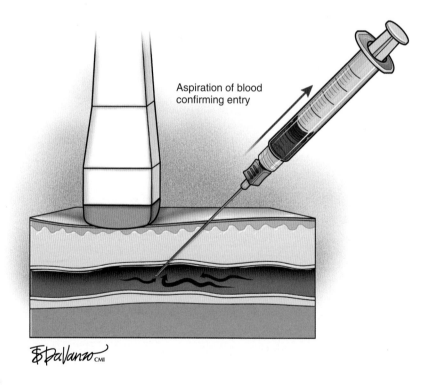

Aspiration of blood
confirming entry

A

■ Fig. 5.6

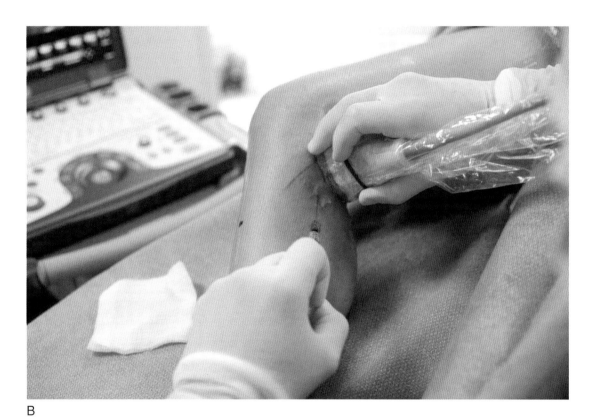

B

■ **Fig. 5.6, cont'd**

HEMOSTASIS AND ANTICOAGULATION

Hemostasis at the entry site is obtained with manual pressure. As a general rule, thromboprophylaxis with anticoagulation is not required unless the patient has an underlying thrombophilia.

Patients should be stratified into mild-risk, moderate-risk, or high-risk classes to determine whether thromboprophylaxis (mechanical, pharmaceutic) is required perioperatively.

As demonstrated in Fig. 5.7, we believe that on-table activation of the calf pump is very effective in preventing thromboembolic complications during thermal ablation procedures. After the ablation and before the ambulatory phlebectomy portion of the procedure (discussed in Chapter 10), we simply ask the patient to actively dorsiflex and plantarflex the foot 20 times.

OPERATIVE STEPS

Once the patient has entered the operating suite, a brief examination of the leg is performed. The skin overlying all areas of bulging varicose veins is marked with a magic marker. The patient is then placed in the supine position on the operating table. A detailed duplex ultrasound report should be readily available so that the operator can review it before beginning the procedure. Our preference is to then perform a rapid scan of the leg with the ultrasound probe for the purpose of obtaining a high-level understanding of the venous anatomy. The operator should note areas of tortuosity, aneurysmal dilatation, and location of tributaries and perforators before beginning the procedure. I call this "reading" the vein; its importance is discussed later.

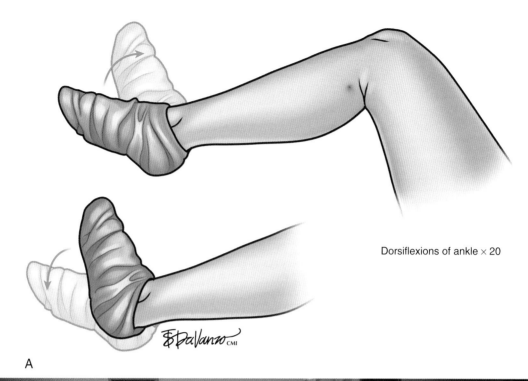

Dorsiflexions of ankle × 20

A

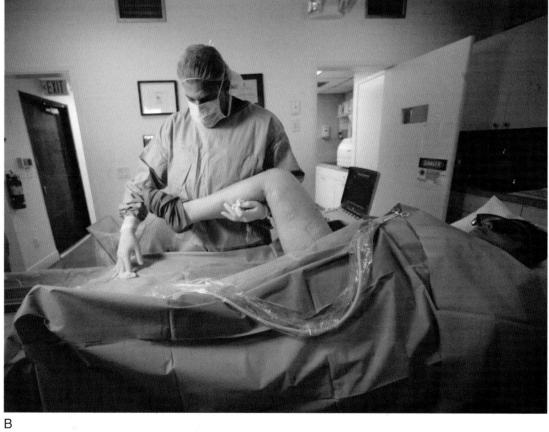

B

■ Fig. 5.7

The ultrasound scan begins at the groin, and the course of the vein is followed distally until the straight segment terminates as it begins to divide and produce varicosed tributaries. These varicosed tributaries are the escape points for saphenous incompetence. This transition zone is usually found just below the knee, although many anatomic variants exist. Therefore percutaneous access is usually obtained immediately below the knee. However, the operator must be prepared to access anywhere from thigh to ankle.

Once the optimal access site is chosen, preparations for entry begin. The intraluminal space of the target vein must be accessed to place a guidewire. The preferred technique is percutaneous access under ultrasound guidance. The surgeon and patient must both be comfortable. The surgeon should rest his or her forearms somewhere in the operative field so that both hands are stable.

The ultrasound probe is held perpendicular to the skin to demonstrate the target vein in either the short or long access on the ultrasound screen. Once venous entry is confirmed, a guidewire is chosen. The micropuncture needle accepts a 0.018-inch (0.045-cm) wire followed by a 4-Fr coaxial microsheath and its intraluminal dilator. Usually a small stab incision with a no. 11 blade scalpel is required at the wire entry site to widen the incision for the microsheath. Confirmation that the 0.018-inch (0.045-cm) wire is in the endoluminal space is performed with ultrasound (Fig. 5.8).

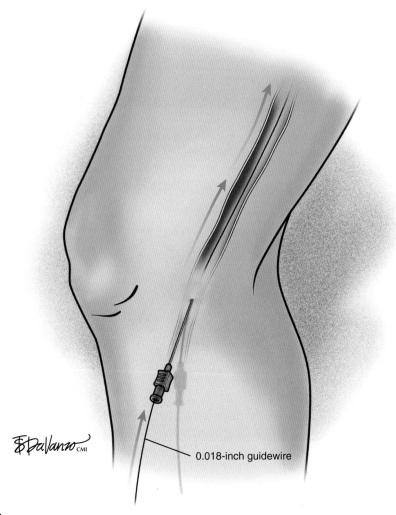

0.018-inch guidewire

A

■ Fig. 5.8

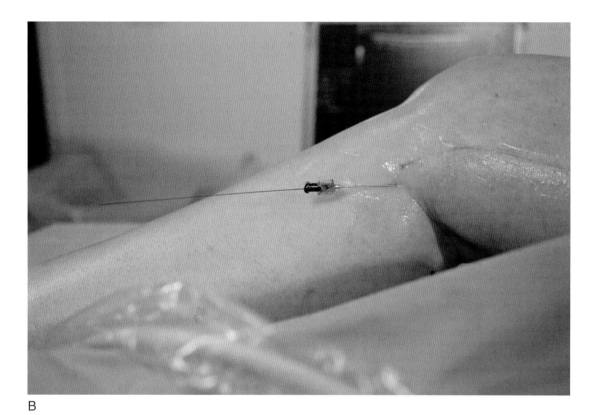

B

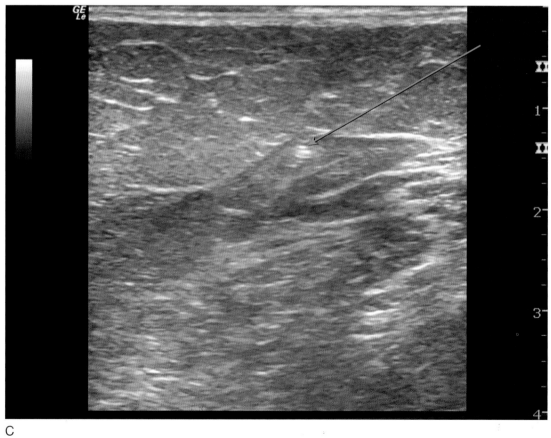

C

■ **Fig. 5.8, cont'd** (C) Cross-sectional ultrasound image demonstrating intraluminal placement of 0.018-inch (0.045-cm) guidewire *(arrow)*.

The microsheath assembly is placed, the microdilator and 0.018-inch (0.045-cm) guidewire are removed, and the remaining microsheath is used to place a 0.035-inch (0.088-cm) guidewire (Fig. 5.9A). The 0.035-inch (0.088-cm) guidewire is then navigated to the SFJ using ultrasound control (see Fig. 5.9B and C).

Some operators prefer to deliver the wire with the J-tip at the lead, but we prefer to send the straight end of the wire up first, especially in smaller veins. J-tipped wires may cause distention of the vein and induce friction with the inner lining of the vein wall during passage. This generally will cause pain secondary to venous distention, which activates the adrenergic sympathetic nerve fibers residing in the adventitia (Fig. 5.10).

Once the tip of the wire is positioned at the SFJ, a larger coaxial sheath is placed (Fig. 5.11). Many systems now allow passage of the fiber directly through the microsheath and the step of exchanging over a 0.035-inch (0.088-cm) platform is avoided.

Text continued on p. 144

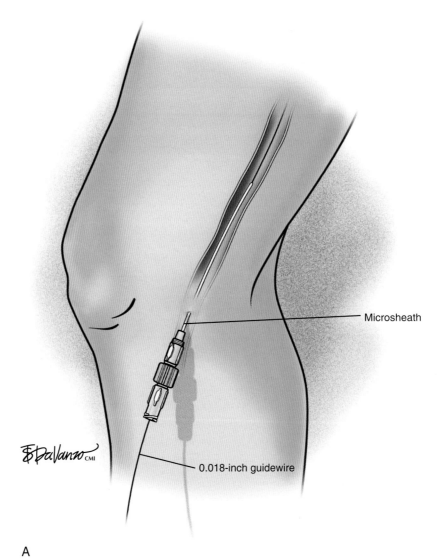

Microsheath

0.018-inch guidewire

A

■ **Fig. 5.9** (A) A 0.018-inch (0.045-cm) guidewire and dilator will be removed, leaving microsheath in place.

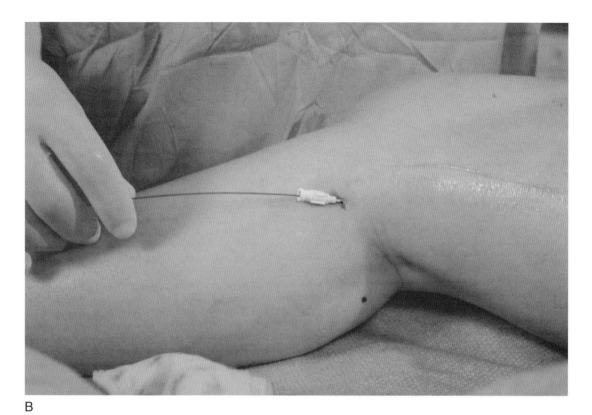

B

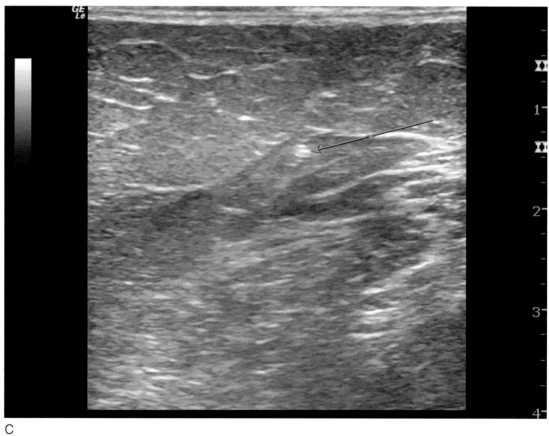

C

■ **Fig. 5.9, cont'd** (B) A 0.035-inch (0.088-cm) guidewire inserted into microsheath. (C) Cross-sectional ultrasound image demonstrating intraluminal placement of 0.035-inch (0.088-cm) guidewire *(arrow).*

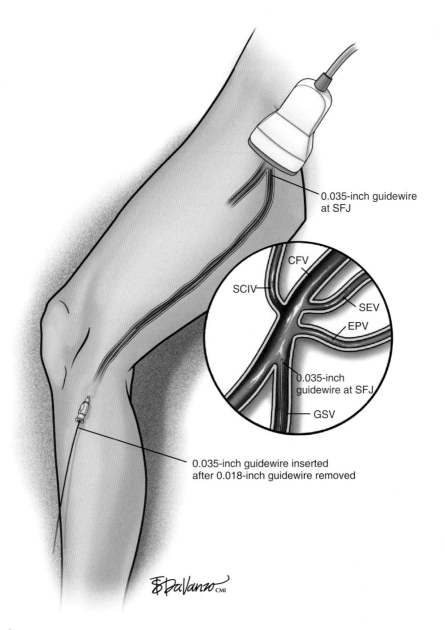

0.035-inch guidewire
at SFJ

CFV

SCIV

SEV

EPV

0.035-inch
guidewire at SFJ

GSV

0.035-inch guidewire inserted
after 0.018-inch guidewire removed

A

■ **Fig. 5.10** (A) *CFV,* Common femoral vein; *EPV,* external pudendal vein; *GSV,* great saphenous vein; *SCIV,* superficial circumflex iliac vein; *SEV,* superficial epigastric vein; *SFJ,* saphenofemoral junction.

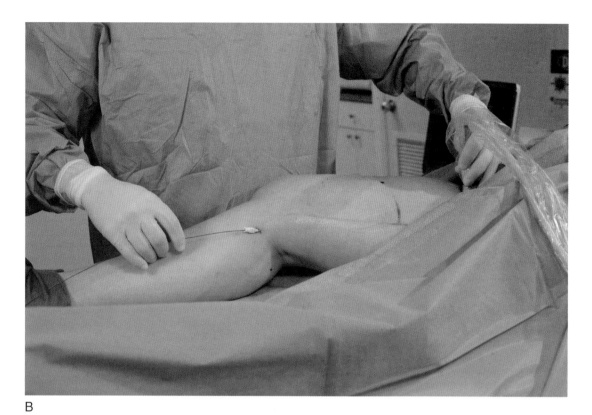

B

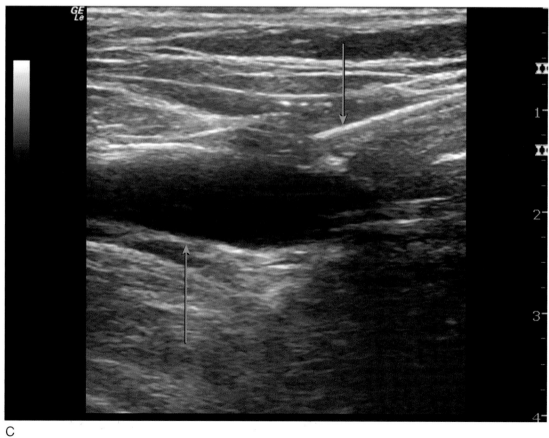

C

■ **Fig. 5.10, cont'd** (C) Long-access ultrasound image of saphenofemoral junction (SFJ). *Top arrow* points to guidewire tip at SFJ. *Bottom arrow* points to common femoral vein.

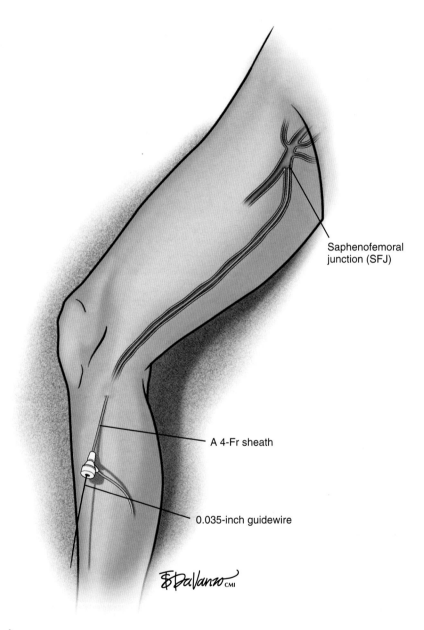

Saphenofemoral junction (SFJ)

A 4-Fr sheath

0.035-inch guidewire

A

■ Fig. 5.11

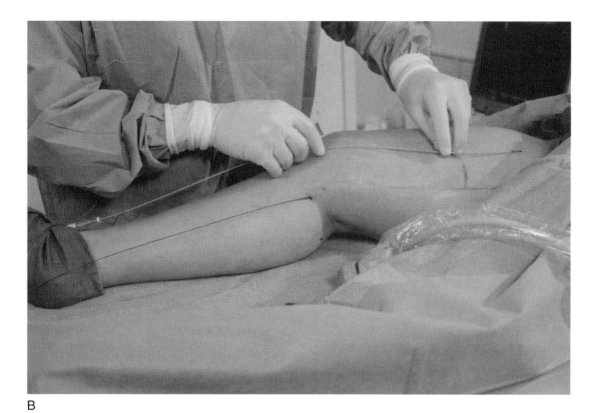

B

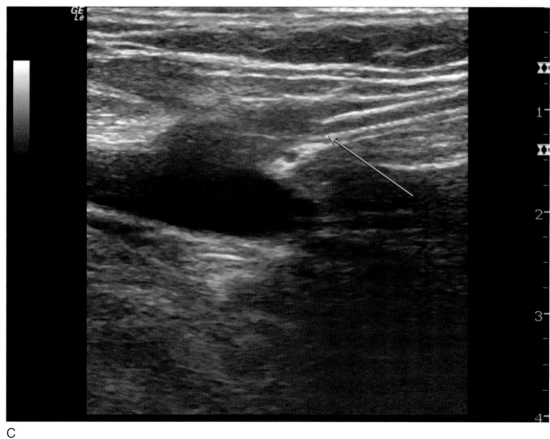

C

■ **Fig. 5.11, cont'd** (B) Outside of the legs, the surgeon measures the estimated sheath length. (C) *Arrow* points to tip of braided sheath at saphenofemoral junction. *Black dot* to the left of *arrow tip* is the external pudendal artery.

Placement of Perivenous Tumescent Anesthesia

The placement of a generous volume of a dilute anesthetic solution into the saphenous canal often causes these tissues to swell; therefore one will often see this procedure referred to as *tumescent anesthesia placement* (Figs. 5.12 and 5.13). Most operators will use a 0.1% lidocaine solution with epinephrine. The solution is easily mixed by placing 50 mL of 1% lidocaine with 1:100,000 epinephrine in a 500-mL reservoir bag of normal saline. Bicarbonate may be added as a buffer if it is the preference of the physician. Alternatively, 50 mL of 1% lidocaine with 1:100,000 epinephrine can be mixed into 500 mL of lactated Ringer solution, which is already buffered. Once the solution is prepared, it can be injected around the circumference of the target vein at various locations.

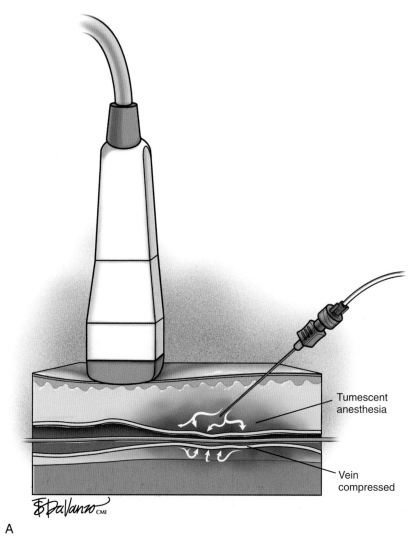

Tumescent
anesthesia

Vein
compressed

A

■ **Fig. 5.12**

Perivenous tumescent anesthesia offers several benefits. First, it acts as a heat sink. By circumferentially surrounding the target vein with fluid, any heat transferred to the vein wall from the thermal ablation catheter will be effectively neutralized by the cool anesthetic fluid. Therefore heat will not be transferred to nontarget tissues, such as nerves, and damage will be localized to the vein wall. Second, perivenous tumescent anesthesia compresses the vein. The ClosureFAST radiofrequency device works by conducting heat to the vein wall. In the case of laser, heat transfer works by a combination of direct contact and convection. Regardless of the technology used, if the vein wall is brought into closer proximity with the thermal ablation catheter, the energy transfer will be more effective. As one delivers the anesthetic solution under ultrasound control, it is easy to visualize the venous diameter shrinking (by compression) as more anesthetic is injected. The goal is to see good apposition of the vein wall to the catheter shaft. Finally, perivenous tumescent anesthesia also has an analgesic effect. Patients should experience a painless procedure.

Several delivery systems are available for placement of tumescent anesthesia, ranging from an inexpensive syringe with a 25-gauge needle to specialized pumps for more rapid delivery.

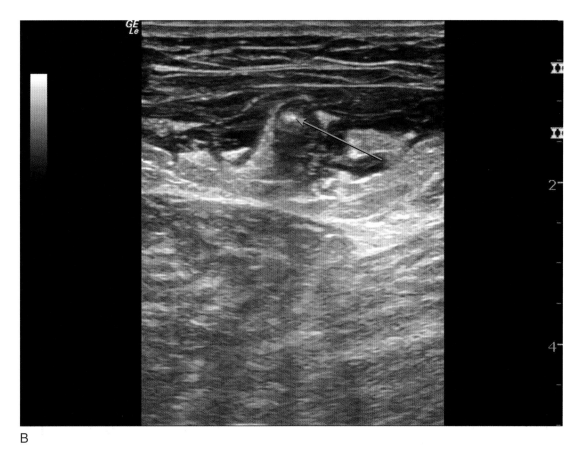

B

■ **Fig. 5.12, cont'd** (B) *Arrow* points to great saphenous vein in cross-sectional view, catheter is seen intraluminally, there is good apposition of vein wall to catheter, and vein is surrounded 360 degrees with tumescent anesthesia.

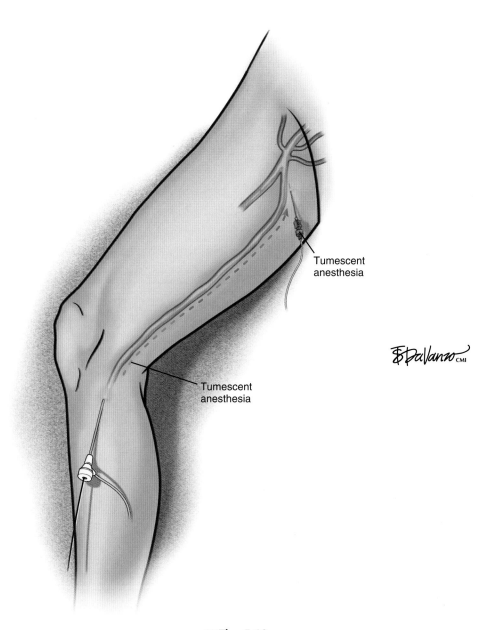

Tumescent
anesthesia

Tumescent
anesthesia

■ Fig. 5.13

Laser

In the case of EVL thermal ablation, a 4-Fr or 5-Fr sheath is preferred. With the early-generation endovenous laser ablation systems, the endovenous sheath for laser had to be long enough to reach the SFJ. The length of the sheath chosen can be estimated by measuring on the outside of the leg from the guidewire entry site to the inguinal crease. In general, this distance is about 40 cm when access is obtained below the knee; therefore a 45-cm-length sheath is most commonly used. Sheaths are commercially available in 25-cm, 35-cm, 45-cm, and 65-cm lengths, although now jacketed fibers can be advanced without sheath. The fiber is navigated to the SFJ. Sometimes the entry site must be widened to allow sheath entry; this is easily accomplished with a no. 11 blade scalpel. If advancing a longer sheath, there are instances in which a patient may feel discomfort during tracking of the sheath, especially when performed in the office setting without conscious sedation. In these situations, the sheath should not be forced. The sheath tracking should be stopped momentarily to allow placement of perivenous tumescent anesthesia. With the guidewire in place, it is easy to identify and to anesthetize the vein. Then tracking of the sheath may be resumed painlessly. Once the sheath has been navigated to its final position, which is about 2 cm distal to the CFV, the inner dilator and 0.035-inch (0.088-cm) guidewire may be removed.

If using a longer sheath, the laser fiber is inserted into the sheath through the hemostatic valve and advanced to the sheath tip. The sheath is then withdrawn 1 cm, to expose the laser fiber tip at the SFJ. Some systems have a locking hub on the fiber to facilitate this process and secure the fiber-sheath components together during withdrawal. Pushing the fiber out of the sheath to expose it should be discouraged because this maneuver can inadvertently penetrate and perforate the vein wall, especially with bare-tipped fibers. Bare-tipped laser fibers are void of cladding, which renders them rather sharp. When working with covered fibers, the tips are smooth and less likely to penetrate the vein wall, therefore "unsheathing" to expose the laser fiber tip is not as critical (Figs. 5.14 and 5.15). As stated earlier, many systems now allow passage of the fiber directly through the microsheath and the step of exchanging over a 0.035-inch (0.088-cm) platform is avoided.

Once the laser fiber tip is exposed, it should be positioned about 2 to 3 cm from the ostium of the CFV. If the superficial epigastric vein is visible, the fiber tip should be positioned distal to this entry of this vessel. There is some empirical evidence that this strategy retards the formation of thrombus extension into the CFV and that it obviates the formation of neovascular channels in the area of the groin, which may lead to recurrence.

After the vein is accessed, the device positioned, and anesthesia given, the patient is treated.

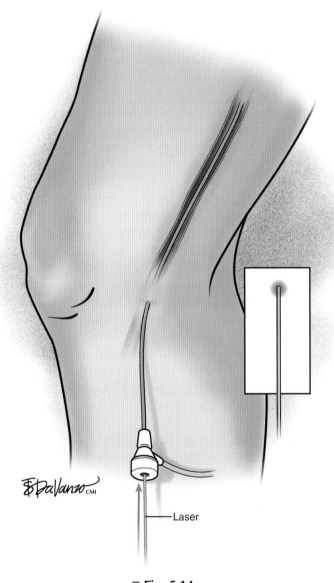

Laser

■ Fig. 5.14

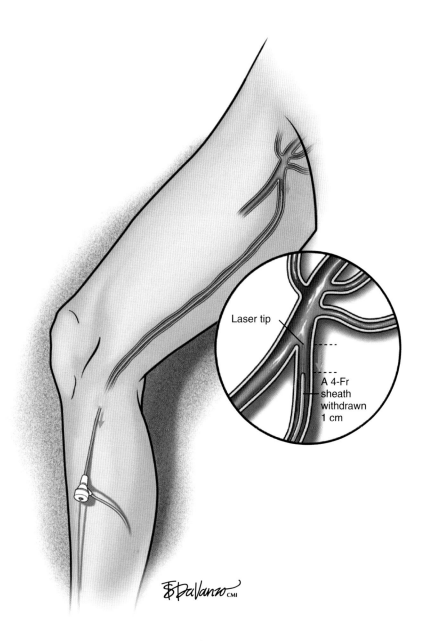

Laser tip

A 4-Fr
sheath
withdrawn
1 cm

■ Fig. 5.15

The Pullback

Laser

The pullback protocol for endovenous laser ablation is not straightforward. Multiple wavelengths are available and no absolute energy protocols have been established. Much of the existing published work in this area is described in Chapter 7. For the three available wavelengths that target the hemoglobin molecule preferentially (810 nm, 940 nm, and 980 nm), the linear endovenous energy density (LEED) should range between 60 J per cm and 100 J per cm. This has produced very satisfactory results with the majority of veins and is a simple formula for the new user. As the operator gains more experience, he or she may want to tailor the therapy to the anatomy of the vein. That is, the presence of aneurysmal segments, large tributaries, or perforators may sway the operator in the direction of delivering higher-energy densities than normal, whereas small-diameter veins and veins near the skin may have improved results with lower-energy densities. The pullback speed measured in millimeters per second is governed by the desired LEED.

The laser has adjustable power outputs. Most laser systems, for purposes of endovenous ablation, will deliver a maximum of 15 W. One watt delivers 1 J of energy per second, and 10 W delivers 10 J per second. With the laser set at 10 W, for most veins the results are very satisfactory. Therefore, if one desires to treat an ordinary incompetent GSV that is 40 cm in length, the following sequence will be used: At a LEED of 60 J per cm, the total energy delivery will be 2400 J. At a power of 10 W, the total time for energy delivery will be 240 seconds. The pullback rate will therefore equal about 0.17 cm per second, 1.7 mm per second, or 10.2 cm per minute.

If the operator does not elect a manual pullback, there is a commercially available motorized pullback device. The motor can be set to produce pullback speeds of 1 mm or 2 mm per second. The advantage of this system is that no human variability is introduced, and when looking at results, the pullback rate is a constant variable. The disadvantage is that all veins are different, and a manual pullback allows for easy adjustment to treat areas of concern, such as aneurysmal segments and segments in close proximity to the skin.

By locating the aiming beam, manual application of pressure at the fiber tip (Figs. 5.16 and 5.17) facilitates the process of bringing the target vein wall in closer proximity to the energy source. Since the advent of covered fiber tips, this maneuver has become controversial. Some small pilot studies have suggested that covered tips may minimize the focal vein perforations seen with bare-fiber laser ablation. The idea of external manual compression during the laser pullback is to bring the vein wall in closer proximity to the energy source. With bare fibers, this translates into areas of direct contact of the vein endothelium with the laser fiber tip (which transfers energy via conduction) and areas of vein not in direct contact with the laser fiber tip (which transfers energy via convection). Gross histologic samples suggest that the venous perforations occur at sites of direct contact. The idea of covered fibers is to not allow any areas of direct contact of the vein wall with the laser fiber, thus minimizing vein perforations.

At termination of the laser pullback, the laser is deactivated by the surgeon removing his or her foot from the foot pedal. The laser and the sheath are removed together in their entirety. A quick on-table duplex scan confirms vein closure. The color flow mode should demonstrate lack of flow, and the greyscale image should demonstrate a thickened, noncompressible vein wall (Fig. 5.18).

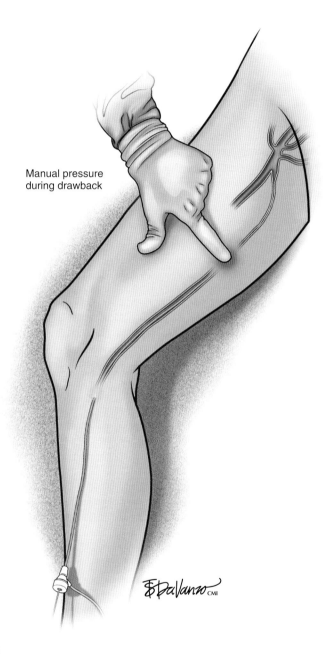

Manual pressure
during drawback

A

■ **Fig. 5.16**

Continued

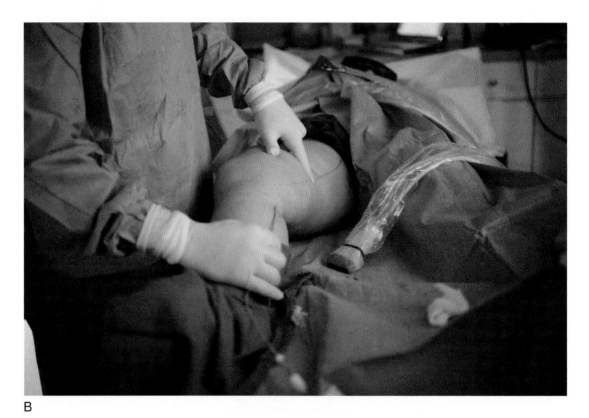

B

■ **Fig. 5.16, cont'd**

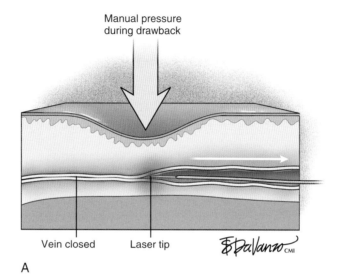

A

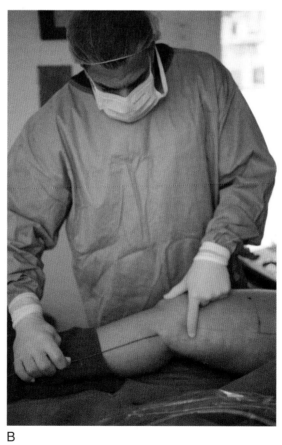

B

■ **Fig. 5.17**

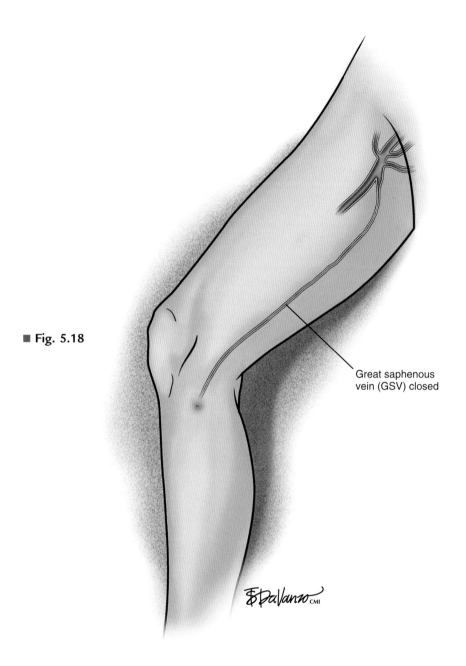

■ **Fig. 5.18**

Great saphenous
vein (GSV) closed

A compression bandage is then placed by the medical assistant (Fig. 5.19). At the Miami Vein Center, we prefer that the patient wear a three-layer bandage for 24 to 48 hours postprocedure. Careful application of the postoperative dressing cannot be overstated; careless dressing placement can lead to hematomas, blisters, nerve injury, ischemia, and bleeding. The limb is wrapped circumferentially from foot to groin with a compression dressing that is removed after 24 to 48 hours. The dressing should be applied with graduated pressure; the amount of pressure should decrease as one proceeds from foot to groin. During placement of the compressive bandage, it is important to pad the lateral fibular head to avoid pressure-induced injury to the deep and superficial peroneal nerves, which can lead to foot drop. Patients are encouraged to ambulate immediately after the procedure to minimize thromboembolic complications.

Application of a compressive dressing in obese patients is especially critical because the dressing tends to unravel. It is important to avoid applying this dressing tightly because this can lead to undue pressure, blistering, and/or skin necrosis.

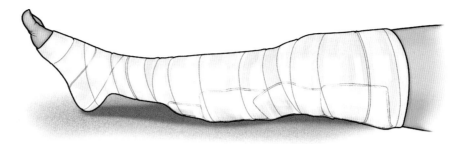

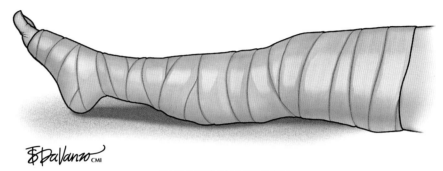

Postoperative leg bandaging

A

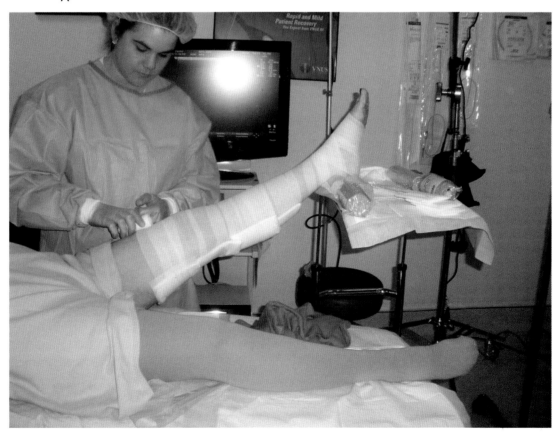

B

■ **Fig. 5.19**

Continued

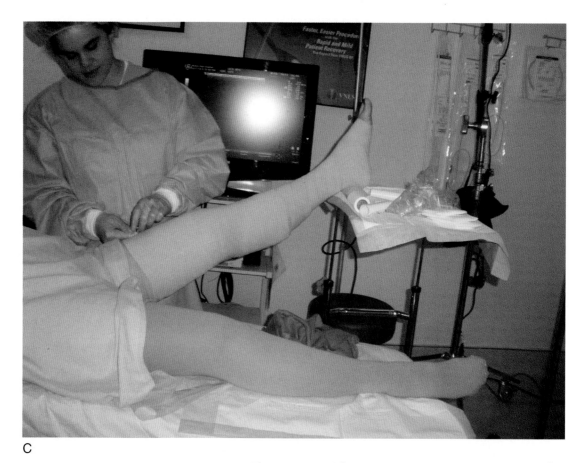

C

◾ **Fig. 5.19, cont'd**

RADIOFREQUENCY ABLATION

The VNUS closure system includes a computer-controlled RF generator and disposable catheters (Figs. 5.20–5.25). RF technology has evolved from a slow, continuous pullback to a rapid segmental pullback. The original device was oriented with an anode and cathode at the catheter tip. When the device was in contact with the vein wall, the vein wall acted as the resistive element of an electrical circuit analogous to a light bulb. In the case of the light bulb, an electrical current passes through a thin tungsten filament, heating it until it produces light. In the case of an incompetent saphenous vein, radiofrequency current passes through the vein, heating it, causing collagen molecules to shrink. Because the heating was only 1 cm in length, a slow, continuous pullback was required to adequately treat a vein. A typical 40-cm vein would take about 20 minutes to treat. Furthermore, coagulum buildup at the tip of the catheter caused an increase in the impedance, which triggered an automatic shutoff of the generator when a threshold number was reached. In this case, catheter removal, cleaning, and reintroduction of the catheter into the vein were required. The device heated the vein wall to 85°C, and studies showed a closure rate of about 85% with 5-year follow-up.

Text continued on p. 166

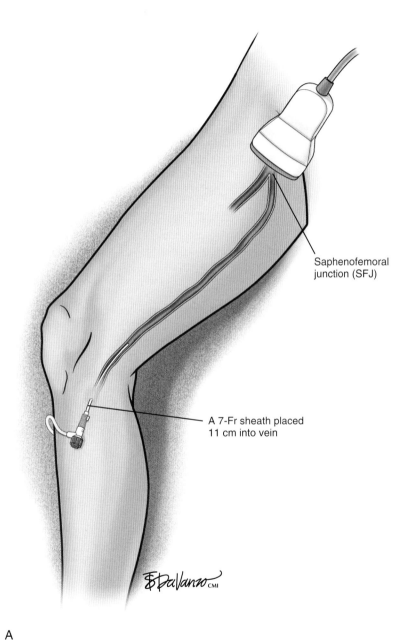

Saphenofemoral
junction (SFJ)

A 7-Fr sheath placed
11 cm into vein

A

■ **Fig. 5.20**

Continued

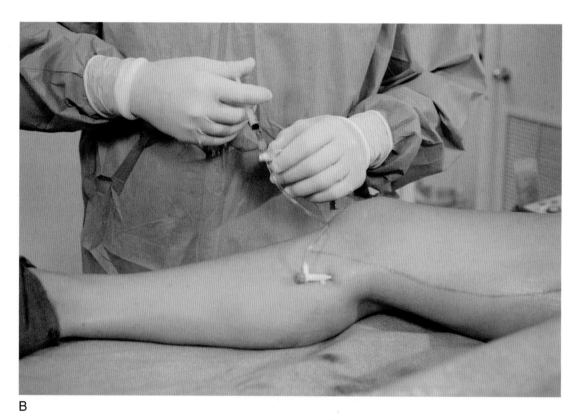

B

■ **Fig. 5.20, cont'd**

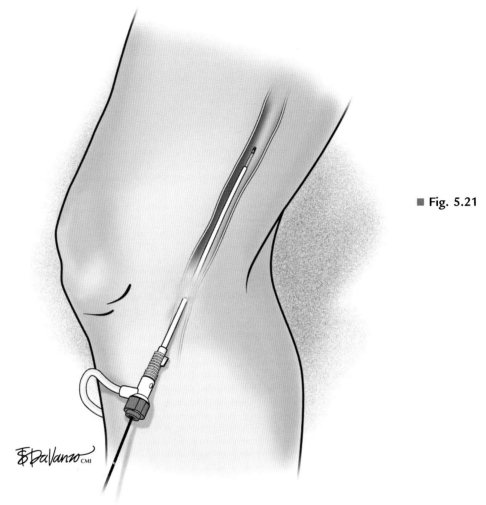

■ Fig. 5.21

Radiofrequency (RF) catheter inserted into sheath

A

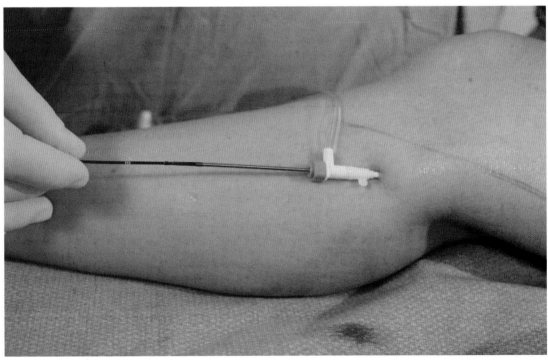

B

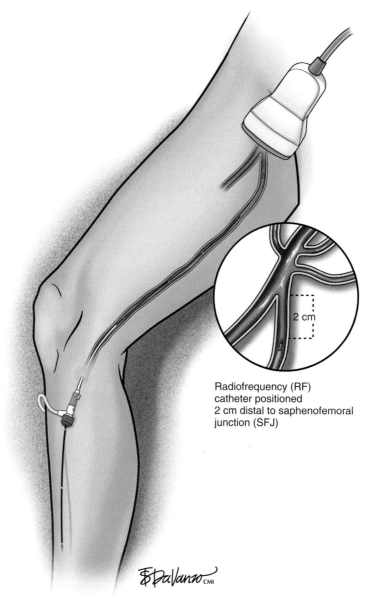

Radiofrequency (RF)
catheter positioned
2 cm distal to saphenofemoral
junction (SFJ)

A

■ Fig. 5.22

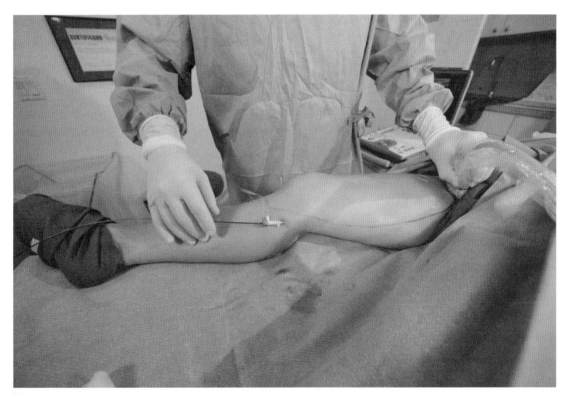

B

■ **Fig. 5.22, cont'd**

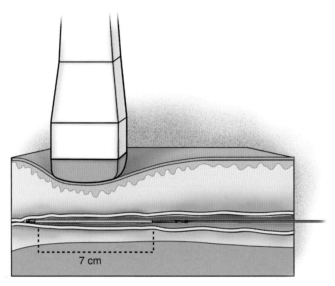

Radiofrequency (RF) catheter treating 7 cm of vein

■ **Fig. 5.23**

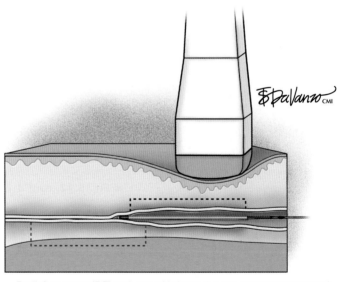

Radiofrequency (RF) catheter withdrawn 6.5 cm, treatment repeated

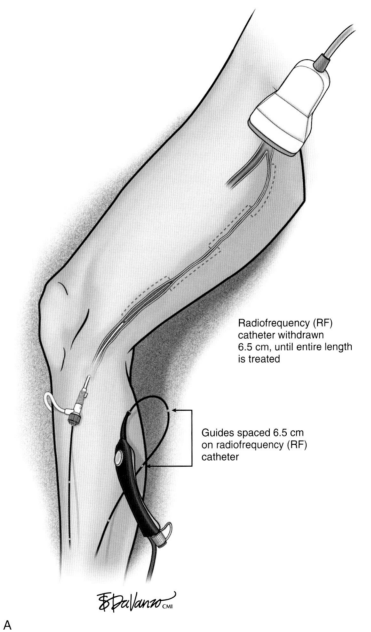

Radiofrequency (RF)
catheter withdrawn
6.5 cm, until entire length
is treated

Guides spaced 6.5 cm
on radiofrequency (RF)
catheter

A

■ **Fig. 5.24**

Continued

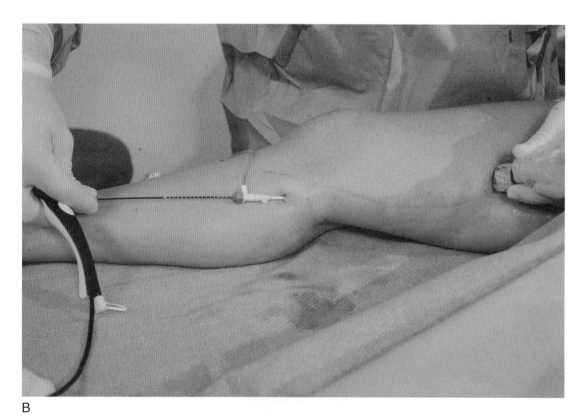

B

■ Fig. 5.24, cont'd

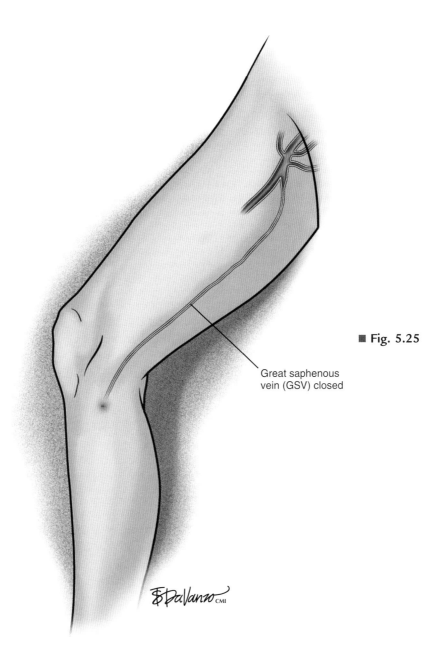

■ **Fig. 5.25**

Great saphenous
vein (GSV) closed

The procedure can be performed under local anesthesia using perivenous tumescent infiltration with or without conscious sedation. An introducer sheath is placed to allow catheter insertion into the target vein. The electrodes are deployed at the SFJ and positioned distal to the entry of the superficial epigastric vein when present, or approximately 2 cm distal to the origin of the common femoral vein in cases where the superficial epigastric vein is not visualized.

The vein must be anesthetized circumferentially along the entire treatment length with a dilute lidocaine solution before treatment is begun.

Upon initiation of RF energy delivery to the electrodes, the catheter is slowly withdrawn while maintaining the treatment temperature at 85°C. The feedback mechanism of the system allows controlled energy delivery and appropriate monitoring of the procedure.

The second-generation device (ClosureFAST) is fitted with a different heating element. The treatment component of the device is 7 cm in length and works with a segmental pullback protocol. That is, once the catheter is in position, activation of the generator delivers 20-second cycles of energy to the catheter tip, which heats the vein wall to 120°C. The catheter is pulled back in increments of 6.5 cm so as to overlap the treatment sites. This segmental pullback strategy with a longer length heating element translates into a treatment time of about 3 minutes for a typical saphenous vein 40 cm in length (see Fig. 5.24B).

SMALL SAPHENOUS VEIN ABLATION

Gibson[10] described the anatomic differences between the SFJ and the thromboprophylaxis, as well as the proximity of the sural nerve to the SSV, correctly noting that endovenous laser ablation of the SSV is slightly different from the GSV. The Gibson anatomic classification is depicted in Fig. 5.26:
- Type A: a saphenopopliteal junction with no significant branches; 43% of limbs
- Type B: a saphenopopliteal junction with a large extension Giacomini vein; 33% of limbs
- Type C: no direct termination into a deep vein (saphenopopliteal or saphenofemoral junction), with the SSV continuing as a Giacomini vein above the popliteal fossa; the Giacomini vein was the sole termination of the SSV in 24% of limbs

In the type A cases where the SSV enters the popliteal vein directly, the concepts remain very similar to those of GSV treatment (Fig. 5.27). The patient is taken to the office operating suite and, in the standing position, all bulging veins are marked on the skin with an indelible marker. Unlike GSV cases, where the patient is placed in the supine position, the prone position is chosen for SSV ablation. The extremity is then prepped and draped in the usual sterile manner (see Fig. 5.27).

Usually, a quick preprocedure scan is performed to select the access site and determine treatment length, so the appropriate sheaths can be readied. A typical length for the SSV is about 15 cm if no cranial extension is present (Fig. 5.28). It is very important to note the anatomy of the SPJ before catheter placement. In the usual arrangement, best visualized with the ultrasound probe in the long axis, the SSV will deepen its course as it approaches its union with the popliteal vein. It will appear as a 45-degree bend, about 2 cm in length. We prefer to leave this 2-cm-length angled segment untreated for two reasons: (1) the gastrocnemius veins enter into this segment and are best preserved; and (2) the tibial nerve comes into proximity to the SSV at this deeper level. Although it is easy to push the tibial nerve away from the vein using tumescent anesthesia, if the anesthetic diffuses onto the nerve, temporary nerve palsy may result and cause unnecessary alarm to both patient and physician.

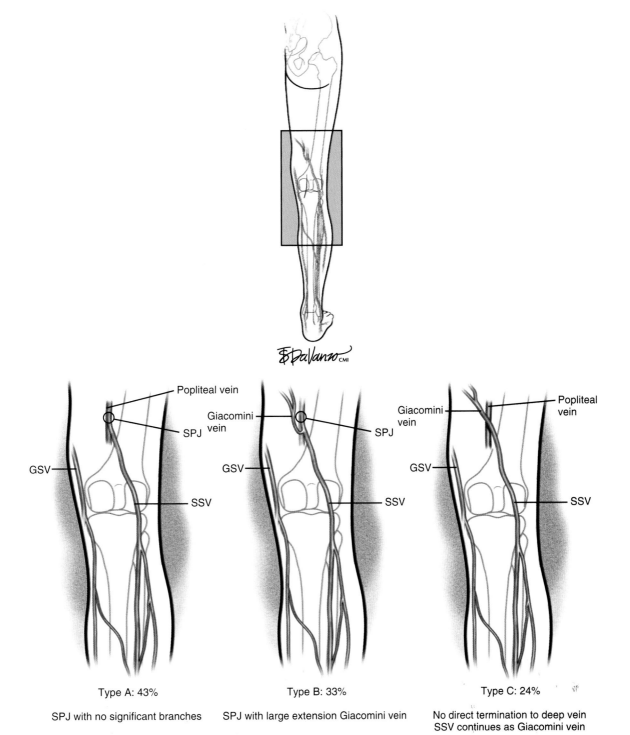

Type A: 43%

SPJ with no significant branches

Type B: 33%

SPJ with large extension Giacomini vein

Type C: 24%

No direct termination to deep vein
SSV continues as Giacomini vein

■ **Fig. 5.26** *GSV,* Great saphenous vein; *SPJ,* saphenopopliteal junction; *SSV,* small saphenous vein.

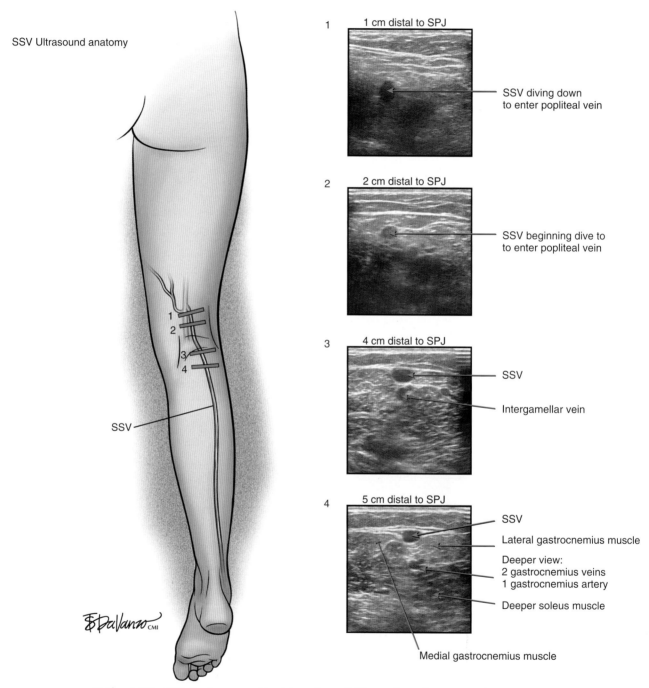

SSV Ultrasound anatomy

SSV

1   1 cm distal to SPJ

SSV diving down to enter popliteal vein

2   2 cm distal to SPJ

SSV beginning dive to to enter popliteal vein

3   4 cm distal to SPJ

SSV

Intergamellar vein

4   5 cm distal to SPJ

SSV

Lateral gastrocnemius muscle

Deeper view: 2 gastrocnemius veins 1 gastrocnemius artery

Deeper soleus muscle

Medial gastrocnemius muscle

■ **Fig. 5.27** *SPJ,* Saphenopopliteal junction; *SSV,* small saphenous vein.

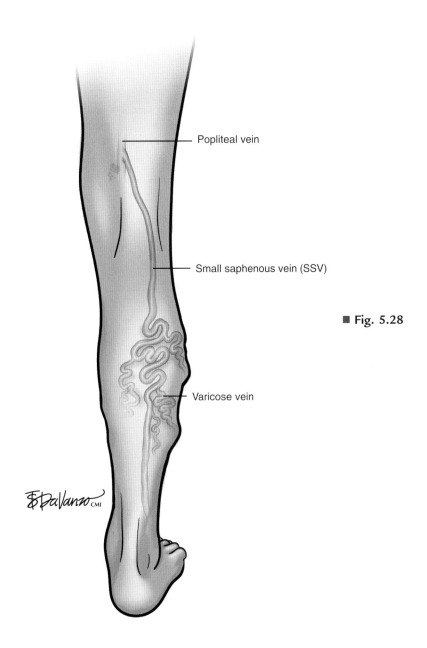

Popliteal vein

Small saphenous vein (SSV)

Varicose vein

■ Fig. 5.28

1. Access

   Percutaneous access (Figs. 5.29–5.31) to the SSV is achieved at midcalf on the inferior aspect of the gastrocnemius muscles. A micropuncture kit with a 21-gauge needle and 0.018-inch (0.045-cm) guidewire is preferred. The 0.018-inch (0.088-cm) wire is advanced through the needle to the SPJ under ultrasound guidance. The microintroducer and sheath are then placed and exchanged for a 0.035-inch (0.088-cm) wire.

   In the case of RF, a 7-cm-length, 7-Fr sheath is placed. A newer heating element of 3-cm length is also available. Keep in mind that once the RF heating element is exteriorized from the end of the sheath, the total length of the device will be about 14 cm. In the typical 15-cm-length SSV, this will translate into one double-treatment cycle at the SPJ, followed by one more cycle of energy delivery after the catheter pullback; three cycles (60 seconds) for total treatment.

   In the case of EVLA, the laser fiber tip governs most of the decision making. Usually the vein is accessed with a 21-gauge needle, followed by microintroducer placement. If using a bare-tipped 600-μm fiber, or a 400-μm fiber, the fiber will fit directly through the microintroducer sheath. However, if working with a 600-μm jacket-tip fiber, the microintroducer will need to be exchanged for a 4-Fr or 5-Fr sheath.

2. Positioning

   The RF and laser fiber tips are positioned at the same location—about 2 cm distal to the popliteal vein opening, where the "bend" of the SSV is usually located (Fig. 5.32). Because there is some forward heating with the RF ClosureFAST device, in general, I prefer laser for SSV ablations, although many operators use RF in this area with success.

3. Anesthesia

   The SSV is also enveloped in a fascial compartment similar to that of the GSV, except that it is more fully developed. This fascial tissue is thicker and serves as a consistent landmark to locate the SSV. The SSV is located in the midline of the posterior calf, at the most superficial location where the medial and lateral heads of the gastrocnemius muscles meet.

   The same principles for tumescent anesthesia apply here. Using ultrasound, the solution is placed in the perivenous plane. Ideally, SSV compression and diameter shrinkage are observed.

4. Pullback (Fig. 5.33)

   In this area, treatment with RF can be challenging. In general, veins of shorter length require more attention from the operator because of the nature of the device with a 7-cm-length heating element (3-cm length may be suitable in these cases). With laser, it is the same technique as for other veins, such as the GSV: one decides the desired LEED, the power is set, and pullback speed is determined. Ablation of Giacomini vein is demonstrated in Fig. 5.34.

Text continued on p. 176

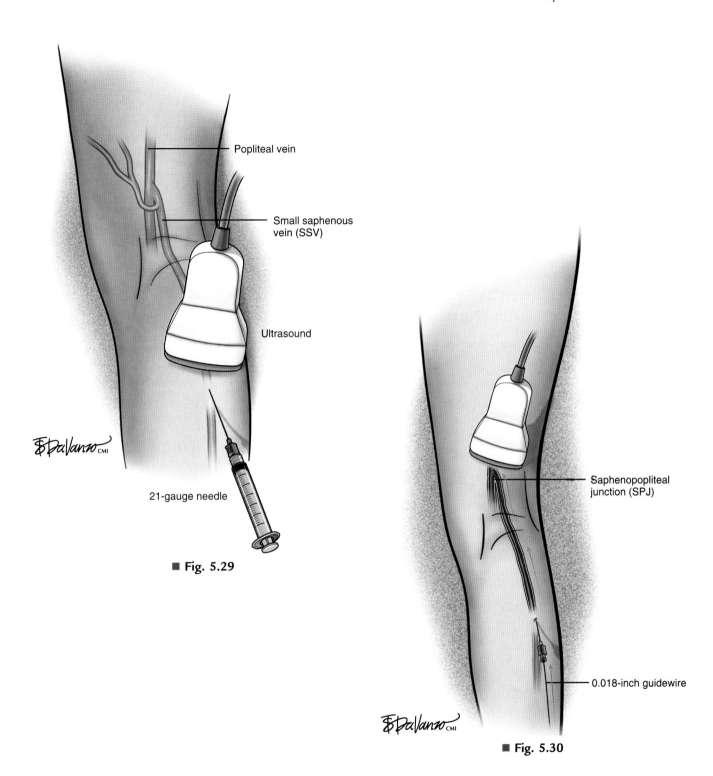

Popliteal vein

Small saphenous
vein (SSV)

Ultrasound

21-gauge needle

■ **Fig. 5.29**

Saphenopopliteal
junction (SPJ)

0.018-inch guidewire

■ **Fig. 5.30**

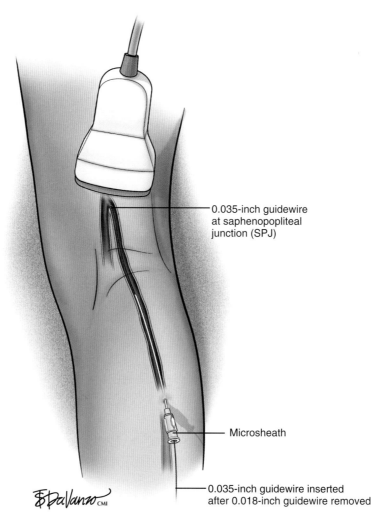

0.035-inch guidewire
at saphenopopliteal
junction (SPJ)

Microsheath

0.035-inch guidewire inserted
after 0.018-inch guidewire removed

■ Fig. 5.31

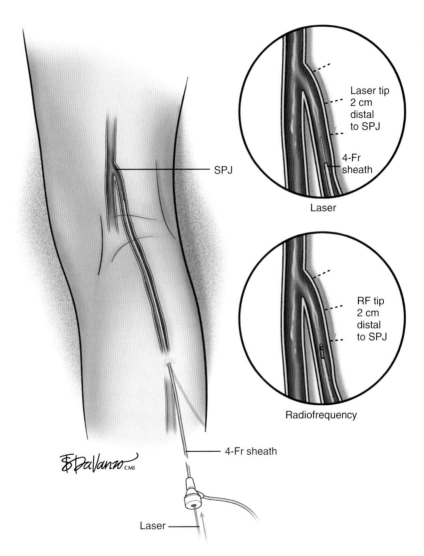

SPJ

Laser tip
2 cm
distal
to SPJ

4-Fr
sheath

Laser

RF tip
2 cm
distal
to SPJ

Radiofrequency

4-Fr sheath

Laser

■ **Fig. 5.32** Laser *(upper panel)* and radiofrequency (RF, *lower panel*) catheter positioning at saphenopopliteal junction (SPJ).

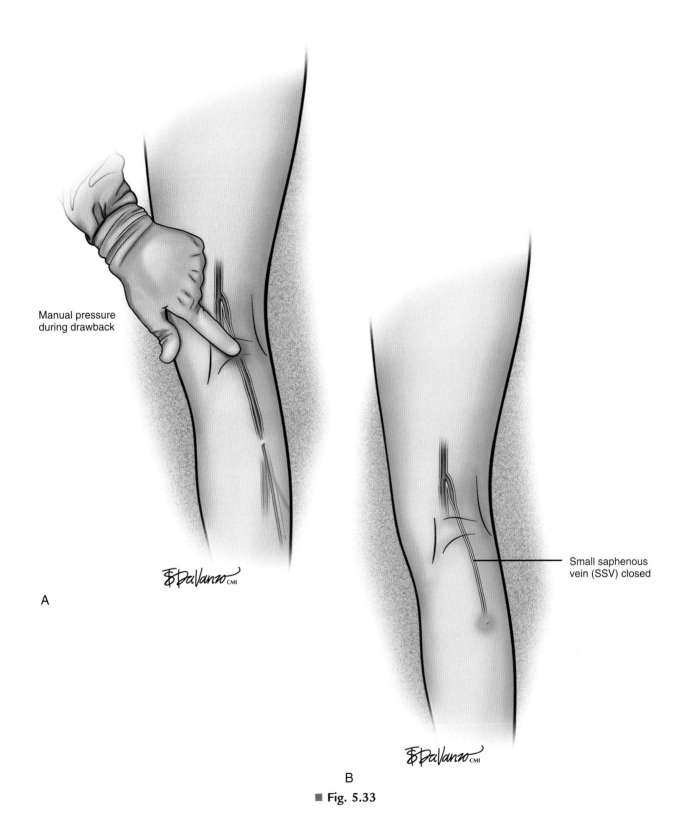

Manual pressure
during drawback

A

Small saphenous
vein (SSV) closed

B

■ **Fig. 5.33**

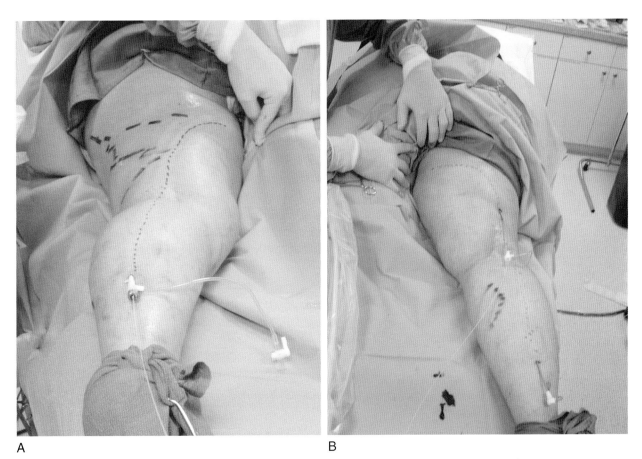

A B

■ **Fig. 5.34** (A) The Giacomini vein can be ablated using standard principles. In this case, a single puncture allowed access to the entire vein. (B) Sometimes two access sites are required.

TREATING ACCESSORY AND CIRCUMFLEX VEINS (FIGS. 5.35–5.37)

The aforementioned principles hold true for incompetent accessory and circumflex veins. The distalmost segment of a straight vein is chosen. For circumflex veins, these access points usually present themselves in the upper third of the thigh; thus treatment lengths tend to be short, in the order of 5-cm to 10-cm lengths. Circumflex veins by definition take oblique angles, and this must be factored in during the hand-eye coordination required for access. Also, because these veins tend to have short treatment lengths, micropuncture exchanges to longer sheaths are often cumbersome. For this reason, I prefer laser for these cases. The laser fiber will fit through a micropuncture access sheath, and the energy is delivered from the tip of the laser fiber. Because the heating element for the RF catheter is 7 cm in length, it is not as versatile when treating circumflex veins; 3-cm length might be more suitable.

Accessory veins are usually longer than circumflex veins but shorter than the GSV. Because they run parallel to the axis of the GSV, access resembles GSV access.

Positioning the tip of the device at the SFJ requires a little more manipulation of the ultrasound probe to obtain an unobstructed view of the junction.

At the groin, the anterior accessory great saphenous vein (AAGSV) is superficial to the CFV, and located lateral to the GSV and medial to the common femoral artery. The alignment sign is useful for tracking the AAGSV. The AAGSV is found directly superior to, and in the same ultrasound plane as, the superficial femoral artery and femoral vein. The AAGSV is found anterior and lateral to the GSV and runs parallel to the GSV; often it is confused with the anterior thigh circumflex vein, which takes an oblique course to the GSV (see Fig. 5.35A).

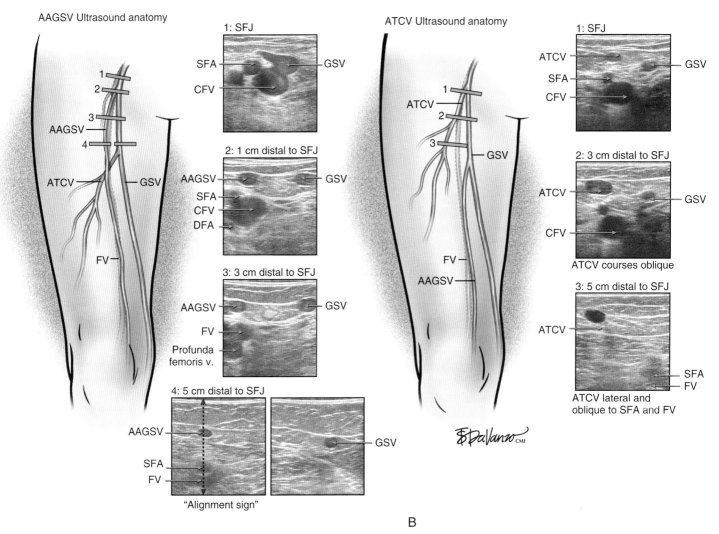

■ **Fig. 5.35** (A and B) *AAGSV,* Anterior accessory great saphenous vein; *ATCV,* anterior thigh circumflex vein; *CFV,* common femoral vein; *DFA,* deep formal artery; *FV,* femoral vein; *GSV,* great saphenous vein; *SFA,* superficial femoral artery; *SFJ,* saphenofemoral junction.

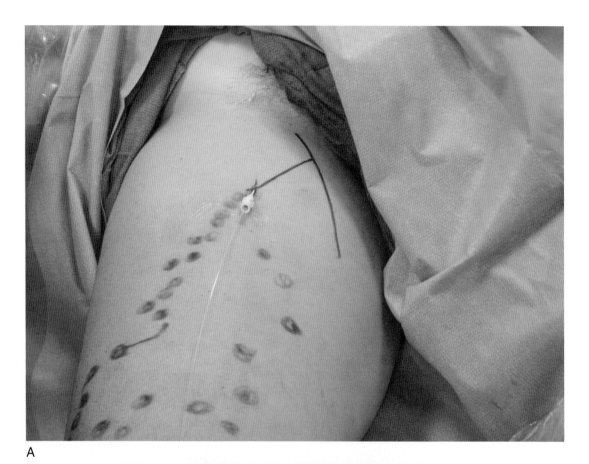

A

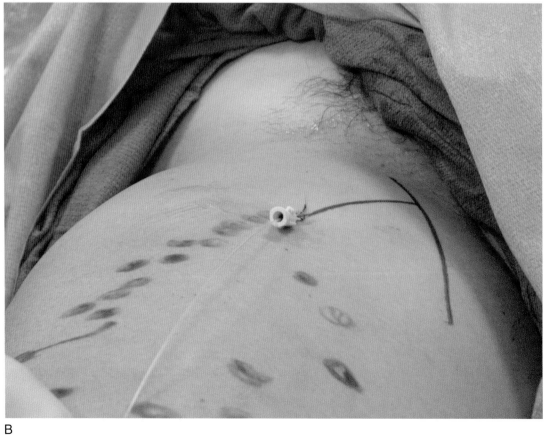

B

■ **Fig. 5.36** (A) Intravenous access of anterior thigh circumflex vein (ATCV) with microsheath (bare laser fiber placed). (B) Close-up of (A).

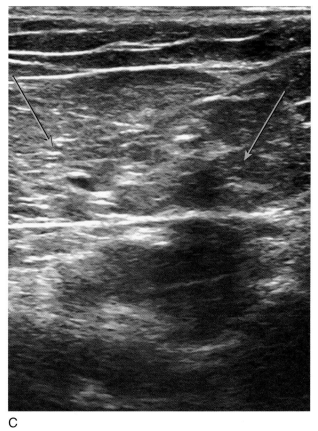

C

■ **Fig. 5.36, cont'd** (C) *Left arrow* points to ATCV. *Right arrow* points to great saphenous vein.

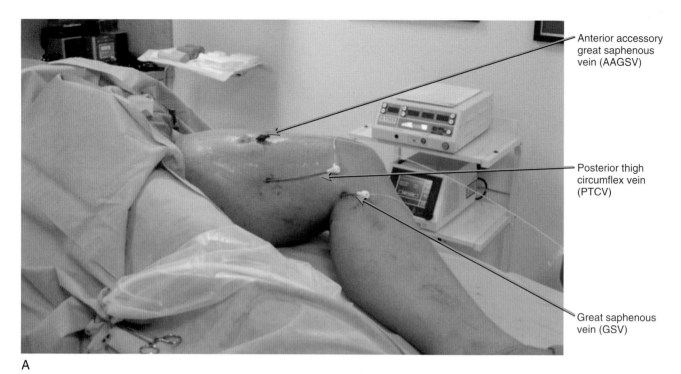

Anterior accessory great saphenous vein (AAGSV)

Posterior thigh circumflex vein (PTCV)

Great saphenous vein (GSV)

A

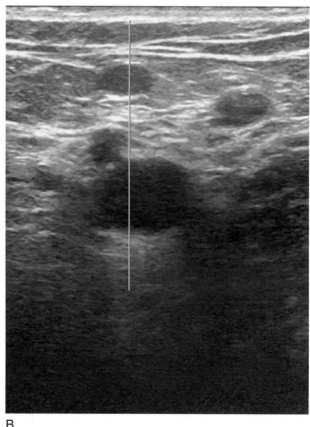

B

■ **Fig. 5.37** (A) Multiple vein access. (B) Line shows alignment of anterior accessory saphenous vein above femoral vessels.

POPLITEAL FOSSA VEIN

Designated the popliteal fossa vein (PFV), it perforates the deep popliteal fascia and empties into the deep system (Fig. 5.38).

With a prevalence of 4.4%, the PFV presents in limbs featuring complex reflux patterns involving all three venous systems proximally and distally, and high venous clinical severity scores. The PFV perforates the deep popliteal fascia, terminating at the deep system (i.e., the popliteal vein in 96%) above the SSV.

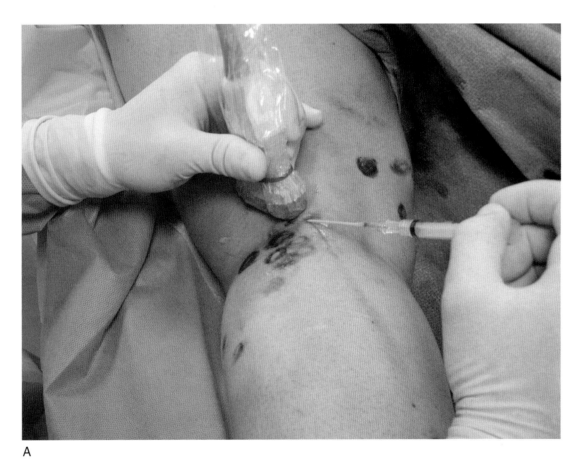

A

■ **Fig. 5.38** (A and B) Percutaneous access of the popliteal fossa vein (PFV) under ultrasound control. Demonstrated is the use of 14-gauge angiocath, through which a bare laser fiber is placed. Note that the treatment length is only 2 cm.

Continued

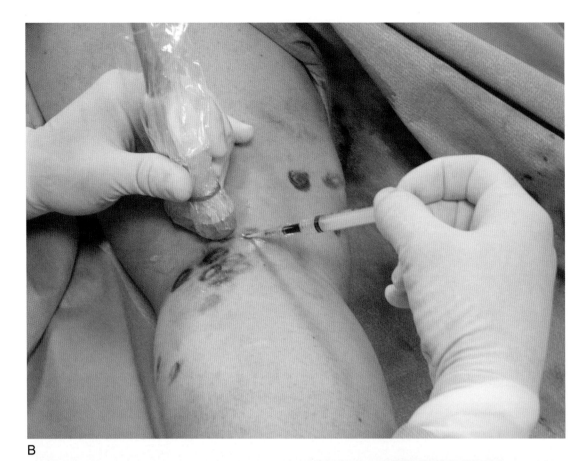

B

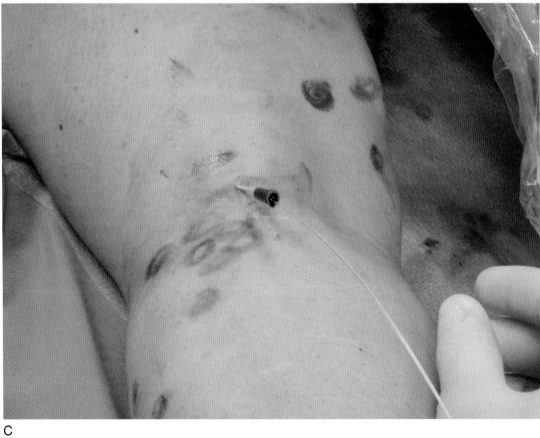

C

■ **Fig. 5.38, cont'd** (C and D) Percutaneous access of the PFV under ultrasound control. Demonstrated is the use of 14-gauge angiocath through which a bare laser fiber is placed. Note that the treatment length is only 2 cm.

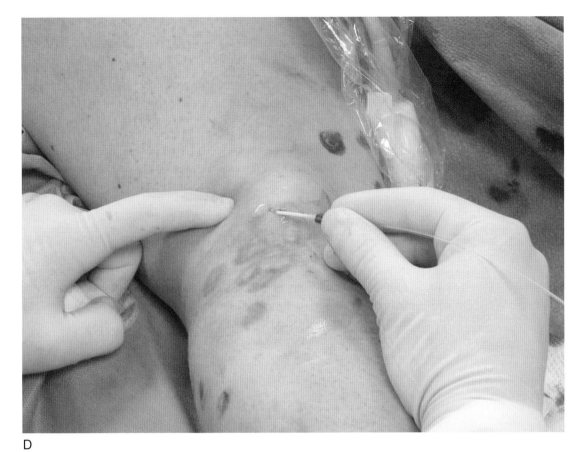

D

E

■ **Fig. 5.38, cont'd** (E) PFV ultrasound. *Bottom left arrow* points to the popliteal vein. *Bottom right arrow* points to the PFV. *Top arrow* points to the small saphenous vein.

LASER-ASSISTED DISTAL SAPHENECTOMY

We also developed a technique referred to as *laser-assisted distal saphenectomy* (LADS). This hybrid technique is useful when the GSV leaves the saphenous canal in the thigh and courses superficially under the skin down the leg (Figs. 5.39–5.45).

The proximal thigh GSV is treated in the usual manner with endovenous laser, but when the superficial course of the vein is identified by the laser-aiming beam, the vein is elevated via a small stab incision and exteriorized. Invagination stripping of the distal saphenous vein is performed by suturing it to the 4-Fr sheath with double-armed 2 Prolene suture. The sheath will serve as an invagination stripping device.

The premise behind the procedure is to avoid the discoloration associated with leaving a thermally ablated vein next to the skin. Thermal ablation causes some carbonization endoluminally, and this pigmentation transilluminates through the skin. The result is a cosmetically unpleasing "dark cord" where the vein courses; therefore it is best removed to avoid this problem.

Text continued on p. 196

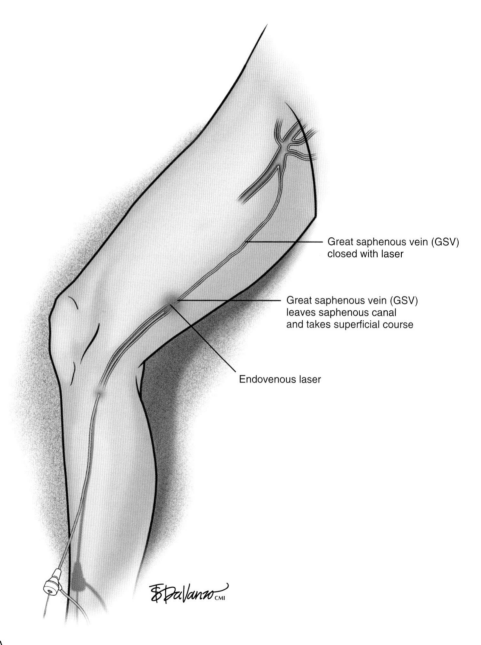

Great saphenous vein (GSV)
closed with laser

Great saphenous vein (GSV)
leaves saphenous canal
and takes superficial course

Endovenous laser

A

■ Fig. 5.39

Continued

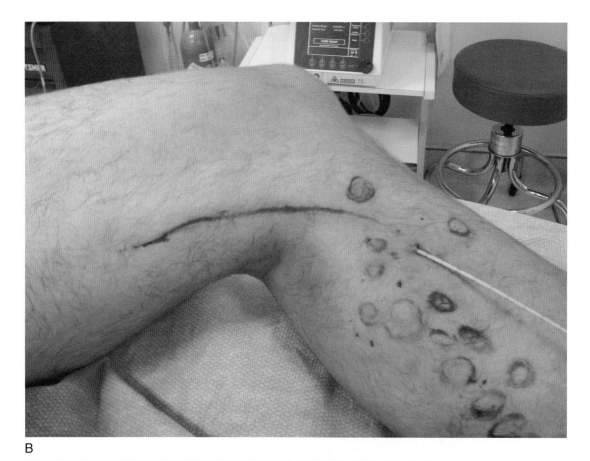

B

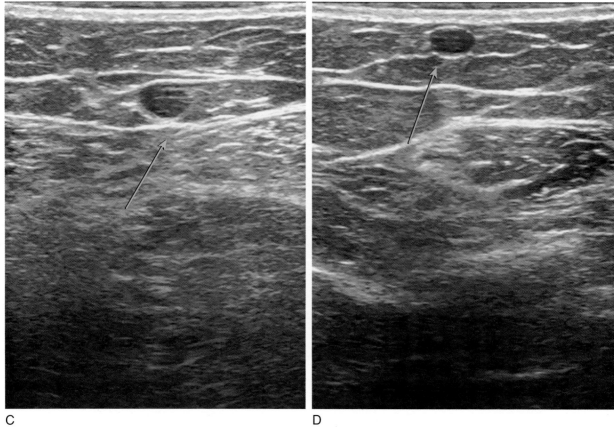

C

D

■ **Fig. 5.39, cont'd** (C) Great saphenous vein (GSV) in saphenous canal *(arrow)*. (D) GSV close to skin; also known as superficial accessory saphenous vein *(arrow)*.

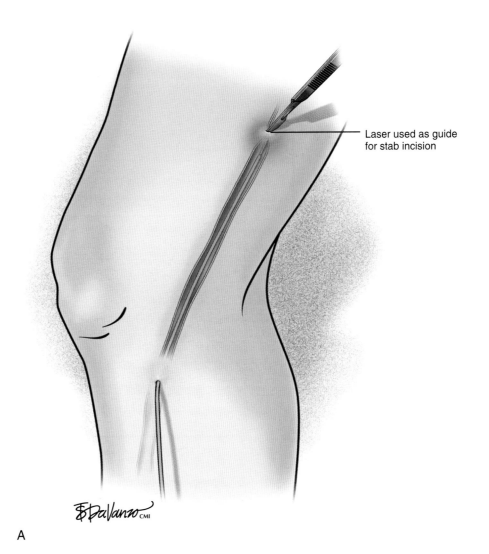

A

Laser used as guide
for stab incision

B

■ **Fig. 5.40**

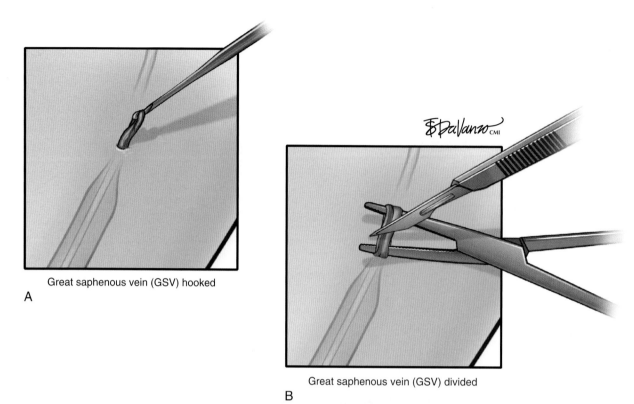

Great saphenous vein (GSV) hooked

A

Great saphenous vein (GSV) divided

B

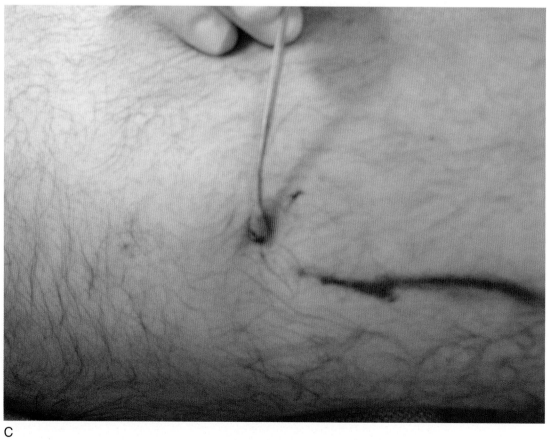

C

■ **Fig. 5.41**

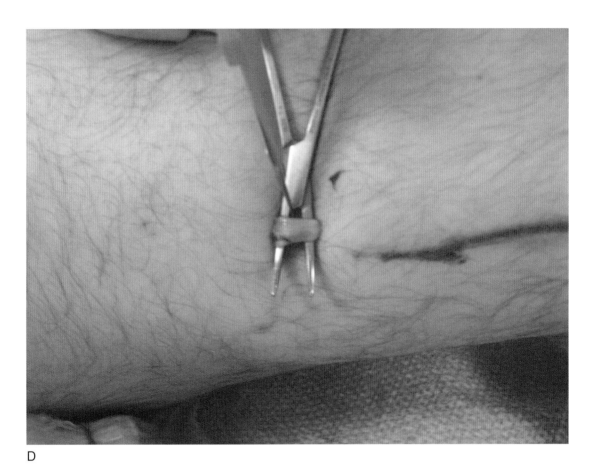

D

■ Fig. 5.41, cont'd

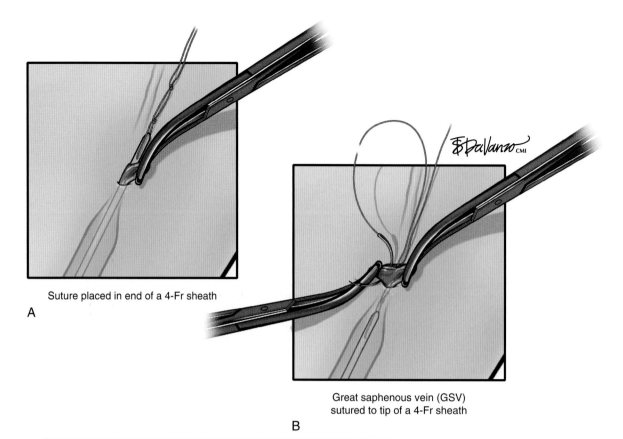

Suture placed in end of a 4-Fr sheath

A

Great saphenous vein (GSV)
sutured to tip of a 4-Fr sheath

B

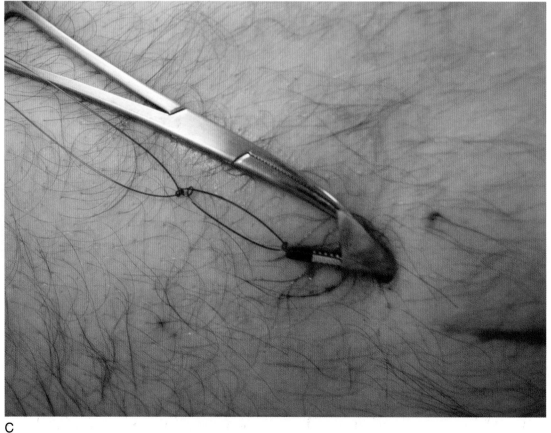

C

■ **Fig. 5.42** (A–C) The endoluminal sheath advanced from below, through the distal vein at midthigh. A braided 4-Fr sheath is preferred because it is more robust. A standard invagination saphenectomy is performed using 2 Prolene double-armed suture. Note that the Prolene suture has been secured through the open end of the 4-Fr braided sheath.

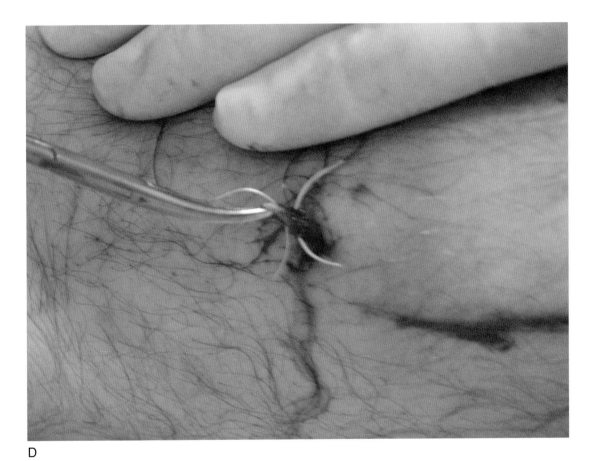

D

■ **Fig. 5.42, cont'd** (D) The endoluminal sheath advanced from below, through the distal vein at midthigh. A braided 4-Fr sheath is preferred because it is more robust. A standard invagination saphenectomy is performed using 2 Prolene double-armed suture. Note that the Prolene suture has been secured through the open end of the 4-Fr braided sheath.

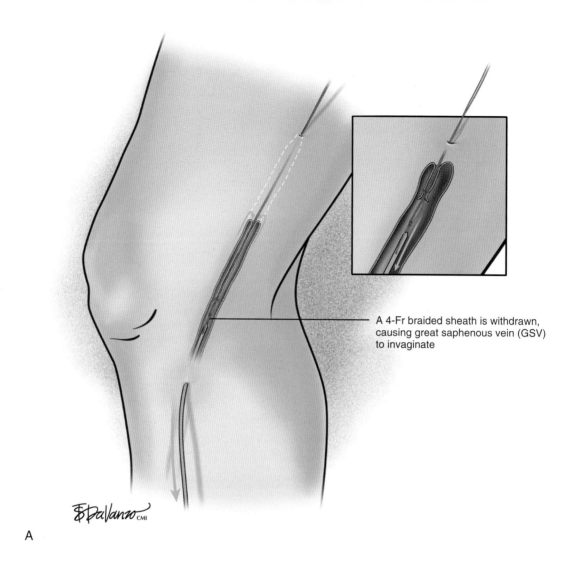

A 4-Fr braided sheath is withdrawn, causing great saphenous vein (GSV) to invaginate

A

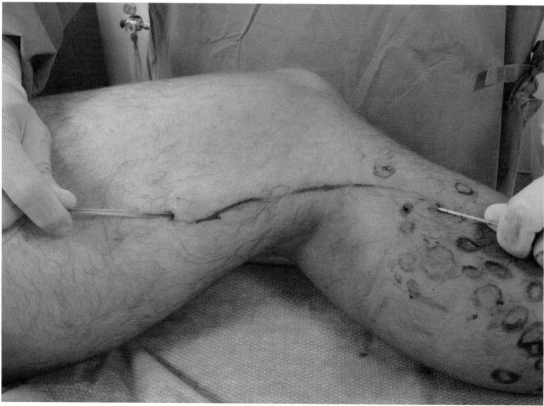

B

■ Fig. 5.43

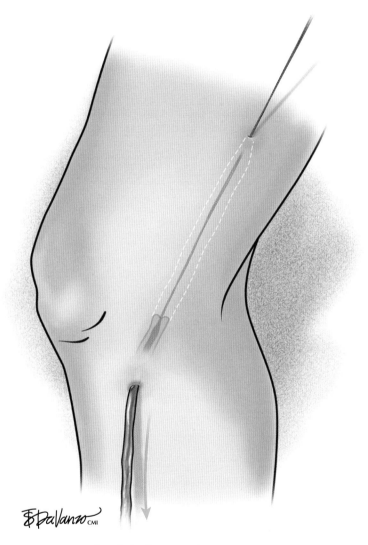

Inverted vein removed

A

■ **Fig. 5.44** (A) The invaginated great saphenous vein (GSV) being harvested from the entry site at the calf. Note how the 2. Prolene suture secured to the 4-Fr braided sheath has nicely invaginated the GSV.

Continued

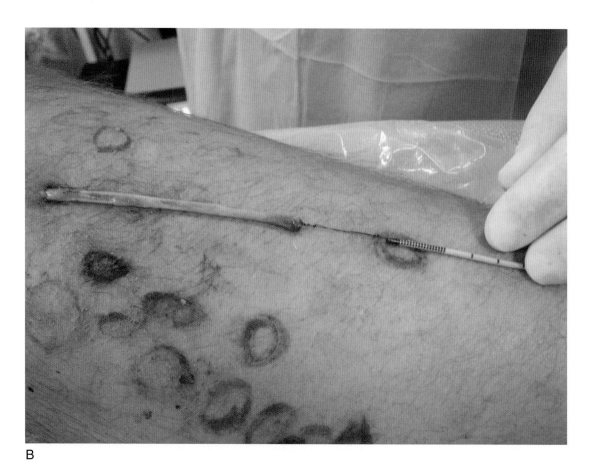

B

■ **Fig. 5.44, cont'd** (B) The invaginated GSV being harvested from the entry site at the calf. Note how the 2 Prolene suture secured to the 4-Fr braided sheath has nicely invaginated the GSV.

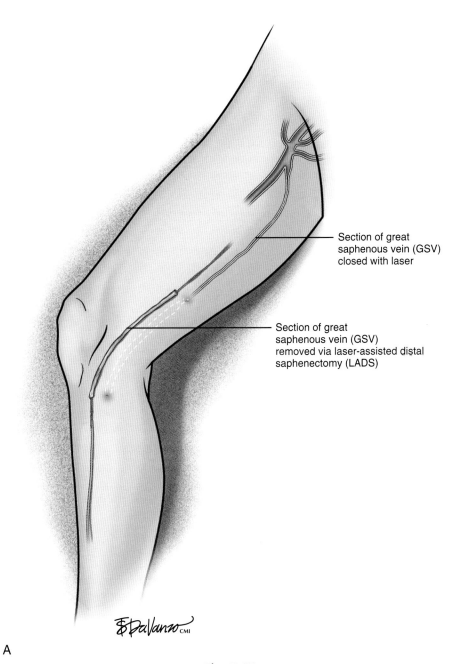

Section of great
saphenous vein (GSV)
closed with laser

Section of great
saphenous vein (GSV)
removed via laser-assisted distal
saphenectomy (LADS)

A

■ **Fig. 5.45**

Continued

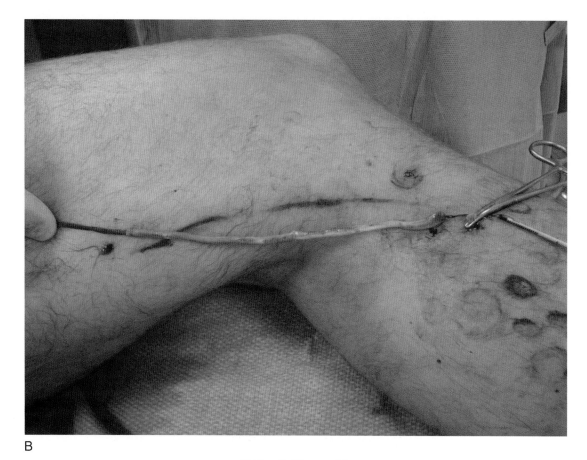

B

■ **Fig. 5.45, cont'd**

MULTIPLE VEINS AND HYBRID PROCEDURES

At the Miami Vein Center, we routinely use multiple modalities or techniques during a procedure, depending on the clinical scenario. In the case of multiple incompetent veins, each is accessed and treated individually using all the aforementioned principles (Figs. 5.46–5.48). In general, to effectively deal with these cases, multimodality therapy is required, along with some creativity on the part of the surgeon. Surgeons skilled in thermal ablation, ambulatory phlebectomy, and ultrasound-guided foam sclerotherapy can tackle in an office-based surgical suite 99% of the cases encountered.

Text continued on p. 202

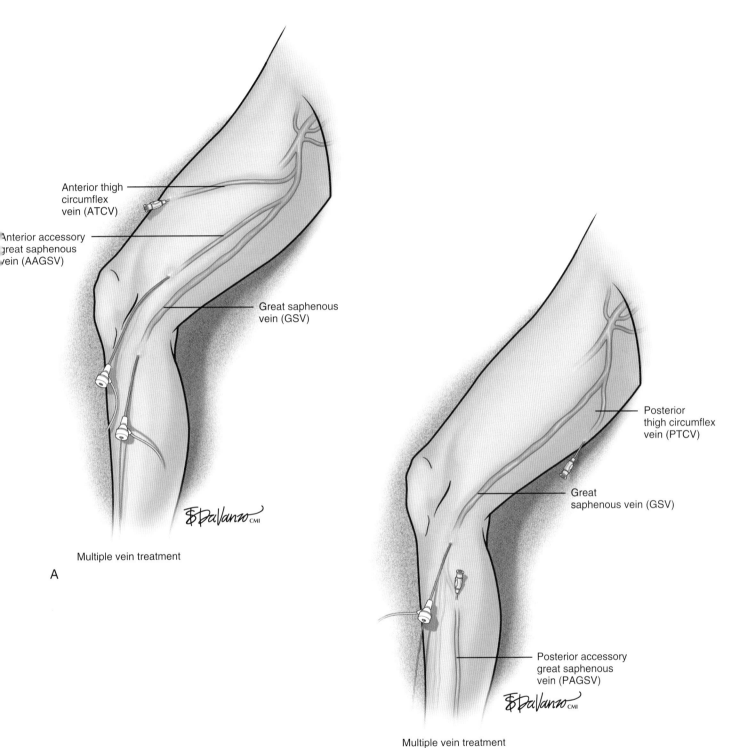

Anterior thigh
circumflex
vein (ATCV)

Anterior accessory
great saphenous
vein (AAGSV)

Great saphenous
vein (GSV)

Multiple vein treatment

A

Posterior
thigh circumflex
vein (PTCV)

Great
saphenous vein (GSV)

Posterior accessory
great saphenous
vein (PAGSV)

Multiple vein treatment

B

■ Fig. 5.46

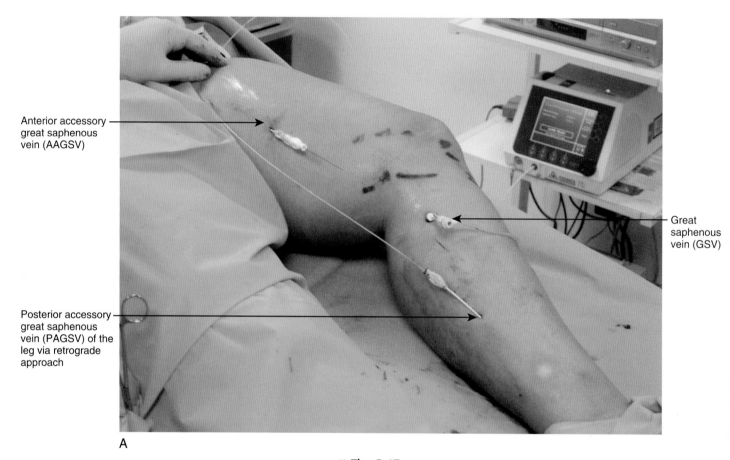

Anterior accessory great saphenous vein (AAGSV)

Great saphenous vein (GSV)

Posterior accessory great saphenous vein (PAGSV) of the leg via retrograde approach

A

■ **Fig. 5.47**

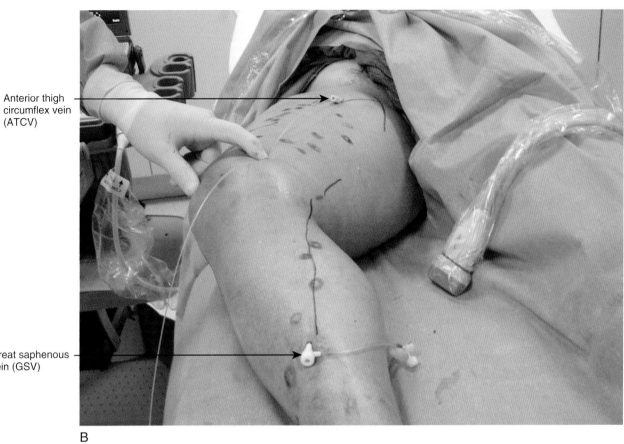

Anterior thigh
circumflex vein
(ATCV)

Great saphenous
vein (GSV)

B

Anterior accessory
great saphenous
vein (AAGSV) of
via retrograde
approach

Great saphenous
vein (GSV)

C

■ Fig. 5.47, cont'd

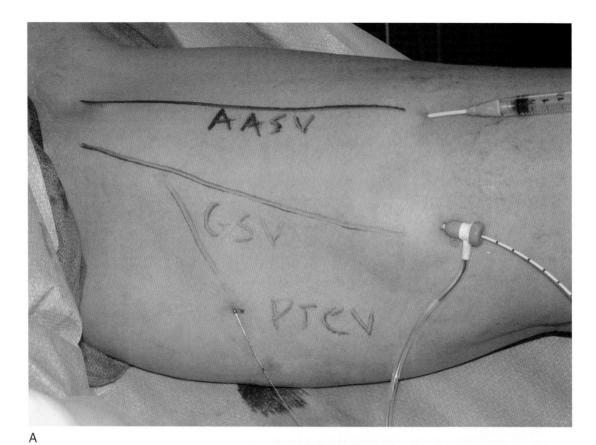

A

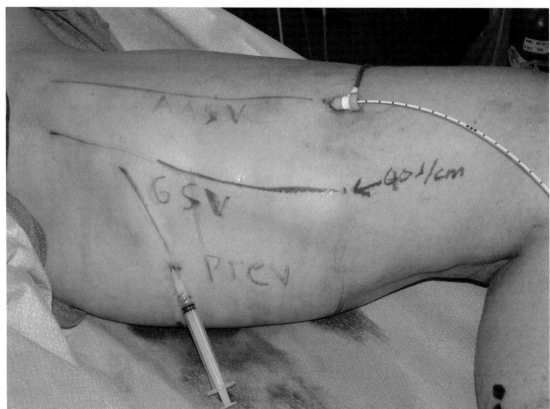

B

■ **Fig. 5.48** (A) Multiple venous access using one kit. Sheath with laser fiber in the great saphenous vein (GSV). Dilator in the anterior accessory saphenous vein (AASV). Wire in the posterior thigh circumflex vein (PTCV). (B) GSV treated with 40 J/cm using 1470-nm wavelength; then the sheath is transferred to the AASV. The PTCV wire was exchanged for 4-Fr microsheath in preparation for laser.

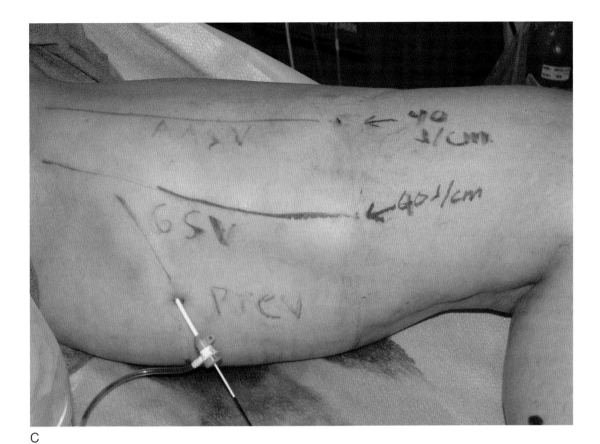

C

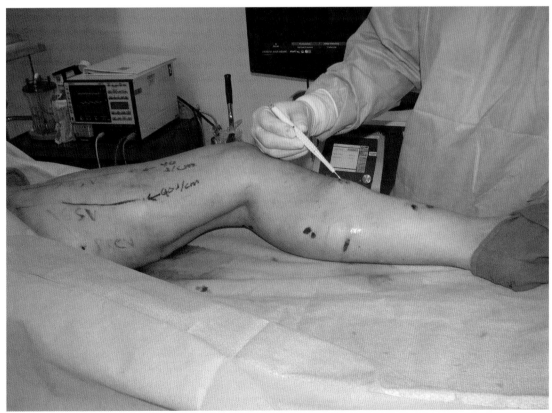

D

■ **Fig. 5.48, cont'd** (C) AASV treatment completed with 40 J/cm of energy, and the same sheath and laser fiber are transferred to the PTCV for treatment. (D) After triple-truncal-vein ablation is complete, ambulatory phlebectomy is performed in the same setting of previously marked bulging varicose veins.

CASE EXAMPLES

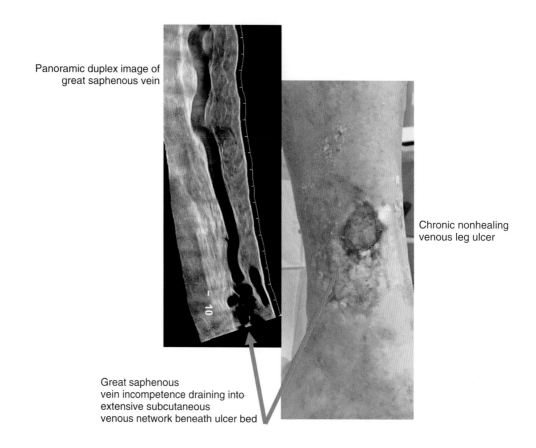

Panoramic duplex image of great saphenous vein

Chronic nonhealing venous leg ulcer

Great saphenous vein incompetence draining into extensive subcutaneous venous network beneath ulcer bed

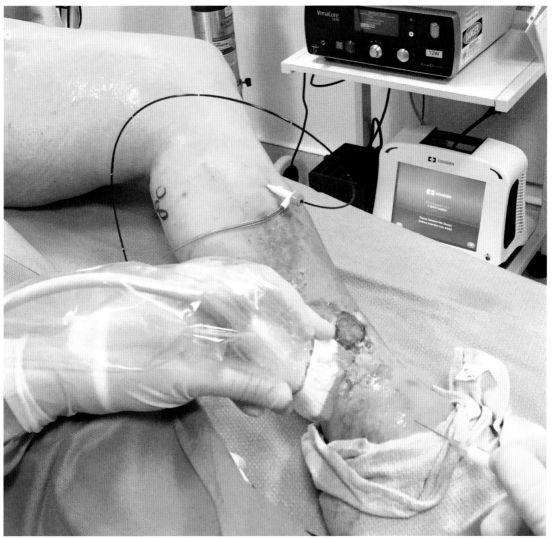

Ultrasound-guided foam sclerotherapy of subcutaneous venous network beneath ulcer with concomitant great saphenous vein ablation

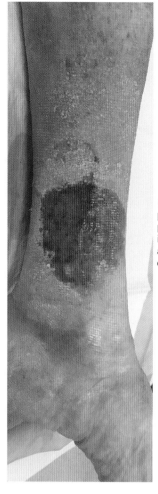

Ulcer healing in progress at 3 months postintervention intervention and weekly application of inelastic compression dressings

Great saphenous vein recanalization and recurrent ulceration 3 years out from original procedure

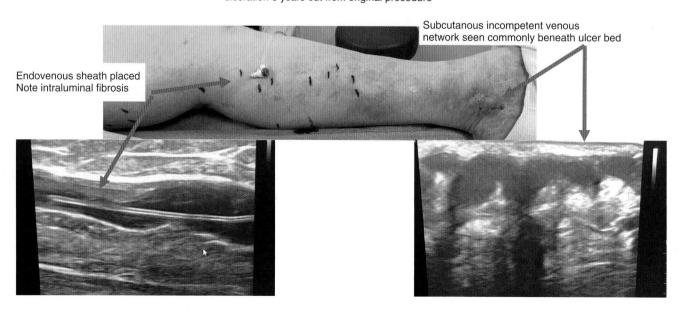

Endovenous sheath placed Note intraluminal fibrosis

Subcutanous incompetent venous network seen commonly beneath ulcer bed

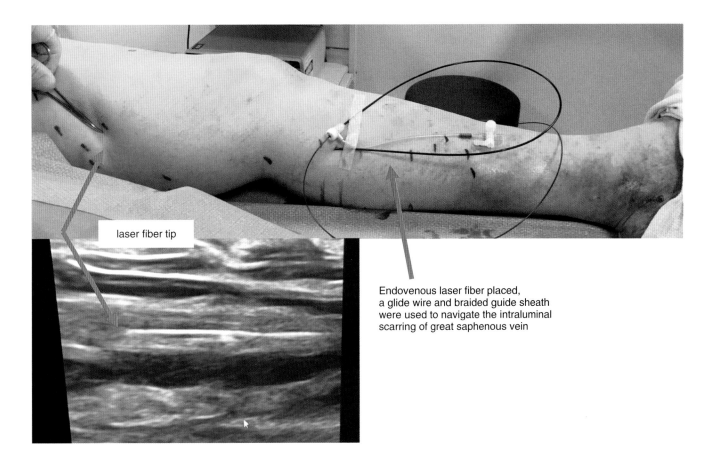

laser fiber tip

Endovenous laser fiber placed,
a glide wire and braided guide sheath
were used to navigate the intraluminal
scarring of great saphenous vein

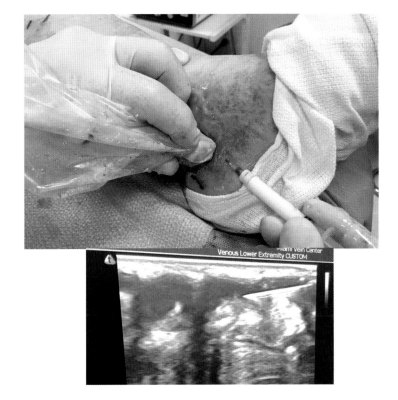

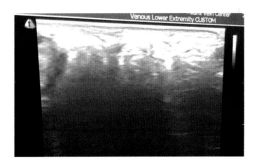

Lateral embryonic vein in patient with
Klippel-Trenaunay syndrome, large lateral thigh perforator visualized with ultrasound imaging

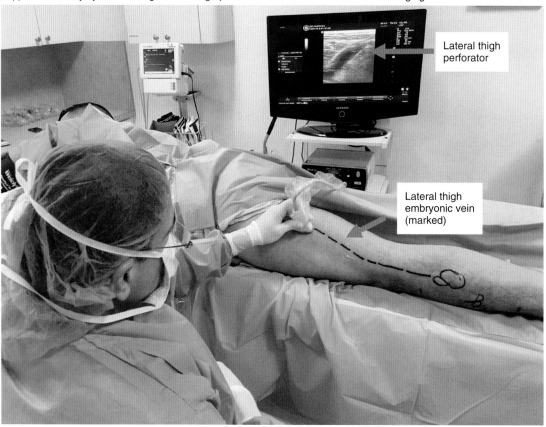

Lateral thigh
perforator

Lateral thigh
embryonic vein
(marked)

Sheath tip visualized in lateral thigh escape perforator

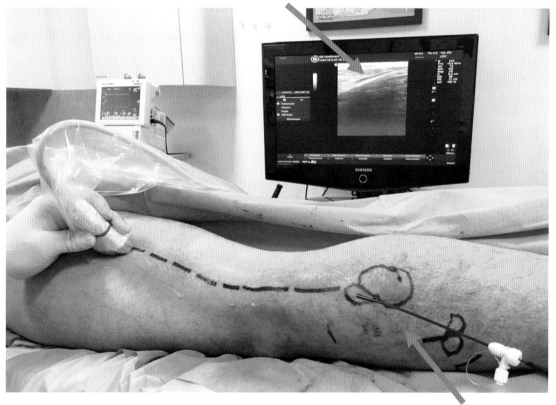

Endovenous placement of braided sheath to deliver laser fiber and server as invagination stripping device

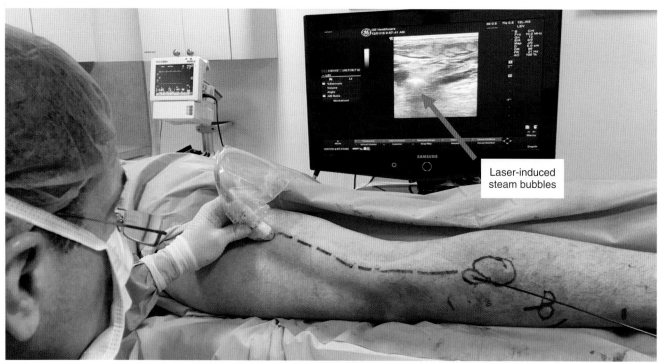

Laser-induced
steam bubbles

Endovenous laser fiber advanced through sheath and positioned midthigh perforator, laser energy delivery begun

Placement of ultrasound guided perivenous tumescent anesthesia

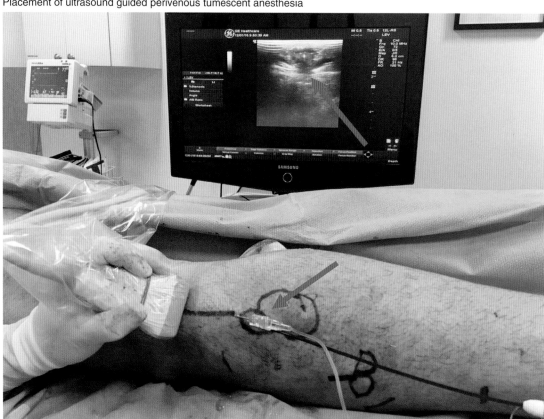

Laser pilot beam used as guide for placement of stab incision needed for vein exteriorization

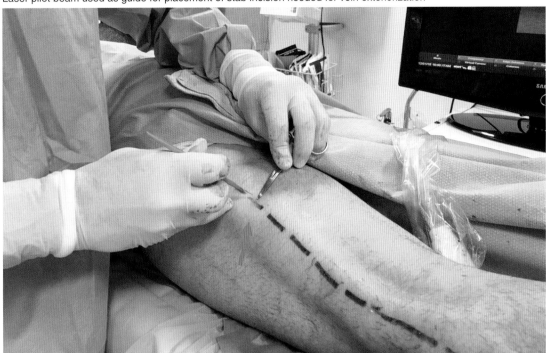

Vein exteriorized and will be divided
(note proximal vein ablated and does not require ligation)

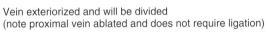

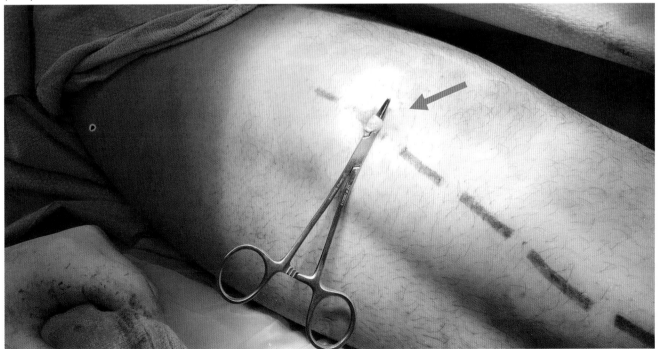

Sheath advanced and will be sutured to vein for invagination

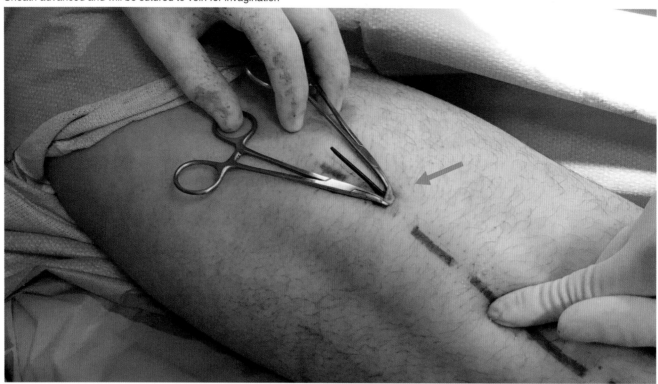

Invagination stripping in progress

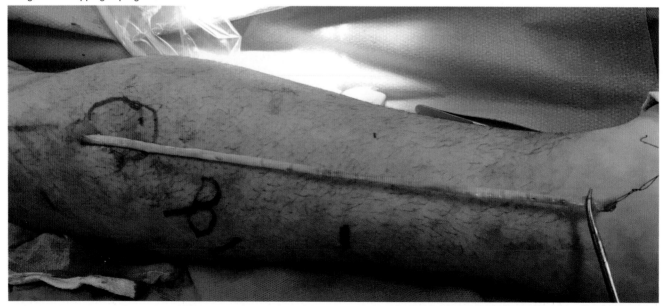

Invagination stripping complete (2 incisions *red arrows*)

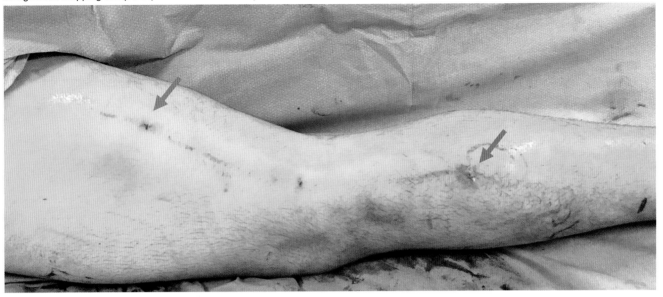

Laser-assisted distal saphenectomy complete with specimen show next to laser fiber

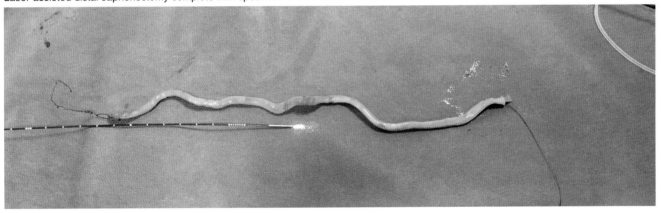

Laser-assisted distal saphenectomy compete with specimen show next to Oesh PIN Stripper

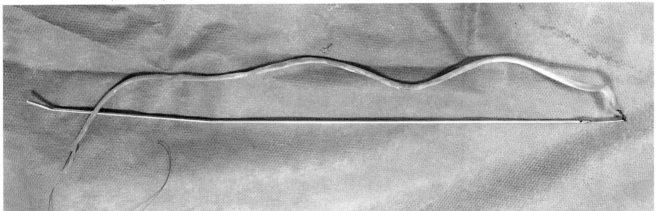

Small saphenous vein ablation with radiofrequency
Note ulcer lateral malleolus

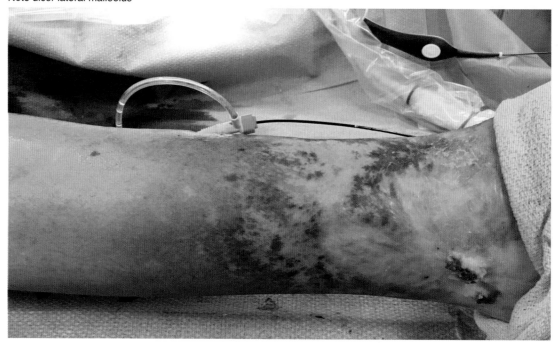

Small saphenous vein ablation with laser
Note lipodermatosclerosis lateral malleolus

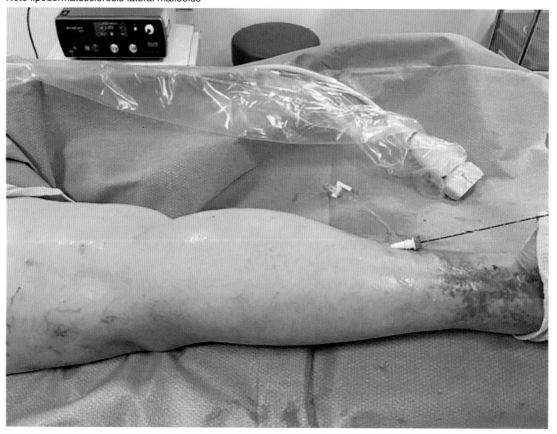

Phlebectomy of massive
varicose veins possible
in the office with tumescent
anesthesia

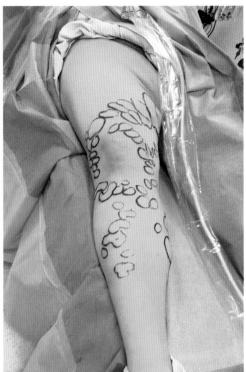
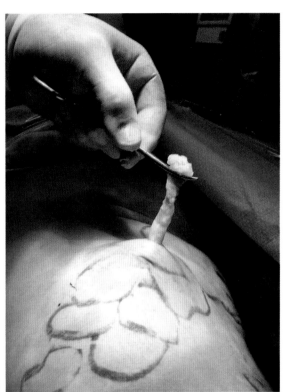

CONCLUSION

Endovenous thermal ablation is elegant by its mere simplicity. It is effective and safe and has acceptable cosmetic results. Ambulatory phlebectomy and ultrasound-guided foam sclerotherapy are perfect complements to endovenous thermal ablation of the saphenous veins. With this combination, virtually all patients with simple, or complex, superficial and perforating vein problems can be dealt with effectively in the comfort of a physician's office.

REFERENCES

1. Trendelenberg F. Uber die Unterbindung der Vena Saphena Magna bie Unterschenkel Varicen. *Beitr Z Clin Chir.* 1891;7:195.
2. Keller WL. A new method of extirpating the internal saphenous and similar veins in varicose conditions. *N Y Med J.* 1905;82:385.
3. Bergan JJ, Pascarella L. Varicose vein surgery. In: Wilmore D, Souba W, Fink M, eds. *ACS Surgery Online.* New York: WebMD, Inc; 2003.
4. Rautio T, Ohinmaa A, Perala J, et al. Endovenous obliteration versus conventional stripping operation in the treatment of primary varicose veins: a randomized controlled trial with comparison of the costs. *J Vasc Surg.* 2002;35:958–965.
5. Lurie F, Creton D, Eklof B, et al. Prospective randomised study of endovenous radiofrequency obliteration (closure) versus ligation and vein stripping (EVOLVeS): two-year follow-up. *Eur J Vasc Endovasc Surg.* 2005;29:67–73.

6. Stotter L, Schaaf I, Bockelbrink A, et al. Radiofrequency obliteration, invagination or cryo stripping: which is the best tolerated treatment by the patients? *Phlebologie.* 2005;34:19–24.

7. Hinchcliff RJ, Ubhi J, Beech A, et al. A prospective randomized controlled trial of VNUS Closure versus surgery for the treatment of recurrent long saphenous varicose veins. *Eur J Vasc Endovasc Surg.* 2006;31:212–218.

8. Min RJ, Khilnani N, Zimmet SE. Endovenous laser treatment of saphenous vein reflux: long-term results. *J Vasc Interv Radiol.* 2003;14:991–996.

9. Almeida JI, Raines JK. Radiofrequency ablation and laser ablation in the treatment of varicose veins. *Ann Vasc Surg.* 2006;20:547–552.

10. Gibson KD, Ferris BL, Polissar N, et al. Endovenous laser treatment of the small saphenous vein: efficacy and complications. *J Vasc Surg.* 2007;45:795–801.

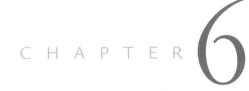

CHAPTER 6

Radiofrequency Thermal Ablation: Current Data

Alan M. Dietzek, Rima Ahmad, and Michele N. Richard

HISTORICAL BACKGROUND

Investigators in the 1960s and 1970s observed third-degree skin burns and saphenous nerve injuries after thermal ablation of the saphenous vein.[1,2] Low-wattage, bipolar current, and specific electrode designs, coupled with algorithms governed by frequent sampling of wall temperature and impedance, were expected to mitigate thermal damage to adjacent tissues. The use of bipolar electrodes, which concentrate current density along minimal impedance paths between the poles, helped resolve these problems.[3] In addition, early experiences demonstrated that procedural modifications were also needed to minimize complications and early failures.

First-Generation Device

In an industry-sponsored feasibility study (1) the Restore catheter (VNUS Medical Technologies, Inc., Sunnyvale, CA) induced a short subvalvular constriction to improve the competence of valve leaflets, and (2) the Closure catheter applied resistive heating over long vein lengths to cause maximum wall contraction for permanent obliteration.[4] Treatment with Restore catheters resulted in recurrent or persistent reflux in 81% of patients followed up for 6 to 12 months. Treatment with Closure catheters resulted in a 6% recurrent reflux rate and a 4% incidence of recurrent varicosities at a mean follow-up of 4.7 months. The authors concluded that treatment with Closure catheters was an effective, less invasive option than saphenous stripping, with complications and early failures that could be mitigated through further procedural modifications.

215

In 1999, VNUS Medical Technologies, Inc. (Sunnyvale, CA) received approval from the US Food and Drug Administration to market and sell a new device for closure of incompetent saphenous veins. The first-generation device, known as the Closure Procedure, used bipolar electrodes mounted on the end of a catheter to deliver radiofrequency (RF) energy to the inner vein wall. The catheter's collapsible bipolar electrodes included a temperature sensor, which provided feedback to a dedicated RF generator. When deployed, the electrodes made direct contact with the endoluminal surface of the vein wall, and RF energy was delivered. The resistive effects of the vein wall tissue caused conversion of RF energy into heat. The principal mechanism of RF ablation has been demonstrated in animal studies.[5] Vein wall collagen contraction, in response to thermal energy, causes immediate vein wall thickening and reduction in the lumen diameter. Endothelial destruction causes an inflammatory response, which results in fibrosis and permanent vein occlusion.

The thermal effect on the vein wall is directly related to both the treatment temperature and the treatment time, the latter being a function of catheter pullback speed. The treatment protocol called for a treatment temperature of 85°C at a pullback speed of 3 cm per minute. The thermal effect produces sufficient collagen contraction to occlude the lumen while limiting heat penetration to perivenous tissue.[6,7] To assess the potential of perivenous tissue damage, the adventitial temperature was recorded in an in vitro model.[8] With the standard treatment protocol, the average peak adventitial temperature was 64.4°C and usually lasted for approximately 10 seconds at any given position along the length of the vein. Peak adventitial temperature was decreased to 51.3°C in the presence of a 2-mm perivenous saline layer.

There are several different modes of endovenous radiofrequency (EVRF) ablation in commercial use around the world. These include the Celon RFITT (radiofrequency induced thermal therapy) procedure which uses bipolar RF, the monopolar FCare Systems EVRF procedure, and VNUS ClosureFast (now Medtronic Venefit) segmental ablation procedure (Fig. 6.1).

Second-Generation Device (VNUS ClosureFast)

With the introduction of the ClosureFast RF ablation (RFA) catheter, the elimination of the slow pullback and the implementation of stationary (segmental) treatment at 120°C markedly improved the procedure. Controlled heating by conduction avoids vein perforations even with high dosing of thermal energy. The postprocedure inflammatory consequences often seen after endovenous laser ablation (EVLA) are relatively absent with ClosureFast.

The linear endovenous energy density (LEED) is frequently used to compare energy dosing in endovenous procedures. With the first-generation (bipolar) RF device, the catheter pullback velocity had to be slow enough to allow resistive heating of the vein wall to a target temperature of 85°C. Measurements of the delivered energy dose to the vein were not displayed to the operator because the power delivered by the generator was subject to regulation by a feedback loop to maintain a constant temperature of 85°C. With ClosureFast, the temperature is kept stable at 120°C during a 20-second treatment cycle. At the saphenofemoral junction (SFJ), two cycles of RF energy are delivered, averaging a LEED of 116.2 ± 11.6 J per cm for the first 7 cm of vein juxtaposed to the SFJ to ensure good vein closure at this critical site.[9] Distal to the SFJ, 68.2 ± 17.5 J per cm is delivered to each 7-cm treatment site. Thus this aggressive double energy cycle at the zone of the SFJ is supported by Almeida and Raines' retrospective analysis.[10]

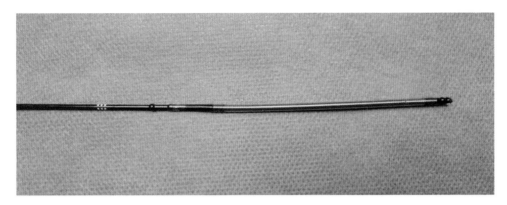

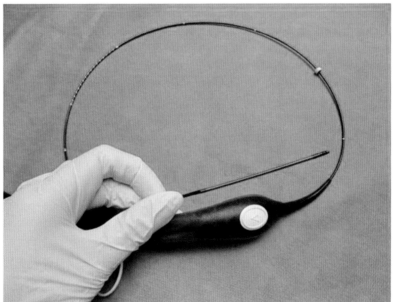

■ **Fig. 6.1** ClosureFast (renamed Venefit) radiofrequency ablation catheter demonstrating gradations along the shaft to help guide withdrawal, as well as the 7-cm heating element at the tip.

Proebstle reported outcomes following ClosureFast in early 2008. The occlusion rate following segmental RFA was 99.6% at 2 years, and 70% of treated patients did not require any analgesia postprocedure.[9]

Quality-of-Life Changes

Studies of quality of life are becoming more important; significant improvements in disease-specific quality-of-life following RFA were reported in the EVOLVeS (Endovenous Radiofrequency Obliteration [Closure] versus Ligation and Vein Stripping) study using the CIVIQ (Chronic Venous Insufficiency Quality of Life)-2 questionnaire.[11,12] Moreover, these quality-of-life statistics were improved compared with patients treated with traditional venous surgery.

ETIOLOGY AND NATURAL HISTORY OF DISEASE

Treatment Efficacy

Duplex ultrasound examination has significantly advanced our understanding of venous disease and provides both anatomic and pathophysiologic information. The morphologic and hemodynamic outcomes following RFA have been described in detailed ultrasound studies by Pichot et al.[13] The pathologic sequelae of a treated vein are reflected by its sonographic progression. Occluded veins were initially hypoechogenic compared with the surrounding tissue and gradually evolved into hyperechogenic and eventually isoechogenic presentations, indicating a healing process. Approximately 60% of veins were hypoechogenic and 40% were hyperechogenic at 1 week. By 6 months, they became either hyperechogenic or isoechogenic.[13] Sonographic disappearance of the saphenous vein, the desired endpoint, was observed by Weiss and Weiss in 90% of limbs at 2 years.[14]

Failures

Incomplete ablation, either segmental or total length of the vein, constitutes anatomic failure. Veins that are patent after treatment represent initial incomplete treatment or subsequent recanalization. Regardless of the presence of an anatomic failure, clinically, symptom improvement was often demonstrated in patients reported in the registry.

Four types of SFJ morphologies were identified after RFA[15–17]: J-1, defined as complete SFJ obliteration with no SFJ flow; J-2, defined as patent SFJ tributaries draining toward the femoral vein with (J-2b) or without (J-2a) a short patent saphenous stump; and J-3, defined as terminal great saphenous vein (GSV) competence with normal antegrade flow coming from both tributaries and the saphenous vein above a limited GSV obliteration. Two years after RFA, the most common findings were either complete SFJ obliteration or a 5-cm or smaller patent terminal stump connecting prograde tributary flow through the SFJ, accounting for approximately 90% of the limbs treated.[15,17]

The clinical significance of a short patent SFJ stump was analyzed in a study by Merchant et al.[15] A total of 319 limbs in the Clinical Registry were followed at 1 week, 6 months, 1 year, and 2 years, with 2-year data available for 121 limbs. Comparison of symptom improvement and varicose vein absence demonstrated no statistically significant differences between patients with complete SFJ obliteration and those with a short patent SFJ stump at any follow-up time point.

While the distal trunk is occluded, SFJ competence is often restored, even with a short patent stump. A patent stump can serve as a conduit and preserve the normal physiologic flow from one or more patent tributaries, such as those draining blood from abdominal and perineal areas. Preservation of such physiologic flow has been considered to be an advantage of endovenous procedures over traditional vein stripping because it causes less hemodynamic disturbance. Interruption of normal tributaries in the groin is postulated to be one of the factors responsible for stimulating neovascularization following vein stripping.

Merchant and Pichot[18] categorized anatomic failure after an RFA procedure into three types. Type I failure (nonocclusion) refers to a vein that fails to occlude because of suboptimal technique, such as a rapid pullback speed resulting in an insufficient delivery of thermal dose. It has also been observed that in a very small percentage of patients, veins may be nonresponsive to thermal ablation; it has been postulated that the collagen structure might be different in these patients. Of veins that recanalized (type II failure), 23% were associated with either tributary or perforator incompetence, accounting for 70% of the total anatomic failures.

The significance of tributary or thigh perforator incompetence and its relationship to the durability of endovenous ablation is not clear. Proactively addressing tributary and perforator incompetence may further improve long-term RFA treatment outcomes. A thorough preoperative ultrasound study and diligent ultrasound follow-up to identify refluxing tributaries and thigh perforators can enhance a carefully designed treatment plan to address all refluxing sources. In addition to type I and II failure, groin reflux developed in 33 limbs (18% of total failures) despite complete occlusion of the GSV trunk. The reflux often involved an accessory saphenous vein associated with or "feeding" varicosities. This type (type III) of failure likely reflects disease progression associated with persistent hypertension of the venous system, but a contributing factor may also be an undiagnosed accessory vein incompetence that existed at the time of the original GSV treatment.

Risk analysis revealed that the pullback speed was a risk factor for type I and II failures with the first-generation device. A certain level of thermal dose is required to efficiently occlude the vein, and an insufficient thermal dose may result in short-term vein occlusion, probably through formation of thrombus in the treated segment. However, thrombotic occlusions are subject to recanalization (type II), particularly when the segment is associated with incompetent tributaries or perforators. Note that anatomic failure does not necessarily result in clinical recurrence. Most patients experienced clinical improvement, and 70% to 80% were asymptomatic, regardless of anatomic failure, during a 5-year follow-up period. This suggests that the anatomic failure may not be significant enough to cause pressure-related symptoms.

On the other hand, type II and type III failures were risk factors for varicose vein recurrence. Type II failure patients were 3.8 times and type III failures were 4 times as likely to develop varicose vein recurrence compared with patients with anatomic success. Type I failure did not reach statistical significance in this analysis. One possible explanation is lack of follow-up. Most patients had follow-up of less than 3 years. Further, some patients may have been treated with other methods and lost to follow-up. In this setting, the impact of early failure on varicose vein recurrence may not have been identified. Surveillance monitoring, early recognition of anatomic failure, and further corrective action that may include RFA retreatment may prevent or reduce varicose vein recurrence. However, it should be recognized that disease progression is likely to play a key role in type III failure and may also account for some of type II failure. This may contribute to an increase in varicose vein recurrence at 4 and 5 years (Fig. 6.2).

Chandler showed that extended SFJ ligation may add little to effective GSV obliteration.[19]

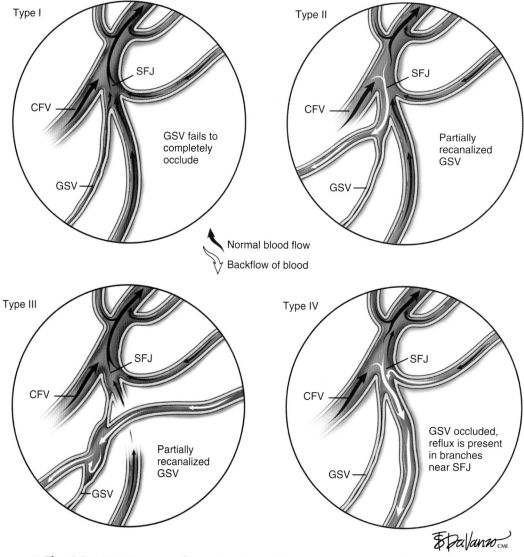

■ **Fig. 6.2** *CFV,* Common femoral vein; *GSV,* great saphenous vein; *SFJ,* saphenofemoral junction.

PROCEDURE

Detailed procedure techniques have been described elsewhere (Chapter 5).

The patient's venous system is mapped using ultrasound and marked before the start of the procedure. Thereafter, the patient is placed on the procedure table in the supine position for GSV ablation and prone position for small saphenous vein (SSV) ablation, as appropriate.

The procedure is started by infiltration of local anesthesia at the site of expected vein entry which should be at the lowest level to which vein incompetence extends. The vein is cannulated under ultrasound guidance with a micropuncture needle and a short 0.018-inch (0.045-cm) wire is introduced. The needle is then removed in exchange for a 7-Fr sheath and the wire is then removed. Once sheath access is established, the RF segmental ablation catheter is advanced through the saphenous vein to a point slightly more than 2 cm from the SFJ (Fig. 6.3).

Any difficulty passing the catheter through the vein is often overcome by slightly repositioning the leg or by manual compression over the proximal or distal catheter. If these maneuvers are unsuccessful in achieving catheter passage, then the use of 0.025-inch (0.063-cm) or 0.018-inch (0.045-cm) guidewires will usually overcome most obstacles. Finally, when even a guidewire will not pass because of a particularly tortuous segment of vein, a second sheath can be placed proximal to the area of disease. The intervening untreated tortuous segment may require surgical removal if it is extensive.

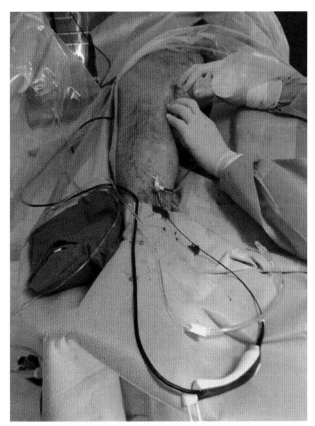

■ **Fig. 6.3** Introduction of the catheter via sheath. The catheter is positioned just over 2 cm away from the saphenofemoral junction to start the ablation.

The use of tumescent anesthesia is a critical aspect of the procedure. It is a dilute anesthetic mixture, usually 0.1% lidocaine, which provides an effective way of delivering anesthesia to large areas of tissue without exceeding a toxic dose of lidocaine. It also creates a heat sink which protects surrounding soft tissues and skin from thermal injury. Finally, if administered properly, it will compress the vein onto the catheter resulting in a more efficient transfer of heat. Once adequate tumescence is infiltrated, the catheter is positioned so that it is no less than 2 cm from the SFJ. In the SSV, the catheter is positioned at the downturn of the vein toward the saphenopopliteal junction (SPJ). Because of forward heating from the catheter tip, a distance less than 2 cm from the SFJ results in a higher incidence of deep venous thrombosis (DVT). The presence of a small, patent SFJ or SPJ stump does not compromise the short-term or long-term results of the procedure. Once in proper position, tumescent anesthetic is applied around the catheter from the entry point to the SFJ/SPJ (Fig. 6.4). Additional approximation of the vessel wall with the catheter is achieved externally by applying firm pressure with the ultrasound probe over the catheter as it is withdrawn from the vein. The catheter is initiated and heats for a total of 20 seconds (Fig. 6.5). At the initial catheter position,

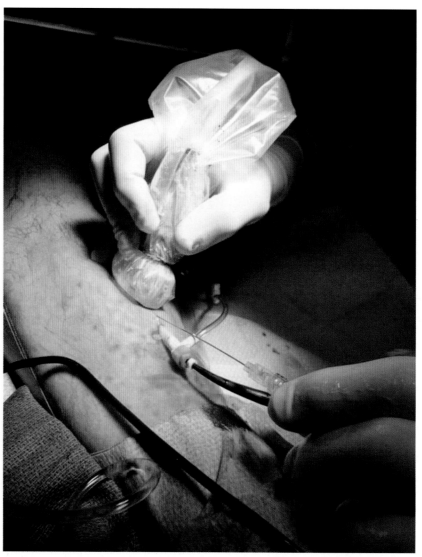

◾ **Fig. 6.4** Infiltration of tumescent anesthesia using ultrasound control.

two treatment cycles are administered. Once a segment has been treated, the catheter is withdrawn 6.5 cm, the ultrasound probe repositioned, and the catheter activated to ablate the next venous segment. Only one treatment cycle is recommended for subsequent segments of vein after the first. The catheter is withdrawn 6.5 cm following each treatment cycle. This results in a 0.5-cm treatment overlap at each vein segment to ensure complete vein ablation. Double treatment cycles can be used for large or dilated vein segments. Once the catheter has been moved distally, it should not be advanced into a previously treated segment of vein.

At the end of treatment, the catheter and sheath are removed, and firm pressure is applied along the length of the treated vein to milk out any excess blood. It is our practice to apply antibiotic ointment to the catheter insertion site and cover it with a dry gauze dressing. The leg is then wrapped with an absorbent gauze such as Kerlix and ACE bandage compression from the foot to the groin followed by a thigh high compression stocking. The dressings are removed by the patient at 24 hours, and they are instructed to wear the compression stocking for an additional 2 days. There is no published evidence that suggests outcomes are improved using compression for any particular time period following any of the thermal ablation procedures, and our practice has been evolving toward shorter periods of postprocedure compression use. Patients are also encouraged to ambulate for 30 minutes following the procedure to minimize the incidence of DVT. At 72 hours, a postprocedure duplex study is performed to confirm vein closure and to assess for evidence of DVT.

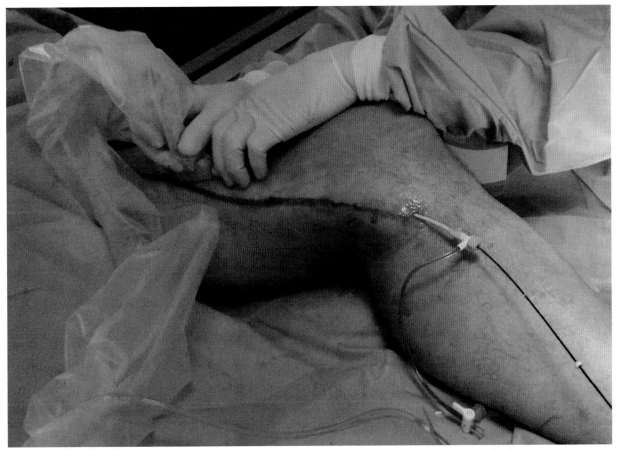

■ **Fig. 6.5** Compression, both manually and with the ultrasound probe, further approximate the catheter to the vein wall during cycle activation.

Potential Hazards and Adverse Events

As with all endovenous interventions, RFA may be associated with technical difficulties in cannulation, guidewire placement, and catheter advancement. These issues are likely to resolve with increasing experience and familiarity with the equipment and technique. Complications, including DVT, skin burns, superficial thrombophlebitis, neuralgia, and bruising, have been reported, but the incidence of these problems appears low. In one study, DVT developed in 12 of 73 limbs (16%) within 30 days of RFA,[20] but the incidence of DVT in the majority of studies is in the range of 1%. Of the 1006 patients recorded in the Closure International Registry, the reported complications were DVT (0.9%), phlebitis (2.9%), and skin burn (1.2%), although the majority of burns occurred in patients who had not received perivenous tumescent anesthesia.[18]

Minor complications such as skin burns and paresthesias were occasionally seen in the early experience with RFA. Contemporary data show virtual elimination of these problems since the advent of subfascial perivenous tumescent anesthesia. Tumescent anesthesia had been used for years by the dermatology and plastic surgery communities for liposuction. Since the concept was applied to veins, heat is no longer transmitted to nontarget tissues. By surrounding the saphenous vein with a dilute lidocaine solution, a heat sink is created. Neighboring structures, such as nerves and skin, are readily cooled as the intraluminal heat rises during passage of the hot catheter tips. Furthermore, the tumescent solution can act as a mechanical barrier to effectively "push" nontarget structures away from veins and other structures.

As is the case for many surgical procedures, DVT is a potential complication. In endovenous ablation, thrombosis can originate from the treated superficial vein and extend into the deep venous system. Attention is drawn to careful tip positioning to ensure treatment begins a short distance from the SFJ and to preserve the physiologic blood flow from the superficial epigastric tributary.

Massive DVT after thermal ablation is almost unheard of, but the surgeon may see a small thrombus extension on the postoperative ultrasound (see Chapter 16).

Small Saphenous Vein and Other Veins

In addition to the GSV, RFA has also been used to treat SSV and anterior accessory saphenous vein (AASV) incompetence in clinical practice. In this series, 4.3% veins treated were SSVs and 1.3% were AASVs. Although there were not enough samples and follow-up to demonstrate their long-term efficacy, one would not expect a dramatic difference between these treatments and GSV treatment. In this series, no serious adverse event such as motor nerve damage was reported with SSV treatment. The paresthesia rate in the SSV group was 8.9% at 1 week and 9.5% at 6 months; this is similar to the results of GSV treatment. The technical aspects of perivenous tumescent infiltration, catheter tip placement, and patient response monitoring during the procedure demand special attention with SSV treatment to protect the sural nerve and other surrounding nerves. When these elements were applied to SSV procedures, the paresthesia incidence dropped to as low as 0.3% (1 of 30) in one center.[11] As has already been emphasized, tumescent infiltration can significantly decrease complications of this procedure.

Treatment efficacy of RFA on large veins was also analyzed by Merchant et al.[21] There were 39 veins with a diameter greater than 12 mm (maximum, 24 mm) in the registry. Vein occlusion rates were 97.4% within 1 week and 96.2% at 6 months and 1 year.

RANDOMIZED CLINICAL TRIAL DATA

Radiofrequency Ablation Versus Open Surgery

Seven randomized controlled trials (RCTs)[11,12,22–24,26–28,33] in nine papers compare RFA with surgery (Table 6.1), and almost all of them conclude that after RFA there was less postoperative pain, faster recovery, earlier return to work and normal activities, and higher patient satisfaction. The longest follow-up is 3 years, and there is no difference in terms of clinical result between classical surgery and RFA. It must be noted that in all series, the bipolar catheter (ClosurePlus) was used, knowing that the new ClosureFast catheter has given better results in published observations. It should, however, be pointed out that modern, less invasive open surgery under tumescent anesthesia in the office setting is showing similar good outcomes.

TABLE 6.1 Radiofrequency Ablation Versus Open Surgery

Operative Procedure	Article	Conclusions
Open surgery versus RFA	Hinchcliffe RJ, Ubhi J, Beech A, et al. A prospective randomised controlled trial of VNUS Closure versus surgery for the treatment of recurrent long saphenous varicose veins. *Eur J Vasc Endovasc Surg.* 2006;31:212-218.[24]	16 patients presenting REVAS with persistent GSV trunk RF VNUS Closure bipolar catheter versus redo-groin surgery + S. Anesthesia: no standardization (local or general) F-U 10 days With RFA Procedure shorter $P = .02$ Less postoperative pain $P = .02$ Less bruising $P = .03$
	Kianifard B, Holdstock JM, Whiteley MS. Diofrequency ablation (VNUS Closure) does not cause neo-vascularisation at the groin at one year: results of a case controlled study. *Surgeon.* 2006;4:71-74.[33]	GSV 55 patients treated by VNUS closure bipolar catheter versus HL+S (control group) Anesthesia: no information F-U 1 year After RFA Absence of neovascularization 11 % after HL+S. $P = .028$
	Lurie F, Creton D, Eklof B, et al. Prospective randomized study of endovenous radiofrequency obliteration (Closure procedure) versus ligation and stripping in a selected patient population (EVOLVES Study). *J Vasc Surg.* 2003;38:207-214.[11]	GSV 86 patients VNUS Closure bipolar catheter versus HL+S Anesthesia: no standardization (local or general) F-U 4 months With RFA Return to normal activity shorter $P = .02$ Return to work shorter $P = .05$ Better health-related QoL

Continued

TABLE 6.1 Radiofrequency Ablation Versus Open Surgery—cont'd

Operative Procedure	Article	Conclusions
	Lurie F, Creton D, Eklof B, et al. Prospective randomized study of endovenous radiofrequency obliteration (Closure) versus ligation and vein stripping (EVOLVeS) Two-year follow-up. *Eur J Vasc Endovasc Surg.* 2005;29:67-73.[12]	GSV 65 patients VNUS Closure bipolar catheter versus HL+S Anesthesia: no standardization (local or general) F-U 2 years With RFA Clinical and DUS results at least equal to those after HL+S Better health-related QoL
	Rautio T, Ohinmaa A, Perala J, et al. Endovenous obliteration versus conventional stripping operating in the treatment of primary varicose veins: a randomized controlled trial with comparison of the costs. *J Vasc Surg.* 2002;35:958-965.[22]	GSV VNUS Closure bipolar catheter ($N = 15$) versus HL+S ($N = 13$) General anesthesia for all procedures F-U 2 months With RFA Less postoperative pain $P = .017–.036$ Shorter convalescence. $P < .001$ Cost saving for society in employed patients
	Perala J, Rautio T, Biancari F, et al. Radiofrequency endovenous obliteration versus stripping of the long saphenous vein in the management of primary varicose veins: 3-year outcome of a randomized study. *Ann Vasc Surg.* 2005;19:1-4.[23]	GSV VNUS Closure bipolar catheter ($N = 15$) versus HL+S ($N = 13$) General anesthesia for all procedures With RFA F-U 3 years No difference in terms of clinical result
	Stötter L, Schaaf I, Bockelbrink A. Comparative outcomes of radiofrequency endoluminal ablation, invagination stripping and cryostripping in the treatment of great saphenous vein. *Phlebology.* 2006;21:60-64.[26]	GSV VNUS Closure bipolar catheter ($N = 20$) versus HL+ invagination S ($N = 20$) versus HL+ cryostripping (20) General anesthesia for all procedures F-U 1 year No difference in the physician-assessed clinical status between the 3 groups With RFA Patients continued to be significantly more satisfied with both their operative procedure $P = .001$ and the cosmetic appearance $P = .006$

TABLE 6.1 Radiofrequency Ablation Versus Open Surgery—cont'd

Operative Procedure	Article	Conclusions
	Subramonia S, Lees T. Radiofrequency ablation vs conventional surgery for varicose veins—a comparison of treatment costs in a randomized trial. *Eur J Vasc Endovasc Surg.* 2010;39: 104-111.[27]	GSV VNUS closure bipolar catheter *(N = 47)* versus HL+S *(N = 41)* General anesthesia for all procedures With RFA Duration procedure was longer $P < .001$ Hospital cost more expensive Earlier return to work $P = .006$
	ElKaffas KH, ElKashef O, ElBaz W. Great saphenous vein radiofrequency ablation versus standard stripping in the management of primary varicose veins—a randomized clinical trial. *Angiology.* 2010;62:49-54.[28]	GSV 180 patients Incompetent SFJ+ saphenous reflux VNUS closure bipolar catheter versus HL+S RFA local anesthesia OS general anesthesia With RFA Lower overall complication rate Shorter hospitalization $P = .001$ More expensive $P + .003$ F-U 2 years No difference in term of recurrence

DUS, Duplex ultrasound; *F-U,* follow-up; *GSV,* great saphenous vein; *HL,* high ligation; *HL+S,* high ligation + saphenous stripping ± perforator ligation ± tributary phlebectomy; *OS,* open surgery; *QoL,* quality of life; *RFA,* radiofrequency ablation; *S,* stripping.

Radiofrequency Ablation Versus Endovenous Laser Ablation

Five RCTs[25,29–32] compare RFA with EVLA (Table 6.2). There was less bruising and less pain with ClosureFast. New laser fibers have been developed, such as radial fibers and jacket-tip fibers. Kabnick has reported on a pilot study comparing RF (ClosureFast in 50 patients) versus EVLA (980 nm jacket-tipped fiber in 35 patients). At 72 hours, there was 100% closure in both groups. At one week, pain and bruising score was identical in the two groups. These results suggest that jacket-tipped laser fibers generate a uniform thermal reaction similar to that generated by ClosureFast. The conclusion was that the most current RF and jacket-tip laser methods and devices are indistinguishable in efficacy and short-term side effects. With procedure time and tumescent anesthesia also equivalent, these procedures present no genuinely significant difference to patients.

TABLE 6.2 Radiofrequency Ablation Versus Endovenous Laser Ablation

Operative Procedure	Article	Conclusions
RFA versus EVLA	Almeida JI, Kaufman J, Göckeritz O, et al. Radiofrequency endovenous ClosureFast versus laser ablation for the treatment of great saphenous reflux: a multicenter, single-blinded, randomized study (RECOVERY Study). *J Vasc Interv Radiol.* 2009;20:752–759.[25]	69 patients GSV Local tumescent anesthesia for both procedures RFA ClosureFast vs EVLA Diode 980-nm barefiber F-U 2 weeks With RFA All scores referable to pain, ecchymosis, and tenderness were statistically lower in the ClosureFast group at 48 hours, 1 week, and 2 weeks. Minor complications were more prevalent in the EVL group $P = .0210$ Venous clinical severity scores and QoL measures were statistically lower in the ClosureFast group No difference in terms of postoperative vein occlusion and truncal elimination reflux between RFA and EVLA
	Shepherd AC, Gohel MS, Brown LC, et al. Randomized clinical trial of VNUS ClosureFAST radiofrequency ablation versus laser for varicose veins. *Br J Surg.* 2010;97;810-818.[29]	131 patients GSV General anesthesia for both procedures RFA ClosureFast vs EVLA Diode 980-nm, barefiber F-U 6 weeks With RFA Less postoperative pain 3 days, $P = 0.010$; 10 days, $P = 0.001$ Less analgesic tablets 3 days, $P = 0.003$; 10 days, $P = 0.001$ QoL: AVVQ and SF-12 No difference
	Gale SS, Lee JN, Walsh ME, et al. A randomized, controlled trial of endovenous thermal ablation using the 810-nm wavelength laser and the ClosurePlus radiofrequency ablation methods for superficial venous insufficiency of the great saphenous vein. *J Vasc Surg.* 2010;52:645-650.[30]	141 lower extremities GSV Local tumescent anesthesia for both procedures RF ClosurePlus vs EVLA Diode 810-nm barefiber. 24 bilateral, 94 unilateral:49 RFA, 48 EVLA F-U 1–4 weeks to 1 year With RFA Less bruising and discomfort Recanalization more frequent at 1 year $P = .002$

TABLE 6.2 Radiofrequency Ablation Versus Endovenous Laser Ablation—cont'd

Operative Procedure	Article	Conclusions
	Goode SD, Chowdury A, Crockett M, et al. Laser and Radiofrequency Ablation Study (LARA study): a randomized study comparing radiofrequency ablation and endovenous laser ablation (810 nm). *Eur J Vasc Endovasc Surg.* 2010;40:246-253.[31]	70 lower extremities GSV General anesthesia for both procedures CELON RFiTT RFA vs EVLA Diode 810-nm barefiber 17 bilateral, 36 unilateral:19 RFA, 17 EVLA F-U 6 weeks–6 months With RFA Less postoperative pain and bruising in the bilateral group QoL and activity score no difference F-U 9 months Same occlusion rate 74% vs 78%
	Nordon IM, Loftus IM. EVVERT comparing laser and radiofrequency: an update on endovenous treatment options. In Greenhalgh R, editor. BIBA publishing, UK. 2011:381-388.[32]	GSV 80 patients laser (Vari-Lase Bright tip 810 nm laser fiber); 79 patients RFA (ClosureFast) General anesthesia F-U 1 week: all GSVs occluded Pain and bruising significantly less after RFA 3 months: 3/68 laser and 2/70 RFA reopened (*P* = ns)

AVVQ, Aberdeen varicose vein questionnaire; *EVLA*, endovenous laser ablation; *F-U*, follow-up; *GSV*, great saphenous vein; *ns*, not significant; *QoL*, quality of life; *RFA*, radiofrequency ablation.

REFERENCES

1. Politowski M, Zelazny T. Complications and difficulties in electrocoagulation of varices of the lower extremities. *Surgery.* 1966;59:932–934. 4287137.
2. Watts GT. Endovenous diathermy destruction of internal saphenous. *Br Med J.* 1972;4:53. 5078434.
3. Pearce JA. *Electrosurgery.* New York: John Wiley & Sons; 1986.
4. Manfrini S, Gasbarro V, Danielsson G, et al. Endovenous management of saphenous vein reflux. *J Vasc Surg.* 2000;32:330–342. 10917994.
5. Weiss RA. RF-mediated endovenous occlusion. In: Weiss RA, Feied CF, Weiss MA, eds. *Vein Diagnosis and Treatment: A Comprehensive Approach.* New York: McGraw-Hill Medical Publishing Division; 2001:211–221.
6. Weiss RA. Comparison of endovenous radiofrequency versus 810 nm diode laser occlusion of large veins in an animal model. *Dermatol Surg.* 2002;28:56–61. 11991272.
7. Goldman MP, Mauricio M, Rao J. Intravascular 1320-nm laser closure of the great saphenous vein: a 6- to 12-month follow-up study. *Dermatol Surg.* 2004;30:1380–1385. 15522018.

8. Zikorus AW, Mirizzi MS. Evaluation of setpoint temperature and pullback speed on vein adventitial temperature during endovenous radiofrequency energy delivery in an in-vitro model. *Vasc Endovascular Surg.* 2004;38:167–174. 15064848.

9. Proebstle TM, Vago B, Alm J, et al. Treatment of the incompetent great saphenous vein by endovenous radiofrequency powered segmental thermal ablation: first clinical experience. *J Vasc Surg.* 2008;47:151–156. 18178468.

10. Almeida JI, Raines JK. Radiofrequency ablation and laser ablation in the treatment of varicose veins. *Ann Vasc Surg.* 2006;20:547–552. 16791452.

11. Lurie F, Creton D, Eklof B, et al. Prospective randomized study of endovenous radiofrequency obliteration (Closure) versus ligation and stripping in a selected patient population (EVOLVeS study). *J Vasc Surg.* 2003;38:207–214. 12891099.

12. Lurie F, Creton D, Eklof B, et al. Prospective randomised study of endovenous radiofrequency obliteration (Closure) versus ligation and vein stripping (EVOLVeS): two-year follow-up. *Eur J Vasc Endovasc Surg.* 2005;29:67–73. 15570274.

13. Pichot O, Sessa C, Chandler JG, et al. Role of duplex imaging in endovenous obliteration for primary venous insufficiency. *J Endovasc Ther.* 2000;7:451–459. 11194816.

14. Weiss RA, Weiss MA. Controlled radiofrequency endovenous occlusion using a unique radiofrequency catheter under duplex guidance to eliminate saphenous varicose vein reflux: a 2-year follow-up. *Dermatol Surg.* 2002;28:38–42. 11991268.

15. Merchant RF, DePalma RG, Kabnick LS. Endovascular obliteration of saphenous reflux: a multicenter study. *J Vasc Surg.* 2002;35:1190–1196. 12042730.

16. Pichot O, Sessa C, Chandler JG, et al. Role of duplex imaging in endovenous obliteration for primary venous insufficiency. *J Endovasc Ther.* 2000;7:451–459. 11194816.

17. Pichot O, Kabnick LS, Creton D, et al. Duplex ultrasound scan findings two years after great saphenous vein radiofrequency endovenous obliteration. *J Vasc Surg.* 2004;39:189–195. 14718839.

18. Merchant RF, Pichot O, for the Closure Study Group. Long-term outcomes of endovenous radiofrequency obliteration of saphenous reflux as a treatment for superficial venous insufficiency. *J Vasc Surg.* 2005;42:502–509. 16171596.

19. Chandler JG, Pichot O, Sessa C, et al. Defining the role of extended saphenofemoral junction ligation: a prospective comparative study. *J Vasc Surg.* 2000;32:941–953. 11054226.

20. Hingorani AP, Ascher E, Markevich N, et al. Deep venous thrombosis after radiofrequency ablation of greater saphenous vein: a word of caution. *J Vasc Surg.* 2004;40:500–504. 15337880.

21. Merchant RF, Pichot O, Mayers KA. Four-year follow-up on endovascular radiofrequency obliteration of great saphenous reflux. *Dermatol Surg.* 2005;31:129–134. 15762202.

22. Rautio T, Ohinmaa A, Perala J, et al. Endovenous obliteration versus conventional stripping operation in the treatment of primary varicose veins: a randomized controlled trial with comparison of the costs. *J Vasc Surg.* 2002;35:958–965. 12021712.

23. Perala J, Rautio T, Biancari F, et al. Radiofrequency endovenous obliteration versus stripping of the long saphenous vein in the management of primary varicose veins: 3-year outcome of a randomized study. *Ann Vasc Surg.* 2005;19:669–672. 16052388.

24. Hinchcliffe RJ, Ubhi J, Beech A, et al. A prospective randomised controlled trial of VNUS closure versus surgery for the treatment of recurrent long saphenous varicose veins. *Eur J Vasc Endovasc Surg.* 2006;31:212–218. 16137898.

25. Almeida J, Kaufman J, Göckeritz O, et al. Radiofrequency endovenous ClosureFast versus laser ablation for the treatment of great saphenous reflux: a multicenter, single-blinded, randomized study (RECOVERY study). *J Vasc Interv Radiol.* 2009;20:752–759. 19395275.

26. Stötter L, Schaaf I, Bockelbrink A. Comparative outcomes of radiofrequency endoluminal ablation, invagination stripping and cryostripping in the treatment of great saphenous vein. *Phlebology.* 2006;21:60–64.

27. Subramonia S, Lees T. Radiofrequency ablation vs conventional surgery for varicose veins—a comparison of treatment costs in a randomized trials. *Eur J Vasc Endovasc Surg.* 2010;39:104–111.

28. ElKaffas KH, ElKashef O, ElBaz W. Great saphenous vein radiofrequency ablation versus standard stripping in the management of primary varicose veins—a randomized clinical trial. *Angiology.* 2010;62:49–54.

29. Shepherd AC, Gohel MS, Brown LC, et al. Randomized clinical trial of VNUS^R ClosureFAST^TM radiofrequency ablation versus laser for varicose veins. *Br J Surg.* 2010;97:810–818.

30. Gale SS, Lee JN, Walsh ME, et al. A randomized, controlled trial of endovenous thermal ablation using the 810-nm wavelength laser and the ClosurePlus radiofrequency ablation methods for superficial venous insufficiency of the great saphenous vein. *J Vasc Surg.* 2010;52:645–650.

31. Goode SD, Chowdury A, Crockett M, et al. Laser and Radiofrequency ablation Study(LARA study) : a randomized Study comparing Radiofrequency Ablation and Endovenous Laser Ablation (810 nm). *Eur J Vasc Endovasc Surg.* 2010;40:246–253.

32. Nordon IM, Loftus IM. EVVERT comparing laser and radiofrequency: An update on endovenous treatment options. In: Greenhalgh R, ed. *BIBA Publishing.* UK: 2011:381–388.

33. Kianifard B, et al. Radiofrequency ablation (VNUS Closure) does not cause neo-vascularisation at the groin at one year : results of a case controlled study. *Surgeon.* 2006;4:71–74.

CHAPTER 7

Laser Thermal Ablation: Current Data

Mikel Sadek and Lowell S. Kabnick

HISTORICAL BACKGROUND

Endovenous laser ablation (EVLA) therapy arose from a background of managing refluxing truncal veins using open surgical techniques, such as stripping with high ligation. The technology was first introduced in 1999, and following US Food and Drug Administration approval for commercial use in 2002, has exhibited exponential growth in use.[1] This is, in part, because of the ability to perform this endothermal ablation technique in an ambulatory setting using tumescent anesthesia.[2] For the most part, the increased use of EVLA for the treatment of refluxing truncal veins, as well as symptomatic refluxing perforators, is in large part because of an outstanding safety, efficacy, and durability profile.

Increased mitigation of postprocedural symptoms remains the final frontier in improving EVLA treatments. Bruising, transient pain, and induration of the thigh are common adverse events after endovenous laser therapy (EVLT) and are most likely caused by laser-induced perforation of the vein wall, with extravasation of blood into surrounding tissue.[3–5] It is known that conversion of an incompetent vein into a fibrous cord, with subsequent sonographic disappearance, generally leads to permanent occlusion. At the onset of EVLT, little was known about the mechanism of action and durability of treatment after intervention with these devices. Studies have indicated that heat-related damage to the inner vein wall leads to thrombotic occlusion of the treated vein, and this has led to iterative improvements in technology and technique.[6–8]

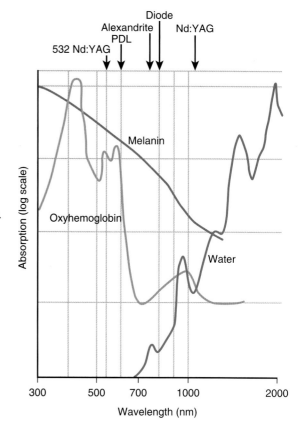

■ **Fig. 7.1** Light absorption curve.

EVLA can be classified into hemoglobin-specific laser wavelengths (HSLWs) and water-specific laser wavelengths (WSLWs) (Fig. 7.1). Wavelengths of 808, 810, 940, 980, 1064, 1319, 1320, 1470, 1510, and 1920 nm have been successfully used for great saphenous vein (GSV) ablation[9] and for other superficial axial and perforating veins.[6,9–15] Hemoglobin and, to a lesser extent, myoglobin in venous smooth muscle cells are the dominant chromophores at the shorter end of this range, whereas in the longer wavelengths, water dominates as the energy-absorbing molecule.[6,11]

Published reports suggest that delivery of higher energy is required to effect secure vein closure; however, with increased energy delivery, pain and bruising after treatment are encountered more frequently. After EVLA, studies have demonstrated that 70% of limbs experience some degree of pain, and 50% require analgesics for pain management.[16] Kabnick reported an average pain score of 2.6 on a scale of 0 to 5 after EVLA.[17] There is increasing focus on reducing perioperative pain and bruising in the field of EVL saphenous ablation. As an example, the 1470-nm laser requires less energy delivery for closure, with concomitant reports of less pain and bruising postprocedure. One report by Shutze et al., compared the 1470-nm laser (295 procedures) with the 810-nm laser (1144 procedures).[18] This study demonstrated that pain, bruising, and quality of life scores were all improved in the 1470-nm cohort. The WSLWs were developed to target the interstitial water in the vein wall and minimize perforations.[11] Trends in the literature suggest that these longer wavelength lasers may produce fewer side effects than HSLW lasers at comparable linear endovenous energy density (LEED). Two comparisons of different wavelengths with similar delivered laser energy have been performed. One study compared 940-nm and 1320-nm wavelengths in a retrospective analysis, and another compared 810-nm and 980-nm wavelengths in a randomized prospective study.[17,19] The two studies demonstrated equivalent safety and efficacy at similar energy dosing. However, EVLA performed at comparable LEED with either the 940-nm (HSLW) or the 1320-nm (WSLW) lasers showed a reduction in postoperative pain and bruising with the 1320-nm device. Also use of less power (5 W) demonstrated a lower rate of side effects than did 8 W, with a laser operating at a wavelength of 1320 nm.[19] A low rate of pain and bruising was reported after GSV treatment for GSV reflux with the 1470-nm wavelength at 5 W, 30 J per cm.[20] To further the concept, Kabnick and Sadek performed a three-way comparison of the 810-nm, 980-nm, and 1470-nm lasers. Essentially, there was a nearly dose-dependent improvement in pain and bruising scores, which correlated directly with increasing wavelength. Efficacy remained equal.[21]

In addition to laser wavelength, fiber type may play an even more pronounced role in the development of postprocedural symptoms. The underlying principle behind this, is the thought that direct contact between the laser fiber and the vein wall may contribute to vein wall perforations and subsequent pain and bruising. Consequently, jacket-tip fibers were developed to minimize this contact. A variety of jacket-tip fibers exist, including ceramic and metallic types, and some are even configured to disperse the emitted energy. In the same three-way comparison of the 810-nm, 980-nm, and 1470-nm laser fibers, concomitant evaluations of the bare versus jacket-tip fibers demonstrated that the fiber type contributed dominantly to whether or not postprocedural bruising/pain would develop. Moreover, this was corroborated by in vitro analysis, which demonstrated decreased thermal injury depths in the jacket-tip fibers as compared with the bare-tip fibers.[21]

ETIOLOGY AND NATURAL HISTORY OF DISEASE

There remains controversy over the mechanism of action of EVL, and most of the investigations were performed with HSLWs. Proebstle found in vitro with an HSLW, that the extensive heat damage of the endothelium and the intima came from steam-bubble formation and induced full-length thrombotic occlusion of the vein.[6] Bush et al., in a histologic study, found that the mechanism of injury with HSLWs is secondary to steam bubbles caused by water evaporation of the blood followed by transmitted heat injury to the tissue.[22] Acutely, there is complete loss of the endothelium and early thrombus formation, followed by the injury response with inflammatory cellular infiltration into the subintimal layers. Eventually, fibroblasts deposit collagen and represent the predominant histologic finding at 4 months postoperatively.

Opposed to the steam-bubble theory, Fan and Rox-Anderson studied existing histologic reports from studies with excellent closure rates using tumescent anesthesia and found that HSLWs produce a transmural, vein wall injury, typically associated with perforations and carbonization.[23] The pattern of injury was eccentrically distributed, with maximum injury occurring along the path of laser contact. The authors concluded that steam production during EVLA accounted for only 2% of applied energy dose (i.e., EVLA causes permanent vein closure through a high-temperature photothermolytic process at the point of contact between the vein and the laser). Precise mechanism-of-action studies with ample histologic information are lacking with WSLWs. Kabnick and Sadek did perform an adjunctive evaluation using a porcine collagen matrix molecule, which demonstrated that thermal injury depths were less in the 1470-nm WSLW as compared with the 810-nm HSLW laser.[21]

Although it is not known exactly how much damage to the individual layers of the vein wall is required, it seems that at a minimum, intimal and medial coagulation are necessary for long-term closure. Technically, the depth of penetration of a 940-nm laser beam into blood is limited to approximately 0.3 mm.[24] Qualitative analysis with optical coherence tomography in an ex vivo model matched with histologic cross-sections showed a symmetric, complete, circular disintegration of intima and media structures, without any transmural tissue defects after radiofrequency ablation (RFA).[25] However, with an HSLW laser, pronounced semicircular tissue ablations and complete vessel wall perforations were detected at 35 J per cm LEED. The quantitative analysis demonstrated a significant ($P < .0001$) increase in intima-media thickness after RFA (38% to 67%) and EVLA (11% to 46%), and a significant ($P < .0001$) reduction in vessel lumen diameter (36% to 42%) after RFA. No linear correlation could be identified between laser energy level and effects on tissue such as ablation/perforation, media thickening, or vein lumen diameter.[26]

Weiss examined the gross tissue effects and tissue temperatures generated during EVLA with an 810-nm diode laser in an in vivo goat model. Using thermal sensors mounted adjacent to the laser optical fiber, they determined the mean temperature at the firing tip was 729°C (peak 1334°C).[27] The intense, thermal-heating zone appeared to be focally situated around the laser tip; the mean temperature decreased to 231°C and 307°C, 2 mm proximal and distal to the fiber tip, respectively. At 4-mm distal from the fiber tip, the mean temperature decreased further to 93°C. Recently, Disselhoff et al., with intravascular temperature measurements in an in vitro system, found that despite the intense heat at the laser tip, the thermal heating zone is predominantly contained within the venous lumen.[9] Zimmet and Min demonstrated in a swine model that during EVLA with an 810-nm diode laser, ear vein outer wall temperatures ranged from 40°C to 49°C. In hind extremity veins, these investigators showed that with tumescent anesthesia, the external vein wall temperatures never exceeded 40°C.[28]

These findings were corroborated in humans by Beale et al., when he inserted thermocouples percutaneously, positioned at 3 mm, 5 mm, and 10 mm from a small saphenous vein (SSV), after administration of tumescent anesthesia.[26] He recorded temperatures during EVL with an 810-nm diode laser, using 1-second pulse application at 12 W, and found peak temperatures of 43°C, 42°C, and 36°C at 3 mm, 5 mm, and 10 mm, respectively, in perivenous tissues.

PEARLS AND PITFALLS

Dosing

Data on the dose-response relationship between laser energy and durability of vein occlusion began to be published in 2004 when parameters describing the LEED and endovenous fluence equivalent (EFE) were introduced.[29] LEED is a linear energy density quantity measured in joules per centimeter, and EFE is an energy parameter that uses a cylindrical approximation of the inner vein surface area expressed in joules per centimeter squared. In addition, the increased specificity of the WSLW for treatment of the vein wall generally requires the use of a lower energy setting to achieve the same LEED.[8]

In a retrospective study, recanalization was reported in 20% of cases treated with administration of less than 80 J per cm and was significantly reduced if laser energy exceeded 80 J per cm at a wavelength of 980 nm.[30] However, in a follow-up prospective study by the same author, 9% of veins treated with LEEDs exceeding 80 J per cm unexpectedly recanalized at 6-month follow-up.[31] Multiple regression analysis determined that EFE was the most significant predictor of recanalization events and, when exceeding 20 J per cm, was associated with durable GSV occlusion after 1-year follow-up.[4,32] Another study reported on 129 GSVs and found that 52 J per cm EFE was ideal to produce long-term occlusion; this author cautioned that recanalization can occur in patients treated with higher fluence.[4,33]

In a study by Almeida and Raines, high rates of vein occlusion and ultimate sonographic disappearance were noted when the thermal dose in each segment of the GSV was tailored to the diameter in that segment.[14] The ranges of energies used fell between 50 J per cm for veins 5 mm in diameter and 120 J per cm for veins 10 mm in diameter at the saphenofemoral junction (SFJ). No increase in complications was seen with any of the higher energy strategies.[34]

Reports from John Hopkins University on low-energy EVL treatment of 34 consecutive GSVs with a 980-nm diode laser at 11 W in continuous mode (mean GSV diameter 12 mm) using mean LEED of 35 J per cm resulted in zero recanalization (100% success) at a mean follow-up of 1 year.[35] Interestingly, the same author reported later in the same year that 60 consecutive GSVs demonstrated a reduced treatment success of 95%; the mean follow-up for this series was 6.8 months and mean LEED for successful and failed treatments was 33 J per cm. The mean maximum diameter of successfully treated GSVs was 11 mm, and that for failed treatments was 21 mm ($P = .008$). The investigators concluded that there were no significant differences in mean unit energy applied for successful, failed, and repeat treatments ($P > .05$); however, larger GSV diameter was associated with early treatment failures.[36] Another trial by Prince et al., indicated that energy density may not be the most important determinant of recanalization. In 471 segments, 11 failures were encountered, including 4 in a group treated with less than 60 J per cm (4%), 2 in a 60 to 80 J per cm group (3%), 4 in an 81 to 100 J per cm group (3%), and 1 in a group treated with more than 100 J per cm (1%). There were no statistically significant differences in failure rates among energy density ranges. The authors concluded that EVLA has a low failure rate and that failure rate is not a function of energy density.[37]

Taking all of the literature into consideration, a reasonable recommendation is to treat patients using LEEDs between 60 and 100 J per cm. Conceivably, this may be achieved using lower wavelengths as the efficiency of the laser increases (i.e., with increased wavelengths).[21,38]

Complications

Significant adverse events reported following EVLA include skin burns, sensory nerve injuries, and deep vein thrombosis (DVT) or endothermal heat-induced thrombosis

(EHIT). Early experience reported skin burn rates as high as 4%; this decreased to almost zero as the use of tumescent anesthesia became the standard of practice.[39] The overall rate for these complications has been shown to be higher in low-volume centers compared with high-volume centers; the rate of skin burns in one series using RFA was 1.7% before, and 0.5% after, the initiation of the tumescent technique.[40] The nerves at highest risk include the saphenous nerve, located adjacent to the GSV below the midcalf perforating vein, and the sural nerve, adjacent to the SSV in the midcalf and lower calf. The most common manifestations of a nerve injury are paresthesias, which are usually transient. The nerve injuries can occur during venous access, the delivery of tumescent anesthesia, or by transfer of thermal energy to perivenous tissues.

Patients treated with EVL, using high rates of energy delivery without tumescent anesthetic infiltrations, demonstrated a high rate of nerve injuries and skin burns.[41] However, in a series using RFA, delivery of perivenous fluid was thought to be responsible for the low rate of cutaneous and neurologic thermal injuries, where the 1-week paresthesia rate was shown to decrease from 15% to 9% after the introduction of tumescent anesthesia.[42] The addition of tumescent anesthesia has been demonstrated to reduce outer vein wall temperatures during EVLA and RFA in animal models.[43,44] In general, complication rates are thought to be reduced dramatically with the effective use of ultrasound guidance and tumescent anesthetic.[45,46] Fortunately, thromboembolic events are uncommon after endovenous thermal ablation.[14] The thrombus extensions at the SFJ, seen occasionally after thermal ablation, are referred to as EHIT, and this is discussed in Chapter 16. Briefly, precautions may be taken to mitigate against the risk of EHIT, and one such technique is to increase the ablation distance from 2 cm to greater than 2.5 cm from the respective deep venous junction.[47]

Small Saphenous Vein

Ablation of the SSV with either laser or radiofrequency is a very attractive alternative to SSV ligation and stripping because open dissection of the popliteal fossa is not required. The popliteal space has traditionally been referred to as "tiger country" in many vascular surgery circles because of the anatomy. Although the usual reason for surgery in this area is for popliteal artery treatment, those who begin an open dissection in this area can injure the popliteal vein and tibial nerve if great care is not taken. Fewer reports of endovenous laser treatment of the SSV than of the GSV have been published.

In a 2003 report on the treatment of SSV in 41 limbs using a 940-nm diode laser, 39 SSVs (95%) were successfully treated with EVLA.[48] During a median follow-up interval of 6 months, no recanalization was observed. Apart from one thrombosis of the popliteal vein in a patient with polycythemia vera, four transient sural nerve paresthesias were reported.

Almeida and Raines reported on 987 treated veins in 2006, 115 of which were SSVs. Most recanalizations occurred in the first 12 months and developed in the SSV proximal to May's perforator.[14] Five of 115 treated SSVs recanalized partially (4%), most likely as a result of cooler blood (37°C) entering the treatment site from a midcalf perforating vein. No thrombus extensions into the popliteal vein or other thrombotic complications of the deep system were identified. Ravi et al. then reported the series in 2006, which consisted of 981 patients and included 101 SSV procedures.[49] There were 9 (9%) failures among the 101 SSVs treated with EVLA.

Gibson et al. published their series of 210 SSVs treated with EVLA.[50] Their data demonstrated that EVLA of the SSV is feasible and safe and has excellent clinical outcomes in combination with concomitant therapies where indicated. All procedures were technically successful; 96% of SSVs remained closed at a mean follow-up of 4 months. The incidence of nerve injury is acceptably low and not clinically significant. Three patients (1.6%) complained of numbness at the lateral malleolus at the 6-week follow-up. In only one of these patients could EVLA alone be implicated in causing numbness, because two of the patients also had microphlebectomy of large varicose vein branches at the lateral malleolus. None of the patients found the numbness to be a significant concern. The incidence of DVT, defined as a tail of thrombus protruding into the popliteal vein, was noted in 12 limbs (5.7%) at the 1-week follow-up examination. The incidence of DVT after treatment of the SSV was 5.7%, higher than in the other reported series. The reason for this difference is unclear; DVT was present in 11.4% of type A anatomy compared with 2.9% of limbs with type B anatomy and 0% of limbs with type C anatomy.

To understand the reason for the high rate of DVT, the authors incorrectly describe the vein of Giacomini as analogous to the inferior epigastric vein in EVLA of the GSV in the case of type A and type B anatomy. That EVLA of the GSV should commence with the tip of the laser distal to the superficial epigastric vein (not the inferior epigastric vein) has become dogma in the endovenous community and is based purely on empirical data. Theoretically, this preserves flow at the SFJ, which in turn may prevent extension of thrombus into the common femoral vein. There is an analogous arrangement at the saphenopopliteal junction (SPJ); however, the similarity exists with drainage of the gastrocnemius veins into the most proximal aspect of the SPJ and not the Giacomini vein as the authors stated. It is correct that patients with type C anatomy may have a reduced risk of DVT because of the absence of communication between the SSV and the popliteal vein. That type B anatomy has the benefit of flow from the Giacomini vein into the SPJ to maintain patency remains to be proved.

In a multicenter prospective study on 229 limbs, the feasibility, safety, and efficacy of EVLA to treat SSVs were evaluated.[51] Duplex ultrasound imaging showed immediate occlusion of the SSV with no thrombosis in the proximal veins. No complications occurred intraoperatively. All patients had postoperative ecchymosis, but it was minimal. Complete occlusion with absence of flow at less than 2 months of follow-up was detected in 226 SSVs (98.7%). It occurred in 22 patients with large SSV diameters. Recanalization was found in one patient at 12 months and in two patients at 24 months. After 1 year, eight limbs developed reflux in new locations and four underwent treatment. Symptoms resolved in most patients soon after the operation. The mean follow-up was 16 months. After 8 to 12 months postprocedurally, the laser-treated veins were fibrotic and almost indistinguishable from the surrounding tissues on duplex ultrasound imaging. In five patients (2.25%), postoperative paresthesia occurred more than 2 to 3 days postoperatively and persisted in the follow-up period.

COMPARATIVE EFFECTIVENESS OF EXISTING TREATMENTS

Nonrandomized Studies

There have been several large case series describing outcomes for EVLA. Most report GSV ablation rates of over 90%, with associated improvement in symptoms and minimal complications (Table 7.1). With regards to long-term outcomes, The International Endovenous Laser Working Group described effective long-term durability rates in a cohort of 1020 limbs treated.[52] Failure rates were 7.7% at 1 year, 5.4% at 2 years, and 0% failures at 3 years.

TABLE 7.1 Published Observational Series of Endovenous Laser for Saphenous Reflux

Study Author, Year	Limbs, (N)	Vein	Anatomic Success (%)	Duplex Ultrasound Scanning Follow-Up (Months)	Major Complication Rate (%)
Navarro et al., 2001[56]	40	GSV	100	4.2	0
Min et al., 2001[5]	90	GSV	97	9	0
Proebstle, 2003[4]	104	GSV	90	12	0
Oh et al., 2003[13]	15	GSV	100	3	0
Min et al., 2003[10]	499	GSV	98	17	0
Proebstle et al., 2003[48]	39	SSV	100	6	2
Perkowski et al., 2004[62]	154	GSV	97	12	0
	37	SSV	97	12	0
Sadick and Waser, 2004[57]	31	GSV	97	24	0
Timperman et al., 2004[30]	111	GSV	78	7	0
Proebstle et al., 2004[29]	106	GSV	90	3	0
Goldman et al., 2004[11]	24	GSV	100	9	0
Proebstle et al., 2005[19]	282	GSV	95	3	0
Timperman, 2005[31]	100	GSV	91	9	1
Puggioni et al., 2005[63]	77	GSV/SSV	94	1	2
Kabnick, 2006[17]	60	GSV	92	12	0
Almeida and Raines, 2006[14]	578	GSV	98	24	0
	115	SSV	96	24	0
Yang et al., 2006[64]	71	GSV	94	13	–
Kim and Paxton, 2006[36]	60	GSV	95	3	–
Kavaturu et al., 2006[65]	66	GSV	97	12	0
Myers et al., 2006[66]	404	GSV/SSV	80	36	0
Sadick and Wasser, 2007[67]	94	GSV	96	48	0
Theivacumar et al., 2007[68]	68	SSV	100	6	4
Gibson et al., 2007[50]	210	SSV	100	1.5	6
Ravi et al., 2006[49]	990	GSV	97	36	0
	101	SSV	90	36	0
Desmyttere et al., 2007[34]	511	GSV	97	48	0
Spreafico et al., 2014[69]	372	GSV/SSV	90	12	0
Mendes-Pinto et al., 2016[70]	90	GSV	94.7	12	0
Jibiki et al., 2016[71]	289	GSV	99.6	24	0.8

GSV, Great saphenous vein; *SSV,* small saphenous vein.

Summary of Randomized Controlled Trials

These randomized studies suggest that abolition of GSV reflux, improvements in quality of life, patient satisfaction, and cosmesis are similar for surgery and EVLA (Table 7.2). Three studies also show that posttreatment discomfort was no different for either technique.

TABLE 7.2 Summary of Outcomes for Randomized Trials of Surgery Versus Endovenous Laser Ablation

	de Medeiros and Luccas[72]	Ying et al.[73]	Rasmussen et al.[53]	Kalteis et al.[54]	Darwood et al.[74]	Roopram et al.[58]	Gauw et al.[59]	Sydnor et al.[60]
No. of limbs (surgery vs. EVLA)	20 vs. 20	80 patients	68 vs. 69	48 vs. 47	35 vs. 79 (1:2 randomization)	57 vs. 118	68 vs. 62	87 vs. 89 (RFA vs. 980 nm)
Anesthesia for EVLA	Regional		Tumescent and LA sedation	General or regional	Tumescent and LA sedation	General or spinal vs. tumescent	Tumescent	Tumescent and LA sedation
Surgical treatment	SFJ ligation, GSV stripping, and phlebectomy		SFJ ligation, GSV stripping, and phlebectomy	SFJ ligation, GSV stripping, and phlebectomy	SFJ ligation, GSV stripping, and phlebectomy	SFJ ligation, GSV stripping, and phlebectomy	SFJ ligation, GSV stripping	N/A
Additional therapy for EVLA patients	SFJ ligation and phlebectomy		Concomitant phlebectomy	SFJ ligation and phlebectomy	Delayed sclerotherapy (6 weeks)	Concomitant phlebectomy	Concomitant phlebectomy	Concomitant phlebectomy/ sclerotherapy
Outcome measures	Bruising, abolition of reflux and pain	Pain, blood loss, hospital stay	Bruising, QoL, normal activity, abolition of reflux, and pain	Bruising, QoL, normal activity, abolition of reflux and pain, and patient satisfaction	QoL, normal activity, abolition of reflux and pain, and patient satisfaction	QoL, normal activity, abolition of reflux and pain, and patient satisfaction	QoL, normal activity, abolition of reflux, and pain	Bruising, QoL, normal activity, abolition of reflux, and pain
Results	EVLA: less bruising; patients preferred EVLA; EVLA: 95% ablation; pain: equivalent	All reduced by EVLA	EVLA: less bruising; QoL: equivalent; NA: equivalent; ablation: 96% vs. 94%; and pain: less with EVLA	EVLA: less bruising; QoL: equivalent; EVLA: delayed NA; ablation: 100% both; pain: equivalent; and cosmesis: equivalent	QoL: equivalent; NA: earlier with EVLA; Ablation: 88% vs. 94%; Pain: equivalent, and satisfaction: equivalent	QoL: equivalent; pain and bruising: equivalent: 81% vs. 99.1%	QoL: equivalent; Surgery 100% vs. 95%; Pain: equivalent	Pain and bruising equivalent; QoL: equivalent; RFA equivalent; RFA 95% vs. EVLA 96%; Satisfaction: equivalent.
Duration of follow-up	60 days		6 months	16 weeks	3 months (limited 12-month data)	1 year	5 years	1 year

EVLA, Endovenous laser ablation; *GSV*, great saphenous vein; *LA*, local anesthesia; *N/A*, nor applicable; *QoL*, quality of life; *RFA*, radiofrequency ablation; *SFJ*, saphenofemoral junction.

Although this may be surprising, it is likely to reflect GSV and adjacent soft tissue inflammation (phlebitis) following the thermal injury inflicted by EVL. Although pain levels appear similar for surgery and EVL, return to normal activity or work is variously reported as occurring earlier after EVL, at the same time following either modality, or delayed after laser therapy.[53-55]

It is evident from these trials that there is no consensus as to the optimum treatment protocol for EVL. Given the results reported by Rasmussen et al.[56] and Darwood et al.,[57] it seems that concomitant saphenofemoral ligation is unnecessary, thus allowing EVLA to be performed without general or regional anesthesia in an outpatient or office setting. The question of simultaneous versus adjuvant treatment for the varicosities has not been answered definitively. At least at this time, there is little differentiation in pain, bruising, or quality-of-life outcomes when it comes to comparing staged versus simultaneous adjunctive therapy.[58-60]

Meta-Analysis

This meta-analysis of randomized controlled trials reviews the current evidence base, comparing open and endovascular treatment of varicose veins.[55] Systematic review of studies reporting duplex scan follow-up after open surgical, laser (EVLT), or radiofrequency (VNUS Closure device, VNUS Medical Technologies, San Jose, CA) treatment of refluxing GSVs was completed. Primary outcome measures were occlusion and complication rates and time taken to resume work. Meta-analysis finds no significant difference in recurrence rates at 3 months between open surgery and EVLA (relative risk [RR], 2.19; 95% confidence interval [CI], 0.99–4.85; $P = .05$) or VNUS (RR, 7.57; 95% CI, 0.42–136.02). Return to work is significantly faster following VNUS (by 8.24 days, 95% CI, 10.50–5.97) or EVLA (by 5.02 days, 95% CI, 6.52–3.52). More recent data comparing EVLA with surgery, compiled for the purposes of a Cochrane review by Nesbitt et al., demonstrated that neovascularization and technical failure were reduced in the EVLA group as compared with the surgery group.[61] No other conclusions could be drawn at this time. Ultimately, endovascular treatment of varicose veins is safe and effective and offers the significant advantage of rapid recovery.

ACKNOWLEDGMENT

This chapter is based in part on a chapter in the previous edition by Jose I. Almeida, MD.

REFERENCES

1. Boné C. Tratamiento endoluminal de las varices con laser de diodo: studio prelimino. *Rev Patol Vasc.* 1999;5:35–46.
2. Theivacumar NS, Dellagrammaticas D, Beale RJ, et al. Factors influencing the effectiveness of endovenous laser ablation (EVLA) in the treatment of great saphenous vein reflux. *Eur J Vasc Endovasc Surg.* 2008;35:119–123.
3. Mundy L, Merlin TL, Fitridge RA, et al. Systematic review of endovenous laser treatment for varicose veins. *Br J Surg.* 2005;92:1189–1194.
4. Proebstle TM, Gul D, Lehr HA, et al. Infrequent early recanalization of greater saphenous vein after endovenous laser treatment. *J Vasc Surg.* 2003;38:511–516.

5. Min RJ, Zimmet SE, Isaacs MN, et al. Endovenous laser treatment of the incompetent greater saphenous vein. *J Vasc Interv Radiol.* 2001;12:1167–1171.

6. Proebstle TM, Lehr HA, Kargl A, et al. Endovenous treatment of the greater saphenous vein with a 940 nm diode laser: thrombotic occlusion after endoluminal thermal damage by laser generated steam bubbles. *J Vasc Surg.* 2002;35:729–736.

7. Proebstle TM, Sandhofer M, Kargl A, et al. Thermal damage of the inner vein wall during endovenous treatment: key role of energy absorption by intravascular blood. *Dermatol Surg.* 2002;28:596–600.

8. Sadek M, Kabnick LS, Berland T, et al. Update on endovenous laser ablation: 2011. *Perspect Vasc Surg Endovasc Ther.* 2011;23(4):233–237.

9. Disselhoff B, Rem AI, Verdaasdonk R, et al. Endovenous laser ablation: an experimental study on the mechanism of action. *Phlebology.* 2008;23:69–76.

10. Min RJ, Khilnani N, Zimmet S. Endovenous laser treatment of saphenous vein reflux: long-term results. *J Vasc Interv Radiol.* 2003;14:991–996.

11. Goldman MP, Mauricio M, Rao J. Intravascular 1320-nm laser closure of the great saphenous vein: a 6- to 12-month follow-up study. *Dermatol Surg.* 2004;30:1380–1385.

12. Goldman MP. Intravascular lasers in the treatment of varicose veins. *J Cosmet Dermatol.* 2004;3:162–166.

13. Oh CK, Jung DS, Jang HS, et al. Endovenous laser surgery of the incompetent greater saphenous vein with a 980-nm diode laser. *Dermatol Surg.* 2003;29:1135–1140.

14. Almeida JI, Raines JK. Radiofrequency ablation and laser ablation in the treatment of varicose veins. *Ann Vasc Surg.* 2006;20:547–552.

15. Maurins U, Rabe E, Pannier F. Does laser power influence the results of endovenous laser ablation (EVLA) of incompetent saphenous veins with the 1470-nm diode laser? A prospective randomized study comparing 15 and 25 W. *Int Angiol.* 2009;28:32–37.

16. Lurie F, Creton D, Eklof B, et al. Prospective randomised study of endovenous radiofrequency obliteration (closure) versus ligation and vein stripping (EVOLVeS): two-year follow-up. *Eur J Vasc Endovasc Surg.* 2005;29:67–73.

17. Kabnick LS. Outcome of different endovenous laser wavelengths for great saphenous vein ablation. *J Vasc Surg.* 2006;43:88–93.

18. Shutze WP, Kane K, Fisher T, et al. The effect of wavelength on endothermal heat-induced thrombosis incidence after endovenous laser ablation. *J Vasc Surg Venous Lymphat Disord.* 2016;4(1):36–43. doi:10.1016/j.jvsv.2015.08.003. [Epub 2015 Nov 11].

19. Proebstle TM, Moehler T, Gul D, et al. Endovenous treatment of the great saphenous vein using a 1,320 nm Nd:YAG laser causes fewer side effects than using a 940 nm diode laser. *Dermatol Surg.* 2005;31:1678–1683.

20. Almeida JI, Mackay EG, Javier JJ, et al. Saphenous laser ablation at 1470 nm targets the vein wall, not blood. *Vasc Endovascular Surg.* 2009;43:467–472.

21. Kabnick LS, Sadek M. Fiber type as compared to wavelength may contribute more to improving postoperative recovery following endovenous laser ablation. *J Vasc Surg Venous Lymphat Disord.* 2016;4(3):286–292. doi:10.1016/j.jvsv.2015.12.004.

22. Bush RG, Shamma HN, Hammond K. Histological changes occurring after endoluminal ablation with two diode lasers (940 and 1319 nm) from acute changes to 4 months. *Lasers Surg Med.* 2008;40:676–679.

23. Fan CM, Rox-Anderson R. Endovenous laser ablation: mechanism of action. *Phlebology.* 2008;23:206–213.

24. Roggan A, Friebel M, Dorschel K, et al. Optical properties of circulating human blood in the wavelength range 400-2500 nm. *J Biomed Opt.* 1999;4:36–46.

25. Schmedt CG, Meissner OA, Hunger K, et al. Evaluation of endovenous radiofrequency ablation and laser therapy with endoluminal optical coherence tomography in an ex vivo model. *J Vasc Surg.* 2007;45:1047–1058.

26. Beale RJ, Mavor AID, Gough MJ. Heat dissipation during endovenous laser treatment of varicose veins—is there a risk of nerve injury? *Phlebology.* 2006;21:32–35.

27. Weiss RA. Comparison of endovenous radiofrequency versus 810 nm diode laser occlusion of the large veins in an animal model. *Dermatol Surg.* 2002;28:56–61.

28. Zimmet SE, Min RJ. Temperature changes in perivenous tissue during endovenous laser treatment in a swine model. *J Vasc Interv Radiol.* 2003;14:911–915.

29. Proebstle TM, Krummenauer F, Gül D, et al. Non-occlusion and early reopening of the great saphenous vein after endovenous laser treatment is fluence dependent. *Dermatol Surg.* 2004;30:174–178.

30. Timperman PE, Sichlau M, Ryu RK. Greater energy delivery improves treatment success of endovenous laser treatment of incompetent saphenous veins. *J Vasc Interv Radiol.* 2004;15:1061–1063.

31. Timperman PE. Prospective evaluation of higher energy great saphenous vein endovenous laser treatment. *J Vasc Interv Radiol.* 2005;16:791–794.

32. Proebstle TM, Moehler T. and Herdemann S: Reduced recanalization rates of the great saphenous vein after endovenous laser treatment with increased energy dosing: definition of a threshold for the endovenous fluence equivalent. *J Vasc Surg.* 2006;44:834–839.

33. Vuylsteke M, Liekens K, Moons P, et al. Endovenous laser treatment of saphenous vein reflux: how much energy do we need to prevent recanalizations. *Vasc Endovascular Surg.* 2008;42:141–149.

34. Desmyttere J, Grard C, Wassmer B, et al. Endovenous 980-nm laser treatment of saphenous veins in a series of 500 patients. *J Vasc Surg.* 2007;46:1242–1247.

35. Kim HS, Nwankwo IJ, Hong K, et al. Lower energy endovenous laser ablation of the great saphenous vein with 980 nm diode laser in continuous mode. *Cardiovasc Intervent Radiol.* 2006;29:64–69.

36. Kim HS, Paxton BE. Endovenous laser ablation of the great saphenous vein with a 980-nm diode laser in continuous mode: early treatment failures and successful repeat treatments. *J Vasc Interv Radiol.* 2006;17:1449–1455.

37. Prince EA, Ahn SH, Dubel GJ, et al. An investigation of the relationship between energy density and endovenous laser ablation success: does energy density matter? *J Vasc Interv Radiol.* 2008;19:1449–1453.

38. Pannier F, Rabe E, Maurins U. First results with a new 1470-nm diode laser for endovenous ablation of incompetent saphenous veins. *Phlebology.* 2009;24:26–30.

39. Merchant RF, dePalma RG, Kabnick LS. Endovascular obliteration of saphenous reflux: a muticenter study. *J Vasc Surg.* 2002;35:1180–1186.

40. Merchant RF, Pichot O, Meyers KA. Four-year follow-up on endovascular radiofrequency obliteration of great saphenous reflux. *Dermatol Surg.* 2005;31:129–134.

41. Chang C, Chua J. Endovenous laser photocoagulation (EVLP) for varicose veins. *Lasers Surg Med.* 2002;31:257–262.

42. Merchant RF, Pichot O. Long-term outcomes of endovenous radiofrequency obliteration of saphenous reflux as a treatment of superficial venous insufficiency. *J Vasc Surg.* 2005;42:502–509.

43. Zikorus AW, Mirizzi MS. Evaluation of setpoint temperature and pullback speed on vein adventitial temperature during endovenous radiofrequency energy delivery in an in-vitro model. *Vasc Endovascular Surg.* 2004;38:167–174.

44. Dunn CW, Kabnick LS, Merchant RF, et al. Endovascular radiofrequency obliteration using 90°C for treatment of great saphenous vein. *Ann Vasc Surg.* 2006;20:625–629.

45. Dexter D, Kabnick L, Berland T, et al. Complications of endovenous lasers. *Phlebology.* 2012;27(suppl 1):40–45.

46. Van den Bos R, Neumann M, De Roos KP, et al. Endovenous laser ablation–induced complications: review of the literature and new cases. *Dermatol Surg.* 2009;35:1206e14.

47. Sadek M, Kabnick LS, Rockman CB, et al. Increasing ablation distance peripheral to the saphenofemoral junction may result in a diminished rate of endothermal heat-induced thrombosis. *J Vasc Surg Venous Lymphat Disord.* 2013;1(3):257–262. doi:10.1016/j.jvsv.2013.01.002. [Epub 2013 May 17].

48. Proebstle TM, Gul D, Kargl A, et al. Endovenous laser treatment of the lesser saphenous vein with a 940-nm diode laser: early results. *Dermatol Surg.* 2003;29:357–361.

49. Ravi R, Rodriguez-Lopez JA, Traylor EA, et al. Endovenous ablation of incompetent saphenous veins: a large single-center experience. *J Endovasc Ther.* 2006;13:244–248.

50. Gibson KD, Ferris BL, Polissar N, et al. Endovenous laser treatment of the small saphenous vein: efficacy and complications. *J Vasc Surg.* 2007;45:795–801.

51. Kontothanassis D, Di Mitri R, Ferrari Ruffino S, et al. Endovenous laser treatment of the small saphenous vein. *J Vasc Surg.* 2009;49:973–979.

52. Spreafico G, Kabnick L, Berland TL, et al. Laser saphenous ablations in more than 1,000 limbs with long-term duplex examination follow-up. *Ann Vasc Surg.* 2011;25:71–78.

53. Rasmussen LH, Bjoern L, Lawaetz M, et al. Trial comparing endovenous laser ablation of the great saphenous vein with high ligation and stripping in patients with varicose veins: short term results. *J Vasc Surg.* 2007;46:308–315.

54. Kalteis M, Berger I, Messie-Werndl S, et al. High ligation combined with stripping and endovenous laser ablation of the great saphenous vein: early results of a randomised controlled study. *J Vasc Surg.* 2008;47:822–829.

55. Brar R, Nordon IM, Hinchliffe RJ, et al. Management of varicose veins: meta-analysis. *Vascular.* 2010;18:205–220.

56. Navarro L, Min RJ, Bone C. Endovenous laser: a new minimally invasive method of treatment of varicose veins—preliminary observations using an 810 nm diode laser. *Dermatol Surg.* 2001;27:117–122.

57. Sadick NS, Waser S. Combined endovascular laser with ambulatory phlebectomy for the treatment of superficial venous incompetence: a 2-year perspective. *J Cosmet Laser Ther.* 2004;24:149–153.

58. Roopram AD, Lind MY, Van Brussel JP, et al. Endovenous laser ablation versus conventional surgery in the treatment of small saphenous vein incompetence. *J Vasc Surg Venous Lymphat Disord.* 2013;1(4):357–363. doi:10.1016/j.jvsv.2013.05.005.

59. Gauw SA, Lawson JA, van Vlijmen-van Keulen CJ, et al. Five-year follow-up of a randomized, controlled trial comparing saphenofemoral ligation and stripping of the great saphenous vein with endovenous laser ablation (980 nm) using local tumescent anesthesia. *J Vasc Surg.* 2016;63(2):420–428. doi:10.1016/j.jvs.2015.08.084.

60. Sydnor M, Mavropoulos J, Slobodnik N, et al. A randomized prospective long-term (>1 year) clinical trial comparing the efficacy and safety of radiofrequency ablation to 980 nm laser ablation of the great saphenous vein. *Phlebology.* 2016; pii: 0268355516658592. [Epub ahead of print].

61. Nesbitt C, Bedenis R, Bhattacharya V, et al. Endovenous ablation (radiofrequency and laser) and foam sclerotherapy versus open surgery for great saphenous vein varices. *Cochrane Database Syst Rev.* 2014;(7):CD005624, doi:10.1002/14651858.CD005624.pub3. Review.

62. Perkowski P, Ravi R, Gowda RCN, et al. Endovenous laser ablation of the saphenous vein for treatment of venous insufficiency and varicose veins: early results from a large single-center experience. *J Endovasc Ther.* 2004;11:132–138.

63. Puggioni A, Kalra M, Carmo M, et al. Endovenous laser therapy and radiofrequency ablation of the great saphenous vein: analysis of early efficacy and complications. *J Vasc Surg.* 2005;42:488–493.

64. Yang CH, Chou HS, Lo YF. Incompetent great saphenous veins treated with endovenous 1,320-nm laser: results for 71 legs and morphologic evolvement study. *Dermatol Surg.* 2006;32:1453–1457.

65. Kavuturu S, Girishkumar H, Ehrlich F. Endovenous laser ablation of saphenous veins is an effective treatment modality for lower extremity varicose veins. *Am Surg.* 2006;72: 672–675.

66. Myers K, Fris R, Jolley D. Treatment of varicose veins by endovenous laser therapy: assessment of results by ultrasound surveillance. *Med J Aust.* 2006;185:199–202.

67. Sadick NS, Wasser S. Combined endovascular laser plus ambulatory phlebectomy for the treatment of superficial venous incompetence: a 4-year perspective. *J Cosmet Laser Ther.* 2007;9:9–13.

68. Theivacumar NS, Beale RJ, Mavor AI, et al. Initial experience in endovenous laser ablation (EVLA) of varicose veins due to small saphenous vein reflux. *Eur J Vasc Endovasc Surg.* 2007;33:614–618.

69. Spreafico G, Piccioli A, Bernardi E, et al. Endovenous laser ablation of great and small saphenous vein incompetence with a 1470-nm laser and radial fiber. *J Vasc Surg Venous Lymphat Disord.* 2014;2(4):403–410. doi:10.1016/j.jvsv.2014.04.012.

70. Mendes-Pinto D, Bastianetto P, Cavalcanti Braga Lyra L, et al. Endovenous laser ablation of the great saphenous vein comparing 1920-nm and 1470-nm diode laser. *Int Angiol.* 2016;35(6):599–604.

71. Jibiki M, Miyata T, Futatsugi S, et al. Effect of the wide-spread use of endovenous laser ablation on the treatment of varicose veins in Japan: a large-scale, single institute study. *Laser Ther.* 2016;25(3):171–177.

72. de Medeiros C, Luccas G. Comparison of endovenous treatment with an 810 nm laser versus conventional stripping of the great saphenous vein in patients with primary varicose veins. *Dermatol Surg.* 2005;31:1685–1694.

73. Ying L, Sheng Y, Ling H, et al. Random, comparative study on endovenous laser therapy and saphenous veins stripping for the treatment of great saphenous vein incompetence. *Zhonghua Yi Xue Za Zhi.* 2007;87:3043–3046.

74. Darwood R, Theivacumar N, Dellagrammaticus D, et al. Randomised clinical trial comparing endovenous laser ablation with surgery for the treatment of primary great saphenous varicose veins. *Br J Surg.* 2008;95:294–301.

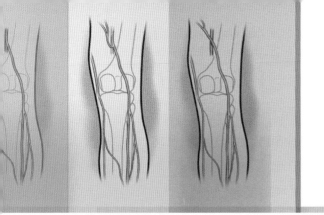

CHAPTER 8

Nonthermal Ablation of Saphenous Reflux

Steve Elias

All endovenous technologies can be classified under two general categories: thermal tumescent (TT) or nonthermal nontumescent (NTNT).[1] The TT technologies include radiofrequency, laser, and steam. NTNT technologies encompass: mechanical occlusion chemically assisted (MOCA), cyanoacrylate closure (CAC), and polidocanol injectable microfoam (PIM), with others emerging. These newer NTNT technologies have some real-world advantages: minimal nerve or skin injury, safety when treating disease to the ankle, decreased patient discomfort as a result of decreased needle sticks by avoiding tumescence, and the elimination of any capital equipment (generator). As with TT techniques, all NTNT techniques can be performed in an office setting in under an hour. Patients can return to normal activity almost immediately.[2,3]

The aforementioned advantages of NTNT techniques do not sacrifice safety, efficacy, or clinical outcomes when compared with TT techniques. All technologies have been shown to significantly improve quality-of-life (QoL) measures.[4,5] We know that successful occlusion of an axial superficial vein (great saphenous vein [GSV], small saphenous vein [SSV], anterior accessory great saphenous vein [AAGSV] etc.) improves a patient's QoL no matter what technology is used.[6] In fact, the evidence is so compelling for improved QoL, societal and government health agencies have recommended that endovenous ablation be the first modality of choice for symptomatic axial vein incompetence.[7,8] Successful ablation is not about treating the vein, it is about treating the patient. The idea of occlusion rate being the primary endpoint has faded in recent years. The question, "Did we improve the patient's QoL?," is now at the forefront, as it should be. Physician-derived and patient-reported outcome measures are now what academics and third-party payers consider to be primary endpoints. We treat patients, not veins. With these concepts in mind, we can better understand where the NTNT technologies of MOCA, CAC, and PIM can be best used when caring for patients with vein disease.

MECHANICAL OCCLUSION CHEMICALLY ASSISTED ABLATION

Overview

MOCA (ClariVein) has the longest follow-up and was the first of the new NTNT technologies to be reported. The device was developed by Michael Tal and John Marano (Fig. 8.1).[9] First human cases were performed in February 2009.[10] There are two components to the device/technique: (1) a mechanical component, which is a rotating wire (Figs. 8.2 and 8.3) that breaks down the surface tension barrier between sclerosant/blood and vein wall; and (2) chemical installation of a detergent liquid sclerosant sodium tetradecyl sulfate (STS) or polidocanol (PLD) simultaneously. The mechanical disruption allows for penetration of the sclerosant so that medial damage and scarring can occur leading to occlusion.[11] The wire rotates at 3500 rpms, which also causes vein spasm, so sclerosant

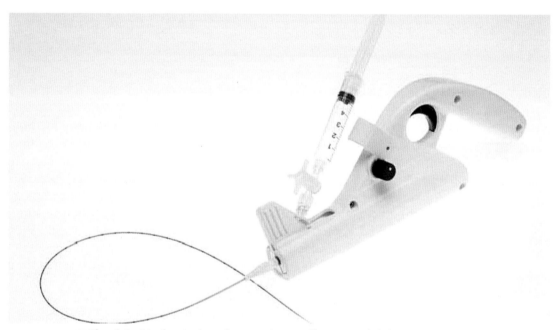

◾ **Fig. 8.1** Mechanical occlusion chemically assisted (ClariVein) device.

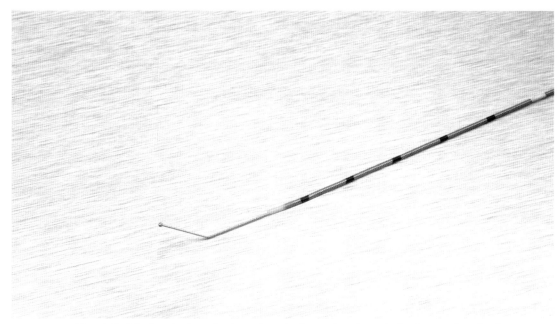

■ **Fig. 8.2** Mechanical occlusion chemically assisted angled wire unsheathed.

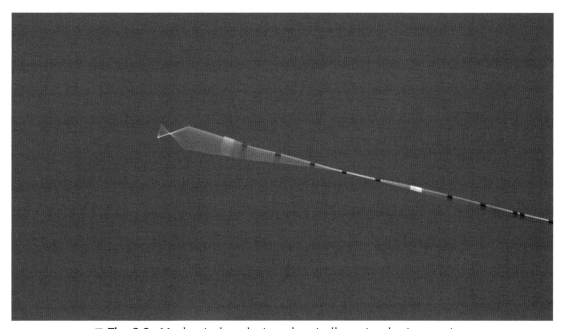

■ **Fig. 8.3** Mechanical occlusion chemically assisted wire rotating.

is not being injected into a vein filled with blood (Figs. 8.4 and 8.5). The technique is not sclerotherapy. Each component, mechanical and chemical, is essential for good results. Alone, each component yields poor results.[12] The sclerosant exits the catheter sheath about 2 cm from the tip of the rotating wire, it is pulled up the rotating shaft of the wire and is released from the tip thus directly "injecting" sclerosant into the damaged vein wall (see Fig. 8.5). This action allows for penetration of sclerosant subendothelial to aid in media damage. One can think of the rotating wire as a sprinkler releasing sclerosant from the tip. In the original trial, all veins received 12 mL of 1.5% STS liquid. A pullback rate of 1.5 mm per second or 1 cm every 7 seconds was used. This was chosen because of the similarity to the existing laser pullback rates at that time. The volume of sclerosant used was irrespective of the length of the vein being treated. Occlusion rate was 96% at 1 year with minimal complications; no deep venous thrombosis (DVT), nerve, or skin damage. Venous clinical severity score (VCSS) improved, as expected with an occluded GSV. Greater than 2-year follow-up was reported by the same group[13] with 96% occlusion rate.

Technique

The technique has undergone some modifications since the original report as all new techniques or technologies do. Here are the current recommendations.
1. Micropuncture access with ultrasound guidance
2. Placement of a 4-Fr or 5-Fr micropuncture sheath into the vein
3. No further wire or sheath exchanges required, no tumescence required
4. Passage of the angled catheter portion of the device up the targeted vein
5. Attachment of the motor unit and unsheathing of the wire placement of the wire tip 2 cm from the saphenofemoral junction (SFJ) or just at the fascial curve of the saphenopopliteal junction (SPJ)
6. Volume of sclerosant determined by diameter and length treated (table available) 8 to 10 mL GSV, 4 to 5 mL SSV
7. Begin rotation only, no injection for the first centimeter of pullback to induce vein spasm, that is, from position 2 cm to 3 cm from SFJ
8. After 1 cm of rotation, begin drip infusion of the sclerosant while continuing pullback; the patient only feels a vibration
9. Maintain constant rate of pullback (1.5 mm/s) with continuous drip infusion; reload syringe when needed
10. Posttreatment, have patient flex ankles to wash out any sclerosant in deep system
11. Wrap legs as per your protocol; this author uses 4-inch and 6-inch ACE from midthigh overnight and then no further compression unless a concomitant phlebectomy
12. Have patient ambulate; may resume normal activity next day

Technical Pearls

Pearl 1: The pullback rate is much more important for success than sclerosant volume. When failures are analyzed, the operator pulled too fast and did not allow enough time for elimination of the sclerosant vein wall surface tension. In the original study, all veins received 12 mL of 1.5% STD, regardless of length treated. No DVT occurred. Obviously, some veins received a little too much and some got a little too little, yet a 96% occlusion rate was achieved with no DVT/skin/nerve injury. The technique is

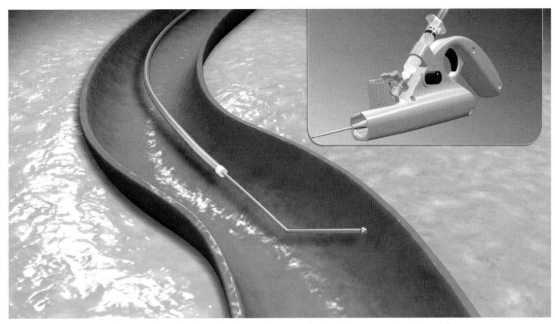

■ **Fig. 8.4** Mechanical occlusion chemically assisted mechanism of action.

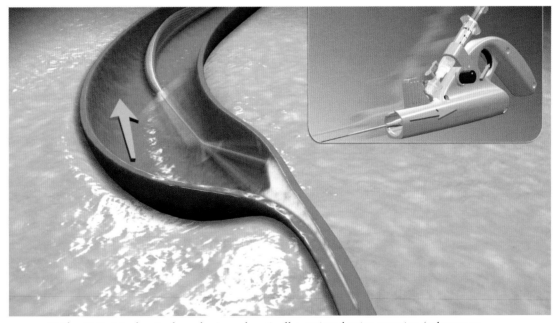

■ **Fig. 8.5** Mechanical occlusion chemically assisted wire rotating/sclerosant injection.

forgiving for volume but not forgiving of pullback rate. It is better to pull too slowly and give too much sclerosant than the contrary. The type of detergent sclerosant does not affect outcomes. Researchers from the Netherlands have reported comparable results with PLD 2% combined with 1%.[14]

Pearl 2: Confirm placement of the wire before starting treatment with ultrasound; ultrasound visualization is not routinely needed during the pullback. If there is a larger segment of vein (> 8–10 mm), then the ultrasound probe is used to partially compress that section to improve vein wall contact. However, routine pressure may lead to the rotating wire getting caught on the vein wall. If in fact it ever does, as happens in around 5% of cases, a quick jerk of the wire will free the catheter. This is akin to pulling a bandage quickly off the skin. During the procedure, one needs to listen to the motor rotating because the first sign of the catheter getting caught is a change in pitch of the motor, and the second sign is the patient having a pulling sensation. The wire cannot be broken by pulling it.

Pearl 3: If doing concomitant phlebectomy, this author recommends access and placement of the MOCA device, but no treatment until the phlebectomy segment is completed. The axial superficial vein is then treated. This sequence minimizes the potential dwell time of sclerosant in the deep system, and thus minimizing the risk of DVT. There are no studies to demonstrate this theoretic issue. The reported DVT rate worldwide is less than 0.5%.[15]

Pearl 4: When imaging posttreatment, it is important to not only use ultrasound greyscale but color flow duplex as well. With MOCA, the vein is immediately occluded, but it takes 3 to 6 months longer to contract (Fig. 8.6).

Therefore any early ultrasound with greyscale will show a dilated vein. This finding is in contrast with TT ablation. The additional use of color flow duplex will document absence of flow.

As with most other endovenous treatments, the postprocedure compression and activity instructions have become less onerous. This author uses compression for 24 hours post-MOCA which is similar for any endovenous procedure. Any and all activity is allowed the next day. These instructions apply only when phlebectomy is not included.

Results

To date, more than 20 articles have been published regarding MOCA (ClariVein) in peer-reviewed literature, and over 100,000 cases have been done worldwide. The results are overwhelmingly coincident with occlusion rates greater than 90% and significant improvement in QoL measures.[16] Some detailed studies, which address specific topics, will be discussed.

One of the longest follow-up has been reported by this author of the original clinical trial[13] at greater than 2 years. Witte et al. found similar improvement in QoL measures and occlusion at 3 years.[16] van Eekeren et al. reported equal results at 1 year when using PLD instead of STS. In addition, all the QoL measures improved at 1 year.[17]

One of the advantages of any NTNT technology is safety and no risk of nerve injury when treating any below-the-knee (BK) segment of vein. Boersma et al.[18] reported 1-year results for MOCA when treating SSV. No nerve injury occurred, and the occlusion rate was 94%. These results are encouraging in that SSV treatment has the concern of potential injury to three nerves; sural, tibial, and peroneal. Many physicians have been loath to treat the SSV because of nerve risk and DVT. This study did not have either issue.

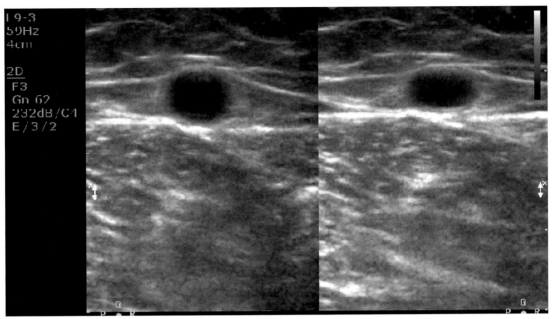

■ **Fig. 8.6** Ultrasound postmechanical occlusion chemically assisted at 6 months.

The management of more advanced disease states, such as C6 ulcer patients, is another advantage of NTNT technologies. In C6 patients, if the axial disease reflux is to the ankle, it is desirable to treat the entire pathologic segment. Tumescence is hard to place in an area of ulceration and significant lipodermatosclerosis. This author has used retrograde cannulation of the GSV in these circumstances with good results. Moore et al.[19] have reported the use of MOCA in a C6 patient with SSV incompetence with good results. Finally, three studies compared MOCA with radiofrequency ablation (RFA). van Eekeren et al.[20] concluded that MOCA yielded less postoperative pain, faster recovery, and faster return to work than RFA. Bootun et al.[21] randomized 119 patients to MOCA or RFA. MOCA had lower intraoperative pain scores, with equal occlusion rate and QoL improvement compared with RFA. Finally, Lane et al. published the final results of a trial comparing MOCA with RFA, which showed equivalent improvement in QoL measures.[22]

The mechanism of action of MOCA has been better understood in recent years. Two articles, one by Boersma[23] and one by Whiteley,[24] illustrate that both components (mechanical and chemical) are needed for successful treatment with MOCA.

Summary

MOCA currently has the longest follow-up of any NTNT technology. Studies support its use for the great majority of incompetent superficial axial veins. All studies comparing MOCA with RFA show as good, if not better, results regarding patient pain during and after, return to normal activities, and any other QoL scores. There are unique advantages of the NTNT techniques and of MOCA specifically. At the conclusion of this chapter, a summary of the benefits, indications, and contraindications of all the TT and NTNT technologies will be discussed.

CYANOACRYLATE CLOSURE (VENASEAL)

Overview

CAC is another NTNT technology that has similar advantages to MOCA: minimal nerve injury, no tumescence, and results equal to or better than TT techniques. The technology was developed by Rodney Raabe. A specially formulated cyanoacrylate (CA) adhesive is extruded into the target vein using a catheter that does not allow solidification of the glue within it. Once in the vasculature, the glue sets and causes immediate occlusion. A foreign body reaction incites an inflammatory response in the vessel, which ultimately involves media damage leading to fibrotic occlusion.[25] The system consists of a delivery catheter/sheath and a delivery gun (Fig. 8.7). First human cases were conducted by Almeida et al.[26] The initial technique involved the extrusion of CA starting 2 cm from the SFJ. This proved to be a little too close because there was an egress of material into the common femoral vein (CFV) in almost 20% of cases. The current technique has some modifications to minimize complications.

Current Technique

1. Access vein percutaneously, pass a long 0.035-inch (0.088 cm) guidewire to the SFJ or SPJ
2. Insert the supplied long 7-Fr sheath to within 5 cm of the SFJ
3. The supplied 5-Fr delivery catheter is placed through the 7-Fr sheath and positioned 5 cm from SFJ (Fig. 8.8)
4. The delivery gun is attached and loaded with CA
5. With each click of the delivery gun 0.1 mL of CA is delivered
6. The first injection begins 5 cm from SFJ and the second is 1 cm distal (6 cm)
7. Pressure is applied for 3 minutes with the ultrasound probe over this area
8. The catheter is moved distally 3 cm and another 0.1 mL is delivered
9. Pressure is applied for 30 seconds to this segment
10. Catheter is segmentally moved 3 cm, 0.1 mL placed, and pressure is applied for 30 seconds each time
11. The entire vein is segmentally treated to the insertion site
12. Postprocedure compression is optional
13. An average of 1.3 to 1.5 mL of CA is used

Technical Pearls

Pearl 1: Being too close to the SFJ or SPJ can lend to glue extrusion into the common femoral/popliteal vein. The glue does not break down over time, so theoretically, this can be a permanent nidus for clot formation. Catheter position needs to be confirmed.

Pearl 2: Air pockets have been incorporated into the catheter for improved visualization and echogenicity at the tip.

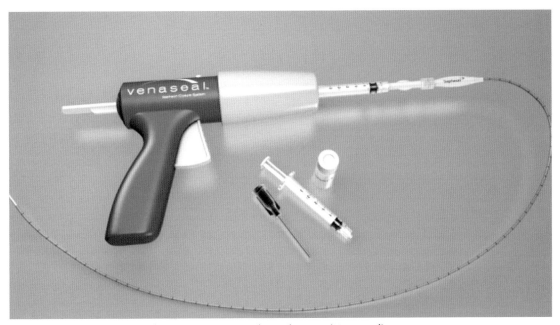

■ **Fig. 8.7** Cyanoacrylate closure (Venaseal) system

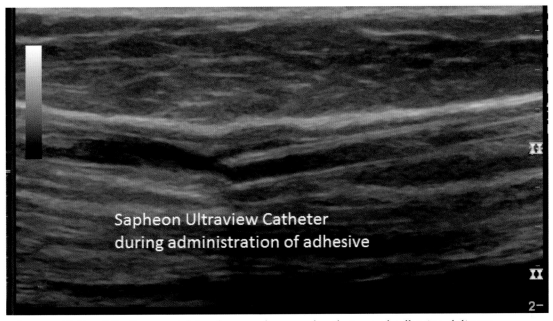

■ **Fig. 8.8** Cyanoacrylate closure ultrasound catheter and adhesive delivery

Pearl 3: The initial 3-minute compression time is important to allow sufficient setting of the glue so that the SFJ/SPJ is thoroughly protected. Doing nothing for 3 minutes can seem like a long time for the operator. Be patient.

Pearl 4: Nick Morrison, the principal investigator for the pivotal US VeClose trial offers two other technical thoughts. In the US trial epifascial veins were not treated. The thought process being that the inflammatory reaction could cause skin damage and the cord of glue might be felt through the patient's skin. Morrison also feels that one should avoid placement of glue immediately at the ostium of a large perforating vein to decrease the risk of deep system damage.

From a technique perspective, this NTNT method is analogous to the TT method of radiofrequency; it is a segmental ablation. The variable of pullback rate is eliminated. This enables a more consistent and predictive delivery of glue to the vein. The operator places the CA, pulls the premeasured trigger, compresses, and moves to the next segment. Eliminating pullback-rate concerns, and removing tumescence, simplifies the technique for both patient and physician.

Results

Initial studies were done in a swine model and reported in 2011.[27] The first human study followed and 2-year follow-up has been reported.[26] Some 38 patients were done initially, and 24 were available for 2-year follow-up. An occlusion rate of 92% was achieved (Fig. 8.9). Importantly, VCSS was still significantly improved from baseline, and edema and pain were positively improved. These procedures were conducted without tumescent anesthesia, and no postoperative compression was used.

The European multicenter eSCOPE (European Sapheon Closure System Observational Prospective) trial reported a 92.9% occlusion rate at 12 months.[28] The VCSS and Aberdeen Varicose Vein Questionnaire showed subsequently improved scores. This highlights the importance of QoL measures as outcomes and not solely occlusion rates. As with all NTNT techniques, no nerve injury occurred. There was some type of phlebitis reaction in about 11% of patients. This study was conducted without postoperative compression.

A more recent trial is the US pivotal trial, VenaSeal Sapheon Closure System Pivotal Study (VeClose).[29] This trial was a noninferiority trial comparing CAC with RFA. All centers had significant RFA technique experience, and there was a roll-in period for CAC before trial entry, so that investigators were over the learning curve. This trial did use postoperative compression as a fair comparison with RFA. Six-month occlusion rates were essentially the same; RFA 94% and CA 99%. Importantly, all measures of QoL were equal: pain during procedure, ecchymosis, VCSS, Euro QOL-5D, and Aberdeen Varicose Vein Questionnaire, highlighting once again that a successfully closed GSV positively impacts patients.

The WAVES trial[30] is a postmarket study that included incompetent GSVs, AASVs, and SSVs. The average diameter of veins in this trial was greater than the VeClose trial. This is the first trial to include veins other than the GSV. Results were comparable with the VeClose trial. Patients were followed to 1 month, and improvements in VCSS were seen in all including those with phlebitis. Return to all normal activities occurred either on the day of procedure or the next day. An analysis of the initial roll-in of patients from the VeClose trial was published by Kolluri et al.[31] They evaluated the fate of those patients who were treated during the learning curve for the VeClose trial. Occlusion was

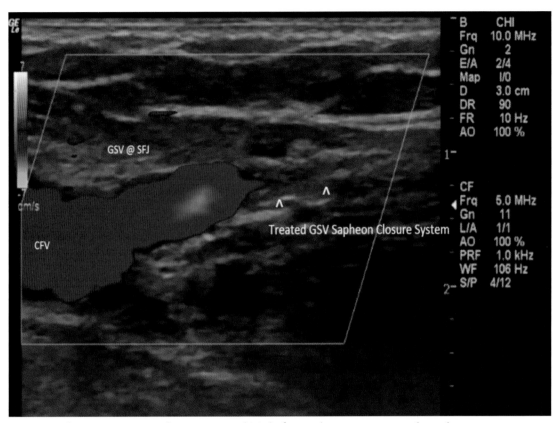

■ **Fig. 8.9** Great saphenous vein (GSV) 6 months postcyanoacrylate closure. *CFV,* Common femoral vein; *SFJ,* saphenofemoral junction.

100%. Although the procedure time was longer for the roll-in patients, all other parameters were parallel to the VeClose trial. This points to the short learning curve for CAC in physicians who already have experience with endovenous procedures.

Other studies have reported the use of CA (VariClose). This is a proprietary n-butyl CA manufactured in Turkey.[32] Results are quite similar, and safety and efficacy mirrors other reported parameters for VenaSeal.

Summary

CAC has similar results to MOCA with similar advantages. It further simplifies an NTNT procedure by eliminating the variable of pullback rate as alluded to earlier. It may have the theoretic benefit in ulcer patients that MOCA has been shown to have regarding being able to treat the full extent of disease even below an ulcer. To date, this has not been reported for CAC. The noninferior VeClose study indicates that CAC is as good, if not slightly better, than RFA in terms of closure and patient experience. Superficial veins may not be ideal for CAC because of the phlebitic reaction. Yet, despite some of these theoretic issues, the real-life patient experience is also very positive with CAC, as it is with MOCA.

POLIDOCANOL INJECTABLE MICROFOAM (VARITHENA)

Overview

PIM is a proprietary foam (Varithena), which has been in development for more than 10 years. A significant amount of research has been done to obtain US Food and Drug Administration (FDA) approval. Some of the issues surrounding physician-made foam historically have been the neurologic incidents that have occurred,[33] stability and uniformity of the foam, and the efficacy in terms of vein closure.[34] PIM was developed to minimize complications and improve efficacy. Suffice it to say, the exhaustive premarket studies showed minimal neurologic complications and good safety profile.[35]

It is indicated for the treatment of: GSV, AASV, and varicose veins. The SSV is not included in the indications for use because the initial VANISH-2 (Ventricular Tachycardia Ablation versus Escalated Antiarrhythmic Drug Therapy in Ischemic Heart Disease-2) study did not include these patients. However, postmarket use has included SSV treatment by practitioners.

Technique

Access to the target vein is ultrasound guided with either a 4-Fr or 5-Fr micropuncture sheath or an 18-gauge angiocath around the knee level if incompetence occurs at that level or lower. If incompetence goes to the BK level, a second access site is made. The reason for not accessing at the lowest point of reflux if it is BK, is that foam can be diluted or lost by the time it travels a long length to the junction. This author prefers the micropuncture sheath with a longer shaft to minimize loss of access. As with the MOCA device, no further wires or sheaths are needed. The foam is then obtained from the storage canister (Fig. 8.10) and injected through the sheath either directly or with extension tubing attached (Fig. 8.11). A second person is needed to visualize the superficial axial vein-deep vein junction (SFJ, SPJ) to be able to see the ascending foam from the insertion site. As soon as foam is detected, injection is halted and compression is applied with the ultrasound probe at the junction for 3 to 5 minutes until spasm is documented. This ends the procedure unless, as mentioned earlier, BK incompetence requires treatment or branch varicosities need treatment. The limb is then wrapped with an eccentric bandage with special roll provided by the manufacturer for 2 weeks.

Technical Pearls

Although this is a relatively straightforward technique, there are some key points that involve planning before, during, and after treatment.

Pearl 1: As mentioned previously, access site depends on extent of disease. If a second access site is contemplated, it should be done before any treatment because of spasm, which can occur in the entire target vein.

Pearl 2: It is recommended that any significantly large perforators in the thigh that attach to the GSV should be identified and marked on the skin, so that manual pressure can be applied to minimize foam entry into the deep system. Although theoretically correct, this author and others find this cumbersome, ineffectual, and unnecessary.

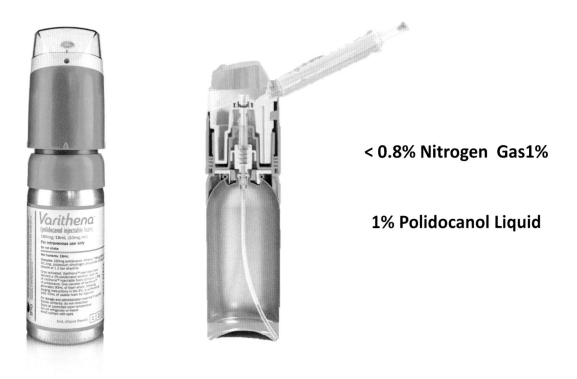

< 0.8% Nitrogen Gas1%

1% Polidocanol Liquid

■ **Fig. 8.10** Varithena cannister

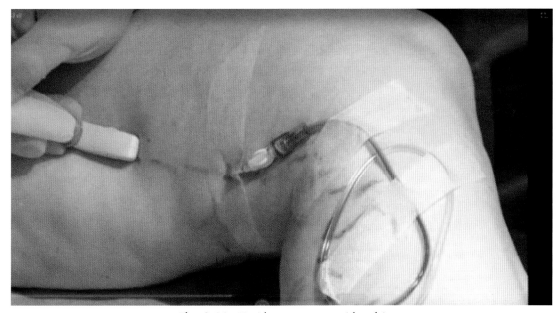

■ **Fig. 8.11** Varithena access with tubing

Pearl 3: To be done safely and with the best results, the procedure really requires two people. This is also recommended in the instructions for use and with PIM training. It is hard for one person to inject at the knee level and view the junction at the same time.

Pearl 4: There is a learning curve when drawing up microfoam from the canister. In early cases, a fair amount of foam may be lost. Pay careful attention to this part of the procedure.

Pearl 5: Although eccentric and continual compression is advised for 2 weeks, in the real world (i.e., not during a study), this does not occur 100% of the time and yet results seem to be good.

Results

One of the most interesting aspects of the results of the pivotal VANISH-2 study[36] is that the primary endpoint was not vessel occlusion but rather patient QoL measures. This was one of the first trials in superficial venous disease in which the FDA requested that patient outcomes be the primary endpoint. Some 221 patients were enrolled and followed to 8 weeks and then revaluated at 1 year. The metrics are listed subsequently:

– VVsymQ: Patient reported assessment of symptoms using electronic diary
– IPR-V3: Independent Physician Review Panel assessment of appearance
– PA-V3: Patient assessment of appearance

All scores improved and maintained improvement to 1 year. Interestingly, the occlusion rate was around 86%. This underscores the concept that one is treating patients and not saphenous veins. Adverse events were within the range of all other types of endovenous procedures and no major neurologic events or pulmonary emboli occurred.

Another study looked at the simultaneous use of axial thermal ablation and PIM for branch varicosities.[37] The same reported outcomes as the VANISH-2 study were used and patients receiving both endovenous ablation thermal and PIM did significantly better with no more adverse events. PIM can be combined with thermal ablation safely and with good outcomes.

Summary

PIM is another NTNT option with good data showing improvement in QoL. It is also the only NTNT or TT technology that can treat axial and branch varicosities. As of this writing, there are not any comparative studies with other technologies and not many published studies in general. More will be forthcoming.

DISCUSSION

Currently the NTNT category is undergoing similar issues that the disruptive TT technologies experienced in the early 2000s. The NTNT technologies are the next wave of disruptive technology regarding the treatment of superficial venous disease. The use of tumescence is the most discomforting aspect of endovenous ablation for patients and physicians. Accurate placement of tumescence is the longest part of the learning curve. It is also

TABLE 8.1 Nonthermal Nontumescent Advantages and Disadvantages

	Advantages	Disadvantages
MOCA	No foreign body left	Need to pullback/inject
	Uses approved liquid sclerosant	simultaneously
	Longest follow-up of all NTNT tortuous veins—angled	Longer learning curve
	wire	
	Perforator treatment	
	90,000 patients worldwide	
CAC	Segmental ablation	Foreign body left
	Pullback rate variable eliminated	Phlebitic reaction
	Second longest follow-up	Tortuous veins—difficult
	No postprocedure compression	
	Perforator treatment?	
PIM	Pullback rate variable eliminated	Requires 2 people for procedure
	Tortuous veins—foam traverses	IFU—2-weeks compression
	Treat branch varicosities also	Not indicated for SSV
	Perforator treatment	Cannister usable for 1 month

CAC, Cyanoacrylate closure; *IFU*, instructions for use; *MOCA*, mechanical occlusion chemically assisted; *NTNT*, nonthermal nontumescent; *PIM*, polidocanol injectable microfoam; *SSV*, small saphenous vein.

the part of the procedure that patients find most uncomfortable. Eliminating tumescence is a laudable goal as long as outcomes are similar to TT results. As illustrated earlier, the literature does support similar outcomes with TT and NTNT, at least in the midterm.

It is this author's belief that any vein specialist needs to be familiar with at least one TT and one NTNT technique. There are certain clinical scenarios when one is more advantageous than the other. Most BK pathology is better treated with NTNT technique to minimize nerve and skin issues. As stated previously, if pathology and reflux includes the ankle level, the NTNT techniques can safely accomplish this. This is even more advantageous with advanced C5 or C6 disease when tumescence is difficult to place in an area of skin changes, lipodermatosclerosis, or ulcer. Access can also be made retrograde from the knee level. MOCA can be safely used for epifascial veins as well because there is a minor phlebitic reaction.

Almost any TT or NTNT technology can be safely used in the above knee axial vein. However, this author feels that for large veins greater than 10 to 12 mm, TT options may be a better choice. Veins greater than 10 to 12 mm have been treated with success with NTNT, but large veins in general require more energy and a thermal mode of action. Recanalized veins from previous thrombophlebitis or previous failed ablations are better treated with TT for similar reasons.

Specifically within the NTNT category, each technology has its own unique advantages and disadvantages (Table 8.1).

These modalities may also have applications in other aspects of venous disease. For example, MOCA, CAC, or PIM with some modification have the potential for treating ovarian vein incompetence or internal iliac vein branch incompetence causing pelvic congestion syndrome. Varicose veins are already treated with foam sclerotherapy, but CAC can also theoretically be used, with perhaps some change in chemical structure.

Which NTNT technique is best? There is not one best technology. Many factors need to be considered: cost, reimbursement, vein specialist comfort with technique, patient's experience, and the unique clinical/anatomic scenario. One thing is clear: all NTNT technologies positively impact patients' QoL.

OVERALL SUMMARY

All new technologies and techniques undergo evolution from initial development, to early adopters, to general use. MOCA, CAC, and PIM are no exceptions. Techniques have been modified as more experience occurs. This new class of ablation will persist and grow. The removal of tumescence from endovenous procedures is a goal that is laudable for patients and treating-vein specialists. Any time a technique can be made simpler with equal or better results, everyone benefits.

The main challenge as of this writing is reimbursement for MOCA, CAC, and PIM. This story is familiar to all of us who began using the TT technologies of laser and radiofrequency in the early 2000s. If technologies show safety and efficacy and improve patients' lives, they ultimately are reimbursed. There is no question that this will follow for the NTNT group as well.

Once the reimbursement hurdle is overcome, this author feels that 80% to 85% of axial vein reflux will be treated by NTNT methods and 15% to 20% will require TT methods. The data does support a positive impact on patient's QoL for NTNT methods. They allow us to more than adequately treat superficial, axial disease. They enable us to safely help patients with vein disease. Any new technology needs to be held to the gold standard of helping patients and not just treating their veins. These technologies achieve this. For now, the future of endovenous ablation is the future of NTNT technologies. We await the next disruptive technology.

REFERENCES

1. Elias S. Emerging endovenous technologies. *Endovasc Today*, March 2014;42–46.
2. Van Eekeren R, Boersma D, deVries JP, et al. Update on endovenous treatment modalities for insufficient saphenous veins – a review of the literature. *Semin Vasc Surg.* 2014;27:117–135.
3. Siribumrungwong B, Noorit P, Wilarusmee C, et al. A systematic review and meta-analysis of randomized controlled trials comparing endovenous ablation and surgical intervention in patients with varicose vein. *Eur J Vasc Endovasc Surg.* 2012;44:214–223.
4. Almeida JI, Kaufman J, Gockeritz O, et al. Radifrequency endovenous ClosureFast versus laser ablation for the treatment of great saphenous reflux: a multicenter, single-blinded, randomized study (RECOVERY study). *J Vasc Interv Radiol.* 2009;20:752–759.
5. Biemans AAM, Kockaert M, Akkersdiijk GP, et al. Comparing endovenous laser ablation, foam sclerotherapy, and conventional surgery for great saphenous veins. *J Vasc Surg.* 2013;58:727–734.
6. Rasmussen LH, Lawaetz M, Bjoern L, et al. Randomized clinical trial comparing endovenous laser ablation, radiofrequency ablation, foam sclerotherapy and surgical stripping for great saphenous varicose veins with clinical and duplex outcome after 5 years. *J Vasc Surg.* 2013;58:421–426.
7. Gloviczki P, Comerota AJ, Dalsing MC, et al. The care of patients with varicose veins and associated chronic venous diseases: clinical practice guidelines of the Society for Vascular Surgery and the American Venous Forum. *J Vasc Surg.* 2011;53:2S–48S.
8. Marsden G, Perry MC, Kelly K, et al. NICE guidelines on the management of varicose veins. *BMJ.* 2013;347:f4279.

9. Tal MG, Dos Santos S, Marano JP, et al. Histologic findings after mechanochemical ablation in a caprine model with use of ClariVein. *J Vasc Surg Venous Lymphat Disord.* 2015;3:81–85.

10. Elias S, Raines JK. Mechanochemical tumescentless endovenous ablation: final results of the initial clinical trial. *Phlebology.* 2012;27:67–72.

11. Whiteley MS, et al. Mechanochemical ablation causes endothelial and medial damage to th vein wall resulting in deeper penetration of sclerosant compared with sclerotherapy alone in extrafascial great saphenous vein using an ex vivo model. *J Vasc Surg Venous Lymphat Disord.* 2017.

12. Boersma D, et al. Macroscopic and histologic vessel wall reaction after mechanochemical endovenous ablation using ClariVein OC device in an animal model. *Eur J Vasc Endovasc Surg.* 2017;53:290–298.

13. Elias S, Lam YL, Wittens CHA. Mechanochemical ablation: status and results. *Phlebology.* 2013;0:1–5.

14. Van Eekeren RR, Boersma D, Holewijn S, et al. Mechanochenical endovenous ablation for the treatment of great saphenous insufficiency. *J Vasc Surg Venous Lymphat Disord.* 2014;28:282–288.

15. Van Eekeren R, Boersma D, Elias S, et al. Endovenous mechanical ablation of great saphenous vein incompetence using the ClarVein device: a safety study. *J Endovasc Ther.* 2011;18:328–334.

16. Witte ME, van Eekeren EJP, Boersma, et al. Mechanical endovenous ablation for the treatment of great saphenous vein insufficiency. *J Vasc Surg Venous Lymphat Disord.* 2014;28:2–8.

17. Van Eekeren RR, Hillebrands JL, van der Sloot K, et al. Histological observations one year after mechanochemical endovenous ablation of the great saphenous vein. *J Endovasc Ther.* 2014;21:429–433.

18. Boersma D, van Eekeren RR, Werson DA, et al. Mechanochemical ablation of small saphenous vein insufficiency using the ClariVein device: one year results of a prospective series. *Eur J Vasc Endovasc Surg.* 2013;45:299–303.

19. Moore HM, Lane TR, Davies AH. Retrograde mechanochemical ablation of the small saphenous vein for the treatment of a venous ulcer. *Vascular.* 2014;5:375–377.

20. Van Eekeren RR, Boersma D, Konijn V, et al. Post operative pain and early quality of life after radiofrequency ablation and mechanochemical ablation of incompetent great saphenous veins. *J Vasc Surg.* 2013;57:445–450.

21. Bootun R, Lane T, Dharmarajah B, et al. Intraprocedural pain score in a randomized controlled trial comparing mechanochemical ablation to radiofrequency: the Multicentre Venefit versus ClariVein trial. *Phlebology.* 2016;31:61–65.

22. Lane T, Boontun R, Dharmarajah B, et al. A multicenter randomized controlled trial comparing radiofrequency and mechanical occlusion chemically assisted ablation of varicose veins – final results of the Venefit vs. ClariVein for varicose veins trial. *Phlebology.* 2017;32:89–98.

23. Boersma, et al. Morphologic and histologic vessel wall rection after mechanochemical endovenous ablation using ClariVein OC device in an animal model. *Eur J Vasc Endovasc Surg.* 2017;53:290–298.

24. Whiteley MS, et al. Mechanochemical ablation causes endothelial and medial damage to the vein wall resulting in deeper penetration of sclerosant compared with sclerotherapy alone in extrafascial saphenous vein using an ex vivo model. *J Vasc Surg Venous Lymphat Disord.* 2017.

25. Vinters HV, Galil KA, Lundie MJ, et al. The histotoxicity of cyanoacrylates: A selective review. *Neuroradiology.* 1985;27:279–291.

26. Almeida JI, Javier JJ, Mackay E, et al. First human use of cyanoacrylate adhesive for treatment of saphenous vein incompetence. *J Vasc Surg Venous Lymphat Disord.* 2013;1:174–180.

27. Almeida JI, Min RJ, Raabe R, et al. Cyanoacrylate adhesive for the closure of truncal veins: 60 day swine model results. *Vasc Endovasc Surg.* 2011;45:631–635.

28. Proebstle TM, Alm J, Dimitri S, et al. The European multicenter cohort study on cyanoacrylate embolization of refluxing great saphenous veins. *J Vasc Surg Venous Lymphat Disord.* 2015;3:2–7.

29. Morrison N, Gibson K, McEnroe S, et al. Randomised trial comparing cyanoacrylate embolization and radiofrequency ablation for incompetent great saphenous veins (VeClose). *J Vasc Surg Venous Lymphat Disord.* 2015;4:485–494.

30. Gibson K, Ferris B. Cyanoacrylate closure of incompetent great, small, and accessory saphenous veins without the use of post procedure compression: Initial outcomes of a post-market evaluation of the VenaSeal system (the WAVES Study). *Vascular.* 2016;25:149–156.

31. Kolluri R, et al. Roll-in phase analysis of clinical study of cyanoacrylate closure for incompetent great saphenous veins. *J Vasc Surg Venous Lymphat Disord.* 2016;4:407.

32. Koramaz I, El Kilic H, Gokalp F, et al. Ablation of the great saphenous vein with non-tumescent n-butyl cyanoacrylate versus endovenous laser therapy. *J Vasc Surg Venous Lymphat Disord.* 2017;5:210–213.

33. Ceulen RP, Sommer A, Vernooy K. Microembolism during foam sclerotherapy for varicose veins. *N Engl J Med.* 2008;359:656–657.

34. Carugo D, Ankrett DN, Zhao X, et al. Benefits of polidocanol endovenous microfoam (Varithena) compared with physician compounded foam. *Phlebology.* 2016;31:283–293.

35. Regan JD, Gibson KD, Rush JE, et al. Clinical significance of cerebrovasculargas emboli during polidocanolendovenous ultra-low nitrogenmicrofoam ablationand correlation with magnetic resonance imaging in patients with right-to-left shunt. *J Vasc Surg.* 2011;53:131–137.

36. Todd KL 3rd, Wright DI, Group V-I. Durability of treatment effect with polidocanol endovenous microfoam on varicose vein symptoms and appearance (VANISH-2). *J Vasc Surg Venous Lymphat Disord.* 2015;3(3):258.e1–264.e1.

37. Vasquez M, Gasparis A. A multicenter, randomized, placebo-controlled trial of endovenous thermal ablation with or without polidocanol endovenous microfoam treatment in patients with great saphenous vein incompetence and visible varicosities. *Phlebology.* 2017;32:272–281.

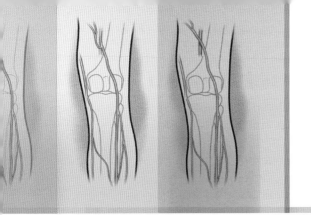

 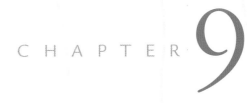

Treatment of Perforating Veins

Jose I. Almeida

HISTORICAL BACKGROUND

Although the role of perforator veins (PVs) in the development of signs and symptoms remains unclear, the number of incompetent PVs and the size of both competent and incompetent PVs have been shown to increase with worsening chronic venous disease (CVD).[1-4] Furthermore, it was recently reported that the duration of outward flow in these veins was longer in patients with ulcers compared with those in lower classes of CVD.[2]

Clinical practice guidelines of the Society for Vascular Surgery and the American Venous Forum (2014) recommend treatment of perforating veins with reflux greater than 500 ms and a vein diameter greater than 3.5 mm located near healed or active venous ulcers (clinical, etiology, anatomy, and pathophysiology [CEAP] class 5 and class 6). In contrast, these guidelines recommend against perforator treatment in CEAP class 1 and class 2 patients. The value of perforator treatment in CEAP class 3 and class 4 disease remains unclear.[5]

ETIOLOGY AND NATURAL HISTORY OF DISEASE

Reflux in PVs is defined as outward flow from the deep to the superficial veins. It has been suggested that high flow from the deep veins during muscular contraction eventually renders the PVs incompetent.[6] The etiology of venous reflux in superficial veins and PVs is unknown. The most predominant theory is that the weakening of the venous wall eventually leads to valve failure.[7] During early stages of the disease, reflux is most prevalent in the superficial veins.[8-10] Others have also suggested that reflux in the PVs is caused by volume overload at the reentry points of incompetent superficial veins.[11,12]

However, direct evidence for both theories is lacking because most investigations have been cross-sectional, population studies without sufficient longitudinal study regarding disease progression.

Labropoulos et al.[12] identified two other patterns by which previously competent PVs become incompetent; these were ascending development and new sites becoming incompetent. The ascending development of reflux into PVs from previously competent segments of superficial veins was more prevalent. A smaller number of incompetent PVs were detected in new locations that previously did not have reflux in any system. PV reflux was always associated with reflux in an adjacent superficial vein and underscores the important role of superficial vein reflux in the development of PV incompetence. Because most limbs in the early stages of CVD exhibit reflux in the superficial veins only, it can be assumed that one of the mechanisms for development of PV insufficiency involves the presence of reflux in an adjacent, superficial vein segment that acts as a capacitor for the refluxing PV. As local hemodynamic conditions change, and as intravenous pressure increases, the diameter of the PV increases, and the PV valve becomes incompetent. This may be in combination with, or separate from, primary venous wall disease.

Deep vein reflux is not required for development of PV incompetence in primary venous disease. Rather, deep vein reflux can develop as a result of increased flow from the incompetent superficial veins through the PV, the diameter of which has increased. Labropoulos et al.[12] showed that only five new incompetent PVs were seen in association with juxtaposed reflux in the deep vein. At all five sites, deep vein reflux was not present at the time of the initial duplex study when the adjacent PV was still competent; the deep venous incompetence developed simultaneously with PV incompetence. Superficial vein reflux was present at all sites.

Finally, this study also suggested that the development of reflux in previously normal PVs was seen in association with worsening of the clinical stage of CVD in 40% of limbs. Although the worsening of the clinical stage cannot be attributed to extension of reflux in the PVs alone, one can assume that the natural history of long-standing reflux in the superficial veins is that of progressive deterioration, with extension of reflux to other previously competent segments of the superficial veins and their associated PVs.[13]

PATIENT SELECTION

In general, PVs should be reserved for specific situations:
1. When they are found in continuity with the areas of axial (or neovascular) reflux in recurrent varicose vein cases
2. When found beneath an ankle ulcer
3. When there are large incompetent midthigh PVs serving as escape points and represent the highest point of reflux

ENDOVASCULAR INSTRUMENTATION

- For chemical ablation, a 25-gauge or 27-gauge needle is used under ultrasound guidance
- Radiofrequency (RF) catheters are dedicated devices and enter without sheath support
- A 16-gauge angiocath (for a 600-μm laser fiber) or a 21-gauge micropuncture needle (for a 400-μm laser fiber) can be used for laser ablation
- If the anatomy of the PV allows, a wire may be placed into the deep system for better control during access

OPERATIVE STEPS

Percutaneous ablation of perforators (PAPs) was coined by Elias and Peden.[13] The basic method involves: (1) ultrasound-guided intraluminal access; (2) introduction of some ablative element (chemical or thermal); (3) confirmation of initial treatment success; and (4) follow-up of treatment success. Thus far, the techniques used have been either chemical (sodium tetradecyl sulfate [STS], aethoxysklerol, or sodium morrhuate)[14,15] or thermal (RF or laser).[16–18]

After access is obtained, the thermal ablation device should be placed at, or just below, the fascia to minimize deep vessel and nerve injury. This is analogous to subfascial endoscopic perforator surgery (SEPS), where clips are placed just below the fascia level.

The patient is placed in a reverse Trendelenburg position to fully dilate the vein for access. After access, the various modalities differ in energy application. Therefore each technique is discussed separately so that key technical points can be elucidated.

Percutaneous Ablation of Perforators Technique: Chemical Ablation

Ultrasound-guided sclerotherapy (UGS) (Fig. 9.1) is an effective and durable method of eliminating incompetent PVs and results in significant reduction of symptoms and signs as determined by venous clinical scores. As an alternative to open interruption or SEPS, UGS may lead to fewer skin and wound-healing complications. Little has been published regarding the outcomes following UGS for PVs.

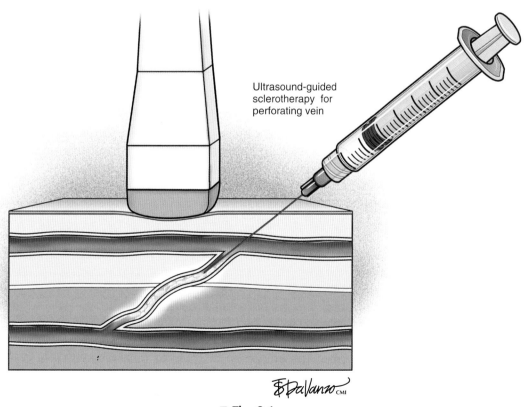

Ultrasound-guided sclerotherapy for perforating vein

■ **Fig. 9.1**

In a series by Masuda et al.,[14] patients primarily had isolated perforator disease (83%) without concomitant axial reflux from the thigh to the calf in the saphenous or deep systems. Clinical improvement following UGS was suggested by improvement of the Venous Clinical Severity Score (VCSS) and Venous Disease Severity (VDS) and lack of perforator recurrence with a mean follow-up of 20 months. In this study, successful obliteration of PVs with no recurrent symptoms was 75%. Perforator recurrence occurs particularly in those with ulcerations, and therefore surveillance duplex scanning after UGS and repeat injections may be needed. This study suggests that patients with perforator disease without axial reflux appear to benefit from injection sclerotherapy.

In 1992 Thibault and Lewis[18] reported their early experience with injection of incompetent PVs by using ultrasound guidance and showed that PVs remained successfully obliterated in 84% at 6 months after treatment. In 2000 at the Pacific Vascular Symposium in Hawaii, Jerome Guex[19] from France reported his experience with direct perforator treatment with ultrasound guidance. The sclerosing agent used was STS (Sotradecol) (3%) (Bioniche Life Sciences Inc., Belleville, Ontario, Canada) or polidocanol (3%) for veins larger than 4 mm, and a more-dilute solution was used for veins smaller than 4 mm. He estimated that 90% of PVs could be eliminated after one to three sessions of injections.

This method also involves ultrasound-guided access and confirmation with aspiration of blood. Many types of sclerosants have been used: sodium morrhuate, STS, and aethoxysklerol. Some advocates use the sclerosant in a liquid state. More recently, foam sclerotherapy has been advocated as being more efficacious. Most studies use STS 3% in the liquid form, injecting 0.5 to 1 mL of sclerosant or sodium morrhuate 5% in a similar manner, with care being taken not to inject the accompanying artery.[15,20] After infusion of the sclerosant, compression is applied with wraps or stockings and direct pressure over the treated PV.

Percutaneous Ablation of Perforators Technique Using the Radiofrequency System

Ultrasound-guided access can be made by needle, angiocath, or specialized probe. Confirmation of access with ultrasound visualization of the device intraluminally and aspiration of blood are the sine qua non of successful entry. The radiofrequency stylet (RFS) catheter (VNUS Medical, Inc.) also has the ability to measure impedance in ohms.

There are times when the device appears to be intraluminal by duplex imaging, but impedance readings indicate an extraluminal location. An impedance value between 150 and 350 ohms is indicative of intraluminal placement. If the RF device is in soft tissue, then higher values are registered. This feature complements ultrasound visualization. After attaining good placement and good location level relative to the fascia and the deep system, a small amount of tumescent anesthesia is infiltrated around the PV with ultrasound guidance. The patient is placed in the Trendelenburg position. Energy is then applied using a target temperature of 85°C, and pressure is applied with the overlying ultrasound transducer. These maneuvers, tumescence, pressure, and Trendelenburg, are done to exsanguinate the vein and improve device-to-vein wall contact.

The RF energy is applied to all four quadrants of the vein wall for 1 minute each. The catheter is then withdrawn 1 to 2 mm, and a second level of vein is treated. Theoretically, the longer the segment of the vein is treated, the better. After energy delivery, pressure is applied to compress the walls of the treated PV for 1 minute. Immediately posttreatment, a duplex scan should show no flow in the treated section of the PV, with normal flow in the deep-paired posterior tibial veins and arteries. If too much anesthetic is infiltrated into the tissues, the PV becomes very difficult to visualize.

Percutaneous Ablation of Perforators Technique Using the Laser System

As with RF, intraluminal access into the target PV is the key step. There are two methods of laser access: a 21-gauge micropuncture needle or a 16-gauge angiocath. A direct puncture is made using ultrasound guidance with the patient in the reverse Trendelenburg position. Intraluminal placement is confirmed by ultrasonography and aspiration of blood. If a micropuncture needle is used (21 gauge), a 400-μm fiber can be passed directly through the needle into the PV with ultrasound visualization and positioned at, or just below, the fascial level; this is similar to RF. If a 600-μm fiber is used, then a 16-gauge angiocath or the sheath from the micropuncture access kit is used (Figs. 9.2–9.5). A 600-μm fiber diameter is too large to traverse the 21-gauge micropuncture needle.

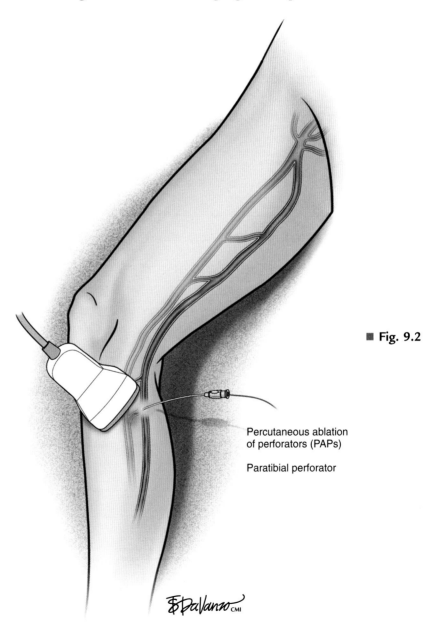

■ **Fig. 9.2**

Percutaneous ablation of perforators (PAPs)

Paratibial perforator

A

Continued

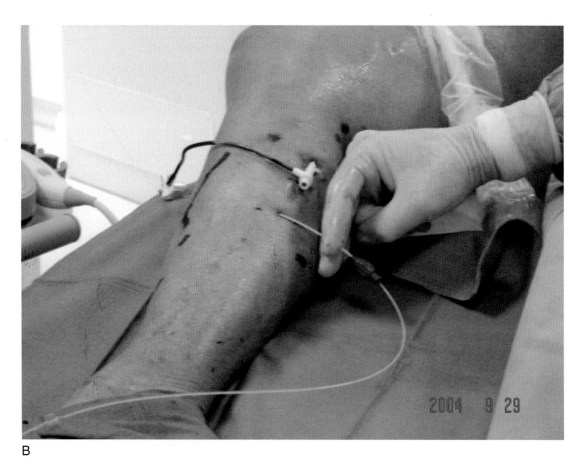

B

■ **Fig. 9.2, cont'd** (B) Percutaneous ablation of perforators: access to Boyd perforator vein (live).

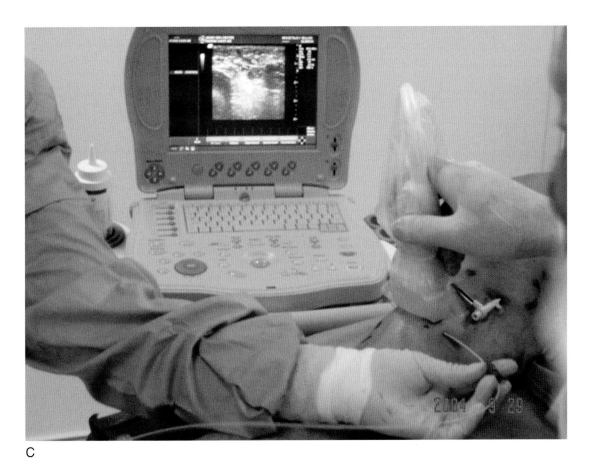

C

■ **Fig. 9.2, cont'd** (C) Percutaneous ablation of perforators: ultrasound-guided positioning of laser fiber tip at deep muscular fascia.

Tumescent anesthesia is infiltrated around the catheter, and the patient is placed in the Trendelenburg position. Energy is then applied to the segment, with pressure being applied with the ultrasound transducer to ensure fiber-to-vein wall contact. It is advisable to treat as long a segment as possible. Therefore areas approximately 1 to 2 mm apart should be treated as the fiber is withdrawn with a total of two or three segments.

Pulsed or continuous delivery methods of energy can be used. If pulsed, the laser is set for 15 W with a 4-second pulse interval during laser pullback. Each segment of vein is treated twice, thus administering 120 J to each segment; three segments are usually treated. At Miami Vein Center, we use 10 W in the continuous mode and deliver 60 to 80 J per cm (see Figs. 9.2–9.5). Often, we approach an ankle PV in a retrograde fashion (see Fig. 9.3).

■ Fig. 9.3

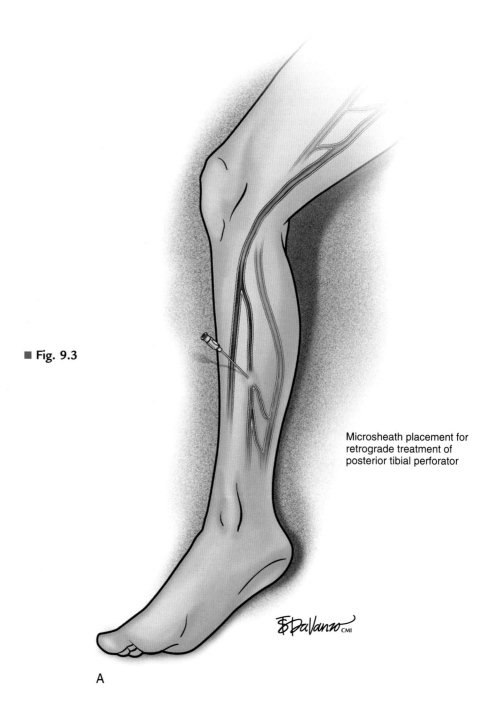

Microsheath placement for retrograde treatment of posterior tibial perforator

A

Proebstle and Herdemann[17] also attempt to treat three locations within the PV (just below the fascia, at the fascia level, and just above). Each treated segment receives between 60 and 100 J. After energy delivery, an eccentric pressure dressing is applied for 1 minute over the PV, as is done with RF. During wrapping, a pressure bandage is applied with direct pressure over each PV with a cotton ball or something similar. They reported on a total of 67 PVs treated with 1320 nm at 10 W (median of 250 J) or with 940 nm at 30 W (median of 290 J). With the exception of one vein, all others were occluded on postoperative day 1. Side effects were moderate. They concluded that ultrasound-guided endovenous laser ablation of incompetent PVs is safe and feasible.[17]

Text continued on p. 278

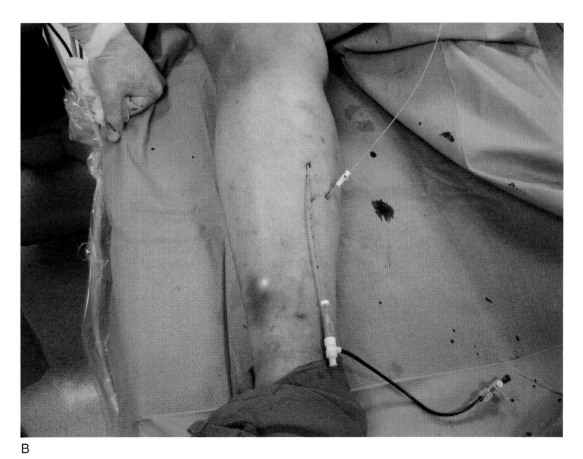

B

■ **Fig. 9.3, cont'd** (B) Retrograde approach to posterior tibial perforating vein (live).

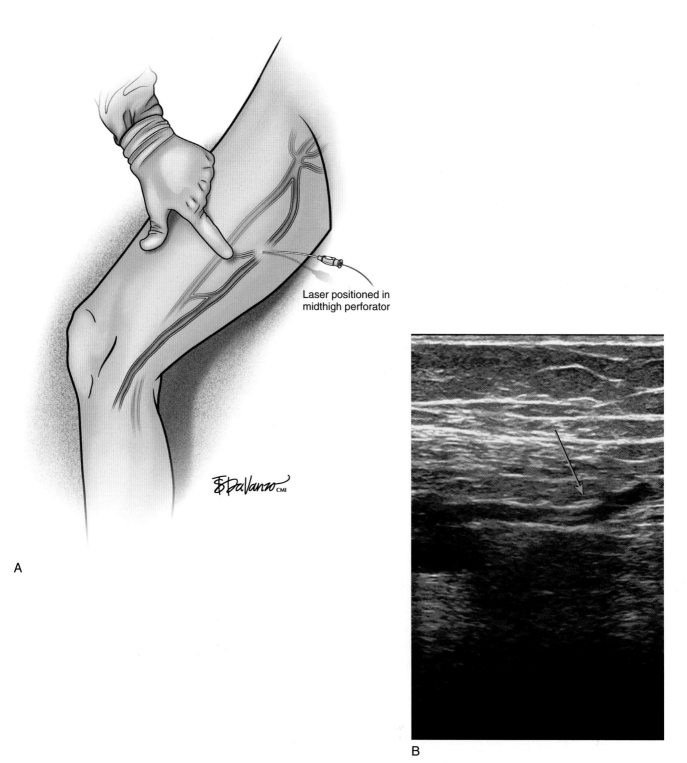

Laser positioned in
midthigh perforator

A

B

■ **Fig. 9.4** (B) Midthigh perforator vein ultrasound image.

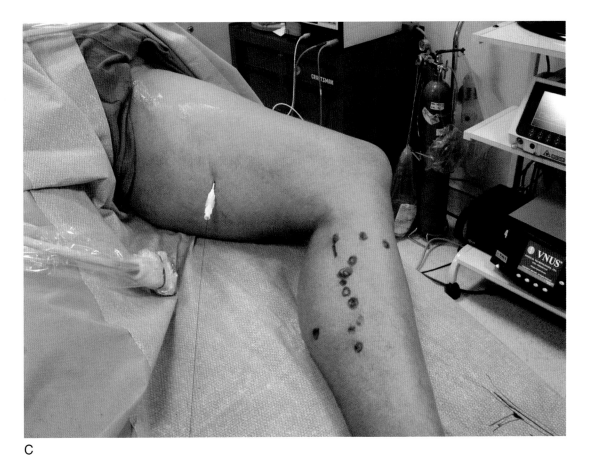

C

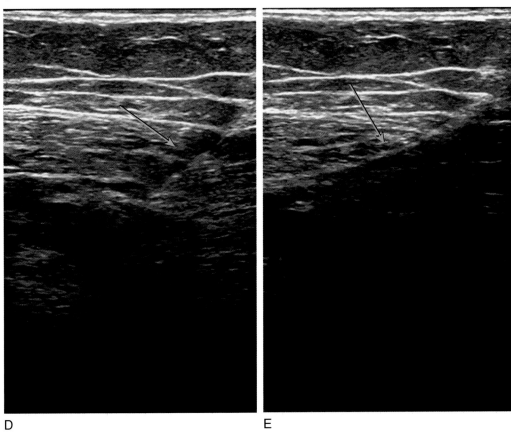

D   E

■ **Fig. 9.4, cont'd** (C) Percutaneous ablation of perforators: midthigh perforator vein (access). (D) Percutaneous ablation of perforators: percutaneous access with 21-gauge needle (ultrasound view). (E) Percutaneous ablation of perforators: midthigh perforator vein (microsheath placement–ultrasound view).

Continued

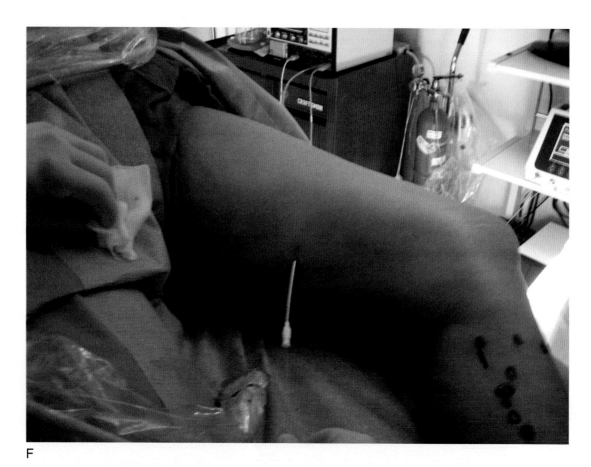

F

■ **Fig. 9.4, cont'd** (F) Laser pullback.

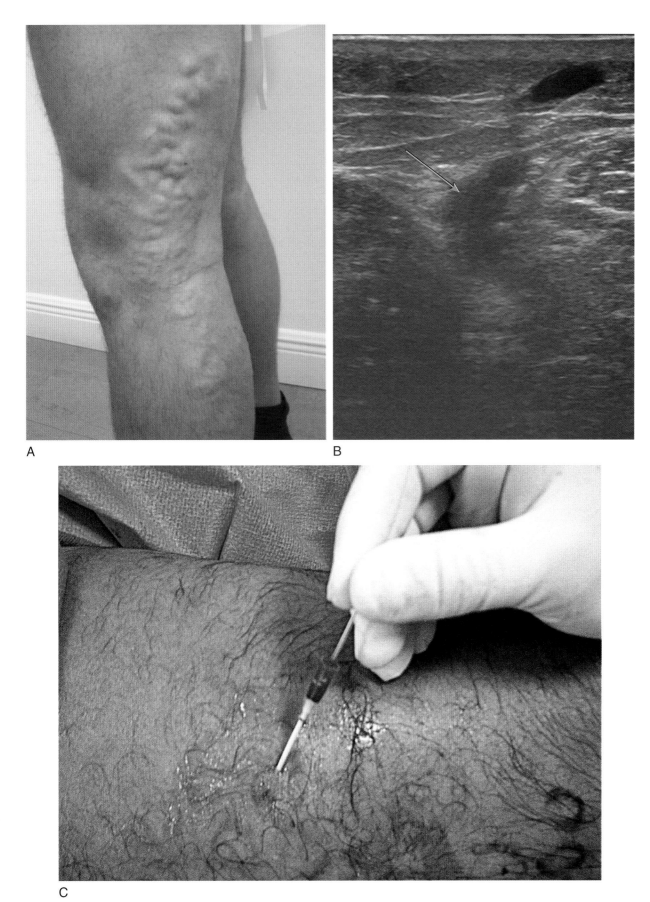

A

B

C

■ **Fig. 9.5** (A) Lateral thigh varicose veins originating from lateral thigh perforator vein. (B) Ultrasound view, lateral thigh perforator vein. (C) Percutaneous access to lateral thigh perforator vein.

Rarely, a small incision is made with the patient under local anesthesia to access larger-diameter PVs to ligate them (Fig. 9.6). Confirmation of occlusion is documented with duplex imaging, and patency of the deep vessels is also confirmed. The results have been quite good.

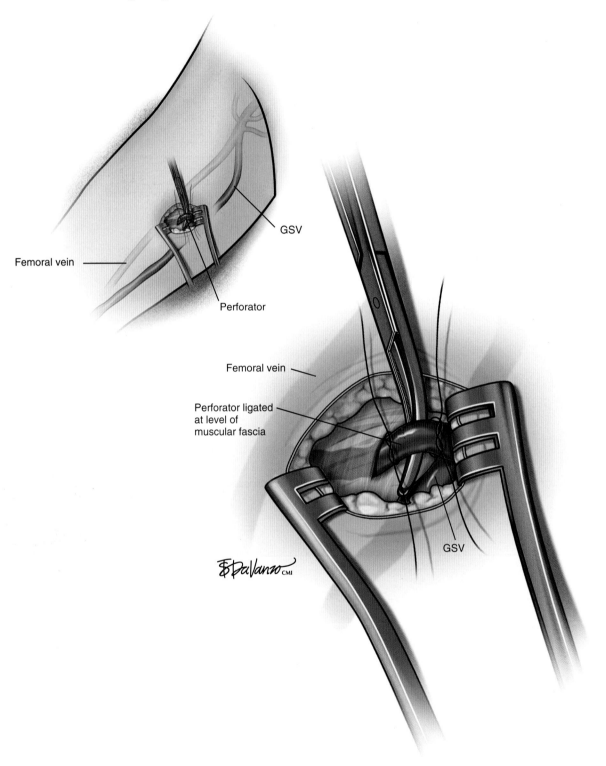

A

■ **Fig. 9.6**

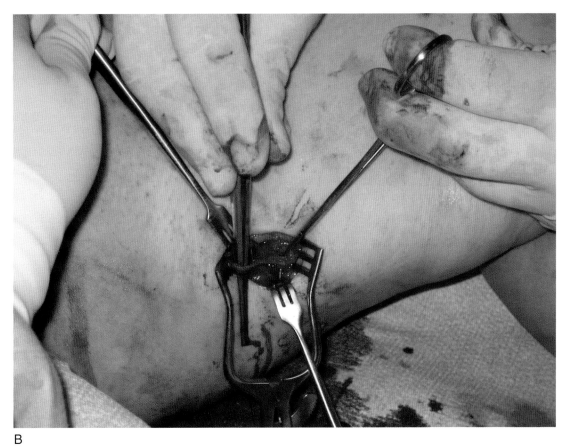

B

■ **Fig. 9.6, cont'd** Continued (B) Open ligation of midthigh perforator vein (live). *GSV*, Great saphenous vein.

PEARLS AND PITFALLS

The question still exists as to which PVs need treatment. Incompetent PVs are usually associated with superficial venous reflux, and therefore incompetent PVs may not require specific surgical interventions after saphenous truncal ablation. Some 90% of patients with C5 to C6 disease have incompetent PVs, whereas less than half of the patients with C2 disease have incompetent PVs. Therefore incompetent PVs are clearly associated with venous ulcers, and the question is whether these incompetent PVs have any hemodynamic significance, and whether they really contribute to the inflammatory changes in these limbs.[21]

COMPLICATIONS

Complications are rare. Wound complications, such as previously seen with the Linton procedure, are virtually nonexistent. Thromboembolic and nervous complications are rare with percutaneous techniques.

COMPARATIVE EFFECTIVENESS OF EXISTING TREATMENTS

In reference to the controversial topic of the role of PV incompetence causing nonhealing venous stasis ulcers, the Effect of Surgery and Compression on Healing and Recurrence (ESCHAR) trial[21] establishes a grade 1A recommendation that ligation and stripping of the great saphenous vein (GSV) are associated with the prevention of ulcer recurrence. More traditional methods, such as the Linton procedure and its modifications of open perforator ligation, have a relatively high incidence of wound complication ranging from 20% to 40%.[22–24] At present, there is no compelling level 1 evidence to provide a grade A recommendation that the treatment of incompetent PVs alone affects venous ulcer healing or recurrence.

Unfortunately, the treatment of incompetent PVs is blurred by concomitant treatment of GSV incompetence in the two randomized controlled trials (RCTs) that putatively explored the role of incompetent PV treatment.[25,26] Moreover, surrogate hemodynamic outcomes, which assess the treatment of incompetent PVs alone, as well as the effect of GSV treatment alone on perforator competence, also argue against the importance of treating incompetent PVs. This observation emphasizes the need for a properly designed trial in CEAP C5 and C6 patients. Based on the RCTs cited and the results of studies with surrogate endpoints of restoring perforator competence, the current role of incompetent PV treatment can be considered a grade 2B recommendation.

There is currently no established role for treatment of perforators in CEAP class 2 and class 3 patients; however, patients with venous ulcers should have consideration given to the treatment of pathologic perforators after superficial reflux and compression have failed. Thermal ablation has a technical success rate of 60% to 80%, with better occlusion rates when treatment is repeated. UGF sclerotherapy has a lower thrombosis rate but may be easier to perform and easier to close varicosities near the ulcer bed in addition to the feeding perforator. Successful closure of pathologic perforators with these technologies may improve ulcer healing and decrease recurrence. Studies with adequate power and proper design are needed to better define the role of PVs in ulcer healing and recurrence. Trials reporting the technical success of percutaneous perforator procedures are listed in Table 9.1, and the effects of perforator treatment on ulcer healing are depicted in Table 9.2.[27]

TABLE 9.1 Technical Success of Radiofrequency Ablation, Endovenous Laser Ablation, and Ultrasound-Guided Foam Sclerotherapy

Primary Author (Year)	Perforator Treatment Modality	Patients/ Procedures (N)	Mean Follow-Up (Months)	Method and Timing of Evaluating Procedure Success	Overall Success Rate (%)
Rueda[28] (2013)	RFA and SEPS	64	37	DUS, 1 week	100
Kiguchi[29] (2014)	UGFS	62	30	DUS, 2 weeks	54
Harlander-Locke[30] (2012)	RFA	20/28	25	DUS, 48–72 hours	96
Harlander-Locke[31] (2012)	RFA	88/140	12	DUS, 48–72 hours	82
Dumantepe[32] (2012)	EVLA	13/23	14	DUS, 12 months	87
Köroglu[33] (2011)	EVLA and UGFS	24	6	DUS, 24 hours	75
Lawrence[34] (2011)	RFA	45/51	13	DUS, 48–72 hours	71
Corcos[35] (2011)	EVLA	303/534	28	DUS; mean, 28 months	72
Nelzén[36] (2011)	SEPS	37	12	DUS, 6–9 months	87
Hissink[37] (2010)	EVLA	28/33	3	DUS, 3 months	78
Marrocco[38] (2010)	RFA	241	5	DUS, 1-7 days	100
Marsh[39] (2010)	RFA	53	14	DUS; mean, 14 months	82
van den Bos[40] (2009)	RFA	12/14/17	3	DUS, 3 months	64
Hingorani[41] (2009)	RFA	38/48	2	DUS, 3–7 days	88
Bacon[42] (2009)	RFA	37	60	DUS, 5 years	81

DUS, Duplex ultrasound; *EVLA,* endovenous laser ablation; *RFA,* radiofrequency ablation; *SEPS,* subfascial endoscopic perforator surgery; *UGFS,* ultrasound-guided foam sclerotherapy.

A MEDLINE search using the keywords *vein perforator surgery, perforator obliteration, perforator ablation, endovenous perforator ablation, subfascial endoscopic perforator surgery,* and *perforator ligation* yielded a total of 109 publications, excluding case reports or case series that contained only one patient with perforator treatment. Of the 109 studies in which radiofrequency, laser, foam sclerotherapy, or subfascial endoscopic perforator surgery was used for perforator treatment, 15 were published between January 1, 2009, and January 1, 2014, and included outcomes of perforator treatment technical success that was objectively confirmed through imaging modalities performed by an independent investigator or vascular laboratory specialist.

All percentages have been rounded to the nearest percentile.

(From Dillavou ED, Harlander-Locke M, Nicos Labropoulos N. Current state of the treatment of perforating veins. *J Vasc Surg Venous Lymphat Disord.* 2016;4:131-135.)

TABLE 9.2 Effects of Perforator Treatment on Ulcer Healing and Recurrence

Primary Author (Year)	Perforator Treatment Modality	Patients/ Procedures (N)	Mean Follow-Up (Months)	Outcomes, (%)	
				Ulcer Healing	Ulcer Recurrence
Alden[43] (2013)	UGFS	86	12	78	23
Rueda[28] (2013)	RFA and SEPS	64	37	92	20
Abdul-Haqq[44] (2013)	EVLA	17	2.5	71	0
Bush[45] (2013)	UGFS	35	4	100	
Kiguchi[29] (2014)	UGFS	62	34	52	
Harlander-Locke[30] (2012)	RFA	20/28	25		5
Harlander-Locke[31] (2012)	RFA	88/140	12	76	
Dumantepe[32] (2012)	EVLA	13/23	6	80	
Lawrence[34] (2011)	RFA	45/51	13	90	4
Hissink[37] (2010)	EVLA	28/33 limbs	3	80	
Marrocco[38] (2010)	RFA	24	5	84	16
Marsh[39] (2010)	RFA	53	14	100	0
Hingorani[41] (2009)	RFA	38/48	2	63	

EVLA, Endovenous laser ablation; *RFA*, radiofrequency ablation; *SEPS*, subfascial endoscopic perforator surgery; *UGFS*, ultrasound-guided foam sclerotherapy.

A MEDLINE search using the keywords *vein perforator surgery, perforator obliteration, perforator ablation, endovenous perforator ablation, subfascial endoscopic perforator surgery,* and *perforator ligation* yielded a total of 109 publications, excluding case reports or case series that contained only one patient with perforator treatment. Of the 109 studies in which radiofrequency, laser, foam sclerotherapy, or subfascial endoscopic perforator surgery was used for perforator treatment, 13 were published between January 1, 2009, and January 1, 2014, and included objective end points of ulcer healing or ulcer recurrence.

All percentages have been rounded to the nearest percentile.

(From Dillavou ED, Harlander-Locke M, Nicos Labropoulos N. Current state of the treatment of perforating veins. *J Vasc Surg Venous Lymphat Disord.* 2016;4:131-135.)

REFERENCES

1. Pascarella L, Schmid Schonbein GW. Causes of telangiectasias, reticular veins and varicose veins. *Semin Vasc Surg.* 2005;18:2–4.
2. Labropoulos N, Mansour MA, Kang SS, et al. New insights into perforator vein incompetence. *Eur J Vasc Endovasc Surg.* 1999;18:228–234.
3. Lees TA, Lambert D. Patterns of venous reflux in limbs with skin changes associated with chronic venous insufficiency. *Br J Surg.* 1993;80:725–728.
4. Pierik EG, Wittens CH, van Urk H. Subfascial endoscopic ligation in the treatment of incompetent perforating veins. *Eur J Vasc Endovasc Surg.* 1995;9:38–41.
5. O'Donnell TF, Passman MA, Marston WA, et al. Management of venous leg ulcers: clinical practice guidelines of the Society for Vascular Surgery and the American Venous Forum. *J Vasc Surg.* 2014;60(suppl):3S–59S.
6. Cockett FB, Elgan-Jones DE. The ankle blow-out syndrome. *Lancet.* 1953;1:17–23.
7. Kistner RL, Eklof B, Masuda EM. Diagnosis of chronic venous disease of the lower extremities: the "CEAP" classification. *Mayo Clin Proc.* 1996;71:338–345.
8. Labropoulos N. CEAP in clinical practice. *Vasc Surg.* 1997;31:224–225.

9. Labropoulos N, Delis K, Nicolaides AN, et al. The role of the distribution and anatomic extent of reflux in the development of signs and symptoms in chronic venous insufficiency. *J Vasc Surg.* 1996;23:504–510.

10. Delis K. Leg perforator vein incompetence: functional anatomy. *Radiology.* 2005;235:327–334.

11. Zamboni P. Pathophysiology of perforators in primary chronic venous insufficiency. *World J Surg.* 2005;29(suppl 1):S115–S118.

12. Labropoulos N, Tassiopoulos AK, Bhatti AF, et al. Development of reflux in the perforator veins in limbs with primary venous disease. *J Vasc Surg.* 2006;43:558–562.

13. Elias S, Peden E. Ultrasound-guided percutaneous ablation for the treatment of perforating vein incompetence. *Vascular.* 2007;15:281–289.

14. Masuda EM, Kessler DM, Lurie F, et al. The effect of ultrasound-guided sclerotherapy of incompetent perforator veins on venous clinical severity and disability scores. *J Vasc Surg.* 2006;43:551–557.

15. Guex JJ. Ultrasound guided sclerotherapy (UGS) for perforating veins (PV). *Hawaii Med J.* 2000;59:261–262.

16. Peden E, Lumsden A. Radiofrequency ablation of incompetent perforator veins. *Perspect Vasc Surg Endovasc Ther.* 2007;19:73–77.

17. Proebstle TM, Herdemann S. Early results and feasibility of incompetent perforator vein ablation by endovenous laser treatment. *Dermatol Surg.* 2007;33:162–168.

18. Thibault PK, Lewis WA. Recurrent varicose veins. Part 2: injection of incompetent perforating veins using ultrasound guidance. *J Dermatol Surg Oncol.* 1992;18:895–900.

19. Guex JJ. Ultrasound guided sclerotherapy (USGS) for perforating veins (PV). *J Vasc Surg.* 2000;31:1307–1312.

20. Stuart WP, Lee AJ, Allan PL, et al. Most incompetent calf perforating veins are found in association with superficial venous reflux. *J Vasc Surg.* 2001;34:774–778.

21. Barwell JR, Davies CE, Deacon J, et al. Comparison of surgery and compression with compression alone in chronic venous ulceration (ESCHAR study): randomized controlled trial. *Lancet.* 2004;363:1854–1859.

22. Sato DT, Goff CD, Gregory RT, et al. Subfascial perforator vein ablation: comparison of open versus endoscopic techniques. *J Endovasc Surg.* 1999;6:147–154.

23. Pierik EG, Van Urk H, Hop WC, et al. Endoscopic versus open subfascial division of incompetent perforating veins in the treatment of leg ulceration: a randomized trial. *J Vasc Surg.* 1997;26:1049–1054.

24. Stacey MC, Burnand KG, Layer GT, et al. Calf pump function in patients with healed venous ulcers is not improved by surgery to the communicating veins or by elastic stockings. *Br J Surg.* 1988;75:436–439.

25. van Gent WB, Hop WC, van Pragg MC, et al. Conservative versus surgical treatment of venous leg ulcers: a prospective, randomized, multicenter trial. *J Vasc Surg.* 2006;44:563–571.

26. O'Donnell TF. The present status of surgery of the superficial venous system in the management of venous ulcer and the evidence for the role of perforator interruption. *J Vasc Surg.* 2008;48:1044–1052.

27. Dillavou ED, Harlander-Locke M, Labropoulos N, et al. Current state of the treatment of perforating veins. *J Vasc Surg Venous Lymphat Disord.* 2016;4(1):131–135.

28. Rueda CA, Bittenbinder EN, Buckley CJ, et al. The management of chronic venous insufficiency with ulceration: the role of minimally invasive perforator interruption. *Ann Vasc Surg.* 2013;27:89–95.

29. Kiguchi MM, Hager ES, Winger DG, et al. Factors that influence perforator thrombosis and predict healing: perforator sclerotherapy for venous ulceration without axial reflux. *J Vasc Surg.* 2014;59:1368–1376.

30. Harlander-Locke M, Lawrence P, Jimenez JC, et al. Combined treatment with compression therapy and ablation of incompetent superficial and perforating veins reduces ulcer recurrence in patients with CEAP 5 venous disease. *J Vasc Surg.* 2012;55:446–450.

31. Harlander-Locke M, Lawrence PF, Alktaifi A, et al. The impact of ablation of incompetent superficial and perforator veins on ulcer healing rates. *J Vasc Surg.* 2012;55:458–464.

32. Dumantepe M, Tarhan A, Yurdakul I, et al. Endovenous laser ablation of incompetent perforating veins with 1470 nm, 400 mm radial fiber. *Photomed Laser Surg.* 2012;30:672–677.

33. Köroglu M, Eris HN, Aktas AR, et al. Endovenous laser ablation and foam sclerotherapy for varicose veins: does the presence of perforating vein insufficiency affect the treatment outcome? *Acta Radiol.* 2011;52:278–284.

34. Lawrence PF, Alktaifi A, Rigberg D, et al. Endovenous ablation of incompetent perforating veins is effective treatment for recalcitrant venous ulcers. *J Vasc Surg.* 2011;54:737–742.

35. Corcos L, Pontello D, De Anna D, et al. Endovenous 808-nm diode laser occlusion of perforating veins and varicose collaterals: a prospective study of 482 limbs. *Dermatol Surg.* 2011;37:1486–1498.

36. Nelzén O, Fransson I; Swedish SEPS Study Group. Early results from a randomized trial of saphenous surgery with or without subfascial endoscopic perforator surgery in patients with a venous ulcer. *Br J Surg.* 2011;93:495–500.

37. Hissink RJ, Bruins RM, Erkens R, et al. Innovative treatments in chronic venous insufficiency: endovenous laser ablation of perforating veins a prospective short-term analysis of 58 cases. *Eur J Vasc Endovasc Surg.* 2010;40:403–406.

38. Marrocco CJ, Atkins MD, Bohannon WT, et al. Endovenous ablation for the treatment of chronic venous insufficiency and venous ulcerations. *World J Surg.* 2010;34:2299–2304.

39. Marsh P, Price BA, Holdsotck JM, et al. One year outcomes of radiofrequency ablation of incompetent perforator veins using the radiofrequency stylet device. *Phlebology.* 2010;25: 79–84.

40. van den Bos RR, Wentel T, Neumann MHA, et al. Treatment of incompetent perforating veins using the radiofrequency ablation stylet: a pilot study. *Phlebology.* 2009;24:208–212.

41. Hingorani AP, Ascher E, Marks N, et al. Predictive factors of success following radio-frequency stylet (RFS) ablation of incompetent perforating veins (IPV). *J Vasc Surg.* 2009;50:844–848.

42. Bacon JL, Dinneen AJ, Marsh P, et al. Five-year results of incompetent perforator vein closure using TRans-Luminal Occlusion of Perforator. *Phlebology.* 2009;24:74–78.

43. Alden PB, Lips EM, Zimmerman KP, et al. Chronic venous ulcer: minimally invasive treatment of superficial axial and perforator vein reflux speeds healing and reduces recurrence. *Ann Vasc Surg.* 2013;27:75–83.

44. Abdul-Haqq R, Almaroof B, Chen BL, et al. Endovenous laser ablation of great saphenous vein and perforator veins improves venous stasis ulcer healing. *Ann Vasc Surg.* 2013;27: 932–939.

45. Bush R, Bush P. Percutaneous foam sclerotherapy for venous leg ulcers. *J Wound Care.* 2013;22(suppl 10):S20–S22.

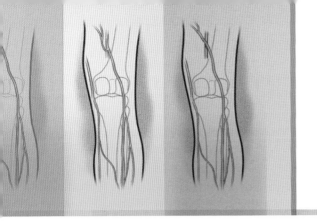

CHAPTER 10

Treatment of Varicosed Tributary Veins

Jose I. Almeida

HISTORICAL BACKGROUND

Ambulatory phlebectomy (AP) is a minor surgical procedure designed to remove varicose vein clusters located close to the skin surface. Originally performed in ancient Rome, the technique was published by Robert Muller in 1966.[1] In many office-based, venous surgery practices in the United States, AP is performed with the use of local tumescent anesthesia. The six basic features of the technique are as follows:

1. Absence of venous ligatures
2. Exclusive use of local infiltration anesthesia
3. Immediate ambulation after surgery
4. Incisions of 2 mm
5. Absence of skin sutures
6. Postoperative compression bandage kept in place for 2 days, then replaced with daytime compression stockings for 3 weeks

Complete surgical removal of varicose veins may be achieved in a single session or in separate sessions. Endovenous ablation and AP are suitable for the office and, in the author's practice, are routinely performed together. All procedures are guided with duplex ultrasound to get a "roadmap underneath the skin." The advantage of this combination technique is that patients can expect all varicose veins to disappear after a 1-hour procedure.

ETIOLOGY AND NATURAL HISTORY OF DISEASE

Bulging varicose veins on the surface of the skin can originate from diverse sources. Identification of these sources is important because the source influences the treatment plan. Varicosities on the medial aspect of the thigh and calf are usually the result of great saphenous vein (GSV) incompetence. To minimize the chance for recurrence, the incompetent GSV must be eliminated from the circulation. This concept has been substantiated in several prospective randomized clinical trials involving patients who were treated with or without saphenectomy by conventional vein stripping.[2-5] The recurrence rates for limbs without saphenectomy were much higher than those for limbs with saphenectomy. Of course, now thermal ablation techniques, with either radiofrequency or laser, have proved to be the methods of choice for eliminating the GSV from the circulation.[6,7]

Varicosities on the anterior thigh usually result from anterior, accessory saphenous vein incompetence. These veins usually course over the knee and into the lower leg. Small saphenous vein (SSV) reflux produces varicosities on the posterior calf. When also present on the posterior thigh, the surgeon must consider a cranial extension of the SSV, which can be identified with duplex ultrasound imaging. Cranial extensions may enter the GSV (Giacomini vein) or enter the femoral vein directly.

In cases where no "feeding source" is found, phlebectomy of the varicosities may be all that is required. Labropoulos et al.[8] have shown that varicose veins may result from a primary vein wall defect and that reflux may be confined to superficial tributaries throughout the lower limb. Without great and small saphenous trunk incompetence, perforator and deep vein incompetence, or proximal obstruction, their data suggest that reflux can develop in any vein without an apparent feeding source. This is often the case when bulging reticular veins are seen along the course of the lateral leg. This lateral subdermic complex and its vein of Albanese are often dilated and bulging in elderly patients. The underlying source of venous hypertension is usually perigeniculate, perforating veins, not easily identifiable with duplex imaging. AP using an 18-gauge needle stab incision and a small crochet hook for exteriorization of the vein is an excellent procedure for this clinical problem.

PATIENT SELECTION

AP is indicated for the removal of varicosed venous tributaries when visible and palpable on the surface of the skin. AP is simple to perform and well tolerated and can be used in conjunction with other treatment modalities. As stated earlier, it is critical to recognize that bulging veins are usually associated with an underlying source of venous hypertension, and treatment of the source is as important as the vein removal. Before AP, the treating physician must perform a thorough evaluation with duplex ultrasound imaging to determine whether a source is present for venous hypertension. The source of venous hypertension should be eliminated before, or in conjunction with, AP.

Before placing the patient in the supine position on the operating table, the veins of interest must be marked in the standing position with an indelible marker. This is critical. Marking is performed in the standing position because hydrostatic pressure is elevated, and the pressurized veins become visible and palpable. Bulging veins literally disappear when patients lie supine because the venous pressure drops to near 0 mm Hg. Without the marking, the surgeon will surely leave disease behind, which of course will result in an unsatisfied patient.

ENDOVASCULAR INSTRUMENTATION

AP is not truly endovascular in the purist sense; rather, it is an adjunct to an endovascular procedure. The following are tools needed to perform AP:
1. Tumescent anesthesia
2. Small blade (or needle)
3. Hook
4. Hemostat

IMAGING

We prefer mapping these veins using visual inspection and palpation; other investigators might prefer transillumination mapping using specialized vein lights.[9] Ultrasound-guided vein hooking is useful for deeper veins.

HEMOSTASIS AND ANTICOAGULATION

Avulsion of venous segments treated by AP is relatively hemostatic when tumescent anesthesia with epinephrine is used. Hemostasis is augmented by applying gentle pressure over the incision site. The epinephrine in the anesthetic preparation enhances the hemostasis process through vasoconstriction. When extracting larger veins with the stab-avulsion technique, significant force may be required, and some minor bleeding may be encountered. Placing the patient in the Trendelenburg position may also reduce venous pressure and help control bleeding if there is more than usual.

Klein[10] has shown through clinical studies that a dose of 35 mg per kg of dilute lidocaine solution is well tolerated and safe. Infiltrating solutions should contain epinephrine in appropriate concentrations to induce vasoconstriction and more gradual absorption of lidocaine into the bloodstream.

Infections are rare after liposuction and venous procedures with tumescent anesthesia and are usually confined to the incision site.[11] The reason for the low rate of infection is not clear, although there are reports of lidocaine concentration–dependent bacteriostatic and bactericidal activity. Pathogens commonly found on the skin may be sensitive to this activity.[12]

Careful application of the postoperative dressing cannot be overstated because improper dressing placement can lead to bleeding and hematoma, blistering, nerve injury, and ischemia. The limb is wrapped circumferentially from foot to groin with a bulky compression dressing that is removed after 48 hours. The dressing should be applied with graduated pressure; the amount of pressure should decrease as one proceeds from foot to groin. It is critical to place extra padding over the lateral fibular head to avoid pressure-induced injury to the deep and superficial peroneal nerves.

Deep peroneal nerve injury is quite serious because it is a motor nerve. A patient who develops a foot drop after venous surgery will be impaired and have a decreased quality of life—a common source of litigation.

All patients are encouraged to ambulate immediately after the procedure to minimize thromboembolic complications.

OPERATIVE STEPS

Tumescent anesthesia (Fig. 10.1) allows large areas of the body to be anesthetized with minimal effect on intravascular fluid status, avoidance of general anesthesia, and short postoperative recovery. Tumescent anesthesia provides a safe, easy-to-administer technique for use with AP. The technique of tumescent anesthesia involves infiltration of the

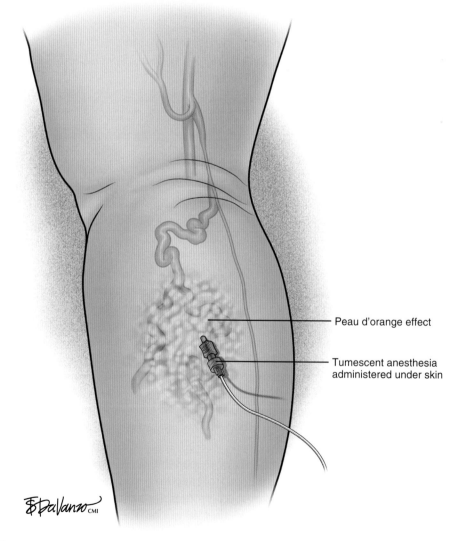

Peau d'orange effect

Tumescent anesthesia administered under skin

A

■ **Fig. 10.1**

subdermal compartment with generous volumes of a 0.1% solution of lidocaine with epinephrine. The anesthetic preparation is administered subdermally under pressure. The doctor pushes the fluid until a characteristic peau-d'orange effect is visualized on the skin. The tumescent fluid hydrodissects the subcutaneous fat from the venous tissue as it enters, thus facilitating vein extraction afterward.

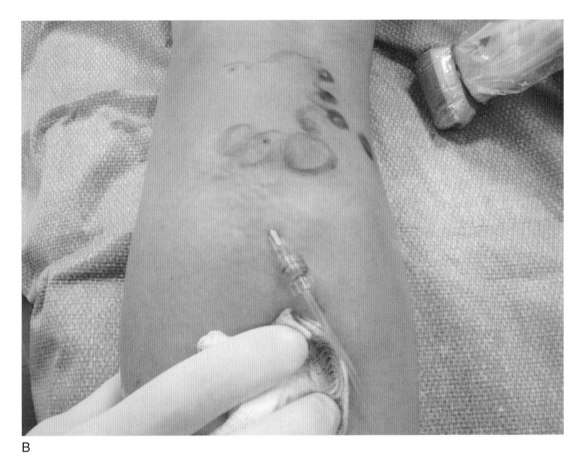

B

■ Fig. 10.1, cont'd

The most popular instruments for creating incisions (Figs. 10.2 and 10.3) are no. 11 scalpel blades, 18-gauge needles, and 15-degree ophthalmologic Beaver blades. Incision length should correspond to vein size but is usually in the range of 1 to 3 mm. The author removes small varicose veins through an 18-gauge needle hole, whereas larger veins require slightly larger incisions made with a no. 11 scalpel blade.

Widening of incisions with a hemostat is tempting but should be avoided because this traumatizes wound margins and may lead to increased pigmentation in the

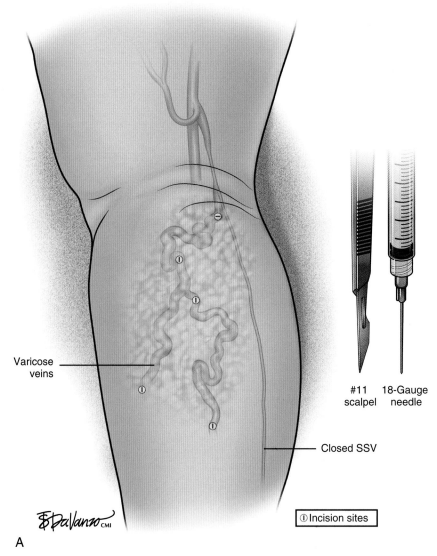

Varicose veins

#11 scalpel   18-Gauge needle

Closed SSV

① Incision sites

A

■ **Fig. 10.2** *SSV*, Small saphenous vein.

postoperative scar. There have been anecdotal reports of tattooing the skin when the incision is placed through the indelible ink mark made preoperatively, which is why many operators mark the veins preoperatively with a circle and incise inside the inkless area.

The incisions are oriented vertically because this allows wound edges to close solely with the force of a circumferentially placed compression dressing. That is, the dressing approximates the wound edges without the need for sutures or adhesive tapes. Horizontal incisions are preferred around Langer's lines at the knees and ankles.

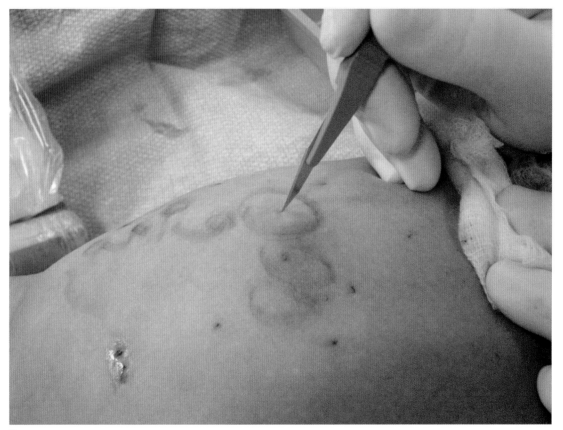

B

■ **Fig. 10.2, cont'd**

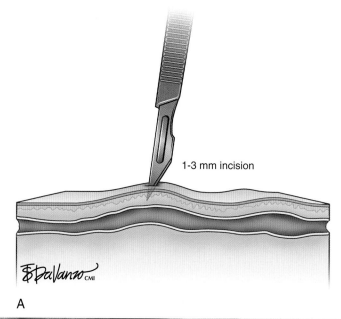

1-3 mm incision

A

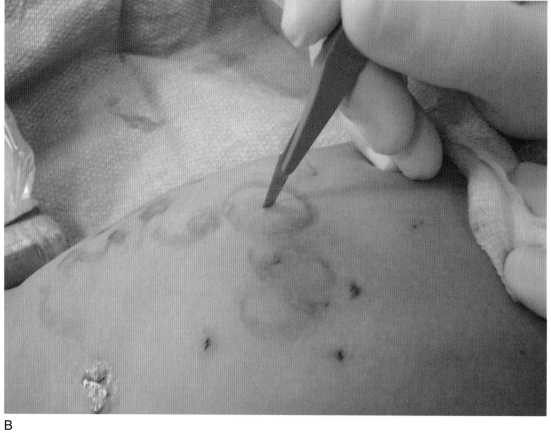

B

■ **Fig. 10.3**

Hooking the target vein (Fig. 10.4) through the small incision is the next step. There are multiple instruments available. Some are medical, and others are manufactured for crochet. The latest available device is disposable and mounts the blade and hook on the same instrument.

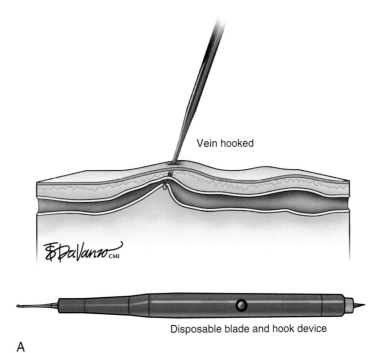

A

B

■ **Fig. 10.4**

Using a hook of choice, the vein is exteriorized from the wound. Hooks need not be introduced into the wound deeper than 2 to 3 mm, and they should be inserted gently and deliberately to avoid unnecessary trauma to the wound margins. Gentle probing and searching for the target vein with the hook are routinely necessary and should be done with great care. Once a segment of vein is exteriorized from the wound,

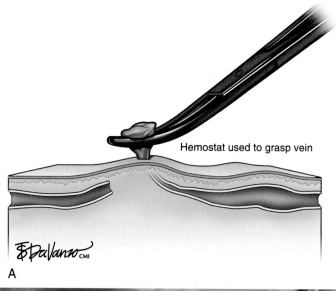

Hemostat used to grasp vein

A

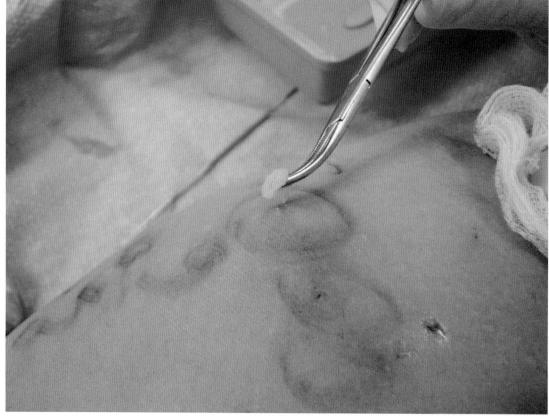

B

■ **Fig. 10.5**

it is grasped with fine hemostatic clamps (Fig. 10.5). With the use of gentle traction in a circular motion, the vein is teased out of the wound (Fig. 10.6).

With experience, one learns to distinguish between the vein wall, which is elastic, and the connective perivenous tissue, which is not elastic. Dissection of the vein from its perivenous investments greatly facilitates its extraction. Perivenous tissue issuing from

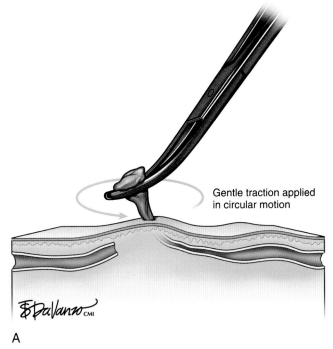

Gentle traction applied in circular motion

A

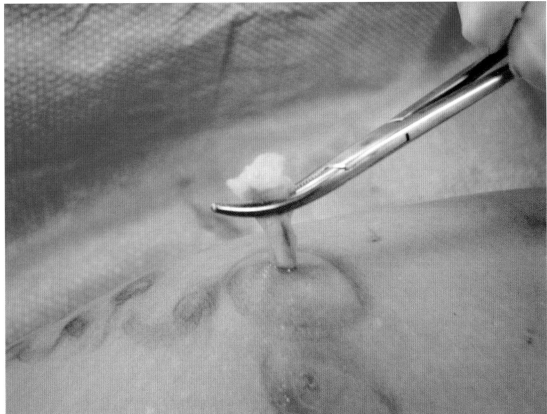

B

■ **Fig. 10.6**

the wound is excised at the skin level. This tissue should never be forcefully pulled out of the wound.

When traction is applied to the vein, the skin juxtaposed to the incision site will momentarily depress downward. Attention to this detail gives the operator an idea of where to place the next incision. The depression represents the point at which the vein will avulse. The next incision is made near the area of depressed skin, and the process is repeated sequentially until all the venous bulges have been addressed. Although all bulges should be marked preoperatively, not all the marks need to be incised if the operator takes care in identifying the skin depressions described earlier. It is very rewarding when a large segment is removed from a single site (Fig. 10.7). On balance,

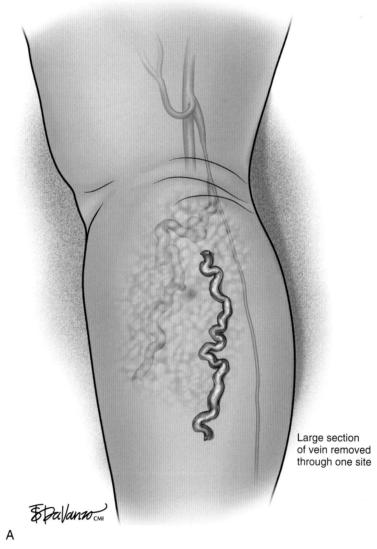

Large section
of vein removed
through one site

A

■ **Fig. 10.7**

in some cases, only small fragments of varicose veins are encountered, which can make the operation quite tedious; this frequently cannot be avoided.

If vein exteriorization proves difficult, it is better to make larger incisions rather than induce ischemia at the wound edges from excessive stretching. For the number of incisions to be reduced, the incisions should be made one at a time (Fig. 10.8). If avulsion proves difficult and the vein breaks, it is more convenient to make more incisions than to waste time trying to retrieve more vein from the same incision (Fig. 10.9).

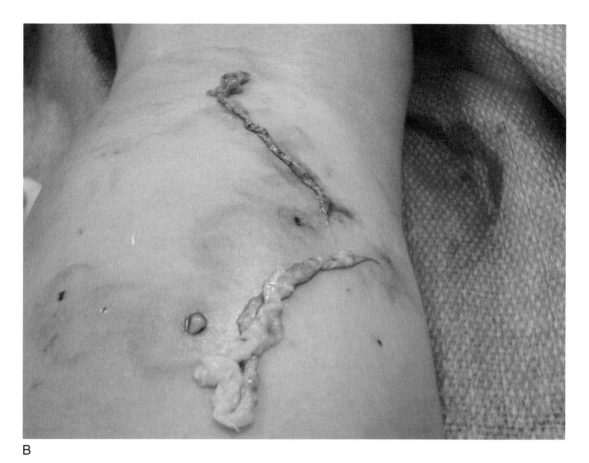

B

■ **Fig. 10.7, cont'd**

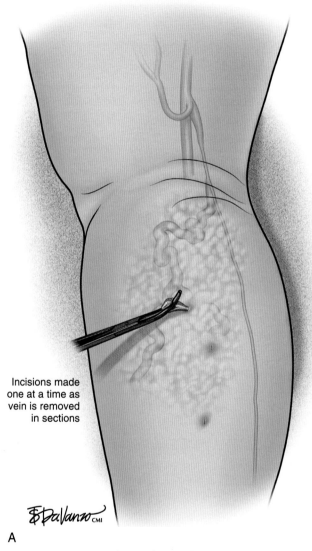

Incisions made
one at a time as
vein is removed
in sections

A

■ Fig. 10.8

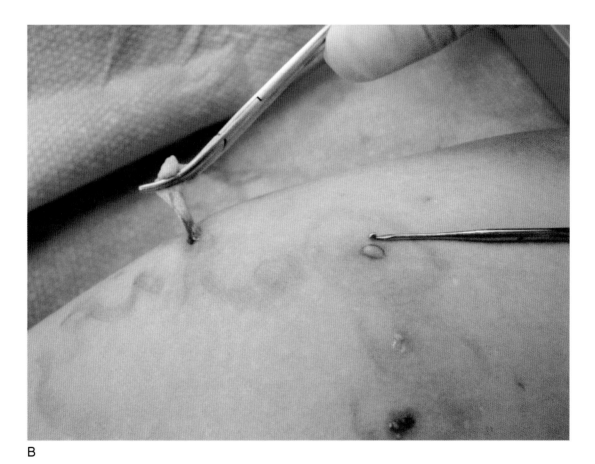

B

■ **Fig. 10.8, cont'd**

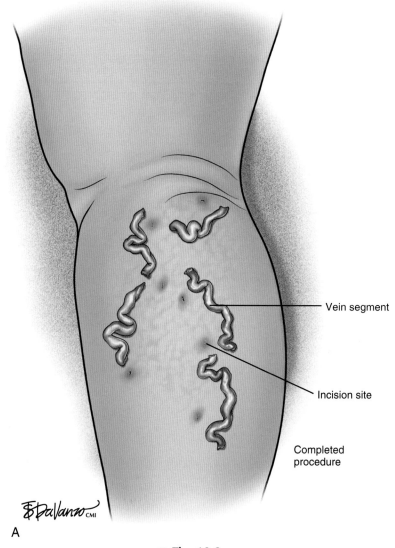

Vein segment

Incision site

Completed procedure

A

■ Fig. 10.9

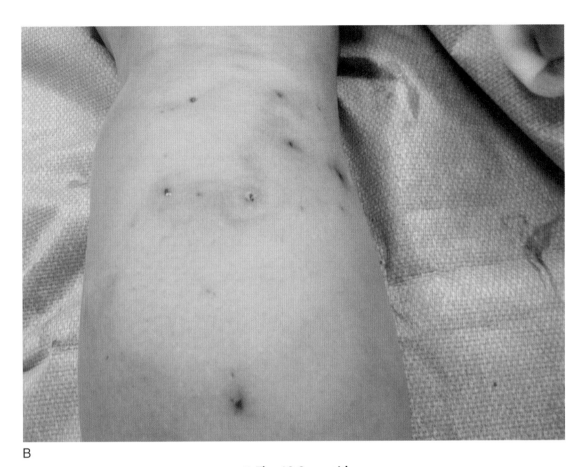

B

■ **Fig. 10.9, cont'd**

Areas where there is minimal subcutaneous fat or inflammatory changes can make the procedure more difficult. Typically, the operator will struggle around the knee, pretibial areas, and dorsum of the feet because these areas do not harbor much fat. Areas involved with previous superficial thrombophlebitis or previous surgery have more fibrosis.

Varicose veins sometimes act as outflow tracts for perforating veins; therefore avulsion of varicose veins can disconnect underlying perforators. A perforator may be recognized by its perpendicular course and by the fact that the patient reports discomfort when traction is applied to the varicosity. The perforator is pulled until it yields, and then avulsed. Bleeding is controlled with digital compression.

Whether to close, or not close, wounds is a matter of judgment. The wounds may be left open or closed with simple sutures or adhesive tape. Most venous surgeons leave the wounds open and allow spontaneous healing. This technique results in little or no scarring and has the advantage of allowing drainage of blood and anesthetic fluid into the overlying compressive dressing, obviating the formation of hematomas.

A single suture to close wounds near the foot and ankle may be required because of the elevated venous pressure at these locations in the upright position. Frequent ambulation will aid in decreasing ambulatory venous pressure in these dependent locations. Adhesive tapes are associated with a high incidence of skin blistering; therefore these must be used with caution.[13]

After 10 minutes of postoperative observation, patients ambulate from the office, with a three-layer compression bandage in place. Minimal postoperative discomfort is the norm, but if it is more intense, it can usually be easily managed with nonsteroidal antiinflammatory agents.

Patients return to the office on postoperative day 2 for dressing removal and for duplex ultrasound to exclude the presence of deep venous thrombosis. Some ecchymosis is to be expected near the treated areas; this rarely results in permanent discoloration of the skin. Some minor leakage of blood and tumescent anesthesia may also drain from the open wounds. Regular adhesive bandages will usually control this satisfactorily. After the compression bandage is removed, patients wear graduated compression stockings (20 to 30 mm Hg) for 2 weeks during the daytime.

Indurated areas are commonly seen at AP incision sites and usually defervesce without incident over a period of several weeks. Firm subcutaneous inflammatory nodules may occasionally form directly under the incision sites; these too are self-limiting after several months.

PEARLS AND PITFALLS

Avoiding nontarget tissues: The venous surgeon must have a thorough command of neurovascular anatomy to avoid injury to nontarget tissues such as arteries and nerves. If the treating physician heeds several important suggestions, complications will rarely be encountered. Knowledge of the course of the common femoral artery, superficial femoral artery, popliteal artery, and anterior and posterior tibial arteries will keep the surgeon from injuring these structures while probing to exteriorize a varicose vein. It would be very difficult, although not impossible, to injure the profunda femoris or peroneal arteries during AP. As stated earlier, the hook rarely needs to plunge deeper than 3 mm to contact the target vein.

The saphenous and sural nerves are particularly prone to injury below the knee because of their proximity to the GSV and SSV. If the saphenous or sural nerves are displaced by the hook, the patient will usually complain of shooting pain into the foot. This is a sign for the surgeon to gently release the structure and replace it in situ. Occasionally, hair-sized sensory cutaneous nerves are encountered and inadvertently avulsed during the course of AP. Patients will experience sharp pain that usually dissipates after 2 to 5 minutes without treatment. If this occurs in the ankle and foot area, chances are that the patient will develop postoperative paresthesia or areas of dysesthesia, which in most cases will be temporary.[14]

The femoral, obturator, sciatic, tibial, and peroneal (common, deep, and superficial) nerves are deep and generally not disturbed in the hands of a competent surgeon.

Foot: The skin of the foot is thin and fibrotic. Further, there is minimal subcutaneous fat, less protection against trauma of the skin, and important underlying tissues such as tendons, tendon sheaths, and joints. There are more small nerve branches that can be damaged by the hook. As in the popliteal space, there is greater risk of injuring an artery.

Eyelid: AP of the periocular vein avoids the concerns regarding thrombotic phenomena within ocular, orbital, or cerebral veins possibly associated with periocular vein sclerotherapy. Weiss and Ramelet[15] reported excellent results on 10 patients who underwent removal of periocular reticular blue veins via AP. A single puncture with an 18-gauge needle sufficed in most cases. It is important to attempt to remove the entire segment because partial resection may lead to recurrence. The use of postoperative compression for 10 minutes reduces the incidence of bruising. The puncture sites typically disappear quickly without scarring.

Hands: In general, inquiries about hand vein treatment come from elderly women who find them unsightly. Often, they have had prior facelift surgery and worry that their hands need rejuvenation to complement the face. Our initial consultation stresses the importance of hand veins for reasons of intravenous access; furthermore, removal of these veins may require central venous access should the patient be hospitalized in the future. The exaggerated hand veins seen in the elderly are from loss of subcutaneous fat in the area, therefore we usually advise fat injections with a cosmetic surgeon. If attempts to dissuade the patient fail, we recommend AP as the procedure of choice for hand vein removal. AP is identical to leg vein treatment and closely resembles treating the dorsum of foot because of the thin skin overlying the area. Results have been excellent; although we rarely do these cases.

COMPLICATIONS

Complications from AP in experienced hands are rare and, when they do occur, are minor.[16] A multicenter study performed in France evaluated 36,000 phlebectomies. The most frequently encountered complications were telangiectasias (1.5%), blister formation (1%), phlebitis (0.05%), hyperpigmentation (0.03%), postoperative bleeding (0.03%), temporary nerve damage (0.05%), and permanent nerve damage (0.02%).

At the Miami Vein Center, we have performed more than 10,000 AP procedures in the office environment, and complications have been limited to hyperpigmentation, telangiectatic matting, seroma, transient paresthesia, superficial phlebitis, blistering, and "missed veins" requiring repeat treatment. Each of these complications occurred in less than 0.5% of cases.

COMPARATIVE EFFECTIVENESS OF EXISTING TREATMENTS

We do not look at AP as a solitary procedure but rather as part of our armada in the treatment of venous disease. We usually perform endovenous thermal ablation of the saphenous trunk in the same setting as AP because bulging varicose veins are usually in continuity with a refluxing axial vein such as the GSV.

Our technique is supported by a well-conducted, randomized trial which compared the 5-year outcomes of endovenous laser therapy with AP (EVLTAP) with concomitant ambulatory phlebectomy, and endovenous laser ablation (EVLA) alone with sequential treatment if required following a delay of at least 6 weeks. Some 50 patients were randomized equally into two parallel groups. The EVLTAP group had lower venous clinical severity score (VCSS) results at 12 weeks (median 0 versus 2; $P < .001$), and lower Aberdeen Varicose Vein Questionnaire (AVVQ) scores at 6 weeks (median 7.9 vs 13.5; $P < .001$) and 12 weeks (2.0 versus 9.6; $P = .015$). VCSS and AVVQ results were equivalent by 1 year, but only after 16 of 24 patients in the EVLA group, compared with one of 25 in the EVLTAP group ($P < .001$), had received a secondary intervention. From 1 to 5 years, both groups had equivalent outcomes. EVLA with either concomitant or sequential management of tributaries is acceptable treatment for symptomatic varicose veins, with both treatments achieving excellent results at 5 years. Concomitant treatment of varicosities is associated with optimal improvement in both clinical disease severity and quality of life.[17]

Other operators delay AP until 4 weeks following endovenous ablation. The argument for this strategy is to allow the bed of varicosities distal to a refluxing axial vein to shrink in size and number. Then fewer incisions will be required for vein removal at the time of AP. It is important to note that Monahan reported during the follow-up period that complete resolution of visible varicose veins was seen in only 13% of limbs after saphenous ablation alone.[18] Therefore about 90% of patients require another intervention after saphenous ablation to fully eradicate their visible varicose veins. This has also been our experience.

If the patient returns in the postoperative period and points out veins that were missed during AP, a redo procedure is generally not required. Sclerotherapy, with or without ultrasound guidance, can be performed 4 to 6 weeks postoperatively to clean-up any missed veins. If redo phlebectomy is required, we permit 3 months to elapse; this allows the inflammatory response to subside at the original AP sites.

AP versus TriVex: In a published prospective comparative randomized trial comparing AP with the new technique of transillumination powered phlebectomy (TriVex), there was no difference in operating time. Although an incision ratio of 7:1 favored TriVex, there was no perceived cosmetic benefit between the patient groups. There was a higher number of recurrences in the TriVex group (21.2%) compared with the AP group (6.2%) at 52 weeks postoperatively. Assessment of pain scores showed no difference between groups.[19]

AP versus compression sclerotherapy: There is one randomized controlled trial on recurrence rates and other complications after sclerotherapy and AP. One year after sclerotherapy, 25% of varicose veins had recurred versus only 2% recurrence after phlebectomy. After 2 years, the difference in recurrence was even larger; 38% recurrence in the sclerotherapy group and only 2% in the AP group.[20]

CONCLUSION

AP is elegant by its mere simplicity. It is effective and safe with acceptable cosmetic results (Fig. 10.10). AP is a perfect complement to endovenous thermal ablation of the saphenous veins. With this combination, patients can expect all varicose veins to vanish following a 1-hour procedure that used only local anesthesia in the comfort of a physician's office.

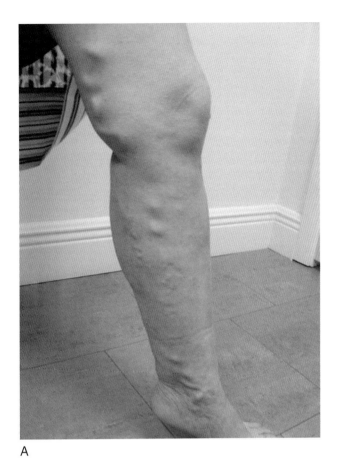

A

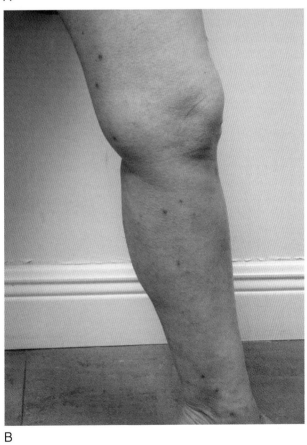

B

■ **Fig. 10.10** (A) Before. (B) After.

REFERENCES

1. Muller R. Traitement des varices par la phlebectomie ambulatoire. *Phlebologie.* 1966;19:277–279.
2. Jones L, Braithwaite BD, Selwyn D, et al. Neovascularisation is the principal cause of varicose vein recurrence: results of a randomized trial of stripping the long saphenous vein. *Eur J Vasc Endovasc Surg.* 1996;12:442–445.
3. Winterborn RJ, Foy C, Earnshaw JJ. Causes of varicose vein recurrence: late results of a randomized controlled trial of stripping the long saphenous vein. *J Vasc Surg.* 2004;40:634–639.
4. Dwerryhouse S, Davies B, Harradine K, et al. Stripping the long saphenous vein reduces the rate of reoperation for recurrent varicose veins: five-year results of a randomized trial. *J Vasc Surg.* 1999;29:589–592.
5. Sarin S, Scurr JH, Coleridge Smith PD. Stripping of the long saphenous vein in the treatment of primary varicose veins. *Br J Surg.* 1994;81:1455–1458.
6. Min RJ, Khilnani N, Zimmet SE. Endovenous laser treatment of saphenous vein reflux: long-term results. *J Vasc Interv Radiol.* 2003;14:991–996.
7. Merchant RF, Pichot O, Myers KA. Four-year follow-up on endovascular radiofrequency obliteration of great saphenous reflux. *Dermatol Surg.* 2005;31:129–134.
8. Labropoulos N, Kang SS, Mansour MA, et al. Primary superficial vein reflux with competent saphenous trunk. *Eur J Vasc Endovasc Surg.* 1999;18:201–206.
9. Weiss RA, Goldman MP. Transillumination mapping prior to ambulatory phlebectomy. *Dermatol Surg.* 1998;24:447–450.
10. Klein JA. Tumescent technique for local anaesthesia improves safety in large-volume liposuction. *Plast Reconstr Surg.* 1993;92:1085–1098.
11. Keel D, Goldman MP. Tumescent anaesthesia in ambulatory phlebectomy: addition of epinephrine. *Dermatol Surg.* 1999;25:371–372.
12. Schmid RM, Rosenkranz HS. Antimicrobial activity of local anaesthetics: lidocaine and procaine. *J Infect Dis.* 1970;121:597.
13. Almeida JI, Raines JK. Principles of ambulatory phlebectomy. In: Bergan JJ, ed. *The Vein Book.* San Diego: Elsevier; 2007:247–256.
14. Ramelet AA. Complications of ambulatory phlebectomy. *Dermatol Surg.* 1997;23:947–954.
15. Weiss RA, Ramelet AA. Removal of blue periocular lower eyelid veins by ambulatory phlebectomy. *Dermatol Surg.* 2002;28:43–45.
16. Olivencia JA. Complications of ambulatory phlebectomy: review of 1,000 consecutive cases. *Dermatol Surg.* 1997;23:51–54.
17. El-Sheikha J, Nandhra S, Carradice D, et al. Clinical outcomes and quality of life 5 years after a randomized trial of concomitant or sequential phlebectomy following endovenous laser ablation for varicose veins. *Br J Surg.* 2014;101(9):1093–1097.
18. Monahan DL. Can phlebectomy be deferred in the treatment of varicose veins? *J Vasc Surg.* 2005;42:1145–1149.
19. Aremu MA, Mahendran B, Butcher W, et al. Prospective randomized controlled trial: conventional versus powered phlebectomy. *J Vasc Surg.* 2004;39:88–94.
20. De Roos KP, Nieman FH, Neumann HA. Ambulatory phlebectomy versus compression sclerotherapy: results of a randomized controlled trial. *Dermatol Surg.* 2003;29:221–226.

CHAPTER 11

Endovenous Approach to Recurrent Varicose Veins

Jose I. Almeida

HISTORICAL BACKGROUND

Recurrence rates of varicose veins of 20% are common, with rates as high as 70% at 10 years.[1-3] Up to 25% of procedures for varicose veins are performed for recurrent disease,[4] thus placing considerable demands on health care resources. Note that recurrent varicose vein surgery carries a much greater morbidity risk to the patient than primary surgery.[3] This risk seems to be reduced with endovenous techniques.

ETIOLOGY AND NATURAL HISTORY OF DISEASE

Patients who have had previous high ligation and stripping (HL/S) typically present with recurrent varicose veins; anatomic distribution of these veins is variable. Neovascularization is commonly seen following traditional stripping procedures and is thought to be secondary to "frustrated" venous drainage from the abdominal wall and perineum.[5] Regardless of the mechanism, the result is recurrent reflux in the thigh or lower leg veins.

Multiple factors contribute in the development of recurrent disease. The weight of each factor has not yet been determined because there are no prospective studies with adequate sample size. The following descriptions are common etiologies seen at Miami Vein Center after clinical and color flow duplex imaging (CFDI) examinations are performed in patients presenting with recurrent varicose veins.

PEARLS AND PITFALLS

Previous High Ligation and Stripping

All patients with recurrent varicose veins should be evaluated with CFDI. Usually, findings include neovascularity in the groin from which one or more tributary veins are found to descend the thigh. The tributary may attach to another tributary, a perforator, or a remnant of the great saphenous vein (GSV) in the thigh or calf (Fig. 11.1). The reflux extends into dilated tributaries of the skin; these vessels bulge and are palpable. In most cases, our approach is to enter any straight, incompetent, axial, venous segments deep to the skin with a micropuncture access kit. These kits usually contain 4-Fr microsheaths, through which we place a 400-μm-diameter or 600-μm-diameter laser fiber. Perivenous,

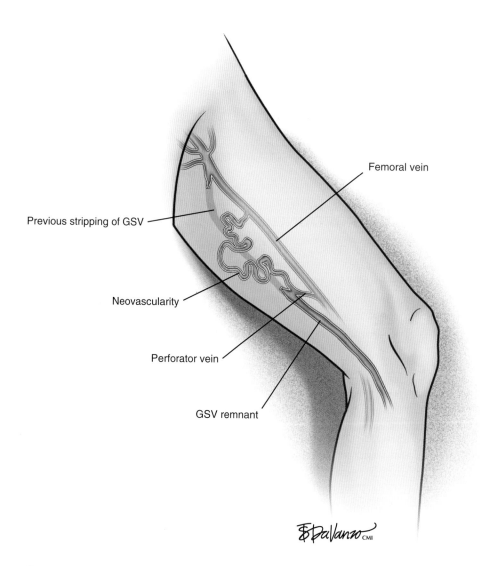

Femoral vein

Previous stripping of GSV

Neovascularity

Perforator vein

GSV remnant

A

■ Fig. 11.1

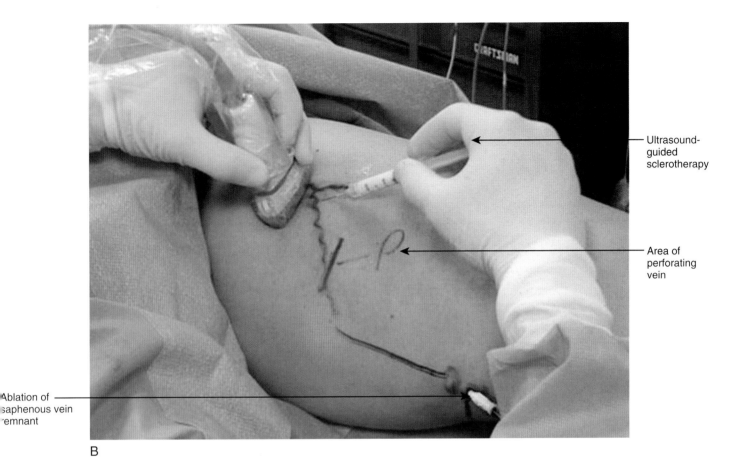

Ultrasound-guided sclerotherapy

Area of perforating vein

Ablation of saphenous vein remnant

B

C

■ **Fig. 11.1, cont'd** (B) Treatment of recurrent varicose vein with the use of combination endovenous laser and foam scleropathy. (C) Cross-sectional view of a subcutaneous tortuous tributary. These tortuous veins are ideal candidates for ultrasound-guided foam sclerotherapy treatment.

Continued

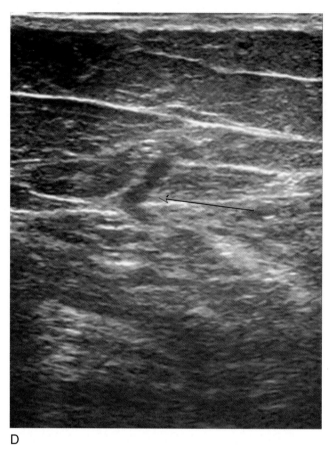

D

■ **Fig. 11.1, cont'd** (D) Incompetent midthigh perforating vein is the source of the recurrent varicose veins, which is most effectively treated with thermal ablation if anatomically in a straight orientation. If oriented in a tortuous manner, however, ultrasound-guided foam sclerotherapy treatment is preferred. *GSV,* Great saphenous vein.

tumescent anesthesia is placed, and the vein or veins are ablated in the usual manner. Because tortuous incompetent venous segments below the level of the skin do not allow the passage of guidewires, these are treated with ultrasound-guided foam sclerotherapy (UGFS) (Fig. 11.2).

Finally, all bulging varicose veins that are palpable on the skin receive treatment with ambulatory phlebectomy. These three techniques, used concomitantly, yield very satisfactory results. These types of patients are told that the treatments are palliative, and they will likely need "touch-up" treatments in the future.

Previous Phlebectomy Without Great Saphenous Vein Stripping

Also common in our practice are patients presenting with recurrent varicose veins previously treated with phlebectomy only at an outside facility. These limbs, once examined with CFDI, usually have a large incompetent GSV descending from the groin and terminating ultimately in the calf at a site where large varicosities are noted. These patients do very well with routine GSV ablation using either radiofrequency or laser and using ambulatory phlebectomy for associated varicosities.

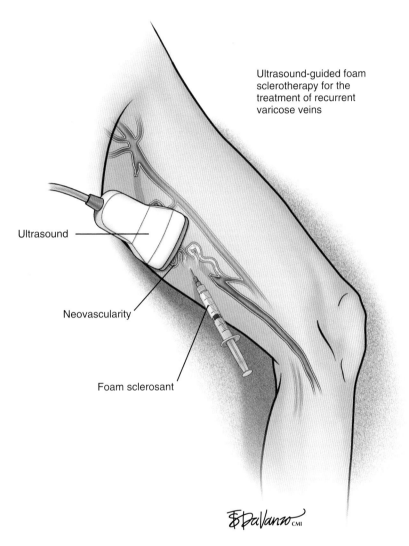

Ultrasound-guided foam sclerotherapy for the treatment of recurrent varicose veins

Ultrasound

Neovascularity

Foam sclerosant

A

■ **Fig. 11.2**

Continued

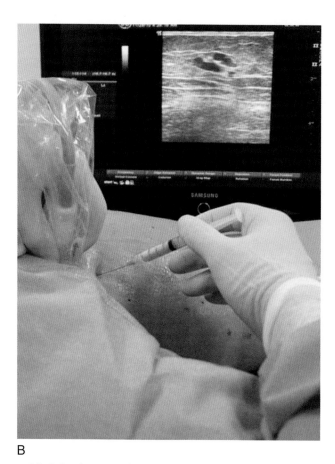

B

■ **Fig. 11.2, cont'd** (B) Ultrasound-guided foam sclerotherapy for the treatment of recurrent varicose veins; tortuous veins seen on ultrasound are in the background.

Previous Laser or Radiofrequency Ablation Without Phlebectomy

There are individuals who have seen other physicians and come to our practice with a history of GSV ablation that "worked temporarily." That is, the venous cluster on the medial calf improved shortly after the procedure, but with time, the same cluster began filling and dilating. CFDI performed in our office usually shows successful ablation of the target GSV. However, the cluster of varicose veins in these cases has found a connection with an incompetent perforating vein. This is usually a Boyd perforating vein in the upper calf. This concept of an untreated "venous reservoir" dictates that other sources of reflux will eventually connect because of low venous resistance. Treatment involves either ultrasound-guided sclerotherapy or thermal ablation of the perforator (function of size) and ambulatory phlebectomy of the varicose clusters.

We have also seen cases in which two sources of venous hypertension from superficial axial vein reflux were identified preoperatively but only one was treated. In these cases, usually only the incompetent GSV was ablated, and the incompetent anterior accessory saphenous vein was left untreated. There may be temporary improvement of the varicosities in direct continuity with the GSV; less direct varicosities may respond with minimal or no improvement. Our approach with these patients is thermal ablation of the anterior accessory saphenous vein, followed by ambulatory phlebectomy at the same stage.

Previous Great Saphenous Vein Ablation With No Improvement

When a patient has a history of previous GSV ablation performed at an outside facility and no improvement was observed by the patient, this should be a red flag that the patient was initially misdiagnosed. The majority of these cases were straightforward, with classic small saphenous vein (SSV) incompetence in the limbs. However, the original physician failed to view the posterior calf with CFDI. Ablation of the SSV with laser or radiofrequency energy in combination with ambulatory phlebectomy will quickly rectify this problem.

Gastrocnemial vein incompetence has a prevalence of up to 30% in patients with varicose veins. Most practitioners do not treat this vein. Also incompetent perforators connecting through this vein at the posteromedial calf may be overlooked or missed. We have seen these as sources of recurrent varicose veins. Depending on the severity of the signs and symptoms of the disease, we may elect to treat gastrocnemius veins with ultrasound-guided sclerotherapy. Obviously, this adds controversy to the dearth of clinical information referable to this vein.

The aforementioned techniques are self-taught techniques, applying standard endovenous principles. The adage developed by the author is "If an incompetent vein is straight—burn it; if it is tortuous—foam it; if the vein is palpable on the skin (straight or tortuous)—remove it with phlebectomy." Depicted in Fig. 11.3 is an endovenous sheath inside a saphenous vein remnant (to deliver laser energy) with a syringe prepared with a foamed sclerosant attached to the sheath side-arm to deliver foam into an area of neovascularization, and the patient is marked for phlebectomy. We have had no complications with this approach in several thousand recurrent varicose vein cases. Recurrences after endovenous treatment develop secondary to progression of disease and are retreatable with the same approach.

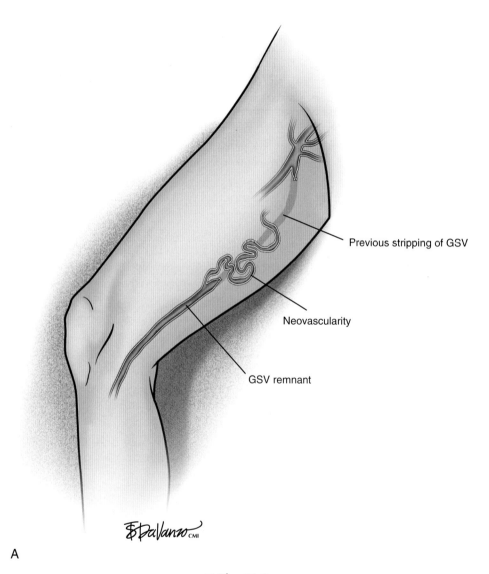

Previous stripping of GSV

Neovascularity

GSV remnant

A

■ Fig. 11.3

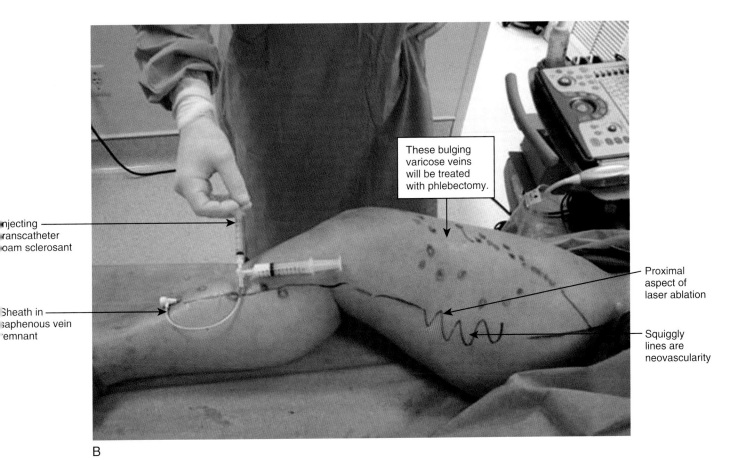

Injecting
transcatheter
foam sclerosant

Sheath in
saphenous vein
remnant

These bulging
varicose veins
will be treated
with phlebectomy.

Proximal
aspect of
laser ablation

Squiggly
lines are
neovascularity

B

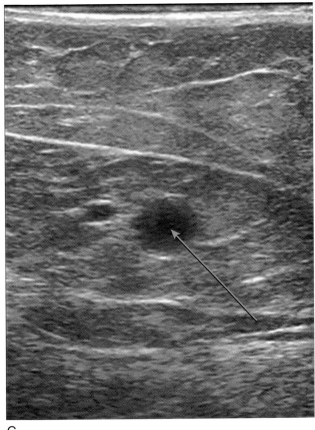

C

■ **Fig. 11.3, cont'd** (B) Recurrent varicose veins from neovascularity in upper thigh and a refluxing saphenous vein remnant. Treatment with a combination of ultrasound foam sclerotherapy, endovenous laser ablation, and ambulatory phlebectomy. (C) *Arrow* points to saphenous vein remnant.

Continued

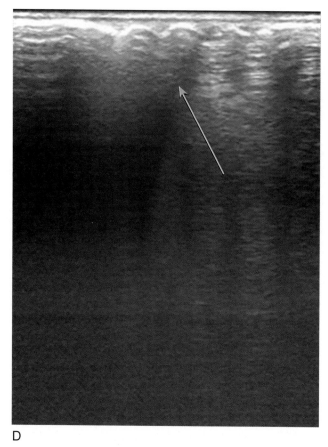

■ **Fig. 11.3, cont'd** (D) *Arrow* points to foam-filled varicose veins just below skin surface. *GSV,* Great saphenous vein.

COMPARATIVE EFFECTIVENESS OF EXISTING TREATMENTS FROM COCHRANE DATABASE

1. Endovenous ablation (radiofrequency and laser) and foam sclerotherapy versus open surgery for great saphenous vein varices.[6]

All randomized controlled trials (RCTs) of UGFS, endovenous laser therapy (EVLT), radiofrequency ablation (RFA), and HL/S were considered for inclusion. Primary outcomes were recurrent varicosities, recanalization, neovascularization, technical procedure failure, patient quality-of-life (QoL) scores, and associated complications. A total of 13 studies with a combined total of 3081 randomized patients were included. Three studies compared UGFS with surgery, eight compared EVLT with surgery, and five compared RFA with surgery (two studies had two or more comparisons with surgery). For the comparison of UGFS versus surgery, the findings may have indicated no difference in the rate of recurrences in the surgical group when measured by clinicians, and no difference between the groups for symptomatic recurrence (odds ratio [OR] 1.74; 95% confidence interval [CI], 0.97–3.12; $P = .06$ and OR, 1.28; 95% CI, 0.66–2.49, respectively). Recanalization and neovascularization were only evaluated in a single study. Recanalization at less than 4 months had an OR of 0.66 (95% CI, 0.20–2.12), recanalization at greater than 4 months an OR of 5.05 (95% CI, 1.67–15.28), and for neovascularization, an OR of 0.05 (95% CI,

0.00–0.94). There was no difference in the rate of technical failure between the two groups (OR 0.44; 95% CI, 0.12–1.57). For EVLT versus surgery, there were no differences between the treatment groups for either clinician noted or symptomatic recurrence (OR 0.72; 95% CI, 0.43–1.22; $P = .22$ and OR 0.87; 95% CI, 0.47–1.62; $P = .67$, respectively). Both early and late recanalization were no different between the two treatment groups (OR 1.05; 95% CI, 0.09–12.77; $P = .97$ and OR 4.14; 95% CI, 0.76–22.65; $P = .10$). Neovascularization and technical failure were both statistically reduced in the laser treatment group (OR 0.05; 95% CI, 0.01–0.22; $P < .0001$ and OR 0.29; 95% CI, 0.14–0.60; $P = .0009$, respectively). Long-term (5-year) outcomes were evaluated in one study so no association could be derived, but it appeared that EVLT and surgery maintained similar findings. Comparing RFA versus surgery, there were no differences in clinician-noted recurrence (OR 0.82; 95% CI, 0.49–1.39; $P = .47$); symptomatic-noted recurrence was only evaluated in a single study. There were also no differences between the treatment groups for recanalization (early or late) (OR 0.68; 95% CI, 0.01–81.18; $P = .87$ and OR 1.09; 95% CI, 0.39–3.04; $P = .87$, respectively), neovascularization (OR 0.31; 95% CI, 0.06–1.65; $P = 0.17$) or technical failure (OR 0.82; 95% CI, 0.07–10.10; $P = .88$). QoL scores, operative complications, and pain were not amenable to metaanalysis; however, QoL generally increased similarly in all treatment groups, and complications were generally low, especially major complications. Pain reporting varied greatly between the studies but, in general, pain was similar between the treatment groups.

Currently available clinical trial evidence suggests that UGFS, EVLT, and RFA are at least as effective as surgery in the treatment of great saphenous varicose veins. Because of large incompatibilities between trials, and different time point measurements for outcomes, the evidence is lacking in robustness. Further randomized trials are needed, which should aim to report and analyze results in a congruent manner to facilitate future metaanalysis.

2. Endovenous ablation therapy (laser or radiofrequency) or foam sclerotherapy versus conventional surgical repair for short saphenous varicose veins.[7]

All RCTs comparing EVLA, endovenous RFA, or UGFS with conventional surgery in the treatment of SSV varices were included. There were three RCTs, all of which compared EVLA with surgery; one also compared UGFS with surgery. There were no trials comparing RFA with surgery. The EVLA versus surgery comparison included 311 participants: 185 received EVLA and 126 received surgery. In the UGFS comparison, each treatment group contained 21 subjects. For the EVLA versus surgery comparison, recanalization or persistence of reflux at 6 weeks occurred less frequently in the EVLA group than in the surgery group (OR 0.07; 95% CI, 0.02–0.22; I2 = 51%; 289 participants, three studies, moderate-quality evidence). Recurrence of reflux at 1 year was also less frequent in the EVLA group than in the surgery group (OR 0.24; 95% CI, 0.07–0.77; I2 = 0%; 119 participants, two studies, low-quality evidence). For the outcome clinical evidence of recurrence (i.e., presence of new visible varicose veins) at 1 year, there was no difference between the two treatment groups (OR 0.54; 95% CI, 0.17–1.75; 99 participants, one study, low-quality evidence). Four participants each in the EVLA and surgery groups required reintervention because of technical failure (99 participants, one study, moderate-quality evidence). There was no difference between the two treatment groups for disease-specific QoL (Aberdeen Varicose Veins Questionnaire) either at 6 weeks (mean difference [MD], 0.15; 95% CI, −1.65–1.95; I2 = 0%; 265 participants, two studies, moderate-quality evidence), or at 1 year (MD, −1.08; 95% CI, −3.39–1.23; 99 participants, one study, low-quality evidence). Main complications reported at 6 weeks were sural nerve injury, wound infection, and deep venous thrombosis (DVT) (one DVT case in each treatment group; EVLA: 1/161, 0.6%; surgery 1/104, 1%; 265 participants, two studies, moderate-quality evidence). For the UGFS versus surgery comparison, there were insufficient data to detect clear differences between the two treatment groups for the two outcomes, recanalization or persistence of reflux at 6 weeks (OR, 0.34; 95% CI, 0.06–2.10; 33 participants, one study, low-quality evidence), and recurrence of reflux at 1 year (OR, 1.19; 95% CI, 0.29–4.92; 31 participants, one study, low-quality evidence). No other outcomes could be reported for this comparison because the study data were not stratified according to saphenous vein.

Moderate-quality to low-quality evidence exists to suggest that recanalization, or persistence of reflux at 6 weeks, and recurrence of reflux at 1 year, are less frequent when EVLA is performed, compared with conventional surgery. For the UGFS versus conventional surgery comparison, the quality of evidence is assessed to be low; consequently, the effectiveness of UGFS compared with conventional surgery in the treatment of SSV varices is uncertain. Further RCTs for all comparisons are required with longer follow-up (at least 5 years). In addition, measurement of outcomes such as recurrence of reflux, time taken to return to work, duration of procedure, pain, and so on, and choice of time points during follow-up should be standardized, such that future trials evaluating newer technologies can be compared efficiently.

REFERENCES

1. Negus D. Recurrent varicose veins: a national problem. *Br J Surg*. 1993;80:823–824.
2. Rivlin S. The surgical cure of primary varicose veins. *Br J Surg*. 1975;62:913–917.
3. Royle JP. Recurrent varicose veins. *World J Surg*. 1986;10:944–953.
4. Hayden A, Holdsworth J. Complications following re-exploration of the groin for recurrent varicose veins. *Ann R Coll Surg Engl*. 2001;83:272–273.
5. Chandler JG, Pichot O, Sessa C, et al. Treatment of primary venous insufficiency by endovenous saphenous vein obliteration. *Vasc Surg*. 2000;34:201–214.
6. Nesbitt C, Bedenis R, Bhattacharya V, et al. Endovenous ablation (radiofrequency and laser) and foam sclerotherapy versus open surgery for great saphenous vein varices. *Cochrane Database Syst Rev*. 2014;(7):CD005624.
7. Paravastu SC, Horne M, Dodd PD. Endovenous ablation therapy (laser or radiofrequency) or foam sclerotherapy versus conventional surgical repair for short saphenous varicose veins. *Cochrane Database Syst Rev*. 2016;(11):CD010878.

Thromboembolic Disease

Timothy K. Liem and Jose I. Almeida

HISTORICAL BACKGROUND AND EPIDEMIOLOGY OF ACUTE VENOUS THROMBOEMBOLIC DISEASE

The incidence of deep venous thrombosis (DVT) ranges from 5 to 9 per 10,000 person-years in the general population, and the incidence of venous thromboembolism (VTE), defined as DVT and pulmonary embolism (PE) combined, is about 14 per 10,000 person-years.[1,2] This equates to more than 275,000 new cases of VTE per year in the United States, with a steady growth in the number of identifiable risk factors that predispose to the development of VTE. This information has allowed physicians to provide more effective thromboembolism prophylaxis that is evidence based and stratified according to the number of risk factors present. In patients with established DVT and PE, the US Food and Drug Administration (FDA) approval of several direct oral anticoagulants has led to a significant expansion in the options available to clinicians and patients, both for the treatment of acute VTE, and for the secondary prevention against recurrence.

This chapter describes risk factors for a first episode of VTE and the options for initial anticoagulation. Risk factors and associated conditions that increase the predilection for VTE recurrence, as well as available prediction models will also be described. The optimal duration and type of longer-term antithrombotic therapy are also covered, and the role of adjunctive vena cava filters is discussed briefly. VTE prophylaxis, modalities for the diagnosis of VTE, and thrombolytic therapy for VTE are beyond the scope of this chapter and are not discussed in detail.

ETIOLOGY AND NATURAL HISTORY OF ACUTE VENOUS THROMBOEMBOLISM

Etiology

Venous thrombosis may develop as a result of endothelial damage, hypercoagulability, and venous stasis (Virchow triad). Of these risk factors, relative hypercoagulability appears most important in the majority of cases of spontaneous DVT, whereas stasis and endothelial damage play a greater role in secondary DVT following immobilization, surgery, or trauma. Identifiable risk factors for VTE may be classified as inherited, acquired, and those with a mixed etiology (Table 12.1).

When multiple inherited and acquired risk factors are present in the same patient, a synergistic effect may occur. Clinically manifest thrombosis most often occurs with the convergence of multiple genetic and acquired risk factors.[3] Hospitalized patients have an average of 1.5 risk factors per patient, with 26% having three or more risk factors.[4] Multiple risk factors often act synergistically to increase risk dramatically above the sum of individual risk factors. For example, patients who are heterozygous for factor V Leiden are at only moderately increased risk for VTE (4-fold–8-fold). However, when combined with the additional risk of oral contraceptive use, the risk for VTE increases to approximately 35-fold, the same order of magnitude as for someone who is homozygous for factor V Leiden. The concomitant presence of obesity, advancing age, and factor V Leiden increases the thrombosis risk associated with hormone replacement therapy alone. In symptomatic

TABLE 12.1 Common Inherited and Acquired Risk Factors for Venous Thrombosis

Acquired	Inherited
Advanced age	Factor V Leiden
Hospitalization/immobilization	Prothrombin 20210A
HRT and OCP	Antithrombin deficiency
Pregnancy and puerperium	Protein C deficiency
Prior VTE	Protein S deficiency
Malignancy	Factor XI elevation
Major surgery	Dysfibrinogenemia
Obesity	
Nephrotic syndrome	**Mixed Etiology**
Trauma/spinal cord injury	Homocysteinemia
Long-haul travel (>6 hours)	Factor VII, VIII, IX, XI elevation
Varicose veins	Hyperfibrinogenemia
Antiphospholipid antibody syndrome	APC resistance without factor V Leiden
Myeloproliferative disease	
Polycythemia	
Central venous catheters	

APC, Activated protein C; *HRT,* hormone replacement therapy; *OCP,* oral contraceptives; *VTE,* venous thromboembolism.

outpatients, the odds ratio for an objectively documented DVT increases from 1.26 for one risk factor to 3.88 for three or more risk factors.[5]

Other factors associated with venous thrombosis include traditional cardiovascular risk factors (obesity, hypertension, diabetes), and there is a racial predilection among Caucasians and African Americans compared with Asians and Native Americans. Certain gene variants (single nucleotide polymorphisms) are associated with a mild increased risk for DVT, and their presence may interact with other risk factors to increase the overall risk for venous thrombosis. However, testing for these polymorphisms is not common in clinical practice.

Natural History

Overt venous injury appears to be neither a necessary nor sufficient condition for thrombosis, although the role of biologic injury to the endothelium is increasingly apparent. Under conditions favoring thrombosis, the normally antithrombogenic endothelium may become prothrombotic, producing tissue factor, von Willebrand factor, P-selectin, and fibronectin.[6] Stasis alone is probably also an inadequate stimulus in the absence of low levels of activated coagulation factors.[7]

The rate of VTE recurrence in patients with untreated isolated calf DVT is approximately 20% to 30%. In contrast, the rate of recurrence in patients with untreated proximal DVT is more difficult to determine because the majority of patients with proximal DVT receive therapeutic anticoagulation. Limited older data suggest that about 50% of patients with inadequately treated proximal DVT will develop symptomatic PE.

Therapeutic anticoagulation stabilizes venous thrombus, prevents propagation, and promotes dissolution by endogenous plasmin and its mediators. However, there is a low rate of VTE treatment failure, even with adequate dosing of any of the currently available antithrombotic regimens. Recent randomized clinical trials demonstrate that the rate of recurrent symptomatic VTE and related death ranges from about 1.5% to 3.5%, during the first 6 to 12 months of therapy.[8–11] The incidence depends, in part, upon the location of the original DVT, with isolated calf DVT having a lower rate of treatment failure when compared with proximal DVT.

Once patients discontinue anticoagulation after 3 to 6 months of therapy, there is also a steady rate of late VTE recurrence, in the range of 2% to 4% per year. Patients with proximal and unprovoked VTE have significantly higher rates than those with distal DVTs and those provoked by significant transient risk factors (major surgery, trauma, or significant immobility).

DIAGNOSIS AND IMAGING

Patient presentation varies widely depending on the extent of the venous thrombosis and the presence of concurrent medical and surgical problems. Patients with superficial venous thrombosis (SVT) often present with pain, induration, and inflammation over the affected region. Many patients with DVT may be asymptomatic, with the thrombosis discovered during routine screening of patients who are at high risk for VTE. However, patients with more extensive or proximal DVT are more likely to present with pain, cyanosis, and edema. In rare situations, patients with phlegmasia alba dolens or cerulean dolens may present with compartment syndrome or even venous gangrene. Those with acute PE may present with chest pain, shortness of breath, hemoptysis, and/or tachycardia, and in severe circumstances, right-heart failure or even sudden death.

Laboratory Testing for Venous Thromboembolism

There are no laboratory tests that independently confirm or exclude the presence of DVT or SVT. D-dimer testing may be useful in two clinical settings. In the first, a negative D-dimer test, in combination with a low probability clinical decision score, using established criteria such as the Wells Rule, has a very good negative predictive value for excluding DVT (<2% in most patients). In contrast, a positive D-dimer test is a poor predictor for the presence of VTE, and further image-based testing is warranted in patients with suspected DVT or PE.

Secondly, in the setting of patients with established VTE who have received a course of anticoagulation, D-dimer testing may be used to guide the duration of anticoagulation. The D-dimer test is one component of most published prediction models that estimate risk for VTE recurrence in patients with *unprovoked* VTE.[12] Our preferred method is the Vienna Prediction Model, which incorporates patient gender, VTE location, and D-dimer to estimate recurrence at up to 10 years (https://cemsiis.meduniwien.ac.at/en/kb/science-research/software/clinical-software/recurrent-vte/#calc-params). Most often, testing is performed about one month after discontinuation of anticoagulation. One factor limiting the usefulness of these prediction models for VTE recurrence is the lack of a validated scoring system that estimates bleeding risk in patients who choose to continue anticoagulation.

Testing for Thrombophilia

Most patients with provoked or unprovoked VTE do not require an evaluation for thrombophilia, and most family members of those with VTE also do not require testing. This more conservative approach is a significant departure from prior recommendations from the American Society of Hematology. It developed after a greater recognition that, although the more common thrombophilias are significant risk factors for initial VTE, they are very weak risk factors for recurrence. More specific clinical guidelines regarding thrombophilia testing are shown in Table 12.2.

In those patients for whom the presence of a hypercoagulable condition might alter the type or duration of anticoagulation, testing should be performed for factor V Leiden mutation, prothrombin G20210A mutation, antiphospholipid antibodies, lupus anticoagulant, and protein C, protein S, and antithrombin activity. Thrombophilia testing should also be performed for patients with thrombosis at unusual sites (cerebral venous sinuses, renal vein, hepatic vein, portomesenteric veins in the absence of portal hypertension). In these patients, testing should also be performed for paroxysmal nocturnal hemoglobinuria (PNH) and myeloproliferative syndromes. PNH is screened for with a flow cytometry assay, and myeloproliferative syndromes are detected with DNA testing for the *JAK2* mutation. Patients who are suspected of having heparin-induced thrombocytopenia (HIT) should be evaluated with the 4Ts scoring system (thrombocytopenia, timing of platelet count fall, thrombosis or other sequelae, other causes of thrombocytopenia), and HIT may be safely excluded in those with a 4Ts score of 3 or lower. Patients with a 4Ts score of 4 or more should receive testing for HIT.[13]

TABLE 12.2 Anticoagulation Forum Guidance Regarding Evaluation of Hereditary and Acquired Thrombophilia

1. Do not perform thrombophilia testing following a provoked venous thromboembolism (VTE). Note: A positive thrombophilia evaluation is not a sufficient basis to offer extended anticoagulation.

2. Do not perform thrombophilia testing following an unprovoked VTE, unless a patient at low risk of bleeding planned to stop anticoagulation, and a positive test would influence this decision. Note: A negative thrombophilia evaluation is not a sufficient basis to stop anticoagulation in a patient with an unprovoked VTE, low-bleeding risk, and willingness to continue therapy.

3. Do not test for thrombophilia in asymptomatic family members of patient with VTE or heritable thrombophilia. Note: Family history of VTE already confers an elevated risk, and a negative thrombophilia evaluation does not eliminate this risk. These relatives should receive prophylaxis in high-risk situations regardless of test results.

4. Do not perform thrombophilia testing in asymptomatic family members of patients with VTE or heritable thrombophilia who are contemplating estrogen. Note: Women contemplating estrogen use who have a first-degree relative with VTE and a known heritable thrombophilia should test for that thrombophilia if it would alter the decision. Family history of VTE itself confers an elevated risk of estrogen-associated VTE, but the absolute risk remains very low, especially in younger women considering oral contraceptive use.

5. Do not perform thrombophilia testing in asymptomatic family members of patients with VTE or heritable thrombophilia who are contemplating pregnancy. Note: Women contemplating pregnancy who have a first-degree relative with VTE and known heritable thrombophilia should test for that thrombophilia if it would alter VTE prophylaxis. If multiple family members are affected by VTE, a more potent thrombophilia (AT deficiency) may be present, potentially altering VTE prophylaxis.

6. Do not perform thrombophilia testing at the time of VTE diagnosis or during the initial 3 months of anticoagulation.

(Adapted from Stevens SM, Willer SC, Bauer KA, et al, Guidance for the evaluation and treatment of hereditary and acquired thrombophilia. *J Thromb Thrombolysis.* 2016;41(1):154–164.)

The timing for the performance of testing for inherited thrombophilia varies widely. Acute thrombosis, inflammation, and a large thrombus burden may cause transient depression of antithrombin, protein C, and protein S levels. Concomitant administration of oral vitamin-K antagonists also decreases protein C and protein S activity. If abnormal results are obtained under these conditions, then repeat testing should be performed once the acute thrombosis has resolved and after discontinuation of any vitamin K antagonist. To avoid the need for repeat laboratory draws, many clinicians do not perform the thrombophilia testing until after the course of therapy has been completed, typically with an interval of about 4 weeks after the discontinuation of anticoagulation. It is also important to remember that many antiphospholipid antibodies are transient, and the official criteria for antiphospholipid antibody syndrome require two positive tests at least 12 weeks apart.

Imaging for Venous Thromboembolism

The venous duplex scan is the most commonly performed test for the detection of infrainguinal DVT. The accuracy of the venous duplex scan depends on the presence or absence of symptoms, and the anatomic location of the thrombosis (Table 12.3). Duplex imaging for patients with symptomatic DVT has a significantly greater sensitivity (89%) when compared with asymptomatic patients (47%). However, the specificity of the examination remains fairly equivalent between the two groups (about 94%). Limited data suggests that sensitivity and specificity also vary based upon anatomic location.[14]

The venous duplex examination is typically performed with the patient supine to assess for venous compressibility (coaptation), spectral Doppler waveform assessment of spontaneous venous flow, phasic variation of flow with respiration, and response of flow to the Valsalva maneuver. Continued improvements in ultrasound technology have also improved the ability to visualize color flow within the tibial veins. However, the primary method of detecting DVT with ultrasound is demonstration of the lack of compressibility of the vein with probe pressure on B-mode imaging. Normally, in transverse section, the vein walls should coapt with pressure (Figs. 12.1 and 12.2). Lack of coaptation indicates thrombus.

Venography is the most definitive test for the diagnosis of DVT in both symptomatic and asymptomatic patients. Diagnostic venography involves placement of a small catheter in the dorsum of the foot with injection of radiopaque contrast to produce projections in at least two views. Venography is not used routinely for the evaluation of lower-extremity DVT because of associated complications. More commonly, it is used for imaging before operative venous reconstruction or catheter-based endovenous therapy.

TABLE 12.3 Duplex Imaging for Deep Venous Thrombosis

Venous Bed	Sensitivity	Specificity
All lower extremity DVT		
Symptomatic patients	89%	94%
Asymptomatic patients	47%	94%
Proximal lower extremity veins		
Symptomatic patients	97%	
Asymptomatic patients	62%	
Isolated calf lower extremity DVT		
Symptomatic patients	73%	
Asymptomatic patients	53%	
IVC and iliac veins	46%	100%
Upper extremity veins	78%–100%	82%–100%

DVT, Deep vein thrombosis; *IVC,* inferior vena cava.
(Adapted from Liem TK. Duplex ultrasound scanning for acute venous disease. In P. Gloviczki (Ed.), *Handbook of venous and lymphatic disorders,* 4th edition (pp. 141–150). Boca Raton, FL: 2017, CRC Press.)

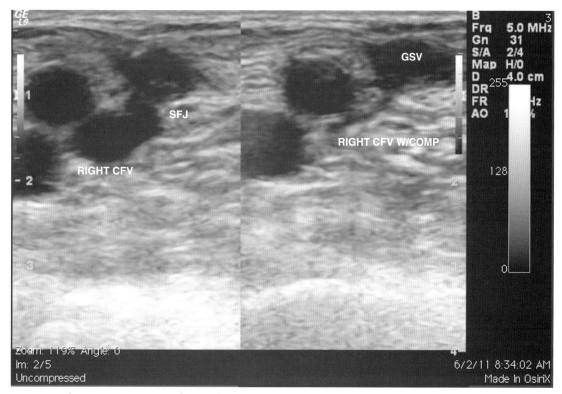

■ Fig. 12.1 Common femoral vein without and with compression. Complete vein wall coaptation indicates absence of deep vein thrombosis. *CFV*, Common femoral vein; *GSV*, great saphenous vein; *SFJ*, saphenofemoral junction; *W/COMP*, with compression.

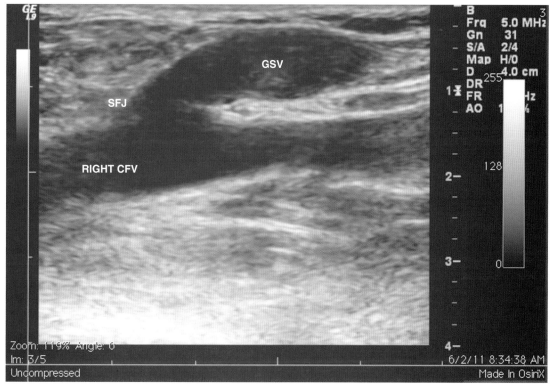

■ Fig. 12.2 Normal saphenofemoral junction. *CFV*, Common femoral vein; *GSV*, great saphenous vein; *SFJ*, saphenofemoral junction.

ANTITHROMBOTIC THERAPY FOR VENOUS THROMBOEMBOLISM

Treatment for Venous Thromboembolism

Once the diagnosis of VTE has been made, antithrombotic therapy should be initiated promptly. The following dosing protocols are the more commonly used treatment regimens, but they are not applicable to all patient populations (Table 12.4). The FDA approval of the oral direct thrombin inhibitors and direct factor Xa inhibitors has significantly increased the treatment options available. Rivaroxaban and apixaban may be initiated as oral monotherapy. Both agents use a higher dosing protocol for the first 21 days and 7 days, respectively.

The other options for anticoagulation require the use of parenteral agents for initial therapy, such as unfractionated heparin, low-molecular-weight heparin (LMWH), or fondaparinux. In this setting, initial anticoagulation should be continued for 5 to 10 days, overlapping with either warfarin, dabigatran, or edoxaban. In patients receiving warfarin, parenteral anticoagulation may be discontinued once the international normalized ratio (INR) is in the therapeutic range (INR goal 2.5, range 2–3) for longer than 24 hours (i.e., two consecutive daily INR values ≥2).

TABLE 12.4 Anticoagulation for Deep Vein Thrombosis/Pulmonary Embolism

Medication	Route	Dose and Duration
Unfractionated heparin (UH)	IV	5000 U or 80 U/kg bolus IV, then 1300 U/h or 18 U/kg/h IV continuous infusion adjusted to prolong the aPTT corresponding to a plasma heparin of 0.3–0.7 IU/mL. Duration 5–10 days, overlapping with a vitamin-K antagonist, dabigatran, or edoxaban.
	SC	Adjusted dose SC UH is an effective alternative.
Low-molecular-weight heparin (LMWH)	SC	Once or twice daily, dose is brand dependent. Duration 5–10 days, overlapping with a vitamin-K antagonist, dabigatran, or edoxaban. No monitoring required (usually), renal excretion.
Fondaparinux	SC	5 mg daily if body weight <50 kg 7.5 mg daily if body weight 50–100 kg 10 mg daily if body weight >100 kg Duration 5–10 days, overlapping with a vitamin-K antagonist, dabigatran, or edoxaban. No monitoring required (usually), renal excretion.
Vitamin-K antagonists	PO	5–10 mg initial dose, titrated to INR 2.0–3.0. Reduce initial dose if age >60 years, impaired nutrition, moderate-to-severe liver disease, coadministration of warfarin potentiating medications.
Rivaroxaban	PO	15 mg twice daily × 21 days, then 20 mg once daily. Contraindicated if CrCl <30 mL/min. Contraindicated for moderate-to-severe liver disease.[a]
Apixaban	PO	10 mg twice daily × 7 days, then 5 mg twice daily. No dose adjustment needed for renal impairment or ESRD. Contraindicated for severe liver disease.[a] Following ≥6 months of therapy, 2.5 mg twice daily for secondary prophylaxis.
Dabigatran	PO	150 mg twice daily, after 5–10 days of parenteral anticoagulation. Contraindicated if CrCl <30 mL/min.[a]
Edoxaban	PO	60 mg daily if body weight >60 kg. 30 mg daily if body weight ≤60 kg, or CrCl 15–50 mL/min. Contraindicated in moderate-to-severe liver disease.[a]

[a]Dose adjustments recommended when coadministering cytochrome P450 and P-glycoprotein inhibitors or inducers.

aPTT, Activated partial thromboplastin time; *CrCl,* creatinine clearance; *ESRD,* end-stage renal disease, *INR,* international normalized ratio; *IV,* intravenous; *PO,* oral; *SC,* subcutaneous.

Duration of Anticoagulation

The recommended duration of anticoagulation depends mainly on the clinical circumstances around the VTE (provoked versus unprovoked), the estimated risk of bleeding while on anticoagulation, and the location of the thrombosis. Abbreviated recommendations from the CHEST Guideline and Expert Panel Report are shown in Table 12.5.[15] In general, patients with unprovoked proximal DVT or PE who are at low risk of bleeding should be considered for extended-duration anticoagulation. At the opposite end of the spectrum, patients with asymptomatic isolated distal DVT (typically found via screening) may safely receive serial duplex imaging, treating only those who develop symptoms or propagation of thrombus.

TABLE 12.5 Recommended Duration of Anticoagulation

Clinical Subgroup	ACCP Treatment Recommendations
First episode LE DVT/surgical or nonsurgical transient risk	Anticoagulation for 3 months
First episode LE DVT/unprovoked	Anticoagulation for at least 3 months
• Proximal DVT/PE with low or moderate bleeding risk	• Extended anticoagulation (no stop date)
• Proximal DVT/PE with high bleeding risk	• Stop anticoagulation at 3 months
• Patients with proximal DVT/PE who stop anticoagulation and have no contraindication to aspirin	• Aspirin (100 mg by mouth daily)
Isolated distal LE DVT	
• With severe symptoms/risk factors for extension	• Anticoagulation for 3 months
• Without severe symptoms/risk factors for extension	• The ACCP suggests serial imaging for 2 weeks, with initiation of anticoagulation if thrombus extends to other distal deep veins or proximal veins
Second episode VTE/unprovoked	
• Low-to-moderate bleeding risk	• Extended anticoagulation (no stop date)
• High bleeding risk	• 3 months of anticoagulation
LE DVT/PE and cancer	LMWH SC for first 3 months, then extended anticoagulation (no stop date)
Superficial vein thrombosis (>5 cm in length)	Fondaparinux 2.5 mg SC daily for 45 days, or LMWH prophylactic dosing SC for 45 days

ACCP, American College of Chest Physicians; *DVT,* deep venous thrombosis; *LE,* lower extremity; *LMWH,* low-molecular-weight heparin; *PE,* pulmonary embolism; *SC,* subcutaneous; *VTE,* venous thromboembolism.
(From Kearon C, Akl EA, Omela J, et al. Antithrombotic therapy for venous thromboembolic disease. Chest Guideline and Expert Panel Report. *Chest.* 2016; 149(2):315–352; Kearon C, Akl EA, Comerota AJ, et al. Antithrombotic therapy for VTE disease: antithrombotic therapy and prevention of thrombosis, 9th ed: American College of Chest Physicians Evidence-Based Clinic Practice Guidelines. *Chest.* 2012;141: e419S–e494S.)

The choice of long-term anticoagulation may also play a role in deciding the duration of therapy. As a group, the direct oral anticoagulants are associated with a lower risk of major bleeding when compared with warfarin. This difference is especially marked for apixaban, which has the lowest annual rate of major bleeding. As a result, this may decrease a clinician's threshold for recommending extended-duration therapy. In patients who have contraindications to anticoagulation, the treatment algorithm will vary depending upon the location of the original DVT (Fig. 12.3).

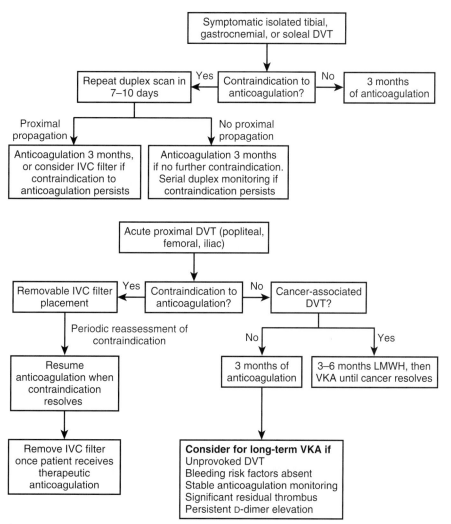

■ **Fig. 12.3** Treatment algorithm for deep venous thrombosis. *DVT,* Deep vein thrombosis; *IVC,* inferior vena cava; *LMWH,* low-molecular-weight heparin; *VKA,* vitamin K antagonists.

SUPERFICIAL VENOUS THROMBOSIS

Acute SVT occurs in approximately 125,000 people in the United States per year.[16] Traditional teaching mistakenly suggests that SVT is a self-limiting process of little consequence and small risk.

Clinical presentation of SVT: approximately 35% to 46% of patients with SVT are males (average age 54 years). The average age for females is about 58 years.[17,18] Factors associated with SVT include varicose veins (most frequent), age older than 60 years, obesity, tobacco use, and a history of DVT or SVT. Factors associated with extension of SVT include age older than 60 years, male gender, and a history of DVT. SVT of the great saphenous vein (GSV) is most common; however, SVT of the small saphenous vein (SSV) should not be overlooked because it may progress to popliteal DVT.

Etiology and Natural History of Superficial Vein Thrombosis

SVT may develop as a result of numerous contributing risk factors. Perhaps the most common of these is chronic venous insufficiency with concomitant varicose veins. Superficial thrombosis is also a common occurrence after stab phlebectomy or sclerotherapy. However, these episodes are self-limited and rarely result in propagation of thrombus. In the absence of chronic venous insufficiency, risk factors include pregnancy and estrogen therapy, intravenous catheters, and inherited or acquired thrombophilia (including malignancy). A hypercoagulable condition may be identified in as many as 40% of isolated SVT patients. However, routine hypercoagulable testing is not likely to be cost effective and may result in overtreating with anticoagulation.

Diagnosis and Imaging of Superficial Vein Thrombosis

The physical diagnosis of superficial thrombophlebitis is based on the presence of erythema and tenderness in the distribution of the superficial veins, with the thrombosis identified as a palpable cord. Duplex ultrasound scanning is the initial test of choice for the diagnosis of SVT as well as DVT. The extent of involvement of the deep and superficial systems may be accurately assessed with this modality because routine clinical examination may not be able to precisely evaluate the proximal extent of involvement. Duplex imaging has shown concomitant DVT to be present in 5% to 40% of patients with SVT.[19-21] Note that up to 25% of these DVTs may not be contiguous with the SVT and may be in the contralateral lower extremity.

Treatment of Superficial Vein Thrombosis

The goals of treatment are 2-fold: reduction in local symptoms and prevention of thrombus propagation into the deep venous system. Symptomatic improvement may be accomplished with nonsteroidal antiinflammatory agents and warm soaks. Compression therapy may not improve clinical symptoms, but it does lead to faster thrombus regression.[22] Resolution of symptoms typically occurs within 1 to 2 weeks, but a palpable cord may persist for many months.

The progression of isolated SVT to DVT has been evaluated. Among 263 patients with isolated SVT by duplex ultrasonography, 30 (11%) patients had documented progression to deep venous involvement.[23] Progression from the GSV in the thigh into the common femoral vein (21 patients) was most common, with 18 of these extensions noted to be nonocclusive and 12 having a free-floating component. Because of the recognized potential for extension into the deep system and embolization, high saphenous ligation with or without stripping often is recommended for SVT within 1 cm of the saphenofemoral junction (SFJ). In a series of 43 patients who underwent ligation of the SFJ with and without local common femoral vein (CFV) thrombectomy and stripping of the GSV, two patients were found with postoperative contralateral DVT, one of whom had a PE[24-27] (Figs. 12.4–12.6).

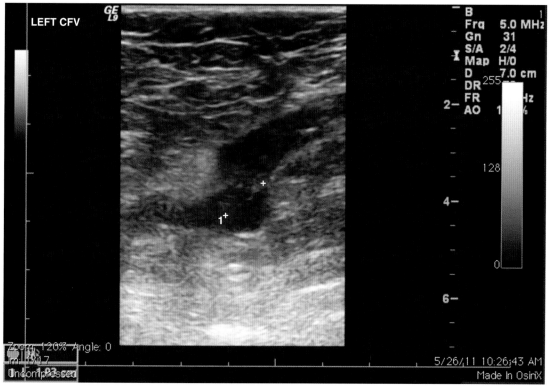

■ **Fig. 12.4** Superficial venous thrombosis: thrombus at saphenofemoral junction extends into common femoral vein. *CFV,* Common femoral vein.

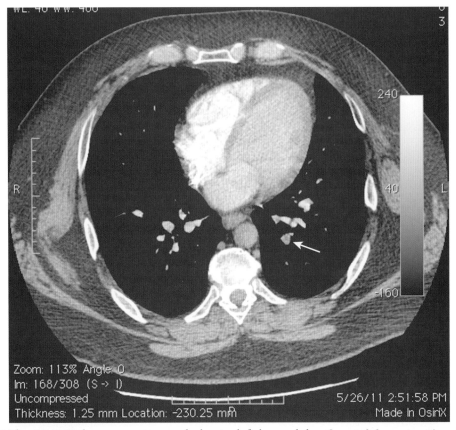

■ **Fig. 12.5** Pulmonary artery embolus to left lower lobe *(arrow)* (cross-sectional view).

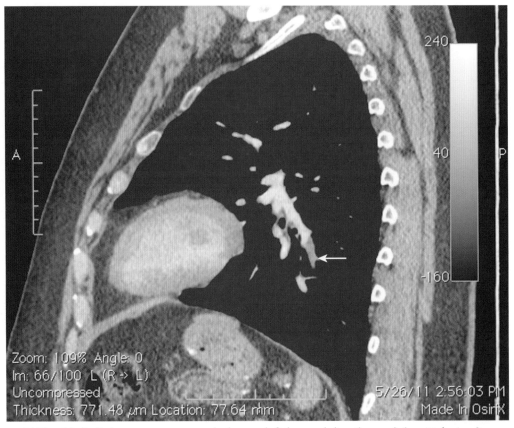

■ **Fig. 12.6** Pulmonary artery embolus to left lower lobe *(arrow)* (sagittal view).

Meta-analysis of surgical versus medical therapy for isolated above-knee SVT has been attempted but has not been feasible because of the paucity of comparable data between the two groups.[28] This review suggested that although stripping provides superior symptomatic relief, medical management with anticoagulants is somewhat superior with respect to minimizing complications and preventing subsequent DVT and PE. Based on these data, the authors suggest that anticoagulation is appropriate in patients without contraindications.

Thus limited-duration anticoagulation has become the mainstay for the prevention of thrombus propagation. In a large, prospective, randomized trial of over 3000 patients who had isolated SVT (≥5 cm in length), fondaparinux (2.5 mg subcutaneously once daily × 45 days) resulted in a 5% absolute reduction (85% relative risk reduction) in the composite endpoint of symptomatic recurrence or superficial extension, symptomatic DVT, symptomatic PE, or death, when compared with placebo.[29] Older trials have found similar benefits with LMWH, and newer trials are underway to evaluate the efficacy of direct oral anticoagulants as well.[30,31] These limited number of studies are the basis for a moderate recommendation in the American College of Chest Physicians (CHEST) guidelines, which suggest that patients with SVT (≥5 cm) receive prophylactic dose fondaparinux or LMWH for 45 days.[32]

Endothermal, heat-induced thrombosis (EHIT) was briefly covered in Chapter 5. The following is a typical example of the natural course of an SFJ thrombosis after thermal ablation treatment. This series of ultrasounds demonstrates a generous thrombus at SFJ retracting over time from postoperative day 3 (initial ultrasound) to postoperative day 5, where retraction has begun. At 3 weeks postoperative, the thrombus extension is no longer visualized. No anticoagulation or platelet therapy was used. Notice that no contiguous thrombotic lesions were identified in the deep system. This situation is very different from the ultrasound and computed tomography scans shown previously (see Figs. 12.4–12.6), in which case the patient presented with spontaneous GSV thrombosis extending into the SFJ and developed a PE (Fig. 12.7).

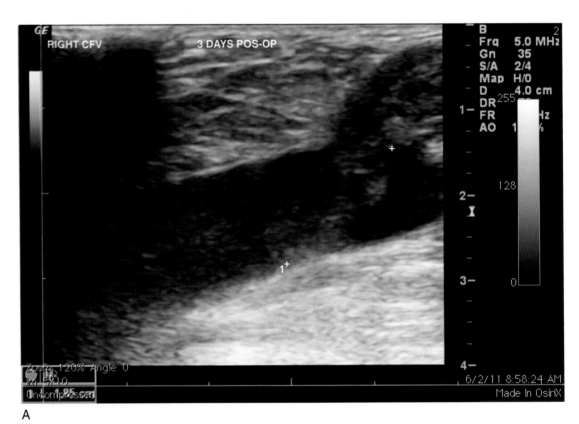

A

■ **Fig. 12.7** (A) Thrombus extension (endothermal heat-induced thrombosis [EHIT]) seen on postoperative day 3 at the saphenofemoral junction.

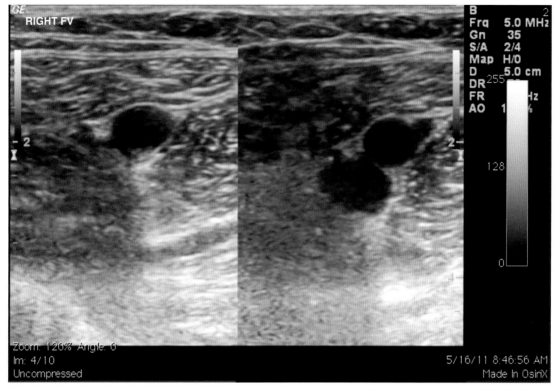

B

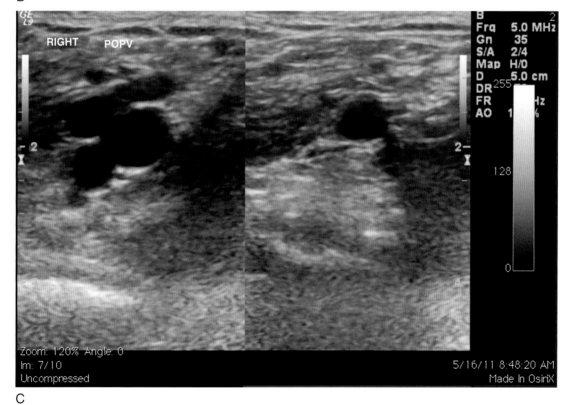

C

■ **Fig. 12.7, cont'd** (B) Fully compressed femoral vein *(left panel)* demonstrating no femoral vein thrombosis. (C) Fully compressed popliteal vein *(right panel)* demonstrating no evidence of popliteal vein thrombosis.

Continued

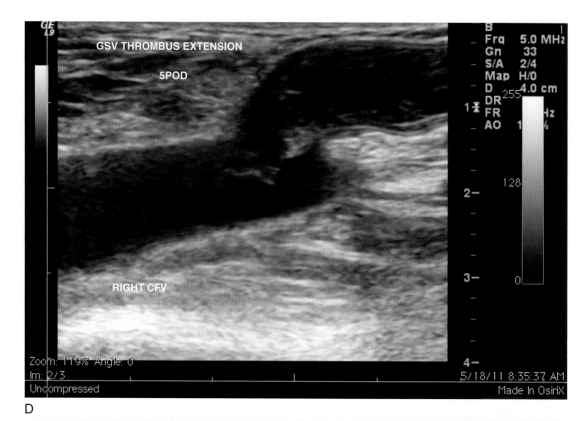

D

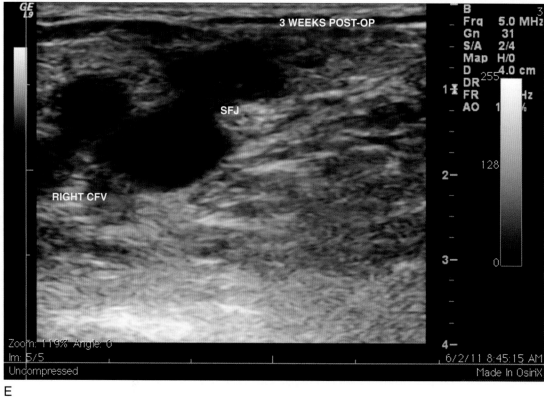

E

■ **Fig. 12.7, cont'd** (D) Onset of thrombus retraction (EHIT) seen on postoperative day 5. (E) Completely retracted thrombus extension (EHIT) seen postoperatively at 3 weeks. *CFV*, Common femoral vein; *FV*, femoral vein; *GSV*, great saphenous vein; *POPV*, popliteal vein; *SFJ*, saphenofemoral junction.

REFERENCES

1. Kearon C, Kahn SR, Agnelli G, et al. Antithrombotic therapy for venous thromboembolic disease. American College of Chest Physicians Evidence-Based Clinical Practice Guidelines. *Chest.* 2008;133:454–545.
2. Kearon C. Natural history of venous thromboembolism. *Circulation.* 2003;107:I22–I30.
3. Rosendaal FR. Venous thrombosis: a multicausal disease. *Lancet.* 1999;353:1167–1173.
4. Anderson FA, Wheeler HB, Goldberg RJ, et al. The prevalence of risk factors for venous thromboembolism among hospital patients. *Arch Intern Med.* 1992;152:1660–1664.
5. Oger E, Leroyer C, LeMoigne E, et al. The value of risk factor analysis in clinically suspected deep venous thrombosis. *Respiration.* 1997;64:326–330.
6. Jacobs B, Obi A, Wakefield T. Diagnostic biomarkers in venous thromboembolic disease. *J Vasc Surg: Venous and Lym Dis.* 2016;4:508–517.
7. Thomas DP, Merton RE, Hockley DJ. The effect of stasis on the venous endothelium: an ultrastructural study. *Br J Haematol.* 1983;55:113–122.
8. Schulman S, Kakkar AK, Goldhaber SZ, et al. Treatment of acute venous thromboembolism with dabigatran or warfarin and pooled analysis. *Circulation.* 2014;129:764–772.
9. The EINSTEIN Investigators. Oral rivaroxiban for symptomatic venous thromboembolism. *N Engl J Med.* 2010;363(24):99–2510.
10. Agnelli G, Buller HR, Cohen A, et al. Oral apixiban for the treatment of acute venous thromboembolism. *N Engl J Med.* 2013;369:799–808.
11. The Hokusai-VTE Investigators. Edoxaban versus warfarin for the treatment of symptomatic venous thromboembolism. *N Engl J Med.* 2013;369:1406–1415.
12. Ensor J, Riley RD, Moore D, et al. Systematic review of prognostic models for recurrent venous thromboembolism (VTE) post-treatment of first unprovoked VTE. *BMJ Open.* 2016;6:e011190.
13. Cuker A, Gimotty PA, Crowther M, et al. Predictive value of the 4Ts scoring system for heparin-induced thrombocytopenia: a systematic review and meta-analysis. *Blood.* 2012;120(20): 4160–4167.
14. Liem TK. Duplex ultrasound scanning for acute venous disease. In: Gloviczki P, ed. Handbook of Venous and Lymphatic Disorders. 4th ed. Boca Raton, FL: CRC Press; 2017:141–150.
15. Kearon C, Akl EA, Omela J, et al. Antithrombotic therapy for venous thromboembolic disease. Chest Guideline and Expert Panel Report. *Chest.* 2016;149(2):315–352.
16. De Weese MS. Nonoperative treatment of acute superficial thrombophlebitis and deep femoral venous thrombosis. In: Ernst CB, Stanley JC, eds. Current Therapy in Vascular Surgery. Philadelphia: BC Decker; 1991:952–960.
17. Lohr JM, McDevitt DT, Lutter KS, et al. Operative management of greater saphenous thrombophlebitis involving the saphenofemoral junction. *Am J Surg.* 1992;164:269–275.
18. Lutter KS, Kerr TM, Roedersheimer LR, et al. Superficial thrombophlebitis diagnosed by duplex scanning. *Surgery.* 1991;110:42–46.
19. Bjorgell O, Nilsson PE, Jarenros H. Isolated nonfilling of contrast in deep vein segments seen on phlebography, and a comparison with color Doppler ultrasound to assess the incidence of deep venous thrombosis. *Angiology.* 2000;51:451–461.
20. Jorgensen JO, Hanel KC, Morgan AM, et al. The incidence of deep venous thrombosis in patients with superficial thrombophlebitis of the lower limbs. *J Vasc Surg.* 1993;18:70–73.
21. Skillman JJ, Kent KC, Porter DH, et al. Simultaneous occurrence of superficial and deep thrombophlebitis in the lower extremity. *J Vasc Surg.* 1990;11:818–823, discussion 823–824.
22. Boehler K, Kittler H, Stolkovich S, et al. Therapeutic effect of compression stockings versus no compression on isolated superficial vein thrombosis of the legs. *Eur J Vasc Endovasc Surg.* 2014;48(4):465–471.
23. Chengelis DL, Bendick PJ, Glover JL, et al. Progression of superficial venous thrombosis to deep vein thrombosis. *J Vasc Surg.* 1996;24:745–749.
24. Gjores JE. Surgical therapy of ascending thrombophlebitis in the saphenous system. *Angiology.* 1962;13:241–243.

25. Husni EA, Williams WA. Superficial thrombophlebitis of lower limbs. *Surgery.* 1982;91:70–74.

26. Lofgren EP, Lofgren KA. The surgical treatment of superficial thrombophlebitis. *Surgery.* 1981;90:49–54.

27. Plate G, Eklof B, Jensen R, et al. Deep venous thrombosis, pulmonary embolism and acute surgery in thrombophlebitis of the long saphenous vein. *Acta Chir Scand.* 1985;151:241–244.

28. Sullivan V, Denk PM, Sonnad SS, et al. Ligation versus anticoagulation: treatment of above-knee superficial thrombophlebitis not involving the deep venous system. *J Am Coll Surg.* 2001;193:556–562.

29. Decousus H, Prandoni P, Mismetti P, et al. Fondaparinux for the treatment of superficial-vein thrombosis in the legs. *N Engl J Med.* 2010;363(13):1222–1232.

30. The Superficial Thrombophlebitis Treated by Enoxaparin Study Group. A pilot randomized double-blind comparison of a low-molecular-weight heparin, a nonsteroidal anti-inflammatory agent, and placebo in the treatment of superficial-vein thrombosis. *Arch Intern Med.* 2003;163:1657–1663.

31. Werth S, Bauersachs R, Gerlach H, et al. Superficial vein thrombosis treated for 45 days with rivaroxiban versus fondaparinux: rationale and design of the SURPRISE trial. *J Thromb Thrombolysis.* 2016;42(2):197–204.

32. Kearon C, Akl EA, Comerota AJ, et al. Antithrombotic therapy for VTE disease: Antithrombotic therapy and prevention of thrombosis, 9th ed: American College of Chest Physicians Evidence-Based Clinical Practice Guidelines. *Chest.* 2012;141:e419S–e494S.

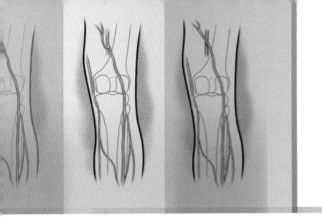

CHAPTER 13

Endovenous Placement of Inferior Vena Caval Filters

Timothy K. Liem

HISTORICAL BACKGROUND

Venous interruption for the prevention of pulmonary embolism (PE) was introduced by Homans in 1934. Although his initial description involved ligation of the femoral vein, surgical techniques soon evolved, focusing on interruption at the level of the inferior vena cava (IVC). Complete ligation of the IVC was performed in 1959, but the resulting cardiovascular complications and venous sequelae led to the development of alternative strategies for either temporary interruption or plication. These included temporary ligation of the IVC using absorbable suture, plication of the IVC using interrupted mattress suture, and partially occluding externally applied polytetrafluoroethylene (PTFE) clips (Moretz clip, Adams-DeWeese clip). These techniques required retroperitoneal exposure and general anesthesia, which are distinct disadvantages, particularly in patients who are often ill with significant comorbidities.

The Mobin-Uddin umbrella, introduced in 1967, was the first IVC filter that could be inserted via a transjugular approach under local anesthesia. The apex of this device was oriented inferiorly, and the original design incorporated a solid, fabric membrane with the intent of causing caval thrombosis. Fenestrations were added later, with the purpose of causing delayed thrombosis, supposedly increasing the development of collaterals. However, some patients maintained a patent IVC, and yet they had a low rate of pulmonary embolization. These observations led to significant design advances, such that IVC thrombosis was no longer the desired outcome. The superior design of the Greenfield filter (Boston Scientific, Natick, MA), with its low rate of caval thrombosis, allowed it to rapidly supplant prior filter designs. The Greenfield (and the ensuing iterations) could be placed via a transjugular or transfemoral approach, and it became the standard caval interruption device to which newer filters were compared for the next few decades.

PATIENT SELECTION

The accepted and relative indications[1] for placement of an IVC filter are shown in Table 13.1. Although anticoagulation is the mainstay of therapy in patients with acute deep venous thrombosis (DVT) or PE, it may be contraindicated for several reasons. Active internal bleeding is an absolute contraindication to therapeutic anticoagulation. However, an increased risk of bleeding caused by recent trauma or major surgery (especially neurologic or ocular surgery) more often is a relative contraindication that is subject to clinical judgment. In the era when unfractionated heparin and vitamin-K antagonists were the only available antithrombotic agents, nonhemorrhagic complications of anticoagulation (e.g., heparin-induced thrombocytopenia, warfarin-induced skin necrosis) were more common indications for IVC filter insertion. However, the greater availability of effective antithrombotic alternatives, such as low-molecular-weight heparin, pentasaccharides, direct thrombin inhibitors, and oral factor Xa inhibitors have curtailed the use of unfractionated heparin and warfarin for the treatment of venous thromboembolism (VTE).

An often-cited indication for IVC filter insertion is "failure of anticoagulation." Significant proximal DVT extension and PE may occur in up to 4% to 11% of patients who receive anticoagulation for acute lower extremity DVT. Over 70% of these failures occur in the first 3 weeks after initiation of therapy. However, there should be a distinction between patients who are receiving adequate antithrombotic therapy versus those receiving inadequate antithrombotic therapy. Patients should be carefully questioned, and the anticoagulation records should be reviewed to determine whether dosages and frequency of antithrombotic medications were adequate (Fig. 13.1 and Table 13.2).

TABLE 13.1 Indications for Placement of an Inferior Vena Cava Filter

Common Indications for IVC Filter Placement

- Contraindication to anticoagulation in a patient with an acute proximal LE DVT or PE
- Recurrent VTE despite adequate antithrombotic therapy; recurrence may include significant proximal DVT extension in an ipsilateral LE, development of a new proximal DVT in a contralateral LE, or PE
- Massive PE with residual LE DVT

Relative Indications for IVC Filter Placement

- Patients with PE and significant pulmonary disease (pulmonary hypertension, cor pulmonale)
- Prophylactic IVC filter placement in a patient at high risk for VTE in whom antithrombotic therapy is contraindicated and in whom adequate diagnostic imaging cannot be performed (e.g., trauma patient with lower extremity injuries)
- During catheter-directed pharmacomechanical thrombolysis
- "Free-floating" thrombus in the proximal deep veins of the lower extremities

DVT, Deep venous thrombosis; *IVC,* inferior vena cava; *LE,* lower extremity; *PE,* pulmonary embolism; *VTE,* venous thromboembolism.

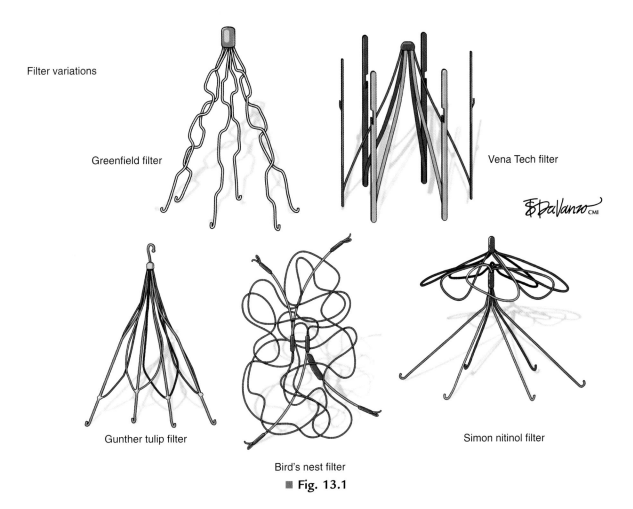

Filter variations

Greenfield filter

Vena Tech filter

Gunther tulip filter

Bird's nest filter

Simon nitinol filter

■ **Fig. 13.1**

TABLE 13.2 Guidewires and Catheters

Name	Diameter	Length
Guidewires		
Bentson/Rosen	0.035 inch	150–180 cm
Angled glide wire	0.035 inch	150–180 cm
Catheters		
Pigtail (with 2-cm calibration)	5-Fr	65–90 cm
Kumpe (or another angled catheter)	5-Fr	65–90 cm
Ancillary Supplies		
Heparinized saline	1000 U/1000 mL of normal saline	
Syringes (2)	20 mL, Luer Lock	
Dilators	5-Fr and 6-Fr	
Injectable nonionic contrast, high-flow power injector		

The routine use of IVC filters in patients with PE who are receiving concurrent anticoagulation is not indicated for most patients.[2] Recent trials have demonstrated that routine filter placement does not decrease the risk for recurrent PE or mortality, but it may increase the risk for lower extremity DVT.[3] Because of the limited number of studies, however, this recommendation against IVC filter placement may not apply to all groups of patients. Those with massive PE (with hypotension) might benefit from an IVC filter.

IMAGING

Venous Duplex Imaging

Most patients who are referred for placement of an IVC filter have had recent ultrasound confirmation of a lower extremity DVT. The proximal extent of the thrombus should be noted because this may affect potential access sites for venography and filter insertion. If the patient has an acute iliofemoral DVT or if the thrombus extends above the level of the proximal femoral vein, then cannulation of the adjacent common femoral vein should be avoided if possible.

Venography

IVC venography should be performed in most patients before insertion of a filter. This imaging is done for several reasons: the location of the renal veins may be determined, the presence of anomalies of the IVC may be detected, the diameter of the IVC may be measured, and the presence of thrombus in the IVC may be visualized. If thrombus is present in the infrarenal IVC, then the filter may need to be placed proximal to the renal veins.

In patients with normal anatomy, the common iliac vein confluence occurs at the L4-L5 vertebral body, and the renal veins insert into the IVC at the L1 vertebral body. Kaufman et al.[4] performed a detailed magnetic resonance imaging analysis of the anatomy of the IVC. The average length of the infrarenal IVC is 94 mm in females and 110 mm in males. However, these lengths vary significantly, especially in patients who have anomalous venous return. Retroaortic and circumaortic left renal veins are found in 7% and 5%, respectively, and multiple right renal veins are present in 8%. Prior literature indicates that the prevalence of duplicate IVCs ranges from 0.7% to 3%, based on radiographic investigations and cadaver dissections. A left-sided vena cava is even less common (0.2%–0.5%). In this latter setting, the infrarenal IVC ascends on the left lateral aspect of the aorta. After insertion in the left renal vein, it then crosses anterior to the aorta to assume its usual anatomic position. A similarly rare anomaly is atresia of the suprarenal IVC, replaced by a hypertrophic azygous vein (0.6%).

ACCESS AND OPERATIVE STEPS

Inferior vena cavography is usually performed via an internal jugular or common femoral approach (right is preferable to left in both instances). The site for access is often left up to the physician. However, certain clinical situations dictate an optimal strategy. A right internal jugular approach is commonly used, and it usually will not disturb thrombi in the iliac or femoral veins. It may also be used to cannulate either of the common iliac veins if further imaging is needed to visualize potential IVC anomalies. All currently available IVC filters may also be inserted via a jugular approach. A common femoral venous approach may be more advantageous in patients who are intubated or have central venous catheters in place. However, the physician should confirm with duplex imaging that the access site is not involved with the venous thrombosis.

Right Internal Jugular Approach

The internal jugular vein should be cannulated using a combination of anatomic landmarks and ultrasound guidance. The internal jugular vein is located deep to the confluence of the two heads of the sternocleidomastoid muscle (SCM). More specifically, it is located deep to the clavicular head of the SCM, about one-third of the distance from the medial border to the lateral border of the muscle. A subcutaneous wheel of local anesthetic is injected, and a no. 11 blade is used to incise the dermis. The subcutaneous tissue is spread gently with a mosquito clamp.

An 18-gauge single-wall puncture needle connected to a 5-mL or 10-mL syringe is used to access the vein with ultrasound guidance. The syringe should freely aspirate dark blood, and a 0.035-inch (0.088-cm) guidewire is passed into the IVC under fluoroscopic guidance. Occasionally, an angled catheter may be required to steer the wire into the IVC. Alternatively, a 21-gauge needle, 0.018-inch (0.045-cm) guidewire, and 5-Fr catheter/dilator set (Micropuncture Introducer Set; Cook Medical, Bloomington, IN) may be used to avoid using the larger needle (Table 13.3; Figs. 13.2–13.10).

Text continued on p. 352

TABLE 13.3 Right Internal Jugular Approach

- Patient supine, slight Trendelenburg positioning if possible
- Slight neck rotation away from the site of access (overrotation beyond 30 to 60 degrees may increase the risk of carotid cannulation)
- Internal jugular access about 2 cm superior to the sternoclavicular junction, between the two heads of the sternocleidomastoid muscle, needle directed laterally
- A standard 5-MHz to 10-MHz ultrasound probe is placed transverse to the jugular vein; the syringe is gently aspirated as the needle is used to indent and puncture the anterior wall of the vein
- The guidewire should pass without resistance and fluoroscopy should be used to confirm wire placement into the superior vena cava

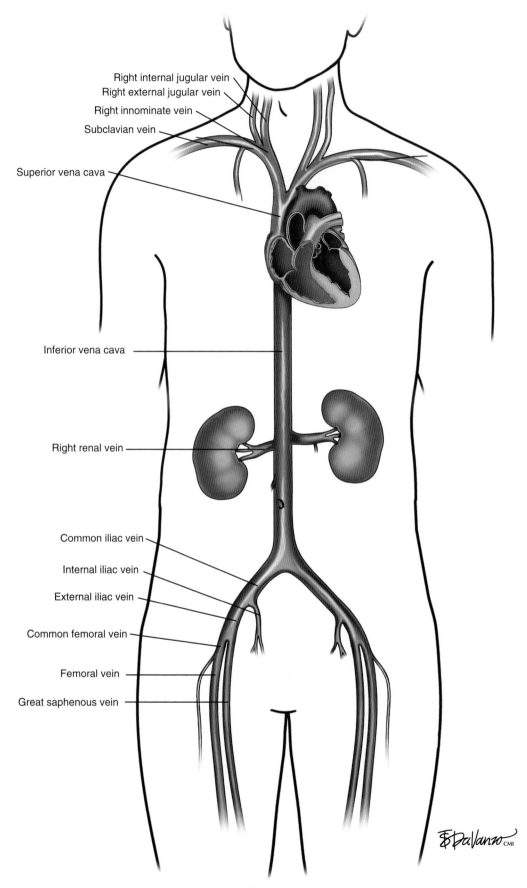

■ Fig. 13.2

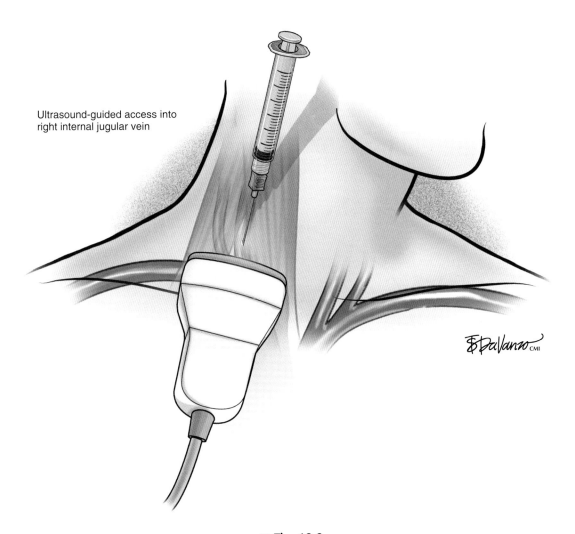

Ultrasound-guided access into
right internal jugular vein

▪ **Fig. 13.3**

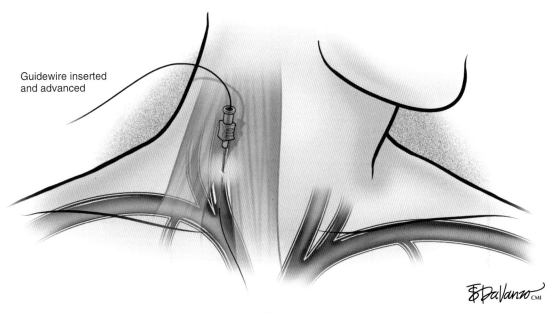

Guidewire inserted
and advanced

▪ **Fig. 13.4**

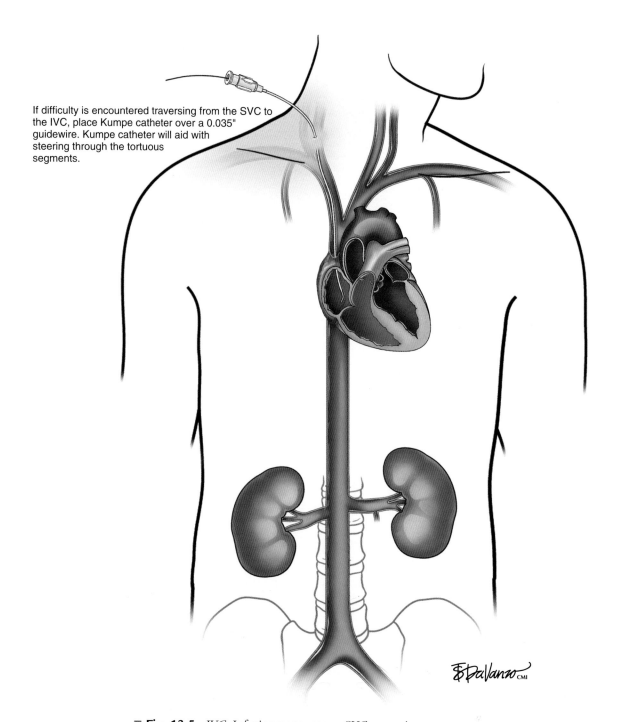

If difficulty is encountered traversing from the SVC to the IVC, place Kumpe catheter over a 0.035" guidewire. Kumpe catheter will aid with steering through the tortuous segments.

■ **Fig. 13.5** *IVC,* Inferior vena cava; *SVC,* superior vena cava.

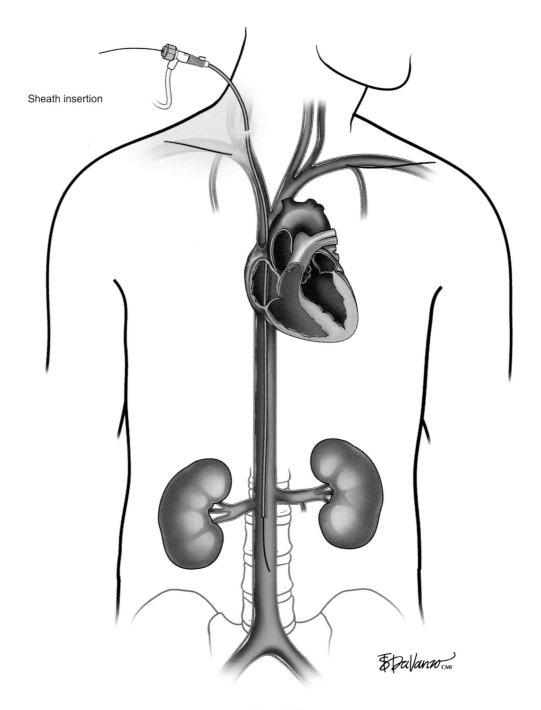

Sheath insertion

■ **Fig. 13.6**

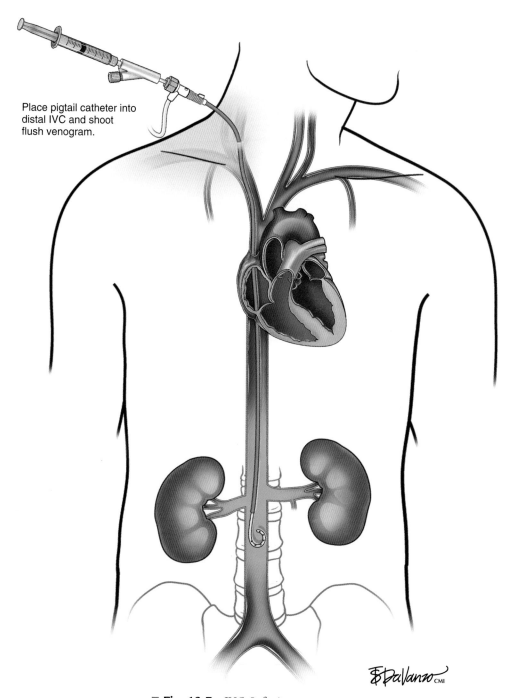

Place pigtail catheter into distal IVC and shoot flush venogram.

▪ **Fig. 13.7** *IVC*, Inferior vena cava.

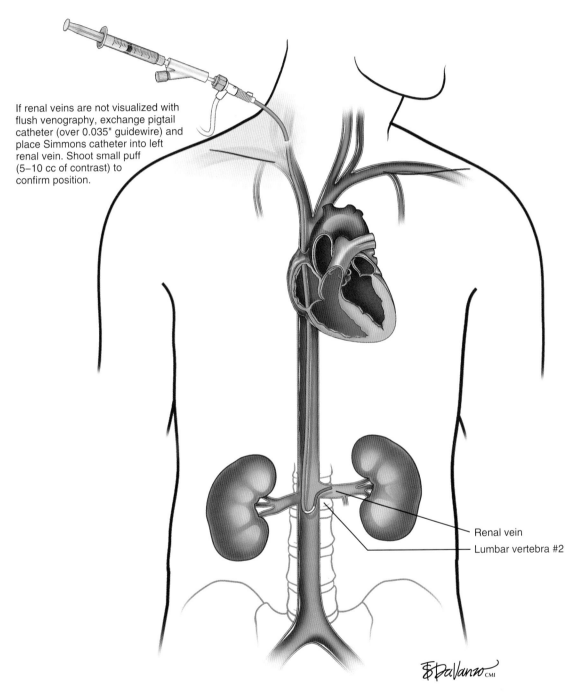

If renal veins are not visualized with flush venography, exchange pigtail catheter (over 0.035" guidewire) and place Simmons catheter into left renal vein. Shoot small puff (5–10 cc of contrast) to confirm position.

Renal vein

Lumbar vertebra #2

■ Fig. 13.8

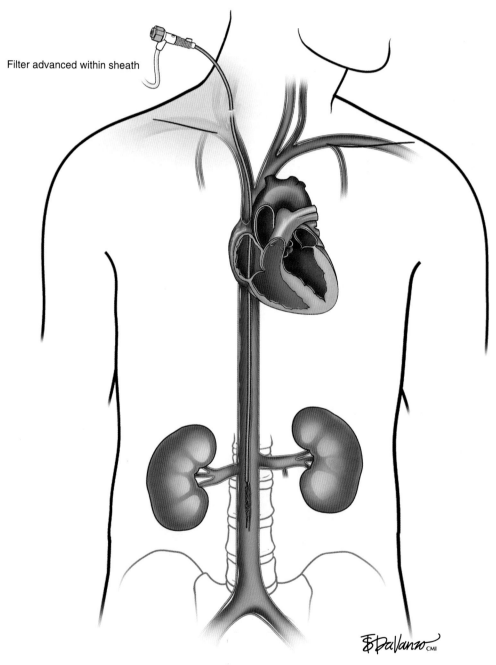

Filter advanced within sheath

■ **Fig. 13.9**

Filter deployed

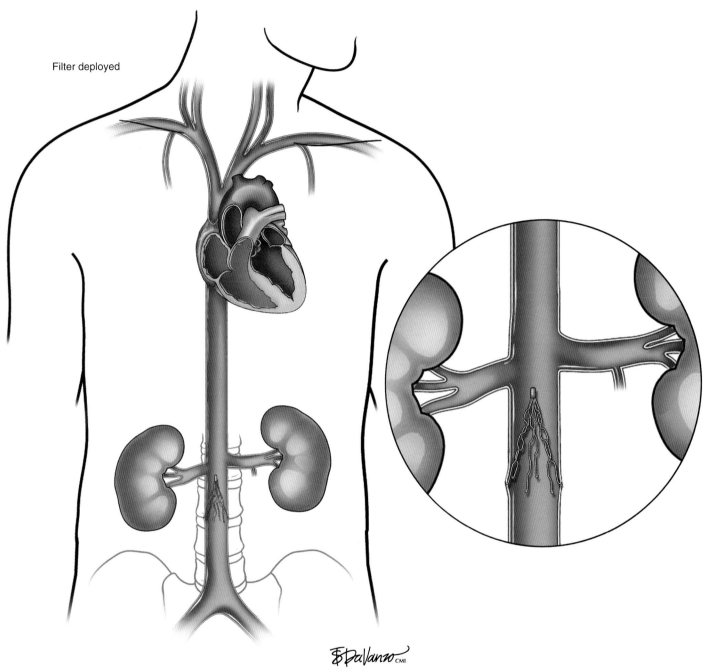

■ Fig. 13.10

Common Femoral Vein Approach

The common femoral vein is usually accessed using anatomic landmarks alone. The femoral pulse is palpated laterally. Ultrasound guidance may be easily applied in circumstances when the patient is obese or if the femoral pulse is absent. The common femoral vein cannulation techniques with an 18-gauge or 21-gauge needle are similar to those described for internal jugular venous access (Figs. 13.11–13.16).

Text continued on p. 358

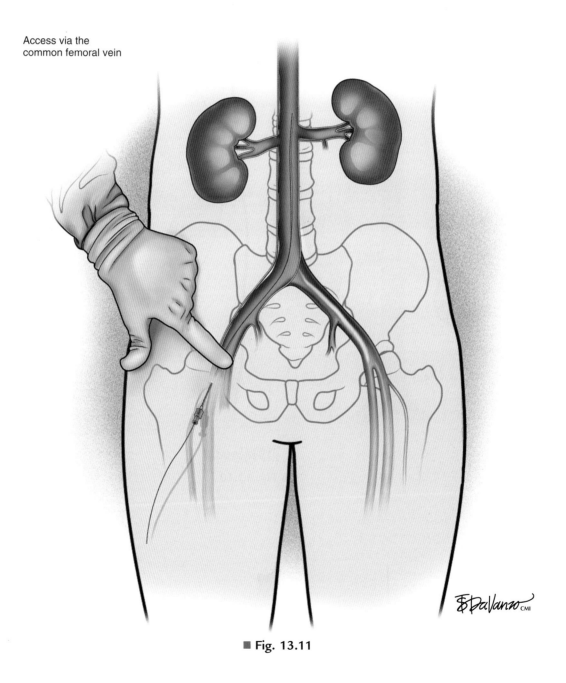

Access via the
common femoral vein

■ **Fig. 13.11**

Sheath placed over
guidewire and advanced
into IVC

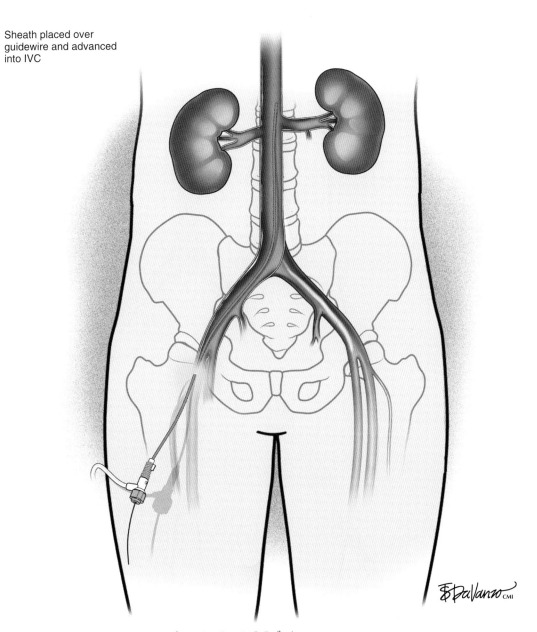

■ **Fig. 13.12** *IVC,* Inferior vena cava.

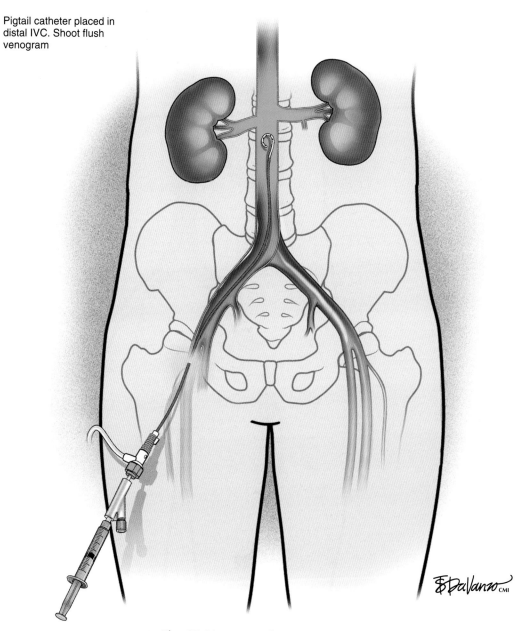

Pigtail catheter placed in distal IVC. Shoot flush venogram

■ **Fig. 13.13** *IVC,* Inferior vena cava.

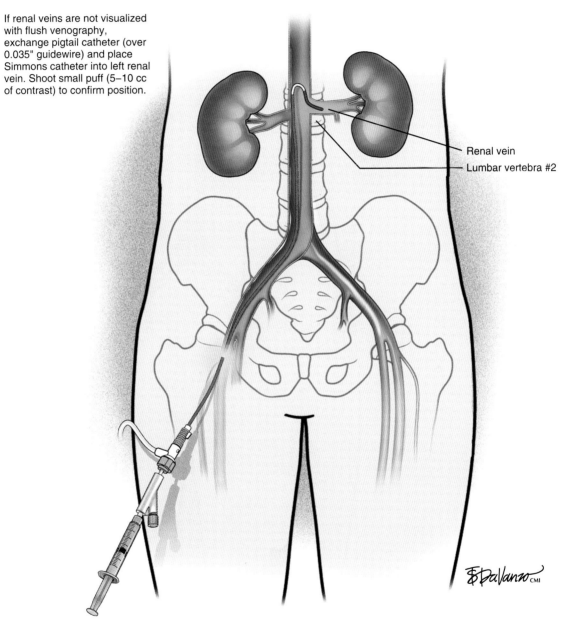

If renal veins are not visualized with flush venography, exchange pigtail catheter (over 0.035" guidewire) and place Simmons catheter into left renal vein. Shoot small puff (5–10 cc of contrast) to confirm position.

Renal vein

Lumbar vertebra #2

■ **Fig. 13.14**

Filter is advanced within sheath

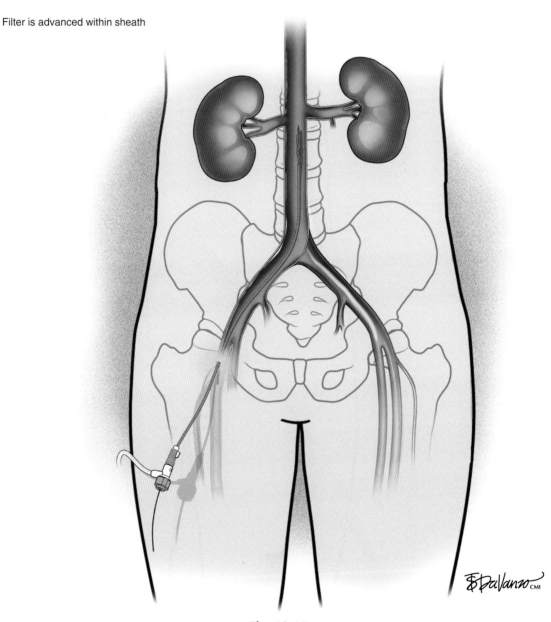

■ **Fig. 13.15**

Filter deployed

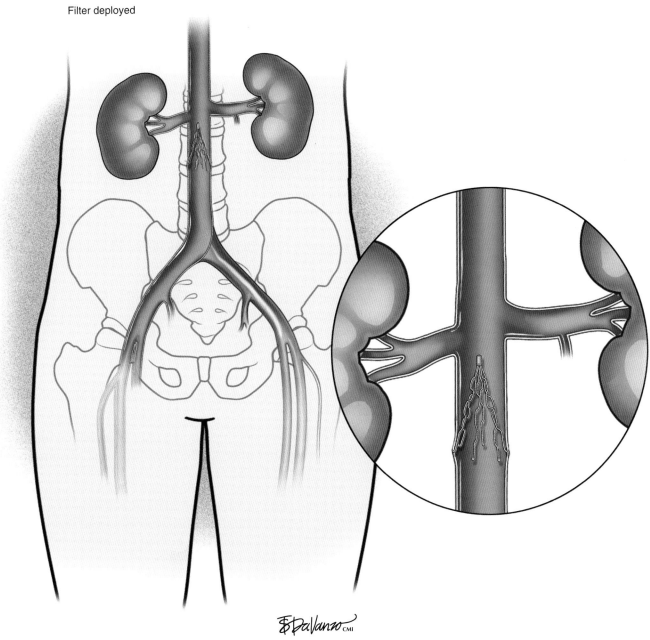

■ **Fig. 13.16**

ANTICOAGULATION MANAGEMENT

The management of anticoagulation around the time of IVC filter insertion will depend on the indication for the filter. If the filter is to be inserted because of a contraindication to anticoagulation (e.g., active internal bleeding, recent major surgery, trauma, anticoagulation-related bleeding), then the IVC filter can be placed without periprocedural anticoagulation. However, if the indication was venous thromboembolism recurrence despite adequate anticoagulation, then the anticoagulation should not be discontinued around the time of the procedure.[5]

PEARLS AND PITFALLS

In patients who receive a filter because of a contraindication to anticoagulation, remember to continually reassess if and when antithrombotic therapy may be reinitiated. Once the patient has safely resumed and remained stable on anticoagulation, the IVC filter should be removed.

In patients who develop recurrent VTE despite adequate anticoagulation, another option is to convert back to low-molecular-weight heparin for more than 1 month.

If the plan is to remove an IVC filter, hospital programs should be instituted to track patients, ensure follow-up, and arrange for filter retrieval in a timely fashion. In patients who receive a permanent filter, yearly follow-up with plain kidney-ureter-bladder films should be obtained to assess for filter fracture or filter migration.

COMPLICATIONS OF INFERIOR VENA CAVA FILTER INSERTION

Complications include pneumothorax, access site thrombosis, filter fracture and migration, filter perforation, vena caval thrombosis, and, rarely, infection or trauma to surrounding structures (aorta, duodenum, pancreas) (Fig. 13.17).

In addition, filter struts or retrieval hooks may become embedded within the caval wall, making retrieval somewhat challenging. A variety of adjunct techniques (snare over looped guidewire, coaxial double sheath, endobronchial forceps, and laser-assisted extraction) may be used for the removal of tilted and embedded filters. When these techniques are ineffective, particularly in patients with symptomatic caval perforations, open surgical retrieval may be performed at specialized centers.

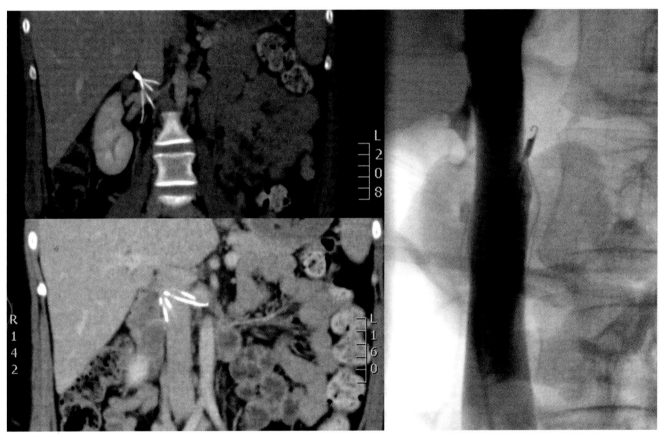

■ **Fig. 13.17**

COMPARATIVE EFFECTIVENESS

Despite the widespread use of IVC filters, there is little high-quality data to support this practice. Most filters gain US Food and Drug Administration (FDA) approval via a 510(k) process whereby manufacturers establish "substantial equivalency" to predicate intravascular filter devices.[6] The FDA approval of the original Mobin-Uddin filter predates the 510(k) process.

A 2010 Cochrane systematic review examined the effectiveness of vena cava filters for the prevention of PE and mortality, and the rate of filter-related complications.[7] At the time of this review, only two controlled or randomized clinical trials had been performed. Both demonstrated a reduction in PE but no difference in mortality. In addition, IVC filters were associated with an increased incidence of DVT. A subsequent 2015 randomized trial compared IVC filters plus anticoagulation versus anticoagulation alone in patients with symptomatic PE.[3] This study demonstrated no reduction in recurrent symptomatic PE or mortality.

These trials were performed in patients who were able to receive standard anticoagulation for at least 3 months. No trials have been performed to evaluate the efficacy of IVC filters in patients who have a contraindication to anticoagulation, and in patients who have failure of anticoagulation therapy. It is unlikely that such studies will be performed. Current recommendations from the American College of Chest Physicians may be summarized as follows[5]:

1. In patients with acute DVT of the leg, we recommend against the use of an IVC filter in addition to anticoagulants
2. In patients with acute proximal DVT of the leg and contraindication to anticoagulation, we recommend the use of an IVC filter
3. In patients with acute proximal DVT of the leg and an IVC filter inserted as an alternative to anticoagulation, we suggest a conventional course of anticoagulant therapy if their risk of bleeding resolves

Regarding the use of prophylactic IVC filters, a recent systematic review suggested that IVC filters were associated with a lower rate or PE and fatal PE in trauma patients. However, the treatment number needed to prevent one additional PE ranged from 109 to 962.[8] The evidence for prophylactic filters is not consistent, with other studies showing that prophylactic filters have no effect on recurrent PE or mortality.[9,10]

RETRIEVABLE FILTERS AND STENTING OF CHRONICALLY OBSTRUCTED INFERIOR VENA CAVA FILTERS

Retrievable filters should be used only when there is a need to prevent PE in a patient with documented venous thromboembolism and when there is a defined retrieval end point. Retrievable filters should not be used as replacements for permanent filters if permanent PE prevention is needed. The FDA recommended that implanting physicians responsible for the ongoing care of patients with retrievable IVC filters consider removing the filter as soon as possible[11]—determined by when anticoagulation can be restarted safely and/or when PE risk has diminished. IVC filters whose dwell times are less than 6 months are usually easily removed with standard commercial retrieval kits via a right internal jugular (RIJ) vein access.

However, an IVC filter incorporated into a chronic postthrombotic caval obstruction requires a different approach. Although filter removal is usually preferred, Neglen et al. reported that stenting across an obstructed IVC filter is safe. Vena cava patency is not influenced by the fact that an IVC filter is crossed by a stent, rather, patency is related to the severity of postthrombotic disease.[12] In our experience, patients presenting with IVC filter induced vena cava occlusions have concomitant iliac vein occlusion (unilateral or bilateral) and limited inflow from chronically obstructed femoral vein postthrombotic disease. The reader is referred to Chapter 18 for case examples of patients treated for IVC filter induced vena cava occlusions:

- Case 2: IVC Filter Induced Vena Cava Occlusion, Extract Filter and Stent Cava—Using a Cloversnare, the IVC filter was controlled. Then slide a 16-Fr sheath downward to collapse the filter and encase with sheath for removal.
- Case 3: IVC Filter Induced Vena Cava Occlusion, Crush Filter and Stent Cava—Permanent filter compressed to vena cava sidewall using high pressure balloon and then stented across it.
- Case 7: Biconical IVC Filter Caval Extraction With Loop Snare and Rigid Bronchial Forceps—Using RIJ access, a 16-FR sheath advanced and parked at IVC confluence. Loop snares from above and below allow counter traction to "cinch down" the filter. Rigid bronchoscopy forceps allow firm grasp of filter. Then slide sheath downward to collapse the filter and encase with sheath for removal.

REFERENCES

1. Robinson ST, Krishnamurthy VN, Rectenwald JE. Indications, techniques, and results of inferior vena cava filters. In: Gloviczki P, ed. Handbook of Venous and Lymphatic Disorders. 4th ed. Boca Raton, FL: CRC Press; 2017:325–342.
2. Kearon C, Akl EA, Ornelas J, et al. Antithrombotic therapy for VTE disease: CHEST guideline and expert panel report. *Chest.* 2016;149(2):315–352.
3. Mismetti P, Laporte S, Pellerin O, et al. Effect of a retrievable inferior vena cava filter plus anticoagulation vs anticoagulation alone on risk of recurrent pulmonary embolism: a randomized clinical trial. *JAMA.* 2015;313(16):1627–1635.
4. Kaufman JA, Waltman AC, Rivitz SM, et al. Anatomical observations on the renal veins and inferior vena cava at magnetic resonance angiography. *Cardiovasc Intervent Radiol.* 1995;18:153–157.
5. Kearon C, Akl EA, Comerota AJ, et al. Antithrombotic therapy for VTE disease: Antithrombotic therapy and prevention of thrombosis, 9th ed: American College of Chest Physicians Evidence-Based Clinical Practice Guidelines. *Chest.* 2012;141:e419S–e494S.
6. https://www.fda.gov/RegulatoryInformation/Guidances/ucm073776.htm Accessed March 1, 2017.
7. Young T, Tang H, Hughes R. Vena caval filters for the prevention of pulmonary embolism. *Cochrane Database Syst Rev.* 2010;(2):Art. No.: CD006212.
8. Haut ER, Garcia LJ, Shihab HM, et al. The effectiveness of prophylactic inferior vena cava filters in trauma patients: a systematic review and meta-analysis. *JAMA Surg.* 2014;149(2):194–202.
9. Cook AD, Gross BW, Osler TM, et al. Vena cava filter use in trauma and rates of pulmonary embolism, 2003-2015. *JAMA Surg.* 2017;152:724–732.
10. Brunson A, Ho G, White R, et al. Inferior vena cava filters in patients with cancer and venous thromboembolism (VTE) does not improve clinical outcomes: a population-based study. *Thromb Res.* 2017;153:57–64.
11. U.S. Food and Drug Administration. MedWatch Safety Information and Adverse Event Reporting Program: Inferior Vena Cava (IVC) Filters: Initial Communication: Risk of Adverse Events with Long Term Use. Posted 8/9/2010. http://www.fda.gov/Safety/MedWatch/Safety Information/SafetyAlertsforHumanMedicalProducts/ucm221707.htm.
12. Neglen P, Oglesbee M, Olivier J, et al. Stenting of chronically obstructed inferior vena cava filters. *J Vasc Surg.* 2011;54:153–161.

CHAPTER 14

Pharmacomechanical
Thrombolysis

Mark J. Garcia

HISTORICAL BACKGROUND

Venous thromboembolism (VTE) remains a significant health problem with over 900,000 new episodes each year in the United States alone.[1] VTE, which comprises both deep venous thrombosis (DVT) and pulmonary embolism (PE), is responsible for up to 300,000 deaths each year and continues to be a leading cause of in-hospital mortality.[2] Post-thrombotic syndrome (PTS) is the most common complication of DVT, with 25% to 50% developing PTS despite anticoagulation (AC) after their first episode of DVT.[3-5] The complications of DVT are well known, yet treatment continues to revolve around conservative therapies (AC and graded compression) aimed primarily at PE prevention while there remains resistance to endovascular treatments. Intravascular thrombus removal however, attempts to prevent both PE and PTS, while focusing on restoring the vein to its prethrombus state. PTS is a chronic condition that adversely affects a patient's quality of life (QoL) while remaining a significant burden socioeconomically.

ETIOLOGY AND NATURAL HISTORY

The pathogenesis of DVT formation is believed to be caused by Virchow's triad, which suggests that thrombosis occurs as a result of alterations in blood flow (stasis), endothelial injury, and hypercoagulability (inherited or acquired).[6] There are several possible outcomes of acute DVT, which include resolution with or without recurrence, propagation, pulmonary embolism, and PTS. PTS develops as a result of venous hypertension from increased resistance and venous obstruction, as well as reflux secondary to valvular incompetence. In fact, those patients who develop both venous reflux and residual obstruction following their DVT have the greatest risk of developing PTS.[7] When considering DVT location, it is important to differentiate those patients with iliofemoral DVT versus those with infrainguinal only (femoropopliteal-tibial) DVT because the former carries a significantly higher risk of developing not only recurrent DVT and PTS but also a more severe PTS.[7] Studies on patients with proximal (iliofemoral) DVT treated with AC showed poorer complete (4%) and partial resolution (14%) respectively.[8] In fact, Raju and Fredericks demonstrated that when venous thrombosis occurs in the common femoral vein (CFV) or above, the more severe the outflow obstruction, the higher the ambulatory venous pressures, and the more severe the PTS.[9] That is not to say that infrainguinal DVT does not cause PTS and QoL issues, particularly in those with residual venous obstruction and valvular damage of the popliteal vein.[10]

TREATMENT OPTIONS

The rationale behind endovascular treatment of acute DVT is for rapid and complete thrombus removal to enhance the possibility of quickly restoring flow and preserving the vein, as well as the valves, and returning them to a normally functioning state. Theoretically, this will help prevent venous hypertension from residual venous obstruction and/or venous incompetence.

There are several categories of intervention, which might be considered after the first line of treatment, therapeutic AC, has been executed. These endovascular options include: catheter directed thrombolysis (CDT), percutaneous mechanical thrombectomy[11] (no thrombolytic agent used), and pharmacomechanical thrombolysis (PMT; thrombolytic agent added to the mechanical device at the time of thrombectomy) also known as pharmacomechanical catheter directed thrombolysis (PCDT). The focus of this chapter will be on pharmacomechanical thrombectomy and the various forms of treatment techniques.

PATIENT SELECTION

In the hopes of preserving complete vein and venous valve function, early and complete resolution or removal of thrombus is important. Given the natural history of proximal DVT and its poor rate of complete resolution with higher risk for PTS, it is an important subset of DVT that warrants early intervention to restore patency. Any patient being evaluated for DVT treatment should undergo rigorous, preprocedural evaluation including a thorough history, physical examination, and appropriate imaging.[12] This includes identifying any contraindications or potential bleeding risks. The Society of Interventional Radiology (SIR) quality improvement guidelines for the treatment of lower extremity DVT recommends thrombus removal in patients with the following[12]:

- Image-proven symptomatic DVT in the inferior vena cava (IVC), iliac, common femoral, and/or femoral vein
- Recent ambulatory patient
- DVT symptoms for less than 28 days or in whom there is a strong clinical suspicion for recently formed (<28 days) DVT.

Variations in patient selection exist, such as those from the recent 2016 CHEST Guidelines, which propose that patients who are most likely to benefit from CDT have the following[13]:

- Iliofemoral DVT
- Symptoms for less than 14 days
- Good functional status
- Life expectancy of 1 year or more
- Low risk of bleeding.

One must keep in mind that this list represents suggested guidelines and that case reports exist on treating patients whose status fell outside these guidelines. A physician's decision to treat any patient with DVT must be made after a number of individual factors, not the least of which is the individual's risk/benefit ratio, as well as the overall clinical status. In my practice, the use of RAPID (<u>r</u>heolytic <u>a</u>ccelerated <u>p</u>harmacomechan<u>i</u>cal directional) lysis[14] PMT has broadened the ability to treat patients suffering from acute DVT because patients previously deemed as having absolute contraindications for CDT have been safely and successfully treated using PMT techniques (Fig. 14.1). This point illustrates one of the theoretic benefits of PMT over CDT in the ability to downgrade absolute contraindications for CDT to relative contraindications for PMT.

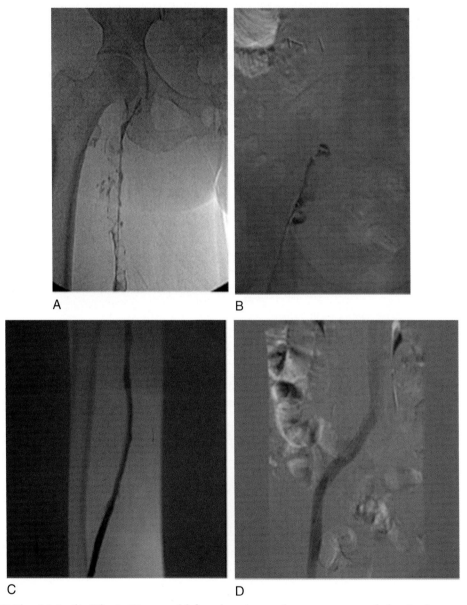

■ **Fig. 14.1** (A–D). A 55-year-old female who underwent recent abdominal surgery and developed a postoperative abdominal wall hematoma that was surgically evacuated. She developed extensive inferior vena cava and low extremity deep venous thrombosis (DVT) with phlegmasia and blistering within 2 days of surgery. Left femoral (A) and iliac (B) venography shows acute and occlusive DVT. Completion venography (C and D) following single session RAPID-lysis treatment (using 10 mg Alteplase in 500 mL normal saline solution and the DVX AngioJet catheter) shows complete resolution of thrombus with restoration of brisk antegrade flow and no need for catheter-directed thrombolysis (contraindicated with recent surgery).

THROMBUS REMOVAL DEVICES

Thrombus removal can occur in a variety of ways. The devices that are US Food and Drug Administration (FDA) approved for mechanical thrombectomy can be categorized by their respective mechanism of action. These include rotational thrombectomy, rheolytic thrombectomy, aspiration thrombectomy, or ultrasound-accelerated thrombolysis. Rotational devices physically macerate the thrombus using a basket or helix configuration that rotates at a high velocity to macerate the clot. These devices include the Trerotola device (Fig. 14.2) (Arrow International, PA), the Cleaner Rotational Thrombectomy System (Fig. 14.3) (Argon Medical, Plano, TX), and the Amplatz thrombectomy device (Microvena, MN).

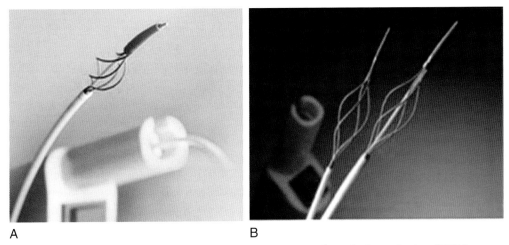

A   B

■ **Fig. 14.2** Teleflex Arrow-Trerotola percutaneous thrombolytic device (PTD). (A) The 5-Fr PTD basket. (B) The 5-Fr PTD basket *(left)* alongside the 7-Fr over-the-wire PTD basket *(right)*.

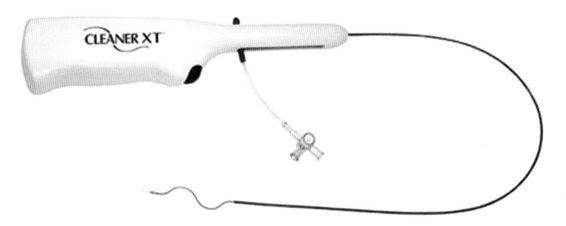

■ **Fig. 14.3** Argon Cleaner XT

The Trellis device (Covidien/Medtronic, MN) is no longer commercially available.

Rheolysis is unique to the AngioJet device (Fig. 14.4) (Boston Scientific, MN), which uses the Bernoulli-Venturi principle and generates high velocity saline jets to create a central, low pressure or vacuum zone within the catheter lumen. At the tip of the catheter, the affluent saline jets also produce a physical maceration or fragmentation of the thrombus, which is then aspirated and evacuated via the catheter through the effluent port. The original rheolytic technique described uses heparin in the affluent saline solution instead of a lytic agent. The PMT or PCDT technique substitutes heparin for a thrombolytic agent added directly into the affluent saline solution. Once the lytic agent has been added to the saline solution, there are several different PCDT techniques that use the AngioJet catheter. The 8-Fr Zelante DVT thrombectomy set is intended for use to break apart and remove thrombus, including DVT, from the iliofemoral and lower extremity veins 6.0 mm or greater in diameter. The 6-Fr AngioJet SOLENT Proxi & Omni thrombectomy sets are intended for use to break apart and remove thrombus from peripheral veins 3.0 mm or greater in diameter.

The first technique to be described is the use of the AngioJet catheter over the guidewire, as its original intended use, while in the thrombectomy mode, allowing for the outflow port to remain open for thrombus evacuation.[11] The second technique is the power pulse technique,[15] which is selected on the console unit. By selecting this technique, the console automatically closes the effluent port while in use. The catheter is advanced through the thrombus at 1 to 2 cm increments while "pulsing" the lytic/saline solution into the clot. The outflow port is closed, allowing for the lytic agent to "dwell" in the clot for an appropriate time, usually 20 to 30 minutes. Once the dwell time is completed, the catheter is again advanced through the thrombus, this time in the thrombectomy mode (selected on the console, which opens the effluent port), where both the combination of the mechanical action and vacuum removes any residual clot. The third technique is called the RAPID lysis technique,[14] which was originated in 1997 and uses an 8-Fr hockey-stick guide catheter with the guidewire retracted inside the AngioJet, allowing the guide catheter to angle the tip of the AngioJet catheter along the

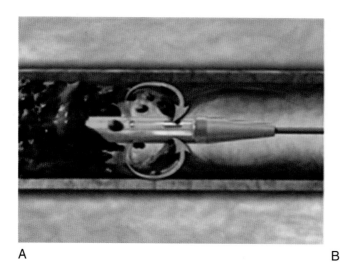
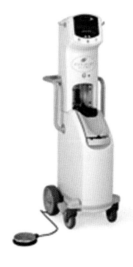

A   B

■ **Fig. 14.4** The AngioJet thrombectomy system. (A) Mechanism of action of the AngioJet catheter demonstrating the Bernoulli-Venturi principle. (B) The AngioJet console drive unit.

periphery of the vessel wall. The operator then slowly retracts the coaxial system from central to peripheral aspects of the DVT, with the device in the thrombectomy mode. While retracting the system through the clot, the operator rotates the guide catheter hub in a slow 360-degree circle, allowing for the AngioJet treatment zone to gain full circumferential coverage of the vessel. This optimizes removal of wall thrombus in addition to luminal clot and, in my opinion, greater overall thrombus removal.

Another thrombectomy technique is termed *aspiration thrombectomy* and is achieved by creating suction in the catheter device once it is placed into the thrombus. Suction created in the closed system is accomplished with the aid of an in-line pump. Two FDA-cleared devices exist, the Indigo device (Penumbra, Alameda, CA) and the Angiovac system (Angiodynamics, Latham, NY).

The EKOS Endowave system (EKOS/BTG, Bothell, WA) combines the use of a thrombolytic agent delivered via a thrombolytic infusion catheter that contains an inner ultrasound core, which emits ultrasound energy or waves that aid in dissolution of the thrombus. This combination technique is termed *ultrasound accelerated thrombolysis* (USAT) or *acoustic pulse thrombolysis*.

RAPID LYSIS TECHNIQUE

The treatment technique of choice for patients presenting with acute to subacute DVT is the RAPID lysis technique.[14] As stated earlier, this technique combines the mechanical and rheolytic properties of the AngioJet system with that of the thrombolytic agent in addition to gaining circumferential, wall-to-wall apposition to enhance the ability for complete clot removal and thrombectomy in a single session. An additional advantage is the opportunity to downgrade absolute contraindications to relative contraindications, as has been established time and again in my practice. Before discussing the details of the technique, one must be prepared with the appropriate imaging equipment and procedural instruments to safely, effectively, and successfully complete the case.

ENDOVASCULAR INSTRUMENTS AND EQUIPMENT

- Imaging Equipment
  - Ultrasound (US) guidance for percutaneous access
  - Angiographic system (C-arm or fixed, mounted)
  - Intravascular ultrasound (IVUS) on an as-need basis
- Procedural Equipment
  - Micropuncture access kit
  - 0.035-inch (0.088-cm) glide wire (180 or 260 cm length depending on clot extent)
  - 0.035-inch (0.088-cm) working guidewire (i.e., 180 or 260 cm Amplatz super stiff)
  - 4-Fr angled catheter
  - 8-Fr sheath (popliteal or above), 6-Fr sheath (tibial access)
  - 8-Fr Hockey stick guide catheter (55 or 90 cm)
  - Appropriate length 6-Fr Solent AngioJet catheter
  - Appropriately sized, standard angioplasty balloons as necessary
  - Appropriately sized, self-expanding stents
  - Optional IVC filter (author does not use one)

PATIENT PREPARATION

Prepping the patient appropriately is perhaps the most important step in ensuring a safe and successful outcome. This includes reviewing all imaging studies, knowing the extent of the thrombus and any patient medically important issues (such as renal function, hypercoagulable states, contraindications, bleeding risks, etc.). The patient should be well hydrated before the procedure and should be tailored based on confounding issues, such as cardiac disease or renal failure. Concerning AC, this operator ensures therapeutic AC before the procedure. If heparin is the agent of choice, then a target partial thromboplastin time (PTT) should be in the range of 70 to 90 seconds, with the goal of being as close to 90 seconds as is safely possible. Early on in our experience, we found that PTTs below 70 seconds led to early rethrombosis despite excellent thrombectomy results and restoration of flow. Remember that "peeling" thrombus off the venous wall will incite a hypercoagulability. I no longer use heparin but rely on enoxaparin (1 mg/kg twice daily dosing, with adjustment for renal insufficiency) because it allows for a more rapid therapeutic AC level and opportunity to treat someone admitted for the sole purpose of their DVT. AC is continued throughout the case and continued postprocedure for 4 weeks, uninterrupted.

PROCEDURAL STEPS

Access

Once deemed prepared, the patient is brought to the angiography suite and typically placed in the prone position, where the access site is prepped and draped in sterile fashion. Access site determination is based upon the goal of restoring direct in-line flow from the ankle to the heart. Therefore if the popliteal vein is free of clot, then that is typically the site used for access. If, however, the popliteal and/or tibial veins are thrombosed, then tibial access is gained with the intent to treat these veins as well. The exact vessel access site is located, and the skin and soft tissues are infiltrated with 1% lidocaine. At a 30-degree to 45-degree angle, the needle is followed under constant and direct US visualization (Fig. 14.5) to avoid puncturing any unwanted structures, such as a geniculate branch of the popliteal artery. Once access is obtained, the 4-Fr micropuncture exchange dilator (catheter) is placed with a gentle hand injection of contrast to ensure proper location and confirm thrombosis. Over a wire, the micropuncture dilator is exchanged for the 8-Fr sheath. As previously, if thrombus extends into the popliteal vein or below, posterior tibial access is obtained in much the same manner with placement of a 6-Fr sheath rather than an 8 Fr.

RAPID Lysis Pharmacomechanical Thrombolysis

Once access has been gained coaxially, an 0.035-inch (0.088-cm) glide wire and angled catheter (4-Fr Berenstein or glide catheter) are advanced, with serial venographic images obtained through the thrombus until the patent central aspect of the DVT is reached. Central venography is performed to ensure the anatomy and to determine the starting

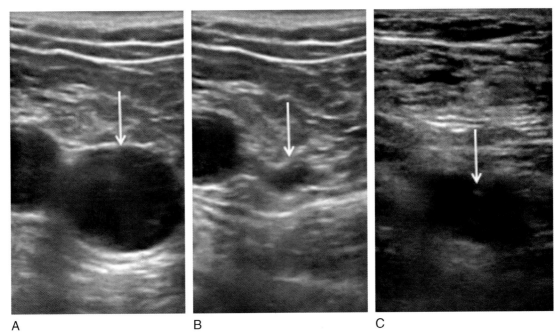

■ **Fig. 14.5** (A) Ultrasound-guided venous access identifying the initial noncompressed vein *(arrow)*. (B) A fully compressed and patent vein *(arrow)*. (C) Under direct visualization, the echogenic micropuncture needle tip *(arrow)* is advanced from skin surface to vein wall, observing it enter the superficial surface of the vein avoiding any unwanted structures.

A   B   C

point for PCDT. Once central location is ensured, the diagnostic catheter is exchanged for the appropriate length 8-Fr hockey-stick guide catheter, which is placed to the central aspect of the clot. The AngioJet system is prepped by adding Alteplase (r-tPA) into the saline solution. The amount of r-tPA added is dependent on the extent of thrombus to be treated. For example, if I am treating a smaller amount of clot burden (common femoral, femoral, and popliteal veins) then I use 10 mg r-tPA in 500 mL normal saline solution (NSS). If I believe I will need a larger volume of solution, such as in treating extensive iliofemoral and popliteal disease or bilateral lower extremity DVT, then I will place 25 mg r-tPA in 1000 mL NSS (this was based on the aliquots previously made by the pharmacy). Once the AngioJet system is prepped and ready for treatment, the 6-Fr Solent Angiojet catheter is placed through the 8-Fr hockey-stick guide, such that the AngioJet catheter tip and full treatment zone extend beyond the tip of the guide catheter. The guidewire is then retracted inside of the AngioJet catheter, which allows the combination of the guide and Angiojet catheters to take the angled shape of the hockey-stick guide. This, in essence, allows for wall-to-wall apposition. Once positioned appropriately at the central aspect of the thrombus, the AngioJet system is placed in the thrombectomy mode, and treatment is initiated. As PMT ensues, the coaxial system is rotated circumferentially in 360 degrees by slowly rotating the hub of the hockey-stick guide while retracting the system through the clot from the central to peripheral aspect of the DVT. Incremental sections are treated approximately 10 cm at a time, at which point reevaluation of that section is made by contrast venography via the outflow port, which contains a stopcock. The system is withdrawn to the next section when venography demonstrates that successful thrombectomy has occurred. This continues throughout the DVT until the most peripheral aspect is successfully treated. If treatment of the popliteal or tibial veins is undertaken, then the angled-guide catheter approach cannot be used because the tibial access is with a 6-Fr sheath. This is not upsized to an 8 Fr for risk of severely damaging the vein. In this case, the AngioJet catheter is advanced over the wire through the tibial and popliteal clot as PMT is performed. Once the popliteal vein has been cleared of thrombus, one can access the popliteal vein if desired. There are many who solely treat from the popliteal access centrally and do not focus on the DVT below the access site. One can also use the micropuncture catheter as a source to give r-tPA into the below-knee veins for thrombolysis. Once PMT has been successfully completed, adjuvant therapies, such as venoplasty and stenting, are undertaken where indicated (Fig. 14.6). The use of IVUS has been helpful in not only identifying underlying lesions and their exact location, but also obtaining optimum results with confirming full expansion and wall apposition of stents as well as complete coverage of the lesion. As a precaution, and because of the hemolysis and hemoglobinuria that can and often does occur, the patient will be continuously hydrated throughout the procedure and postprocedure until discharge. In addition, if more than 500 mL solution is used, I will administer 20 to 40 mg furosemide to ensure optimum renal excretion of hemolytic byproducts.

If there is residual thrombus post-PMT and further thrombolysis is desired, an infusion catheter of appropriate length is placed for CDT. It should be remembered that because of the successful debulking of the thrombus burden, CDT can often be completed in smaller doses and a shorter infusion time than would be seen in a patient who has not undergone PCDT.

Closure

Once the procedure is completed, the catheters and sheath are removed, with hemostasis obtained with manual pressure for 5 to 10 minutes, followed by 4 × 4 gauze rolled up and placed at the site for additional compression, secured in place with microfoam tape stretched around the gauze and site to ensure continuous compression. Keep in mind that the access was made antegrade with flow, and that it is a low-pressure venous stick, so overcompression is to be cautioned against.

INFERIOR VENA CAVA FILTERS AND OTHER ADDITIONAL PROCEDURAL POINTS

If the operator deems it appropriate or necessary, IVC filtration can be performed at the start of the PCDT treatment by placing a retrievable or option filter from an appropriate access. I do not routinely use IVC filters for these procedures and have yet to have a PE occur while performing the RAPID-lysis technique. Obviously, once the procedure is completed, it is at the operators' discretion as to when to retrieve the filter.

When performing CDT, whether or not following PCDT, pneumatic compression boots are applied and kept in place until the patient is discharged.

As mentioned previously, AC with enoxaparin is initiated before the start of the procedure and continued throughout the procedure and postprocedure for 2 to 4 weeks, at which time they are transitioned to an appropriate oral agent.

Patients are discharged with a script for knee-high compression stockings. I will typically order 20 to 30 mm Hg stockings to help ensure they will use them from the time they are out of bed to getting back into bed.

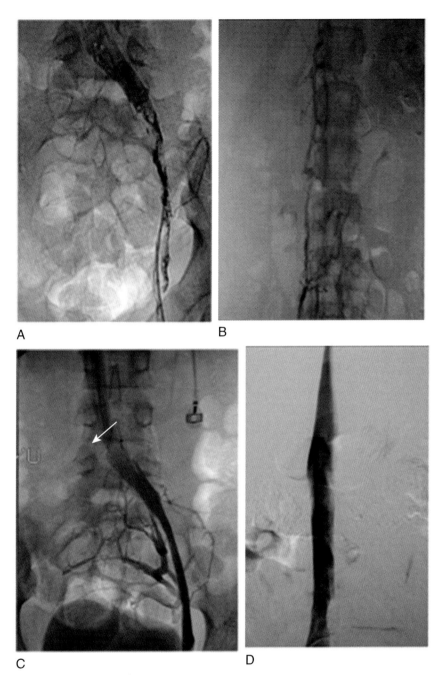

A

B

C

D

■ **Fig. 14.6** Initial left pelvic (A) and inferior vena cava (IVC) (B) venography demonstrates diffuse, acute, and occlusive iliofemoral and IVC thrombosis. Patients presented with acute anuria. Post single session RAPID-lysis pharmacochemical thrombolysis venogram (C and D) shows complete resolution of pelvic and IVC thrombus with underlying "pancake deformity" of the left common iliac vein (C, *arrow*) suggesting May-Thurner compression.

ADJUVANT THERAPIES: ANGIOPLASTY AND STENTING

It is not uncommon to find an underlying iliac lesion compromising flow from the lower extremity to the IVC. This scenario is classically found with May-Thurner compression. It is necessary to treat these lesions because they can potentially lead to rethrombosis, venous hypertension, and/or reflux. To adequately treat these segments, intravascular ultrasound is helpful for both stent sizing and to ensure complete coverage of the diseased segment. Incomplete stent coverage may lead to failure and rethrombosis. Self-expanding stents are recommended for use in the iliofemoral region, as is early stent placement following PMT or CDT (Fig. 14.7). As mentioned earlier, the stent(s) should cover the entire length of the lesion and can safely be placed from the caudal IVC to the greater trochanteric level. In general, I do not advocate stenting into the femoral vein or profunda vein.

PEARLS AND PITFALLS

- Therapeutic AC is obtained preprocedure. I prefer patients to be on enoxaparin (1 mg/kg twice per day dosing) before the procedure and to continue it for 30 days postprocedure. If heparin is used, the PTT should be between 70 to 90 seconds to prevent early rethrombosis. AC is continued throughout the case (not discontinued during thrombolysis or thrombectomy).
- Expect gross hemoglobinuria; this statement is written on post orders to alleviate nursing concerns for acute hematuria. Usually resolves within 24 to 72 hours. Hydrate well until it is resolved.
- Bradycardia and hypotension can be seen during AngioJet activation but are transient and typically resolve by holding rheolysis for 15 to 30 seconds. This phenomenon tends to be short lived and dissipates after a few of these episodes.
- Add lytic agent to normal saline solution bag without heparin (heparin may precipitate the lytic agent).
- The more acute the clot (<4 weeks), the better the result.
- Wall-to-wall apposition leads to more efficient thrombus removal.
- Treat underlying lesions (i.e., iliac vein compression) early with percutaneous transluminal angioplasty (PTA)/stent.
- Aggressively anticoagulate postprocedure (again, I prefer enoxaparin for 30 days, then transition to appropriate oral agent of choice for proper length).
- If lytic therapy is absolutely contraindicated, instead use 3000 to 5000 U of heparin added to normal saline.

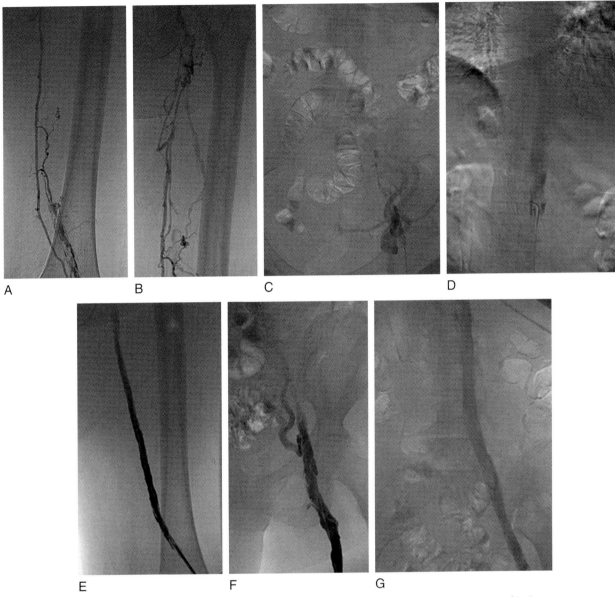

■ **Fig. 14.7** (A–G). Right leg (A and B), pelvic (C) and inferior vena cava (IVC; D) venography shows diffuse extensive deep venous thrombosis to the level of the indwelling IVC filter with patent IVC above the filter. Postpharmacochemical thrombolysis with RAPID-lysis technique, the femoral-popliteal (E) and common femoral (F) veins are patent with chronic occlusion of the common and external iliac veins. Post stenting, the right iliofemoral and IVC are widely patent without residual thrombus.

SINGLE CENTER REGISTRY FINDINGS

During the 2007 Society of Interventional Radiology Annual Scientific Meeting, results of our single center registry entitled ATTACK DVT: Angiojet and TPA Thrombolysis, A Closer Look at Combined Therapy for the Treatment of DVT[16] were presented. Conclusions from that abstract included the following:
- RAPID lysis and PCDT has been seen to:
  reduce overall need for post-PCDT lytic infusion
      increase single-session treatments
  reduce lytic infusion time when CDT performed
  reduce risk of bleeding from lytic infusion by reducing overall use of CDT
  reduce need for intensive care unit bed

RAPID-LYSIS AND LYTIC CONTRAINDICATIONS

RAPID lysis has expanded the population treated and has been used to safely and successfully treat patients with absolute contraindications to catheter-directed thrombolysis who present with acute DVT and phlegmasia. A complete and thorough evaluation and investigation of the patients' medical state with an in-depth discussion of bleeding risks with the patient and family are necessary before undertaking treatment. Situations that have been safely and effectively treated without complication include the following:
- Recent or active bleed
- Cerebral vascular accident (CVA) (within 2 months)
- Major surgery or trauma (within 10 days)
- Pregnancy or recent delivery
- Central nervous system neoplasms

COMPLICATIONS

Complications that can be seen with the RAPID-lysis technique are the same as those encountered with any endovascular procedure and PCDT treatment technique including the following:
- Infection from endovascular entry: essentially nonexistent with standard sterile technique throughout the case. If a patient develops signs or symptoms of infection, then appropriate steps should be taken to exclude a hematogenous infection.
- Minor bleeding or ecchymosis: most commonly seen at the puncture site secondary to supratherapeutic AC or prolonged catheter thrombolysis.
- Major bleeding: rare and requires a blood transfusion. Can occur in the brain, retroperitoneum, muscles, or gastrointestinal/genitourinary tract.
- Vein wall injury: damage to the vessel wall during manipulation of wires, catheters, or thrombectomy procedure or rupture during balloon angioplasty.
- Pulmonary embolism: rare and represents clot dislodgement into the pulmonary arteries during the procedure.

● The Peripheral Use of AngioJet Rheolytic Thrombectomy with a Variety of Catheter Lengths (PEARL) registry[17] demonstrated a significant reduction in the major and minor bleeding rates compared with both the Venous Registry[18] and the long-term outcome after additional catheter-directed thrombolysis versus standard treatment for acute iliofemoral deep vein thrombosis (the CaVenT study).[19]

COMPARATIVE EFFECTIVENESS OF EXISTING TREATMENTS

Comparative effectiveness of existing treatment methods is difficult because there are no trials comparing the different treatment devices or methods. Suffice it to say that surgical thrombectomy is typically not performed in centers that offer the more minimally invasive catheter techniques. Amongst the thrombectomy devices available, there has been no direct head-to-head comparison made. However, most studies reporting on each device demonstrate very good results with safety and efficacy in removing thrombus burden. It does appear, and has been the experience of this author, that debulking of the thrombus burden using PCDT techniques leads to shorter infusion times and improves the risk of bleeding complications. The PEARL registry[17] compared reported findings from the Venous Registry,[18] CaVenT trial[19] with those of the PEARL registry and found significantly reduced infusion times and bleeding complications with PCDT treatments.[17]

A list of the current FDA-approved thrombectomy devices are provided in Table 14.1.

TABLE 14.1 US Food and Drug Administration–Approved Mechanical Thrombectomy Devices

Company Name	Product(s) Name	Sheath Size (Fr)	Guidewire (inch)	Working Length (cm)	Mode of Action	Vessel Diameter (mm)
Argon Medical	Cleaner XT	6	—	65,135	Sinusoidal vortex wire with maceration	9
	Cleaner 15	7	—	65,135		15
Arrow/Teleflex	Trerotola PTD	5	—	65	Fragmentation basket macerates clot	9
	OTW-PTD	7	0.025	65,120		9
Boston Scientific	AngioJet AVX	6	0.035	50	Rheolysis: high velocity saline jets cause fragmentation and removal	≥3
	AngioJet Solent	4, 6, 8	0.014–0.035	90,120,145		≥1.5, ≥3
	AngioJet Zelante	8	.035	105		≥6
Codman/J & J	Revive PV	≥5	—	205	Self-expanding Nitinol stent thrombectomy with aspiration	1.5–5
Control Medical	Aspire	—	—	—	Mechanical thrombectomy with aspiration	
Penumbra	Indigo CAT 3, 5, 6, 8	3.4, 5, 6, 8	0.014–0.038	85–150	Vacuum aspiration	

FIVE SALIENT REFERENCES

1. Kearon C, Akl E, Ornelas J, et al. Antithrombotic Therapy for VTE Disease CHEST Guideline and Expert Panel Report. *Chest.* 2016;149(2):315–352.
2. Vedantham S, Sista A, Klein SJ, et al. Quality Improvement Guidelines for the Treatment of Lower-Extremity Deep Vein Thrombosis with Use of Endovascular Thrombus Removal. *J Vasc Interv Radiol.* 2014;25:1317–1325.
3. Garcia MJ, Lookstein R, Malhotra R, et al. Endovascular Management of Deep Vein Thrombosis with Rheolytic Thrombectomy: Final Report of the Prospective Multicenter PEARL (Peripheral Use of AngioJet Rheolytic Thrombectomy with a Variety of Catheter Lengths) Registry. *J Vasc Interv Radiol.* 2015;26(6):777–785.
4. Mewissen MW, Seabrook GR, Meissner MH, et al. Catheter-directed thrombolysis for lower extremity deep venous thrombosis: report of a national multicenter registry. *Radiology.* 1999;211:39–49.
5. Haig Y, Enden T, Grøtta O, et al. Post-thrombotic syndrome after catheter-directed thrombolysis for deep vein thrombosis (CaVenT): 5-year follow-up results of an open-label, randomised controlled trial. *Lancet Haematol.* 2016;3:e64–e71.

REFERENCES

1. Heit JA. The epidemiology of venous thromboembolism in the community. *Arterioscler Thromb Vasc Biol.* 2008;28(3):370–372.
2. Society of Hospital Medicine, Maynard GA, Stein JM, et al. Preventing Hospital-Acquired Venous Thromboembolism: A Guide for Effective Quality Improvement. Rockville, MD: Agency for Healthcare Research and Quality, US Dept. of Health and Human Services; 2008.
3. Prandoni P, Lensing A, Cogo A, et al. The long-term clinical course of acute deep venous thrombosis. *Ann Intern Med.* 1996;125:1–7.
4. Prandoni P, Lensing AW, Prins MH, et al. Below knee elastic compression stockings to prevent the post-thrombotic syndrome. *Ann Intern Med.* 2004;141:249–256.
5. Brandjes DP, Buller HR, Heijboer H, et al. Randomized trial of effect of compression stockings in patients with symptomatic proximal-vein thrombosis. *Lancet.* 1997;349:759–762.
6. Bagot CN, Arya R. Virchow and his triad: a question of attribution. *Br J Haematol.* 2008;143(2):180.
7. Prandoni P. Long-term clinical course of proximal deep venous thrombosis and detection of recurrent thrombosis. *Semin Thromb Hemost.* 2001;27:9–13.
8. Comerota AJ, Aldridge SC. Thrombolytic therapy for deep venous thrombosis: a clinical review. *Can J Surg.* 1993;36:359–364.
9. Raju S, Fredericks R. Venous obstruction: an analysis of one hundred thirty-seven cases with hemodynamic, venographic, and clinical correlations. *J Vasc Surg.* 1991;14:305–313.
10. Prandoni P, Frulla M, Sartor D, et al. Vein abnormalities and the post-thrombotic syndrome. *J Thromb Haemost.* 2005;3(2):401–402.
11. Kasirajan K, Gray B, Ouriel K. Percutaneous AngioJet thrombectomy in the management of extensive deep venous thrombosis. *J Vasc Interv Radiol.* 2001;12:179–185.
12. Vedantham S, Sista A, Klein SJ, et al. Quality Improvement Guidelines for the Treatment of Lower-Extremity Deep Vein Thrombosis with Use of Endovascular Thrombus Removal. *J Vasc Interv Radiol.* 2014;25:1317–1325.
13. Kearon C, Akl E, Ornelas J, et al. Antithrombotic Therapy for VTE Disease CHEST Guideline and Expert Panel Report. *Chest.* 2016;149(2):315–352.
14. Garcia MJ. Thrombolytic-assisted rheolytic thrombectomy for DVT. *J Vasc Interv Radiol.* 2004;15(2):72–73.
15. Allie DE, Hebert CJ, Lirtzman MD, et al. Novel simultaneous combination chemical thrombolysis/rheolytic thrombectomy therapy for acute critical limb ischemia: the power-pulse spray technique. *Catheter Cardiovasc Interv.* 2004;63:512–522.

16. Garcia MJ, Dignazio M, Kimbiris G, et al. ATTACK-DVT: Angiojet and TPA Thrombolysis: A Closer LooK at Combined Therapy for the Treatment of DVT. *J Vasc Interv Radiol.* 2007;18(1):S20–S24.
17. Garcia MJ, Lookstein R, Malhotra R, et al. Endovascular Management of Deep Vein Thrombosis with Rheolytic Thrombectomy: Final Report of the Prospective Multicenter PEARL (Peripheral Use of AngioJet Rheolytic Thrombectomy with a Variety of Catheter Lengths) Registry. *J Vasc Interv Radiol.* 2015;26(6):777–785.
18. Mewissen MW, Seabrook GR, Meissner MH, et al. Catheter-directed thrombolysis for lower extremity deep venous thrombosis: report of a national multicenter registry. *Radiology.* 1999;211:39–49.
19. Haig Y, Enden T, Grøtta O, et al. Post-thrombotic syndrome after catheter-directed thrombolysis for deep vein thrombosis (CaVenT): 5-year follow-up results of an open-label, randomised controlled trial. *Lancet Haematol.* 2016;3:e64–e71.

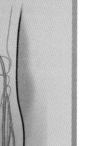

New Concepts in the Management of Pulmonary Embolus

Jason Thomas Salsamendi and Issam Kably

HISTORICAL BACKGROUND

Demographics

Acute pulmonary embolism (PE) continues to be a major cause of morbidity and mortality worldwide. There are approximately 530,000 cases of symptomatic PE, and almost 300,000 deaths each year from acute venous thromboembolisms.[1] The International Cooperative Pulmonary Embolism Registry (ICOPER), a collaboration between 52 European and North American hospitals, was established to better calculate rates of clinical outcomes, such as the reoccurrence of PE and death, because prior studies had reported a large variability in these prognostic measures. The ICOPER data showed that the overall crude mortality rate at 3 months was 17.4% (426 of 2454 deaths), with 45.1% (179 of 387) of the deaths attributed directly to PE and 17.6% (70 of 387) secondary to malignancy.[2] Patients with hemodynamic instability at presentation (108 patients), qualified as a systolic blood pressure less than 90 mm Hg, had a prominently higher mortality rate of 52.4% (95% confidence interval [CI], 43.4–62.1) at 3 months compared with 14.6% (95% CI, 13.3–16.2) in the rest of the cohort.[2,3] Similarly, the Management Strategy and Prognosis of Pulmonary Embolism Registry (MAPPET) revealed an increase in mortality with worsening cardiopulmonary function. Among 1001 patients with acute PE, in-hospital mortality was 8.1% for hemodynamically stable patients, 25% for patients in cardiogenic shock at presentation, and 65% for patients who required cardiopulmonary resuscitation.[3] Conversely, normotensive patients with no evidence of right ventricular (RV) dysfunction who were treated for PE had a short-term mortality rate of 2%.[4]

Prognostic Factors

Overall, the strongest prognostic factor of short-term mortality is hemodynamic status at time of presentation.[2] Poor prognosis in acute PE is also heavily associated with a history of malignancy (hazard ratio 2.3; 95% CI, 1.5–3.5), congestive heart failure (2.4; 95% CI, 1.5–3.7), systolic arterial hypotension (2.9; 95% CI, 1.7–5.0), tachypnea (2.0; 95% CI, 1.2–3.2), and RV hypokinesis on echocardiography (2.0; 95% CI, 1.3–2.9). It is worth noting that patients who are hemodynamically stable at presentation may subsequently destabilize as a result of recurrent thromboembolism or worsening RV dysfunction. Therefore therapy for PE based on initial hemodynamic status may be inappropriate for long-term management. In addition, elevated cardiac troponins, including tropinin I and troponin T, are associated with adverse prognosis in acute PE (odds ratio [OR] of 5.90; 95% CI, 2.68–12.95).[5] Age over 70 years (1.6; 95% CI, 1.1–2.3) and a history of chronic obstructive pulmonary disease (1.8; 95% CI, 1.2–2.7) are also significant prognostic factors.[2] Lastly, cardiac imaging measures seen on transthoracic echocardiography and computed tomography (CT) scan have demonstrated high predictive values for overall mortality.[6] A meta-analysis by Sanchez et al. showed RV dysfunction on echocardiography was prognostic of mortality in both hemodynamically stable and unstable patients (2.53; 95% CI, 1.17–5.50).[7] Likewise, the Prognostic Value of Computed Tomography (PROTECT) study established the reproducibility of multidetector CT scan in verifying RV dysfunction.[8] Considering these factors, the Geneva Score, Pulmonary Embolism Severity Index (PESI), and simplified PESI (sPESI) clinical scoring systems were developed to simplify risk stratification of patients and determine management.[3,6,9]

Categories of Pulmonary Embolism

There are three types of acute PEs defined in the literature: massive, submassive, and nonmassive PE. Massive PE is defined as an acute PE with evidence of hemodynamic instability, or systolic blood pressure lower than 90 mm Hg.[2] Massive PEs are always located centrally and are accompanied by RV dysfunction or myocardial necrosis. The American Heart Association (AHA) defines RV dysfunction as at least one of the following: (1) RV dilatation (RV-to-left ventricular [LV] diameter ratio >0.9 on apical four chamber view) or systolic hypotension on echocardiography; (2) RV dilatation on CT; (3) elevation of brain natriuretic peptide (BNP) (>90 pg/mL); (4) elevation of N-terminal pro-BNP (500 pg/mL); and (5) electrocardiographic changes including new complete or incomplete right bundle branch block, anteroseptal ST elevation or depression, or anteroseptal T-wave inversion.[3,8] Myocardial necrosis is identified by an elevation of either troponin I (>0.4 ng/mL) or troponin T (>0.1 ng/mL).[3] A submassive PE is a central PE accompanied by either RV dysfunction or myocardial necrosis in the absence of systolic hypotension (≥90 mm Hg).[2] Nonmassive PEs are peripherally or segmentally located, and therefore not accompanied by RV dysfunction or hemodynamic instability.[2]

RISK STRATIFICATION

Conventionally, patients with acute, symptomatic PE who present with shock or arterial hypotension warrant thrombolysis. However, in PE patients with preserved hemodynamic function, patient-risk stratification is paramount in dictating therapeutic options. Low thrombus burden, negative D-dimer, or complete lower limb ultrasound testing may identify patients at a lower risk of death when compared with patients with a higher risk. Unfortunately, test standardization and lack of generalizability limit the use of these biomarkers and imaging testing regarding outpatient PE therapy.[3,6]

Identification of patients who are at a higher risk for complications is critical in determining whether escalation of PE therapy is necessary. Some evidence has suggested that high-risk normotensive patients with PE would benefit from thrombolytic therapy.[6] However, markers such as BNP testing, indicating RV strain, or cardiac troponin T or I, indicating myocardial injury, lack positive predictive value for mortality specifically related to PE. No single test has a sufficient positive predictive value for PE-related mortality to direct an escalation of therapy.[6] Studies have suggested that a combination of these prognostic indicators, including both elevated cardiac biomarkers and echocardiographic RV dysfunction, is sufficient to determine which patients are at higher risk for death. However, the combination of normal echocardiographic RV function and normal cardiac biomarkers did not more accurately identify low-risk patients with PE than each test individually.[6,10,11] A meta-analysis of the prognostic value of elevated troponin levels for short-term death and adverse outcome events (overall mortality, mortality from shock, thrombolysis requirement, intubation, vasopressor infusion requirement, cardiopulmonary resuscitation, or recurrent PE), suggests that an elevated troponin had a positive predictive value of 43.6% (95% CI, 36.9–50.3). Lower limb venous compression ultrasound had a positive predictive value for 90-day morality related to PE of 6.6%. Only 9 out of 20 studies included in the analysis had information on the composite endpoint, however.[6]

These data echo the need for reliable risk stratification methods. One such method is the PESI, which stratifies patients into five classes of increasing risk of mortality within 30 days of hospitalization. The PESI score uses 11 clinical parameters at the time of presentation: age, male sex, malignancy, heart failure, chronic lung disease, pulse greater than 110 beats per minute, systolic blood pressure lower than 100 mm Hg, respiratory rate 30 breaths or more per minute, temperature lower than 36°C, altered mental status, and oxyhemoglobin saturation lower than 90%[12] (Table 15.1). A simplified version of the PESI, or sPESI, which uses age (>80 years), history of malignancy, history of chronic obstructive pulmonary disease, heart rate greater than 110 beats per minute, systolic blood pressure lower than 100 mm Hg[6,13] (see Table 15.1 and Table 15.2).

Another stratification method, known as the Geneva Score, uses six parameters at time of presentation: malignancy, heart failure, previous deep venous thrombosis (DVT), systolic blood pressure lower than 100 mm Hg, partial pressure of oxygen (PaO_2) less than 8 kPa, and the presence of DVT on ultrasound. The Geneva Score is based on adverse outcomes that include death, recurrent thromboembolism, and major bleeding in a 3-month follow-up period (see Table 15.1).[6,14]

TABLE 15.1 PESI and sPESI Clinical Models Prognostic Factors and Weighting

PESI (Original and Simplified)		
Parameter	Standard PESI	sPESI
Age	Age in years	1 point is age >80 years
Male sex	+ 10 points	
Cancer	+ 30 points	1 point
Chronic heart failure	+ 10 points	1 point
Chronic pulmonary disease	+ 10 points	1 point
Pulse rate > 109 beats per minute	+ 20 points	1 point
Systolic blood pressure < 100 mm Hg	+ 30 points	1 point
Respiratory rate > 30 breaths per minute	+ 20 points	
Temperature < 36°C	+ 20 points	
Altered mental status	+ 60 points	
Arterial oxyhemoglobin saturation < 90%	+ 20 points	1 point

PESI, Pulmonary Embolism Severity Index; *sPESI,* simplified Pulmonary Embolism Severity Index.

TABLE 15.2 Risk Evaluation by PESI and sPESI Clinical Models

PESI	Risk	sPESI	Risk
Class I ≤65 points	Very low 30-day mortality risk (0%–1.6%)	0 points	30-day mortality risk of 1.0%
Class II 66–85 points	Low mortality risk (1.7%–3.5%)		(95% CI, 0.0–2.1)
Class III 86–105 points	Moderate mortality risk (3.2%–7.1%)	>0 points	30-day mortality risk 10.9%
Class IV 106–125 points	High risk mortality risk (4.0%–11.4%)		(95% CI, 8.5–13.2)
Class V >125 points	Very high mortality risk (10.0%–24.5%)		

PESI, Pulmonary Embolism Severity Index; *sPESI,* simplified Pulmonary Embolism Severity Index.

TREATMENT GUIDELINES

Guidelines for the management of acute PE have been published by several societies, including the American College of Cardiology (ACC), the AHA, and the European Society of Cardiology (ESC).[3,15–17] The ESC suggests that intravenous anticoagulation should be administered to patients with a high or intermediate clinical probability of PE awaiting results of diagnostic tests. Appropriate anticoagulation includes intravenous unfractionated heparin (UFH), subcutaneous low-molecular-weight heparin (LMWH), or subcutaneous fondaparinux.[16] For patients with high-risk PE or with hemodynamic compromise, intravenous anticoagulation with UFH should be initiated immediately. In this same cohort of patients, LMWH or fondaparinux have not been adequately studied.[16] Normotensive patients classified as PESI class III, or sPESI of 1, and who demonstrate either negative RV dysfunction and negative cardiac troponins are classified as intermediate-low risk. For these patients, parenteral anticoagulation followed by a vitamin K antagonist or nonvitamin K antagonist oral anticoagulants can be offered.[16] Low-risk patients, such as those satisfying criteria for PESI class I or II, may be considered for early discharge and outpatient treatment, according to the ESC. The American College of Clinical Pharmacy (ACCP) states that at-home treatment with LMWH of acute-PE in these low-risk patients is adequate.[18] The goal of anticoagulation in patients with PE is to prevent recurrence of venous thromboembolism (VTE). General consensus is to treat patients for at least 3 months. However, the decision to continue treatment beyond this time is based on individual clinical assessment.[16,18]

In patients with high-risk PE, primary reperfusion treatment, particularly systemic fibrinolysis, is the treatment of choice.[3,19] This method can rapidly reduce thrombus burden, RV dysfunction, and pulmonary vascular resistance.[20] In a meta-analysis of 1061 patients treated with fibrinolytic therapy and 1054 patients treated only with anticoagulation, fibrinolytic therapy reduced total mortality (adjusted OR, 0.53; 95% CI, 0.32–0.88) and recurrent PE (adjusted OR, 0.40; 95% CI, 0.22–0.74).[21] Consequently, patients with massive PE and associated hemodynamic instability receive a clear mortality benefit from systemic fibrinolysis compared with anticoagulation alone. For those with submassive PE and major myocardial necrosis or severe RV dysfunction, patients must be considered on a case-by-case basis. Although systemic fibrinolysis in massive PE has been found to decrease mortality compared with anticoagulation alone, it also carries a high morbidity risk. There is a 20% risk of major hemorrhage and a 3% to 5% risk of intracranial hemorrhage. This is primarily caused by the large recombinant tissue plasminogen activator (r-tPA) dosage of up to 100 mg over 2 hours. Conversely, anticoagulation is not without its own risks and has been associated with a 15% chance of minor hemorrhage and a 1% to 5% risk of major bleeding complications.[22] Surgical pulmonary embolectomy has been used in patients with large, centrally-located thromboemboli. This procedure requires a median sternotomy and cardiopulmonary bypass. In patients with submassive PE, surgical embolectomy can be considered when systemic fibrinolysis is contraindicated or has failed, when patients have thrombi in the right atrium or ventricle, or when patients are ineligible for catheter directed therapy.[23]

Catheter Directed Therapy

Percutaneous catheter directed thrombolysis (CDT) has emerged as a viable option for patients with submassive or massive PE who have contraindications to thrombolysis and for whom thrombolysis has not improved hemodynamic compromise.[19] As mentioned earlier, the clinical differentiation between massive and submassive PE is based on the presence or absence of cardiogenic shock, respectively.[24] Utility of CDT in patients with massive PE has been studied thoroughly. In a meta-analysis published by Hofmann et al., clinical success rate of CDT in 594 patients with massive PE was 86.5% with only 7.6% experiencing minor complications and 2.4% of patients experiencing major complications.[19] When compared with systemic fibrinolysis, which has a 20% risk of major hemorrhage and a 3% to 5% risk of hemorrhagic stroke, these risks are minimal. In patients with submassive PE with RV strain, CDT can be used to decrease the rate of recurrent PE, DVT, and PE-related death that is associated with persistent RV dysfunction.[25]

ESTABLISHED CATHETER DIRECTED TREATMENT MODALITIES

Rheolytic Embolectomy

Rheolytic embolectomy devices, such as the Angiojet catheter (Possis, Minneapolis, MN), use the Venturi and Bernoulli principles to create a vortex, which causes fragmentation of the clot allowing for clot aspiration. Angiojet is a double lumen system with a diameter ranging from 4-Fr to 6-Fr. This enables the catheter to be advanced over a wire and placed precisely in the desired vessel (Fig. 15.1). The use of this device has been associated with the occurrence of severe bradyarrhythmias and type III heart block in up to 15% of cases in the literature.[26] This has been attributed to the possibility of hyperkalemia secondary to hemolysis, which can lead to an adenosine-mediated heart block, intraarterial and intraventricular stretch receptor mediated reflex bradycardia, and hemolytic pulmonary vasoconstriction caused by the sequestration of nitric oxide by liberated hemoglobin.[26,27] Because of the risk of cardiac conduction abnormalities, transcutaneous or transvenous pacemakers should be inserted before the procedure.[26] Although human data is lacking, physiology literature has suggested that streptomycin and gadolinium may play a role in preventing arrhythmias by blocking cardiac stretch receptors.[26] The US Food and Drug Administration (FDA) has issued a black-box warning regarding intrapulmonary interventions with the Angiojet catheter system.[28] Previously used rheolytic devices include the Hydrolyser catheter system (Cordis Corporation, Warren, NJ) and Oasis catheter (Boston Scientific, Natick, MA).

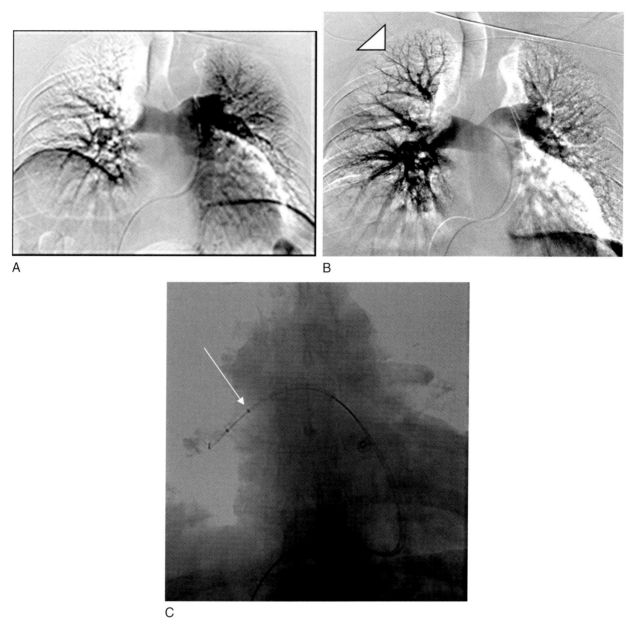

A

B

C

■ **Fig. 15.1** Massive pulmonary embolism requiring immediate catheter directed treatment. (A) Angiogram of the pulmonary arteries demonstrating decreased distal perfusion in the right lung. (B) Angiogram after pharmacomechanical thrombectomy with Angiojet Xpedior catheter shows improved distal perfusion in the right lung *(arrowhead)*. (C) Fluoroscopic image of Angiojet Xpedior catheter *(arrow)* during right main pulmonary artery catheter directed thrombectomy.

Suction Embolectomy

The Greenfield embolectomy device (Boston Scientific; Watertown, MA) was the first suction embolectomy device designed specifically for the treatment of massive PE and has been in use for over four decades. It is a 10-Fr braided, steerable catheter with a funnel shaped tip, measuring 5 mm or 7 mm.[29] The catheter is inserted through the femoral or jugular vein via a venotomy, a large, valveless, vascular sheath. An acute nonorganized thrombus can be removed by manual suction with a large syringe and retrieved with the device as a unit through the access site. The Greenfield embolectomy device has been shown to successfully remove pulmonary embolisms and provide significant hemodynamic improvement in up to 83% of patients.[29]

Balloon Angioplasty-Assisted Clot Disruption

Balloon angioplasty has been in use for several years in the treatment of pulmonary emboli. Angioplasty balloons, which are 6 to 16 mm in size, are used for mechanical fragmentation of clots, thereby improving pulmonary blood flow and decreasing right ventricular pressure.[30] The balloons compress the thrombus to the vessel wall resulting in distal embolization of thrombus fragments.[29] Intraarterial CDT is used as an adjunct to this technique, which results in greater reduction of pulmonary artery pressure over time. If catheter fragmentation and thrombolysis is unsuccessful in clot disruption, rapid clinical improvement is achieved with the use of self-expanding stents such as Wallstent (Schneider Europe AG; Bülach, Switzerland) and Gianturco Z stents (Cook Europe; Bjaerskov, Denmark).[31,32]

Mechanical Embolectomy With Rotating Pigtail

The catheter used for rotating embolectomy is a modified 5-Fr pigtail catheter with a radio-opaque tip. It has ten side holes for contrast injection and an oval side hole in the outer aspect of the pigtail loop, which allows for direct passage of a 0.035-inch (0.088-cm) guidewire through the hole acting as a pivot on which the catheter is rotated manually for clot fragmentation. In a study by Schmitz-Rode et al., rotating pigtail thrombectomy was successful in up to one-third of the patients.[33] Combination of this technique with r-tPA thrombolysis over 48 hours resulted in a greater decrease in pulmonary artery pressure.[34] In this study, treatment had a success rate of 80%; one patient died from right heart failure 1 hour after clot fragmentation. A potential complication of this technique is macroembolization into a previously patent lobar pulmonary artery, which can further compromise cardiopulmonary status. This complication can be managed by continuation of clot fragmentation and the use of adjuvant thrombolytic therapy.[34]

Ultrasound-Assisted Catheter Directed Thrombolysis

Ultrasound-assisted catheter directed thrombolysis (USAT) using an EkoSonic catheter (EKOS Corporation, Bothel, WA) is a new technique that has been FDA approved for pulmonary thrombolysis. The EKOS catheter has multiple side holes used for infusion of thrombolytics such as r-tPA. The catheter also has a filament with numerous small transducers that emit low-power (0.5 W per element), high-frequency (2.2 MHz) ultrasound. The filament is placed in the catheter's central lumen and emits ultrasound along the treatment zone (Fig. 15.2). This technique can disrupt the thrombus and increase its susceptibility to thrombolytic agents. Lower-energy application dissociates fibrin strands, enhancing thrombolysis with lower doses.[35,36]

Venbrux et al., conducted a multicenter case series that demonstrated the complete extraction of thrombus with 24-hour USAT and r-tPA 24 infusion at doses less than 1 mg per hour in 76% of patients, and near complete thrombolysis in 18% of patients.[37] In a retrospective study, Kougias et al. showed that a significantly shorter treatment of 17 hours and a mean r-tPA dose on 0.86 mg per hour effectively reduced the Miller Index (measure of angiographic burden) while still providing similar efficacy when compared with traditional passive infusion catheters at higher rates and with longer infusions times.[38] There were fewer treatment-related complications with USAT because of the lower amounts of administered thrombolytic therapy. The Ultrasound Accelerated Thrombolysis of Pulmonary Embolism (ULTIMA) trial randomized patients with acute main or lower lobe PE and an echocardiographic right-to-left ventricular ratio of 1 or more to receiving either unfractionated intravenous heparin or an USAT regimen of 10 to 20 mg r-tPA over 15 hours.[39] It showed that the USAT regimen was superior to anticoagulation alone in reversing RV dilatation without an increase in bleeding complications.

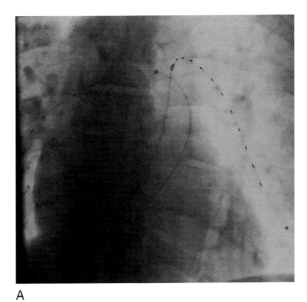

A

■ **Fig. 15.2** Bilateral pulmonary embolisms with submassive presentation. (A) Placement of bilateral pulmonary artery EKOS thrombolysis catheters for 15-hour thrombolysis.

Continued

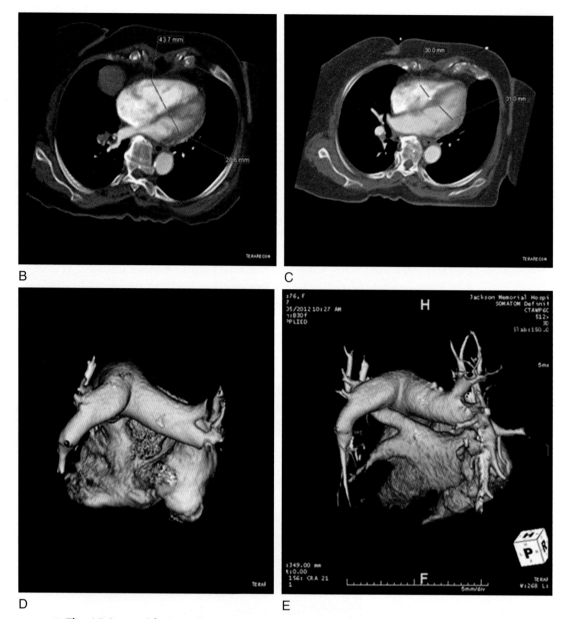

■ **Fig. 15.2, cont'd** (B and C) Prethrombolysis *(upper left)* and postthrombolysis *(upper right)* computed tomography angiograms demonstrating marked improvement in right-to-left ventricular ratio. (D and E) Prethrombolysis *(lower left)* and postthrombolysis *(lower right)* three-dimensional reconstruction of the pulmonary arteries and veins showing recanalization after thrombolysis.

A Prospective, Single-Arm, Multicenter Trial of Ultrasound-Facilitated, Catheter-Directed, Low-Dose Fibrinolysis for Acute Massive and Submassive Pulmonary Embolism (The SEATTLE II Study) was a single arm multicenter study with the purpose of evaluating the efficacy of USAT with EKOS catheter. The study enrolled 150 patients; 31 with acute massive and 119 with submassive PE, with RV/LV ratios of greater than 0.9. Two different administration methods were used: 24 mg of r-tPA was administered either as 1 mg per hour for 24 hours with a unilateral catheter or as 1 mg per hour catheter for 12 hours with bilateral catheters. The result was a mean decrease in RV/LV ratio from 1.55 pre-procedure to 1.13 at 48-hours postprocedure ($P < .0001$). There were no deaths within 30 days and no intracranial hemorrhage or fatal bleeding events. The rates of EKOS catheter assisted r-tPA infusion can vary. They range from 1 mg or less per hour and usually continued for 24 hours and subsequently removed. In stable patients, follow-up of PE is accomplished with bedside echocardiography or CT pulmonary angiography.

COMPLICATIONS OF CATHETER DIRECTED THERAPIES

Overall, CDTs have a favorable safety profile. Complications of CDT for PE include injury to several adjacent structures, such as the pulmonary vessels and the RV outflow tract, which can lead to pericardial tamponade. Perforation of a major pulmonary artery can cause massive pulmonary hemorrhage leading to immediate death. The risk of pulmonary artery injury is increased with treatment of vessels less than 6 mm in diameter.[40] Thus thrombectomy is indicated for use in the main and lobar pulmonary arteries, not in the segmental pulmonary arteries. It should be terminated when there is satisfactory hemo-dynamic improvement, regardless of the angiographic result.[29,41]

Additional concerns include arrhythmias with passage of devices through the right heart, blood loss and mechanical hemolysis leading to hypotension, and acute pancreatitis.[41] Use of thrombolytic therapy, even in low doses, can cause bleeding, albeit rates as low as 2.4 % have been reported.[19] There are also several adverse effects specific to particular devices. Mechanical devices can cause fragmentation and showering of thrombus fragments into distal pulmonary segments, leading to further deterioration in clinical status. As mentioned previously, rheolytic embolectomy with Angiojet carries a risk of bradyar-rhythmias and type III heart block. As with any vascular intervention, CDT carries a risk of contrast-induced nephropathy, anaphylactic reaction to iodinated-contrast media, and vascular access site complications.

ON THE HORIZON

Pulmonary Embolism Response Teams

The treatment of pulmonary embolism is multifaceted and varies based on severity. In the past, surgery was the only treatment option in patients with massive PE and those with contraindication to thrombolytics. In recent years, CDT has played an increasing role in treatment. In the management of patients with massive and submassive PE with RV dysfunction, CDT, especially with EKOS endovascular system, will play an increasing role as the results from ULTIMA and SEATTLE II study are realized.[39,42] Multidisciplinary programs called Pulmonary Embolism Response Teams (PERT) have been created at various hospitals because of the numerous treatment options for PE and the disparities in evidence from various specialties. Once activated, PERT coordinate the efforts of multiple specialties to expedite treatment of patients with intermediate and high-risk PE.[43] Since their inception, PERT have successfully provided a framework for rapid multidisciplinary consultation and mobilization of resources.[44]

Extracorporeal Membrane Oxygenation

In the past decade, medical technologies, such as venoarterial extracorporeal membrane oxygenation (ECMO), have become increasingly useful as adjunctive treatment for massive and submissive PE.[45] ECMO is used to maintain arterial oxygenation as a bridge to more definitive therapies, such as catheter directed thrombolysis or surgery. ECMO should be considered in patients who fail to maintain adequate oxygenation despite mechanical ventilation with a high fraction of inspired oxygen (FiO_2). In this way, ECMO can provide much-needed time for diagnostic and therapeutic measures in cases of massive or submissive PE.[46,47] ECMO is also an effective option with heparin and catheter guided embolectomy for management of high-risk surgical patients.[48] More studies are needed to identify the patients who would receive the most benefit from ECMO therapy.

AngioVac

A promising, emerging device for the treatment of PE is the AngioVac venous drainage catheter (AngioDynamics, Latham, New York). The AngioVac venous drainage catheter is a 22-Fr coil-reinforced cannula and has a balloon actuated, funnel-shaped tip that facilitates high-flow aspiration. The system consists of a vacuum cannula and venous return circuit. The device was originally approved by the FDA for the removal of soft thrombi and emboli, and as a venous drainage catheter for extracorporeal bypass for up to 6 hours, but the AngioVac system has also shown potential for use in the acute management of PE. For the treatment of PE, the catheter is directed through the right heart into the pulmonary artery, clot and blood are then aspirated from the pulmonary artery by the cannula and pulled through an extracorporeal circuit that includes a filtration canister. Blood is then returned to the patient via a reinfusion venous cannula. Two case series and one case report have demonstrated the feasibility of this procedure with mixed technical success.[49–51] Currently, the use of the AngioVac system has been limited to a small number of patients with massive PE and a contraindication to thrombolysis or had previously failed catheter directed or systemic thrombolysis. In one case series of five patients with hemodynamically compromising PE, technical success of aspiration (i.e., retrieval of embolus and reduction in mean pulmonary artery [PA] pressure) was achieved in two patients (40%) (Fig. 15.3). In this same case series, there was one major complication of RV free-wall rupture, which resulted in patient death.[49] The potential for injury to the wall of the myocardium or chordae tendineae is caused by the inherent stiffness of the coil-reinforced AngioVac cannula and the extra-stiff guidewire necessary to navigate it into the right outflow tract. In its current form, AngioVac aspiration cannula is not optimally designed for application within the pulmonary artery. Perhaps future iterations of the concept will result in greater maneuverability, efficacy, and safety.

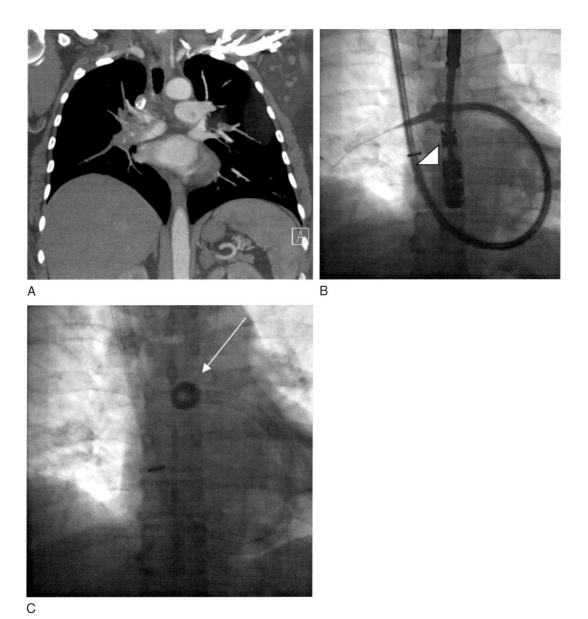

A

B

C

■ **Fig. 15.3** AngioVac aspiration thrombectomy for massive pulmonary embolism (PE). (A) Coronal computed tomography angiography demonstrates near complete occlusion of the right main pulmonary artery secondary to PE. (B) Placement of an AngioVac cannula via a Gore DrySeal sheath into the right main pulmonary artery with transesophageal echocardiography (TEE) *(arrowhead)* and fluoroscopic guidance. (C) AngioVac catheter during active aspiration with balloon activated funnel tip *(arrow)*.

FlowTriever

FlowTriever (Inari Medical, Irvine, California) is a novel device that combines mechanical clot retrieval with suction embolectomy for percutaneous treatment of PE. The device has not yet been approved by the FDA and is currently undergoing clinical trials. The FlowTriever catheter is a nitinol mesh with three self-expanding disks that engage and retrieve a clot. It is delivered by a 20-Fr dual function aspiration guide catheter. Once engaged within the clot, a hand-powered ratcheting mechanism synchronizes retraction and aspiration of the clot into the guide catheter. There is a single case report documenting the successful use FlowTriever, seen as a reduction of clot burden on CTA and decreased RV dilation on echocardiography.[52] Safety and efficacy of the device are pending the results of the FlowTriever Pulmonary Embolectomy Clinical Study (FLARE).

REFERENCES

1. Tapson VF. Acute pulmonary embolism. *N Engl J Med.* 2008;358(10):1037–1052.
2. Goldhaber SZ, Visani L, De Rosa M. Acute pulmonary embolism: clinical outcomes in the International Cooperative Pulmonary Embolism Registry (ICOPER). *Lancet.* 1999;353(9162): 1386–1389.
3. Jaff MR, McMurtry MS, Archer SL, et al. Management of massive and submassive pulmonary embolism, iliofemoral deep vein thrombosis, and chronic thromboembolic pulmonary hypertension: a scientific statement from the American Heart Association. *Circulation.* 2011;123(16): 1788–1830.
4. White RH. The epidemiology of venous thromboembolism. *Circulation.* 2003;107(23 suppl 1):I4–I8.
5. Becattini C, Vedovati MC, Agnelli G. Prognostic value of troponins in acute pulmonary embolism: a meta-analysis. *Circulation.* 2007;116(4):427–433.
6. Jimenez D, Aujesky D, Yusen RD. Risk stratification of normotensive patients with acute symptomatic pulmonary embolism. *Br J Haematol.* 2010;151(5):415–424.
7. Sanchez O, Trinquart L, Colombet I, et al. Prognostic value of right ventricular dysfunction in patients with haemodynamically stable pulmonary embolism: a systematic review. *Eur Heart J.* 2008;29(12):1569–1577.
8. Jimenez D, Lobo JL, Monreal M, et al. Prognostic significance of multidetector computed tomography in normotensive patients with pulmonary embolism: rationale, methodology and reproducibility for the PROTECT study. *J Thromb Thrombolysis.* 2012;34(2):187–192.
9. Quintana D, Salsamendi J, Fourzali R, et al. Ultrasound-assisted thrombolysis in submassive and massive pulmonary embolism: assessment of lung obstruction before and after catheter-directed therapy. *Cardiovasc Intervent Radiol.* 2014;37(2):420–426.
10. Binder L, Pieske B, Olschewski M, et al. N-terminal pro-brain natriuretic peptide or troponin testing followed by echocardiography for risk stratification of acute pulmonary embolism. *Circulation.* 2005;112:1573–1579.
11. Pieralli F, Olivotto I, Vanni S, et al. Usefulness of bedside testing for brain natriuretic peptide to identify right ventricular dysfunction and outcome in normotensive patients with acute pulmonary embolism. *Am J Cardiol.* 2006;97:1386–1390.
12. Jimenez D, Yusen RD. Prognostic models for selecting patients with acute pulmonary embolism for initial outpatient therapy. *Curr Opin Pulm Med.* 2008;14:414–421.
13. Jimenez D, Aujesky D, Moores L, et al. Simplification of the pulmonary embolism severity index for prognostication in patients with acute symptomatic pulmonary embolism. *Arch Intern Med.* 2010;170:1383–1389.

14. Nendaz MR, Bandelier P, Aujesky D, et al. Validation of a risk score identifying patients with acute pulmonary embolism, who are at low risk of clinical adverse outcome. *Thromb Haemost.* 2004;91:1232–1236.

15. Holbrook A, Schulman S, Witt DM, et al. Evidence-based management of anticoagulant therapy: Antithrombotic Therapy and Prevention of Thrombosis, 9th ed: American College of Chest Physicians Evidence-Based Clinical Practice Guidelines. *Chest.* 2012;141:e152S–e184S.

16. Konstantinides SV, Torbicki A, Agnelli G, et al. 2014 ESC guidelines on the diagnosis and management of acute pulmonary embolism. *Eur Heart J.* 2014;35:3033–3069, 3069a–3069k.

17. MacLean S, Mulla S, Akl EA, et al. Patient values and preferences in decision making for antithrombotic therapy: a systematic review: Antithrombotic Therapy and Prevention of Thrombosis, 9th ed: American College of Chest Physicians Evidence-Based Clinical Practice Guidelines.*Chest.* 2012;141:e1S–e23S.

18. Kearon C, Akl EA, Ornelas J, et al. Antithrombotic therapy for VTE disease: CHEST guideline and expert panel report. *CHEST Journal.* 2016;149(2):315–352.

19. Kuo WT, Gould MK, Louie JD, et al. Catheter-directed therapy for the treatment of massive pulmonary embolism: systematic review and meta-analysis of modern techniques. *J Vasc Interv Radiol.* 2009;20:1431–1440.

20. Piazza G. Submassive pulmonary embolism. *JAMA.* 2013;309(2):171–180.

21. Chatterjee S, Chakraborty A, Weinberg I, et al. Thrombolysis for pulmonary embolism and risk of all-cause mortality, major bleeding, and intracranial hemorrhage: a meta-analysis. *JAMA.* 2014;311(23):2414–2421.

22. Lin PH, Chen H, Bechara CF, et al. Endovascular interventions for acute pulmonary embolism. *Perspect Vasc Surg Endovasc Ther.* 2010;22(3):171–182.

23. Leacche M, Unic D, Goldhaber SZ, et al. Modern surgical treatment of massive pulmonary embolism: results in 47 consecutive patients after rapid diagnosis and aggressive surgical approach. *J Thorac Cardiovasc Surg.* 2005;129(5):1018–1023.

24. Clark D, McGiffin DC, Dell'italia LJ, et al. Submassive pulmonary embolism where's the tipping point? *Circulation.* 2013;127(24):2458–2464.

25. Grifoni S, Vanni S, Magazzini S, et al. Association of persistent right ventricular dysfunction at hospital discharge after acute pulmonary embolism with recurrent thromboembolic events. *Arch Intern Med.* 2006;166(19):2151–2156.

26. Dwarka D, Schwartz SA, Smyth SH, et al. Bradyarrhythmias during use of the AngioJet system. *J Vasc Interv Radiol.* 2006;17(10):1693–1695.

27. Nassiri N, Jain A, McPhee D, et al. Massive and submassive pulmonary embolism: experience with an algorithm for catheter-directed mechanical thrombectomy. *Ann Vasc Surg.* 2012; 26(1):18–24.

28. Sobieszczyk P. Catheter-assisted pulmonary embolectomy. *Circulation.* 2012;126(15):1917–1922.

29. Kucher N. Catheter embolectomy for acute pulmonary embolism. *Chest.* 2007;132:657–663.

30. Handa K, Sasaki Y, Kiyonaga A, et al. Acute pulmonary thromboembolism treated successfully by balloon angioplasty—a case report. *Angiology.* 1988;39:775–778.

31. Haskal ZJ, Soulen MC, Huettl EA, et al. Life-threatening pulmonary emboli and cor pulmonale: treatment with percutaneous pulmonary artery stent placement. *Radiology.* 1994;191:473–475.

32. Koizumi J, Kusano S, Akima T, et al. Emergent Z stent placement for treatment of cor pulmonale due to pulmonary emboli after failed lytic treatment: technical considerations. *Cardiovasc Intervent Radiol.* 1998;21:254–255.

33. Schmitz-Rode T, Janssens U, Duda SH, et al. Massive pulmonary embolism: percutaneous emergency treatment by pigtail rotation catheter. *J Am Coll Cardiol.* 2000;36:375–380.

34. Schmitz-Rode T, Janssens U, Schild HH, et al. Fragmentation of massive pulmonary embolism using a pigtail rotation catheter. *Chest.* 1998;114:1427–1436.

35. Sobieszczyk P. Catheter-assisted pulmonary embolectomy. *Circulation.* 2012;126:1917–1922.

36. Braaten JV, Goss RA, Francis CW. Ultrasound reversibly disaggregates fibrin fibers. *Thromb Haemost.* 1997;78:1063–1068.

37. Chamsuddin A, Nazzal L, Kang B, et al. Catheter-directed thrombolysis with the Endowave system in the treatment of acute massive pulmonary embolism: a retrospective multicenter case series. *J Vasc Interv Radiol.* 2008;19:372–376.

38. Lin PH, Annambhotla S, Bechara CF, et al. Comparison of percutaneous ultrasound-accelerated thrombolysis versus catheter-directed thrombolysis in patients with acute massive pulmonary embolism. *Vascular.* 2009;17(suppl 3):S137–S147.

39. Kucher N, Boekstegers P, Muller OJ, et al. Randomized, controlled trial of ultrasound-assisted catheter-directed thrombolysis for acute intermediate-risk pulmonary embolism. *Circulation.* 2014;129:479–486.

40. Biederer J, Charalambous N, Paulsen F, et al. Treatment of acute pulmonary embolism: local effects of three hydrodynamic thrombectomy devices in an ex vivo porcine model. *J Endovasc Ther.* 2006;13:549–560.

41. Kucher N, Goldhaber SZ. Management of massive pulmonary embolism. *Circulation.* 2005;112:e28–e32.

42. G P. A Prospective, single-arm, multicenter trial of ultrasound-facilitated, low-dose fibrinolysis for acute massive and submassive pulmonary embolism (SEATTLE II). Program and abstracts of the American College of Cardiology Scientific Session 2014; Late-breaking clinical trial.

43. Provias T, Dudzinski DM, Jaff MR, et al. The Massachusetts General Hospital Pulmonary Embolism Response Team (MGH PERT): creation of a multidisciplinary program to improve care of patients with massive and submassive pulmonary embolism. *Hosp Pract (1995).* 2014;42:31–37.

44. Kabrhel C, Jaff MR, Channick RN, et al. A multidisciplinary pulmonary embolism response team. *Chest.* 2013;144(5):1738–1739.

45. Omar HR, Miller J, Mangar D, et al. Experience with extracorporeal membrane oxygenation in massive and submassive pulmonary embolism in a tertiary care center. *Am J Emerg Med.* 2013;31(11):1616–1617.

46. Bombino M, Redaelli S, Pesenti A. Newer indications for ECMO: pulmonary embolism, pulmonary hypertension, septic shock and trauma. *ECMO-Extracorporeal Life Support in Adults.* Springer. 2014;179–192.

47. Chon MK, Park YH, Choi JH, et al. Thrombolytic therapy complemented by ECMO: successful treatment for a case of massive pulmonary thromboembolism with hemodynamic collapse. *J Korean Med Sci.* 2014;29:735–738.

48. Malekan R, Saunders PC, Yu CJ, et al. Peripheral extracorporeal membrane oxygenation: comprehensive therapy for high-risk massiv.

49. Al-Hakim R, Park J, Bansal A, et al. Early Experience with AngioVac Aspiration in the Pulmonary Arteries. *JVIR.* 2016;27(5):730–734.

50. Donaldson CW, Baker JN, Narayan RL, et al. Thrombectomy using suction filtration and venovenous bypass: single center experience with a novel device. *Cathet Cardiovasc Interv.* 2015;86(2):E81–E87.

51. Pasha AK, Elder MD, Khurram D, et al. Successful management of acute massive pulmonary embolism using Angiovac suction catheter technique in a hemodynamically unstable patient. *Cardiovasc Revasc Med.* 2014;15(4):240–243.

52. Weinberg AS, Dohad S, Ramzy D, et al. Clot Extraction With the FlowTriever Device in Acute Massive Pulmonary Embolism. *J Intensive Care Med.* 2016;31(10):676–679.

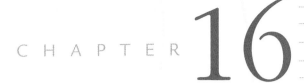

CHAPTER 16

Endothermal Heat-Induced Thrombosis

Mikel Sadek, Jose I. Almeida, and Lowell S. Kabnick

HISTORICAL BACKGROUND

Endothermal ablation techniques used to treat superficial venous reflux, such as endovenous laser ablation (EVLA) and radiofrequency ablation (RFA), use heat to induce endothelial injury. This results in a combination of thrombosis, fibrosis, subsequent vein contracture, and eventual occlusion of the treated vein. As stated, a component of this mechanism involves thrombus formation, which may vary depending on the modality or technique used. The thrombus that forms may propagate into the contiguous deep vein junction, most commonly the saphenofemoral junction, and is thus designated as an endothermal heat-induced thrombosis (EHIT).[1] EHIT is a relatively novel entity that has no equivalent from the era of surgical ligation and stripping.

EHIT is classified according to the extent of central propagation of thrombus into the respective deep vein lumen. The classification scheme was not well delineated initially, and earlier reports used the term *deep venous thrombosis* (DVT) but without clear characterization of the pathology being evaluated. Based on a combination of the previous reports as well as newer information that specifically referred to the concept of EHIT, the incidence has ranged from 0% to 16%.[2–4]

The natural history of EHIT remains poorly defined, particularly when one evaluates the subgroups within the EHIT classification. Moreover, this is further complicated by taking into account the truncal vein that is being treated. Given the poorly defined natural history, there is little consensus regarding postprocedural surveillance or treatment for EHIT. The data will be reviewed in the chapter herein.

DEFINITION OF ENDOTHERMAL HEAT-INDUCED THROMBOSIS

EHIT refers to the central propagation of thrombus relative to the treated refluxing truncal vein. Endothermal heat-induced explicitly states that the entity of EHIT relates to thermal ablation technologies. Traditionally, these would include EVLA and RFA. Other techniques and modalities may be applicable but are not necessarily governed by the same pathophysiology, natural history, or even treatment. These include foam, glue, steam, mechanicochemical ablation (MOCA), and so on. The entity specifically refers to thrombosis as it relates to the respective deep vein. An argument can be made that all thermal ablation techniques result in superficial vein thrombus of the treated superficial vein. Therefore implicit in the definition of EHIT is the involvement of the respective deep vein. Also implicit in the definition is the acute nature of the pathology. It is "heat-induced," and therefore the entity needs to be identified in the periprocedural period. Lastly, because it is also a heat-induced process directly related to a specific modality of treatment, the thrombosis should be contiguous with the treated vein. For example, an isolated gastrocnemius vein DVT following endothermal ablation of the great saphenous vein (GSV) with access obtained in the thigh would not fall under the definition of an EHIT.

CLASSIFICATION OF ENDOTHERMAL HEAT-INDUCED THROMBOSIS

The classification scheme was alluded to in the introduction, and it is predicated on fulfilling the criteria noted in the definition section. The classification scheme was derived because of the potential for differences in outcomes, and therefore treatments, depending on the extent of the central propagation of thrombus.[1] It is also predicated on central propagation of thrombus as measured with the patient in the upright position. This is critical, because the classification level may change when the evaluation is performed in an upright as compared with a supine position, given that the thrombus may retract away from the deep vein when the patient is erect. The classification scheme is as such (Fig. 16.1):

1. Up to and including the respective deep vein junction
2. Propagation into the respective deep vein but comprising less than 50% of the deep vein lumen
3. Propagation into the respective deep vein but comprising more than 50% of the deep vein lumen
4. Occlusive deep vein thrombus, contiguous with the treated truncal vein

The most common forms of EHIT are propagation into the common femoral vein following treatment of the GSV or propagation into the popliteal vein following treatment of the small saphenous vein (SSV). The same would apply to treatment of all the truncal veins emanating from the common femoral vein (e.g., anterior accessory GSV).

With regards to other anomalies or variants, such as a duplicated deep venous system, central propagation into the contiguous vein would be considered an EHIT.

Because of the low reported incidence in the literature, the development of a DVT following endothermal ablation of a perforator vein has not been well described. Moreover, the drainage systems are myriad, and drainage can be into any of the calf muscle veins, as well as the named axial deep veins, and therefore thrombosis, as it relates to treatment of perforator veins, is generally excluded from discussions of EHIT.

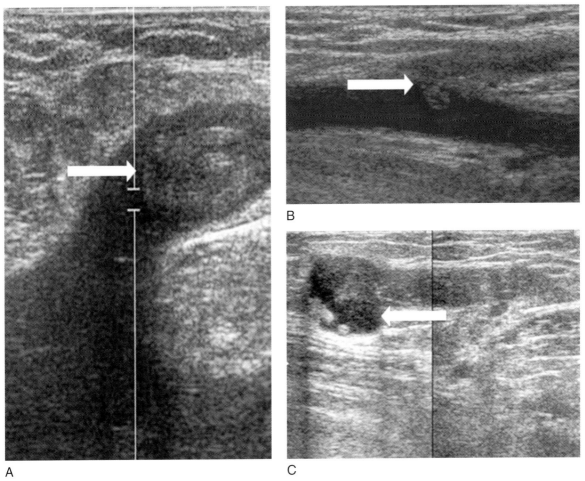

■ **Fig. 16.1** (A) Endothermal heat-induced thrombosis (EHIT) 1: duplex ultrasound demonstrating thrombus that is extending up to and including the respective deep vein junction. *Arrow* points to thrombus that remains peripheral to the deep vein junction. (B) EHIT 2: thrombus that propagates into the respective deep vein but comprises less than 50% of the deep vein lumen. *Arrow* points to the thrombus protruding into the common femoral vein. (C) EHIT 3: thrombus that propagates into the respective deep vein, but comprises greater than 50% of the deep vein lumen. *Arrow* points to the thrombus that is laminating a portion of the wall of the common femoral vein.

PATHOPHYSIOLOGY

Virchow's triad remains central to the development of EHIT. Endothelial injury, stasis, and hypercoagulability all may play a role, either individually or in concert, resulting in the development of an EHIT.

With regards to endothelial injury, endothermal ablation in fact relies on inducing endothelial injury to effect ablation of the refluxing truncal vein. The mechanisms by which EVLA induces endothelial injury varies by laser wavelength with the dichotomy occurring between the hemoglobin specific laser wavelengths and the water specific laser wavelengths, and this is discussed in detail in the EVLA chapter (Chapter 7). The original RFA technology induced endothelial injury by transfer of radiofrequency waves through the vein wall from a catheter tip housing anode and cathode elements, but the more recent iteration of the Venefit procedure, which uses segmental ablation, results in endothelial injury using direct transfer of heat by conduction. Also in some of the early literature there is the possibility that some adjoining deep veins were treated/injured unintentionally by direct contact with the thermal device, and this situation has likely diminished with increased global experience. It is also possible that the heat transmitted at the time of treatment may propagate centrally, possibly contributing to the development of an EHIT. Some evidence suggests that increasing the ablation distance from the respective deep vein junction may result in a reduction in EHIT.[4]

With regards to stasis, there may be a potential stagnant column of blood central to the area of treatment. In certain instances, the central aspect of the truncal vein may be retained patent by inflow of "cool blood" from a patent, superficial epigastric vein (SEV), for example. There is a possibility that this is protective against the development of an EHIT. Earlier recommendations for treatment included specifically identifying the SEV so that one could ensure they are peripheral to this "protective" junctional tributary before initiating treatment. More recent recommendations suggest that starting the ablation 2 cm, or greater than 2.5 cm, peripheral to the deep vein junction produces equally efficacious results without an increased incidence in the development of EHIT.[4] Nonetheless, the generation of any thrombus within a previously open truncal vein would result in some element of stasis.

Lastly, hypercoagulability may contribute to the development of an EHIT. Many patients are treated appropriately without a full preprocedural screening for a hypercoagulability state. Moreover, the treatment may unmask a previously unknown hypercoagulability state. Lastly, it is conceivable that there may be a local hypercoagulability state, in the sense that heat transmitted to components of blood or plasma may result in a prothrombotic state independent of endothelial injury.

EPIDEMIOLOGY

There has been considerable variation in the incidence of EHIT based on a review of the current literature. In general, the trends suggest that the incidence of EHIT has diminished over time with increases in the individual as well as the collective operator experience. As alluded to previously, there is some heterogeneity in tracking the entity of EHIT because of differing definitions, and therefore the epidemiologic data is based on an evaluation of the incidence/prevalence of a combination of DVT and EHIT. In 2004, Hingorani et al. provided one of the initial reports in the literature of DVT development following treatment of GSV reflux with RFA.[2] The study (felt to be an outlier by most) reviewed 73 patients who were followed up at the 1-month time point, and the incidence of DVT was 16% in patients treated under general anesthesia. The EHIT classification scheme was not used for the study; 11 of the 12 DVTs were not occlusive and were most likely consistent with a classification of an EHIT 2 or 3. In addition, there were several limitations and criticisms related to the study design. In particular, the ablations were initiated 1 cm peripheral to the saphenofemoral junction. This is contrary to widely accepted recommendations, which state that the ablation should be initiated 2 cm peripheral to the saphenofemoral junction. This is one of the key arguments explaining the high incidence of DVT in this study, and this has yet to be replicated in numerous subsequent patient cohorts. Other studies arose subsequently that demonstrated significantly lower rates of EHIT. One year later, Puggioni et al. retrospectively reviewed patients treated with either EVLA or RFA.[5] Some 130 procedures were evaluated, and the reported rate of DVT was 2.3%. The DVTs were consistent likely with EHIT 2 or 3, given that they were nonocclusive. Interestingly, the methodology still used a distance of 1 cm from the saphenofemoral junction and the thrombotic events occurred only in the EVLA cohort.

Because of the data put forth by the aforementioned investigators and others, the standard of care with regards to procedural methodology changed, such that ablations were to be performed 2 cm peripheral to the deep venous junction (i.e., saphenofemoral or saphenopopliteal) and peripheral to the SEV. The theoretic reason for attention being paid to the first junctional tributary (i.e., SEV) was that tributary flow through the SEV may help to maintain the patency of the central aspect of the saphenofemoral junction thereby preventing the development of a thrombus propagating into the subjacent deep vein. Because of the lack of data in support of maintaining patency of the SEV, and the tremendous anatomic variation in SEV location, the instructions for use for the Venefit procedure have since evolved to the sole condition of maintaining a 2-cm distance from the respective deep venous junction.

A mixed retrospective evaluation by Marsh et al.[6] of 2470 procedures using the 2-cm distance guideline, with an average follow-up of 2 weeks, showed an EHIT rate of 0.28%. The methodology of treatment (EVLA vs. RFA) did not result in a significant difference, although the incidence was too low overall to allow for a meaningful statistic evaluation. In another trial further illustrating the variegated nature of this pathology, 2-week follow-up ultrasound demonstrated an EHIT rate of 4%.[7] The methodology still consisted of treatment starting 2 cm peripheral to the saphenofemoral junction. Some consider the relatively early follow-up of 2 weeks to be partially contributory to the 4% EHIT rate, given the possibly higher incidence of detection. The natural history of EHIT and its resolution will be described later in this chapter.

The initial ClosureFast data that were collected prospectively by Proebstle and colleagues demonstrated a 0% incidence of thrombosis for EHIT.[8] This has persisted with the latest study update.[3] As has been demonstrated previously, the highly controlled nature of the clinical trial likely contributed to the very low complication rate. Although, the trial failed to demonstrate a risk for DVT, the US Food and Drug Administration (FDA) Adverse Event Database contained 15 reports of DVT in the same year of usage. In addition, four patients developed pulmonary emboli; however, these were asymptomatic.[9]

As clinical experience continued to grow, the data with regards to EHIT remained excellent. Merchant et al. performed a review of 858 limbs whereby eight patients (1%) developed an EHIT or DVT.[10] Interestingly, four patients developed an occlusive DVT, which is one of the highest reported incidences in the literature.

An evaluation of 17 randomized controlled trials comparing a combination of ligation and stripping with RFA or EVLA that encompassed 2624 limbs treated, demonstrated that the overall thrombosis rate was 0.85%.[11] The primary comment noted by the authors was that DVT or EHIT was not reported consistently, or at all, in many instances. Overall, EHITs were detected seven times and occlusive DVTs were detected twice. Again, in the setting of a randomized controlled trial, the results are often better than those seen with real-world experience. Overall, current trials have demonstrated an EHIT rate ranging from 0% to 4%.

NATURAL HISTORY/SURVEILLANCE

Conventional wisdom views the natural history of EHIT as a self-limiting phenomenon in most patients. Therefore the clinical relevance of this entity is constantly in question.

There is some thought that the majority of EHITs are identified only in patients who undergo early surveillance (i.e., within 2 weeks postprocedure). Lawrence et al. evaluated 500 patients who underwent RFA and found that the incidence of femoral extension of the thrombus occurred in 2.6% of patients.[12] With regards to the natural history, all patients exhibited full thrombus retraction to the level of the saphenofemoral junction at an average of 16 days postprocedure. Consequently, most practitioners have adopted the practice of obtaining a postprocedure duplex ultrasound 1 to 2 weeks following intervention.

RISK FACTORS

Although the incidence of DVT or thrombosis is quite low in patients treated using EHIT, some effort has been made in an attempt to identify potential predisposing factors to reduce the risk. Generally speaking, the low incidence of EHIT has made it challenging to convincingly identify risk factors that would predispose to central propagation of thrombus. Most studies are likely underpowered. As stated previously, thrombosis risk in general has been linked to Virchow's triad. Specifically, larger vein diameter, obesity, and increased venous disease severity have all been linked to postprocedural thrombus formation.[12,13]

Lawrence et al. performed an evaluation where thrombus extension was evaluated relative to the saphenofemoral junction as well as the SEV.[12] The study included 500 patients who underwent treatment of the GSV with RFA. Thrombus propagation into the adjacent femoral vein occurred in 2.6% of patients. Age and use of anticoagulation were not identified risk factors. The significant risk factors identified were patients with a prior history of DVT and patients with a GSV diameter that exceeded 8 mm. Having a history of DVT may indeed be a surrogate for a hypercoagulable state, and this is a plausible mechanism for the development of EHIT, although this has not been demonstrated in a reproducible manner. With regards to GSV diameter, one possible mechanism of action is that the ablation is not fully effected, and therefore increased wall separation, particularly at the saphenofemoral junction, may expose damaged but "unsealed" endothelium, thereby resulting in a locally hypercoagulable state resulting in an EHIT. Rhee et al. retrospectively reviewed 519 procedures whereby they identified 21 cases (4%) of EHIT.[14] The evaluation included patients who underwent treatment of truncal reflux using either EVLA or RFA. Multiple variables were evaluated, and of the clinical factors, it did not appear that catheter tip distance from the deep vein junction, vein diameter, concomitant treatments, or the use of perioperative anticoagulation were significant in contributing to the development of an EHIT. As part of the univariate analysis, male gender, increased Caprini score, CEAP (clinical, etiologic, anatomic, and pathophysiologic) classification, and history of thrombosis appeared to contribute. On multivariate analysis, male gender and an increased Caprini score appeared to contribute significantly to the development of an EHIT. Of note, there was some suggestion that EVLA might have a higher incidence of EHIT as compared with RFA; however, the EVLA patients had a higher Caprini score, which is why the finding did not hold with the multivariate analysis. Kane et al. evaluated 528 patients who were treated with EVLA.[15] Moreover, this study included treatment of both the GSV and SSV. The incidence of EHIT was 5.1%. Three patients developed occlusive DVTs. There were no pulmonary emboli, and all EHITs resolved fully. Other risk factors associated with the development of an EHIT that have been recorded in the literature include age greater than 65 years, male gender as stated previously, and even female gender, adjunctive procedures such as microphlebectomy, advanced disease (e.g., stasis ulcers), ablation distance when reviewing the data historically, and the Caprini score as stated previously.[14]

One potentially considerable risk factor that has emerged is the distance of ablation relative the deep venous junction. As stated previously, the collective experience has shown that thrombosis rates declined dramatically once ablation was started 2 cm relative to the saphenofemoral junction as compared with 1 cm relative to the saphenofemoral junction. More recent data has also suggested that increasing the ablation distance to 2.5 cm or greater from the level of the saphenofemoral or saphenopopliteal junction as compared with 2 cm from the respective deep venous junction resulted in a potential for improvement in the rate of EHIT 2.[4] The incidence of EHIT 2 was reduced to 1.3%, down from 2.3%.

PREVENTION

With regards to prevention of EHIT, there is little guidance beyond the consideration of the aforementioned risk factors, and therefore taking empiric steps to mitigate against the risk of EHIT. For example, all male patients, or patients with large veins, should not be treated with preprocedural anticoagulation to reduce the risk of EHIT. Moreover, there has been no prospective evaluation to support the use of any techniques or methods to mitigate against the risk of development of an EHIT. Some of the anecdotal techniques that have been recommended include: (1) performing in ambulatory center (office) with patient awake; (2) adequate tumescence of 1 cm around the entire vein, including paying special attention to the saphenofemoral junction; (3) ablating distal to the SEV in patients with large veins (i.e., >8 mm); (4) administering prophylactic anticoagulation in patients with a history of DVT; (5) remaining superficial to the level of the muscular fascia during treatment of the SSV; and (6) early and brisk ambulation.

Taking the collective literature into account, the only technique based on evidence is increasing the ablation distance from the saphenofemoral or the saphenopopliteal junction. As stated previously, a higher incidence of DVT was noted with the initial endothermal ablation experiences, where a 1-cm distance was used as the treatment protocol.[2,5] The body of literature thereafter, which was based on increasing the ablation distance to 2 cm from the respective deep venous junction consistently, demonstrated a lower EHIT rate. The most recent iteration of this has already been alluded to, and it derives from the authors' data.[4] The authors identified that increasing the ablation distance to greater than 2.5 cm resulted in a decrease in the incidence of EHIT from 2.3% to 1.3%. The impetus for the study was that the incidence of EHIT could not be lowered in the authors' internal data set beyond the 2% threshold regardless of the technique or modality used. Therefore the decision to increase the ablation distance was made in a calculated fashion, and the results were as delineated. To date this remains the only technique with supporting evidence that reduces the risk for EHIT development.

TREATMENT FOR EHIT

The emerging consensus is that EHIT is a low-risk and possibly benign condition. The rationale behind the aforementioned statement is that most reported series have failed to detect the presence of a symptomatic pulmonary embolus or of a symptomatic DVT. Moreover, it appears that the incidence of EHIT is correlated to the timing of postprocedural surveillance duplex, whereby earlier duplex ultrasounds would generally identify a greater number of EHITs, because most would resolve by 2 weeks.

Despite the data that are currently available, there are no randomized controlled trials delineating the appropriate treatment for EHIT. Moreover, because of the low incidence of the development of EHIT 2, achieving the power necessary to conduct a randomized trial may not be practical. The recommendations thus far are based mostly on expert opinion and consideration of the various risks and benefits associated with treatment versus observation. There has also been some informal extrapolation from the literature on the treatment of DVT.

One recommended treatment paradigm is based on the EHIT classification by Kabnick et al.[1] In most instances, treatment choices are ultimately left to the discretion of the practitioner. In the study, which evaluated the effect of ablation distance on the incidence of EHIT, a proposed treatment paradigm emerged based on data.[4] In the study EHIT, one was considered not to be a DVT, and therefore no patients were anticoagulated. There was not a single incidence of central thrombus propagation that was identified on follow-up in this cohort of patients. With regards to EHIT 2, the general trend was to fully anticoagulate the patient with low-molecular-weight heparin (LMWH) until full resolution of the EHIT 2 was confirmed by ultrasound. For the initial phase of the study, only 54% of the patients with an EHIT 2 were treated with LMWH, and in the second phase of the study, 100% of the patients with a detectable EHIT 2 were treated with LMWH. In general, ultrasound surveillance was performed on a weekly basis until the EHIT 2 was no longer detectable. All episodes of EHIT 2 resolved, and there were no EHIT 3 or 4 detected.[4] In a subgroup evaluated from the initial phase of the study, two of nine patients who were screened with computed tomography scans of the chest were found to have asymptomatic pulmonary emboli. Other studies have also demonstrated that the average resolution of an EHIT is on the order of 1 to 2 weeks.[12]

All told, and also taking into consideration the increased ease that has come about with the relatively recent availability of the novel oral anticoagulants such as dabigatran, apixaban, and rivaroxaban, the general recommendation is to treat EHIT 1 as a likely benign condition and EHIT 2 as a relatively benign condition where there is mixed opinion relative to treatment. The authors, for the most part, favor low-dose aspirin or no treatment. The treatment should be limited to resolution of the entity as determined by duplex ultrasound. For EHIT 3, the benefit of anticoagulation may outweigh the risk, and LMWH is recommended; although this rare entity should be taken in isolation (Fig. 16.2). Lastly, EHIT 4 (occlusive DVT) may warrant a full course of therapeutic anticoagulation as would be recommended in the CHEST guidelines for the treatment of a provoked acute DVT[16] (Fig. 16.3). These are only guidelines and practice may vary from practitioner to practitioner. It is unlikely that a randomized controlled trial will be powered adequately to allow for a formal evaluation of this entity.

CONCLUSIONS

The advent of endothermal ablation resulted in significant improvements to the safety and efficacy in the treatment of chronic venous insufficiency. Moreover, it allowed for a transition to the outpatient setting, and this has resulted in the exponential growth of this treatment modality. With increasing usage and experience with endothermal ablation, the distinct clinical entity of EHIT was identified. A classification scheme was developed to standardize the reporting and ultimately the treatment of this entity. Currently, risk factors have been identified, although these have been inconsistently reported. EHIT is

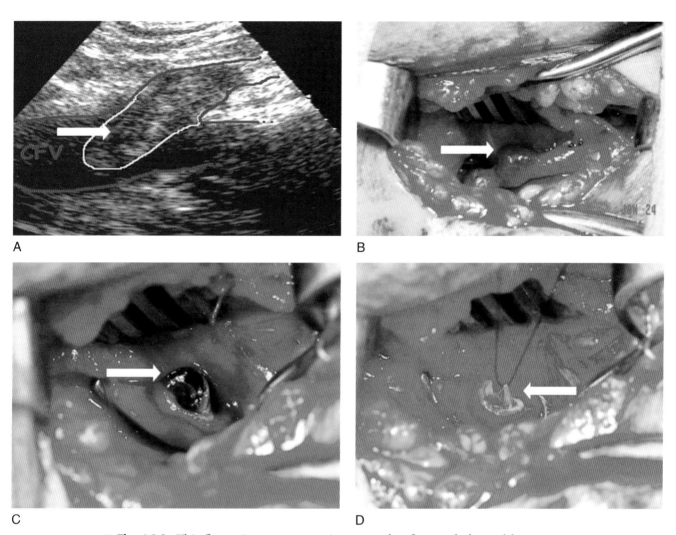

■ **Fig. 16.2** This figure is a representative example of an endothermal heat-induced thrombosis (EHIT) 3, highlighting the variability in the natural history of this pathology. Thrombus persisted at the terminal valve for 3 months postendothermal ablation and ultimately warranted surgical removal. (A) Duplex ultrasound demonstrating EHIT 3 with *arrow* pointing to the thrombus. Yellow outlines the thrombus and blue outlines the saphenofemoral junction. (B) Surgical exposure revealing persistent thrombus at the central-most aspect of the great saphenous vein. *Arrow* points to dilated segment of vein with intraluminal thrombus. (C) Venotomy reveals underlying thrombus *(arrow)*. (D) Terminal valve secured with suture at site of thrombus extraction, with *arrow* pointing towards the terminal valve. *CFV,* Common femoral vein.

usually asymptomatic, and therefore screening ultrasound following every endothermal ablation is required to diagnose the entity. Treatment with anticoagulation is generally reserved for EHIT 2 or greater, and the only preventative measure reported in the literature thus far is to increase the starting ablation distance from 2 to 2.5 cm. Lastly, the clinical relevance of EHIT is still being debated, and this is consequential given the cost associated with postprocedural screening ultrasound. Currently, EHIT remains a well-described clinical entity that warrants identification, proper characterization, and a careful consideration for treatment that is tailored to the individual patient.

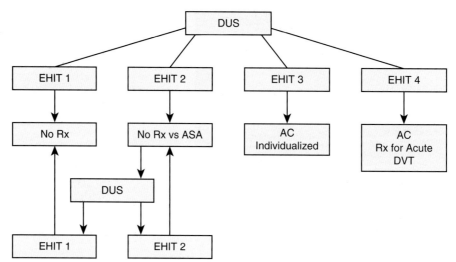

◼ **Fig. 16.3** Suggested treatment algorithm for endothermal heat-induced thrombosis (EHIT) 1 to 4. *AC,* Full anticoagulation with low-molecular-weight heparin, warfarin, or a direct oral anticoagulant, as examples; *ASA,* aspirin; *DUS,* duplex ultrasound; *DVT,* deep venous thrombosis; *Rx,* treatment.

REFERENCES

1. Kabnick LS, Ombrellino M, Agis H, et al. Endovenous heat induced thrombus (EHIT) at the superficial-deep venous junction: a new post-treatment clinical entity, classification and potential treatment strategies. 18th Annual Meeting of the American Venous Forum, Miami, FL; February 2006.
2. Hingorani AP, Ascher E, Markevich N, et al. Deep venous thrombosis after radiofrequency ablation of greater saphenous vein: a word of caution. *J Vasc Surg.* 2004;40:500–504.
3. Proebstle TM, Alm J, Göckeritz O, et al; European Closure Fast Clinical Study Group. Three-year European follow-up of endovenous radiofrequency-powered segmental thermal ablation of the great saphenous vein with or without treatment of calf varicosities. *J Vasc Surg.* 2011;54(1):146–152.
4. Sadek M, Kabnick LS, Rockman CB, et al. Increasing ablation distance peripheral to the saphenofemoral junction may result in a diminished rate of endothermal heat induced thrombosis. *J Vasc Surg.* 2013;1:257e62.
5. Puggioni A, Kalra M, Carmo M, et al. Endovenous laser therapy and radiofrequency ablation of the great saphenous vein: analysis of early efficacy and complications. *J Vasc Surg.* 2005;42:488–493.
6. Marsh P, Price BA, Holdstock J, et al. Deep vein thrombosis (DVT) after venous thermoablation techniques: rates of endovenous heat-induced thrombosis (EHIT) and classical DVT after radiofrequency and endovenous laser ablation in a single centre. *Eur J Vasc Endovasc Surg.* 2010;40:521–527.
7. Rhee SJ, Stoughton J, Cantelmo NL. Procedural factors influencing the incidence of endovenous heat-induced thrombus (EHIT). *J Vasc Surg.* 2011;53:555.
8. Proebstle TM, Vago B, Alm J, et al. Treatment of the incompetent great saphenous vein by endovenous radiofrequency powered segmental thermal ablation: first clinical experience. *J Vasc Surg.* 2008;47:151–156.
9. Food and Drug Administration. Search of the MAUDE adverse event reporting system. Available at: http://www.accessdata.fda.gov/scripts/cdrh/cfdocs/cfMAUDE/search.CFM. Accessed April 13, 2008.
10. Merchant RF, Pichot O, Myers KA. Four-year follow-up on endovascular radiofrequency obliteration of great saphenous reflux. *Dermatol Surg.* 2005;31:129–134.

11. Dermody M, O'Donnell TF, Balk EM. Complications of endovenous ablation in randomized controlled trials. *J Vasc Surg.* 2013;1:427e36.

12. Lawrence PF, Chandra A, Wu M, et al. Classification of proximal endovenous closure levels and treatment algorithm. *J Vasc Surg.* 2010;52(2):388–393.

13. Caprini JA. Risk assessment as a guide for the prevention of the many faces of venous thromboembolism. *Am J Surg.* 2010;199(15):S3–S10.

14. Rhee SJ, Cantelmo NL, Conrad MF, et al. Factors influencing the incidence of endovenous heat-induced thrombosis (EHIT). *Vasc Endovascular Surg.* 2013;47:207e12.

15. Kane K, Fisher T, Bennett M, et al. The incidence and outcome of endothermal heat-induced thrombosis after endovenous laser ablation. *Ann Vasc Surg.* 2014;28(7):1744–1750. doi:10.1016/j.avsg.2014.05.005. [Epub 2014 Jun 6].

16. Kearon C, Akl EA, Ornelas J, et al. Antithrombotic Therapy for VTE Disease: CHEST Guideline and Expert Panel Report. *Chest.* 2016;149(2):315–352. doi:10.1016/j.chest.2015.11.026.

CHAPTER 17

Postthrombotic Syndrome

Rafael D. Malgor and Nicos Labropoulos

HISTORICAL BACKGROUND

Postthrombotic syndrome (PTS) remains an important health care problem in United States. A population-based study showed that the incidence of venous ulcers currently approaches 18 per 100,000 habitants per year.[1] The same study identified that PTS is responsible for economic expenses estimated at least $200 million.[1]

Diagnosis of PTS is based on history and clinical presentation. The syndrome consists of signs and symptoms of heaviness, intolerance to exercises, pain, leg edema, paresthesia, cramps, and pruritus that may evolve to skin damage, such as hyperpigmentation, lipodermatosclerosis, and ulcers (Fig. 17.1). The severity of PTS is measured by different scales and scores assigning points for the presence of each sign and symptom. Although there is a good association with PTS severity, further refinement and validation are necessary.[2–5]

Attention to differential diagnosis should be outlined. Trauma, congenital venous disease (i.e., venous malformations, valve aplasia), and other causes of ulcerative disease, such as rheumatologic (lupus, scleroderma, rheumatoid arthritis), oncologic (squamous and basal cell carcinoma), or infectious disorders (syphilis, lymphangitis) are potential causes of misdiagnosis and inappropriate treatment.[6,7] Table 17.1 shows the location and cause of nonvenous-related ulcers.

Not all patients who have had a documented episode of deep venous thrombosis (DVT) sustain PTS. Recovery with no signs or symptoms of PTS occurs in two-thirds of the patients, and only the rest will eventually develop PTS with variable spectrum and severity.[8] It appears that other factors are involved in the disease process, rendering some patients more vulnerable than others to PTS changes. A list of important clinical

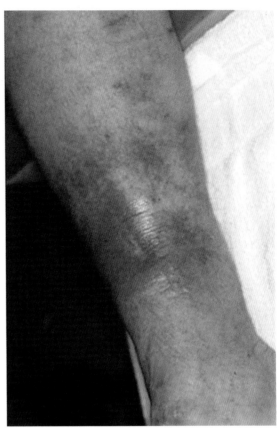

■ **Fig. 17.1** Image of the right leg from a patient with previous venous thrombosis. Features of postthrombotic signs are seen in the medial aspect of the leg (CEAP [clinical, etiologic, anatomic and pathophysiologic] classes 3, 4, and 5). This patient also had pain and an itching and burning sensation.

predictors of PTS is shown in Table 17.2.[4,9–11] Among those predisposing factors, the strongest one for PTS remains ipsilateral recurrent DVT because several prospective studies have shown high odds for skin damage (Fig. 17.2).[12,13] Patients who had unprovoked DVT and are older than 65 years have a higher risk of recurrent DVT and therefore PTS.[14] Residual thrombus was also reported as a cause of recurrent DVT[15] (Fig. 17.3). In addition, patients who had DVT in more than one site, popliteal valve insufficiency, or a calf DVT associated with a proximal DVT also have an increased risk of recurrent DVT (Fig. 17.4).[11,16,17] Notably, the recurrence of DVT is likely to affect the proximal veins and is related to inadequate duration of anticoagulation.[13] In a recent review, the limitations of studies on recurrent DVT are discussed.[10] Most of the studies used a nonstandardized ultrasound analysis, giving limited or inaccurate information on the incidence of fatal pulmonary embolism (PE) as well as having poor documentation of anticoagulation and its monitoring. The effects of thrombolytic therapy and its socioeconomic and quality-of-life impact are also questions that remain unanswered.[10] These are important because ipsilateral recurrent DVT has a significant impact on the development of PTS.

Biomarkers have been used to estimate the odds of developing PTS. In a study of 305 patients with PTS, persistent elevated levels of D-dimer in the course of DVT were investigated. Patients with elevated levels of D-dimer at 4 months following DVT, after stopping anticoagulation, showed a 4-fold risk of PTS.[18] The molecular aspects of chronic postthrombotic changes following an episode of DVT were recently reported by Comerota and colleagues.[19] Their recent study of 16 patients undergoing endovenectomy of common femoral and femoral veins to treat chronic obstruction showed dystrophic calcification

TABLE 17.1 Characteristics of the Ulcers Found on 21 Patients

Sex	Age (Years)	Limb	Location on Calf	Duration (Years)	Duplex	ABI	Medication	Pathology
M	63	L	u-1/med	3	nl	nl	abx	Undetermined
		R	u-1/med	3	nl	nl	abx	Undetermined
F	72	L	1/med	5	nl	nl		Vasculitis
		R	1/med	5	nl	nl		Vasculitis
F	52	L	m-l/med	4	nl	nl	abx	Chronic inflammation
M	73	R	1/med	8	nl	nl	abx	Chronic inflammation
M	54	R	1/ant-lt	2	nl	nl	abx	Chronic inflammation
M	68	L	m/post	1	nl	nl		Kaposi sarcoma
M	79	L	1/med	16		nl		Carcinoma
F	76	R	1/med	18	Venous reflux	nl		Squamous cell carcinoma
F	73	R	1/med	15	Venous reflux	nl		Squamous cell carcinoma
F	64	L	m-1/med	3	nl	nl		Undetermined
		R	m-1/med	3	nl	nl		Undetermined
M	71	L	1/med	4	nl	nl		No histology
F	82	R	m-1/med	7	nl	nl	abx	No histology
F	73	R	1/med	14	nl	nl		Basal cell carcinoma
M	78	L	m/med	2	nl	nl		Pyoderma gangrenosum
	59	L	1/med	0.17	nl	nl		Hydroxyurea
M	17	R	1/med	0.33	nl	nl		Sickle cell
M		L	1/med	0.25	nl	nl		Sickle cell
F	62	R	1/med	0.75	Mild reflux	0.7		Rheumatoid arthritis

ABI, Ankle-brachial index; *abx,* antibiotics; *ant-lt,* anterior lateral; *m,* midcalf; *nl,* normal; *post,* posterior; *u,* upper calf.
(Adapted from Labropoulous N, Manalo D, Patel NP, et al. Uncommon leg ulcers in the lower extremity. *J Vasc Surg.* 2007;45:568–573.)

TABLE 17.2 Important Clinical Predictors of Postthrombotic Syndrome

Clinical Predictors of PTS

1. Recurrent ipsilateral DVT
2. Iliofemoral DVT
3. Higher 1-month Villalta score
4. Nonoptimal anticoagulation
5. Higher BMI

BMI, Body mass index; *DVT,* deep venous thrombosis; *PTS,* postthrombotic syndrome.

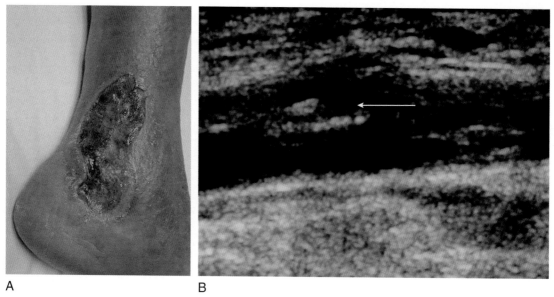

A   B

■ **Fig. 17.2** (A) A 64-year-old male with history of multiple episodes of deep vein thrombosis involving left common femoral vein extending up to the common iliac vein who developed a recalcitrant left distal medial calf ulceration. (B) Chronic postthrombotic luminal changes are noted in the common femoral, which displays trabeculae likely containing collagen but no thrombus *(yellow arrows)*.

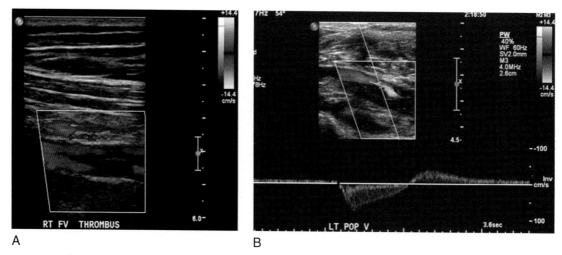

A   B

■ **Fig. 17.3** (A) Chronic postthrombotic luminal changes in a male patient who presented with swelling and pain in the right lower extremity. The femoral vein is partially recanalized as seen by the multiple channels and the intraluminal filling defects. (B) A 55-year-old female patient sustaining leg edema, discoloration, and a venous ulcer. Reflux is seen in a partially recanalized popliteal vein.

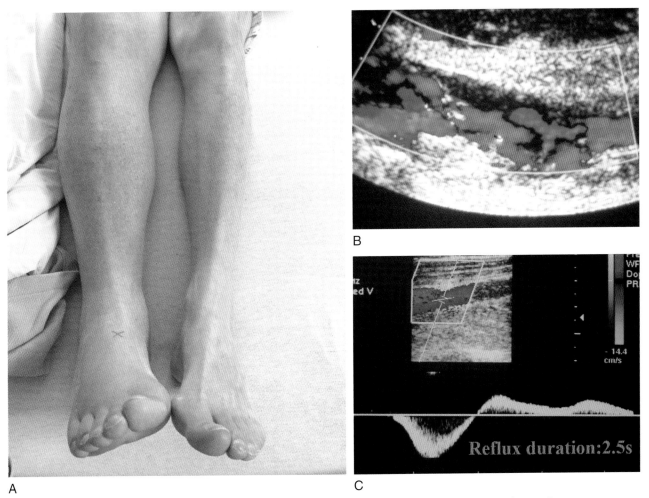

A

B

C

■ **Fig. 17.4** (A) A 70-year-old male with 1-year history of right common femoral, femoral, and calf vein thrombosis presenting with right lower extremity edema and skin damage. (B and C) Near complete recanalization with reflux is noted in the right femoral vein.

and a collagen-rich tissue material on the analyzed specimens. Interestingly, no thrombus or smooth cells were found in the material analyzed (Fig. 17.5). These findings suggest the term ***chronic deep vein thrombosis*** is likely a misnomer.

Patients with asymptomatic DVT are also at risk of developing PTS. A systematic review including 364 patients with asymptomatic DVT showed that abdominal and

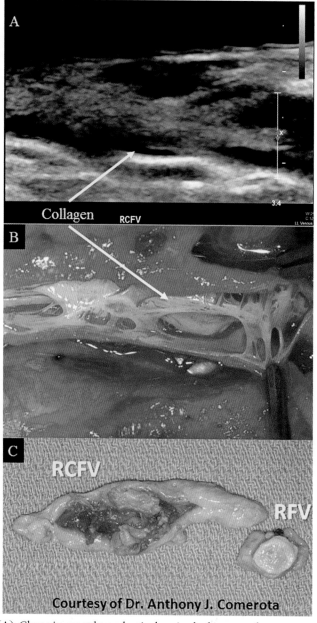

■ **Fig. 17.5** (A) Chronic postthrombotic luminal changes demonstrated on duplex ultrasound in 2015 of a 49-year-old male patient with previous history of right lower extremity deep venous thrombosis in 2008, who presents with signs and symptoms of postthrombotic syndrome. Note the femoral vein has an echogenic intraluminal material, which was found to be rich in collagen with no thrombus. (B) Intraoperative findings showing trabeculae (chronic obstruction) in a partial recanalized right common femoral vein (RCFV) and right femoral vein (RFV). (C) RCFV and RFV specimens obtained from endophlebectomy.

orthopedic surgeries are major predictors for PTS. The drawbacks in the former study were different definitions of PTS according to each author's criteria, random use of anticoagulation upon diagnosis, and different diagnostic methods including venography, duplex ultrasound (DUS), and ^{125}I-fibrinogen uptake test. Regardless of distinct methodology found in the literature, if a poor DVT history is associated with marked PTS findings, it must prompt careful investigation with DUS first, especially following major abdominal or orthopedic surgery.

Progression of secondary cardiovascular disease (CVD) evolving to PTS has been demonstrated. A study of 73 limbs with secondary CVD showed overall progression in clinical CEAP (clinical, etiologic, anatomic, and pathophysiologic) classes in 31% of the limbs. Skin damage (C4–C6) rate strikingly rose from 4% at the first year to 25% in the 5-year follow-up. Other studies also investigated secondary CVD and clinical course of PTS.[15] In an Italian cohort of 355 patients, the incidence of PTS increased from 17% after the first year to 29% at 8 years of follow-up.[15] Development of reflux alone has been associated with PTS.[10–12,14–18] However, a combination of reflux and obstruction is associated with more severe PTS than reflux or obstruction alone.[12]

Patients with a hypercoagulable state, such as carriers of factor V Lieden (FVL), prothrombin gene mutation, or proteins C and S have been investigated for occurrence of PTS. A study comprising 667 patients with DVT, who sustained hypercoagulable state, demonstrated no association with increased risk of PTS. Furthermore, heterozygosis for FVL was even less associated with PTS than in noncarriers.[20] Another study of 387 patients tested for thrombophilia found no increased risk of PTS in carriers of FVL or prothrombin gene mutation.[11] The same study also showed that the intensity of persistent signs and symptoms in the first month after the episode of acute DVT predicted the incidence of PTS in a dose-dependent manner in the first 2 years.[11]

NONOPERATIVE TREATMENT

PTS generates high expenses for government and insurance companies because of disability premiums, loss of labor force, and need for rehabilitation and wound care. Thus prevention should always be contemplated to minimize the socioeconomic impact of the disease. DVT prophylaxis is mandatory in different settings such as major surgeries, critically ill patients, and those with significant risk factors for DVT.[21]

Multiple reports have shown that elastic compression applied in patients with acute DVT may decrease the incidence of PTS by 50% at long term.[22,23] This was evident in two review papers that analyzed all the relevant prospective studies before the release of the SOX trial results.[24–26] In patients with established PTS, a few treatments are available. Initial treatment for all patients with PTS is nonoperative, with compression to the legs in different levels and intensity. The use of compression stockings in 387 patients could not predict the progression or lack of PTS. However, 20% of patients who did use compression stockings had a risk of developing PTS compared with 47% who did not use compression stockings.[15] The Cochrane collaboration review of 39 randomized control trials concluded that compression was more effective than no compression on ulcer healing.[27] It was also shown that multicomponent systems were more effective in ulcer healing compared with single-component systems. The shortcoming of compression therapy is that up to 20% of patients are noncompliant, and compliance with stockings does not change regardless of the symptoms of PTS.[28] Further discussion of compression and its role on preventing PTS is provided later under Pearls and Pitfalls.

Complementary to the compression therapy, wound care is important to improve ulcer healing rates and patients' quality of life. Many techniques have been applied in different settings varying from local care to more extensive surgical debridement.

More recently, in a small prospective randomized study of patients with PTS, exercise training for 6 months was associated with improvement in quality of life and improvement in scores on the Villalta scale.[29] The authors concluded that these results should be confirmed in a large, prospective randomized trial.

INTERVENTIONAL TREATMENT

Surgical and endovascular procedures are indicated when deep venous reflux or obstruction is present, with or without superficial vein involvement, in patients with skin damage or disabling symptoms. Before the endovenous techniques, obstruction used to be treated with bypass grafts. More recently, chronic venous obstruction is treated with balloon angioplasty and stenting. Bypass grafting is reserved for cases in which the endovenous approach is unsuccessful. However, the endovenous treatment for chronic venous obstruction is discussed extensively in Chapter 18. This chapter concentrates on the bypass grafting.

The treatment of proximal occlusion, including iliocaval segment, differs from that for femoropopliteal thrombotic occlusive disease. The higher velocity, significant blood volume, and better outflow of common femoral, iliac veins, and inferior vena cava (IVC) create a more amenable setting for treatment with either vein or prosthetic bypass grafts. An initial study of 44 venous reconstructions for nonmalignant iliofemoral and IVC occlusion was conducted at the Mayo Clinic.[30] A wide variety of possible options for IVC and iliofemoral segment reconstruction were used, including great saphenous vein (GSV) crossover grafts (Palma procedure), supported expanded polytetrafluoro-ethylene (ePTFE), spiral vein grafts, and femoral vein patch angioplasty (Fig. 17.6). The overall primary and secondary patency at 3 years was 54% and 62%, respectively. Conversely, lower primary and secondary patency rates were found for iliocaval and femorocaval bypasses when analyzed separately, reaching only 38% and 54% at 2-year follow-up. The lower patency found in those bypasses was deemed to be related to the ePTFE bypass grafts. A small number of procedures failed to show statistical significance, although a trend toward higher patency rates was shown for GSV bypass grafts. Highest patency was also achieved with GSV crossover grafts, reaching 77% in a 4-year period, similar to other reports in the literature.[30,31] A more recent study including complex, open and hybrid, open endovascular procedures has also been published by the Mayo Clinic.[32] Forty-eight patients had a venous bypass done and 12 had hybrid procedures (endovenectomy, patch angioplasty, and stenting). About 60% of the patients who underwent bypass surgery had no venous claudication and no or minimal swelling when last seen. Despite ulcer healing, half the patients with patent grafts had recurrence of ulceration. A low 2-year secondary patency rate for complex open surgery (COS) and hybrid procedures (HP) was reported (COS, 28% and HP, 30%).[32]

Several open surgical techniques have been used to correct venous reflux reconstructing the valves. The main procedures described are internal or external (transcommissural) valvuloplasty, axillary vein transfer, vein transplantation, or valve transplantation.[28,33,34] Overall, the results vary based on the technique used, the surgeon's expertise, and postprocedure care. A few specialized centers have currently been conducting open venous reconstruction or valvuloplasty.

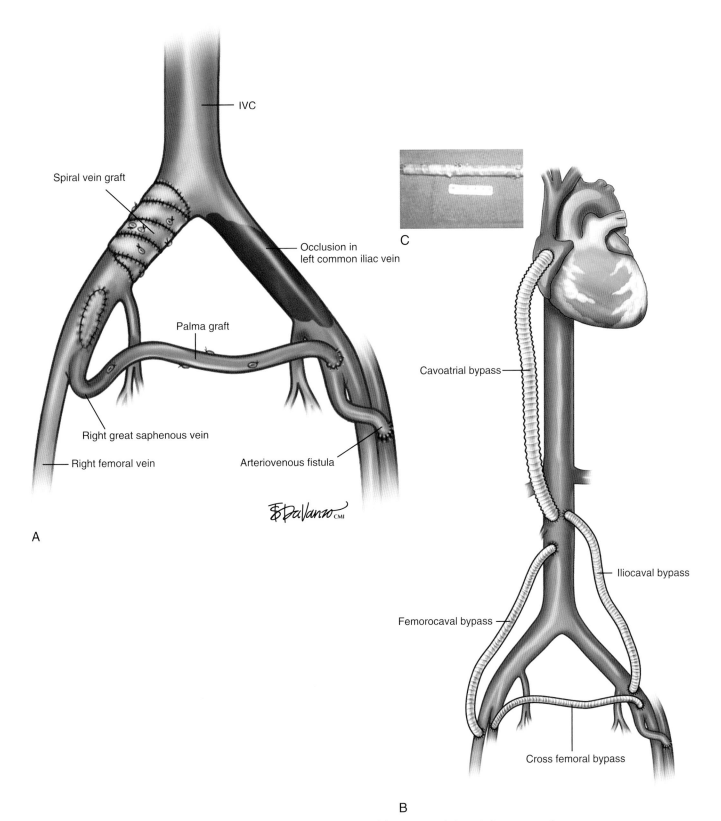

■ **Fig. 17.6** Examples of venous repair and bypasses. (A) A Palma procedure with an arteriovenous fistula, a common femoral vein venoplasty, and a spiral vein graft in the right common iliac vein. (B) Different prosthetic bypasses. (C) Spiral vein graft constructed over a chest tube. *IVC,* Inferior vena cava. *(Modified from Jost CJ, Gloviczki P, Cherry KJ Jr, et al. Surgical reconstruction of iliofemoral veins and the inferior vena cava for nonmalignant occlusive disease.* J Vasc Surg. *2001;33:320–327.)*

The internal valve vein repair is carried out by performing a venotomy to expose the incompetent valve to reapproximate the valve leaflets (Fig. 17.7). In a study of 42 patients (52 limbs), Cheattle and Perrin reported an 85% valve competency and 9% ulcer recurrence rate at 1-year follow-up.[35] A long-term follow-up is provided in another study of 51 cases reported by Masuda and Kistner.[36] In the latter, the authors found better results in patients sustaining primary valve incompetency than secondary CVD and an overall clinical success of 60% in 10-year follow-up. The drawback is that most patients sustained primary valve insufficiency, and therefore the technique may rarely be used for patients with PTS because of possible chronic degenerative changes of the venous wall and valve system damage. In addition, the series comprises a small number of patients. A few other disadvantages of the internal technique include challenging limbs with small narrowed veins and multiple venotomies required in long diseased segments, increasing the operative time and complexity of the repair.

The external valve vein repair is another option that may expedite the operative procedure and simplify the repair (Fig. 17.8). The advantage of this technique is that multiple valves can be repaired in a single procedure. Despite the argument against blind suturing to tighten up the loose intercommissural space, the technique has shown decent results.[37,38] A large experience applying external or so-called transcommissural repair was reported in a study of 141 limbs. The ulcer-free rate when this technique was performed was 63% at 30-month follow-up.[37] Overall early complication rate was 9%, including a low, early vein thrombosis rate of 3%. In contrast with internal valve repair studies,[36,39] the durability achieved with transcommissural valve repair was found to be the same for patients with either primary or secondary CVD.[38]

The use of an external sleeve of Dacron or PTFE wrapped around the incompetent valve has also been applied to correct reflux.[40] It has also been used around axillary vein transplant procedures to prevent dilation of the valve and subsequent reflux.[41] Only a few reports exist, with the external sleeve providing short-term data. In patients with PTS, this procedure will constrict the vein because there are no functioning valves; the reflux may be reduced, but the effect of the obstruction is of concern.

The transfer or transplantation of venous segment with competent valves is a third alternative. The first autologous valved graft transplant used was the ipsilateral GSV.[42–44] The shortcomings of either in situ or transposition of a segment of GSV to the femoral vein are vein mismatch size, degenerative changes with vein incompetence secondary to vein wall dilatation, and the fact that isolated deep vein reflux with competent superficial vein is rare, limiting the use of GSV. Conversely, the axillary vein transfer (AVT) was proposed as another potential conduit to restore the directional venous outflow. The axillary vein is preferred instead of other deep veins because of the quality of the valves, good size match, and low degree of anatomic variation in that region (Fig. 17.9). Furthermore, the upper extremity blood return is mainly done by the superficial veins and therefore not being significantly impaired after axillary vein harvesting. However, a strip test is advocated to assess the axillary vein valve competency before transfer. Some authors reported up to 40% of axillary vein incompetency and advise in favor of valve repair in a bench or in situ procedure.[38] The spatial orientation of the anastomosis with precise trimming of the vein must also be accomplished to avoid reflux. Several authors have reported their experience with valved vein graft transfer.[34,39,45,46] Results are variable, ranging from 18% to up to 70% of recurrence of ulcers based upon follow-up time (1-year to 5-year follow-up) and type of the conduit.[34,39,45,46] A more recent series of AVT reported long-term patency greater than 80% and ulcer-free recurrence greater than 60% at 10-year follow-up.[38]

Another technique of transfer was described by Ferris and Kistner in 1982.[47] It consists of ligation of the femoral vein below the level of valve incompetency and redirection

Internal valve vein repair

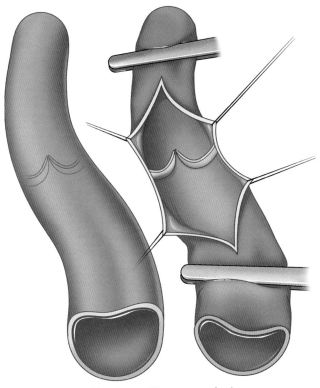

Venotomy with exposure of valve

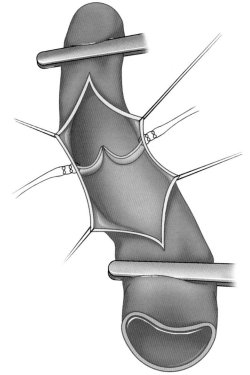

Edge repair with one interrupted suture

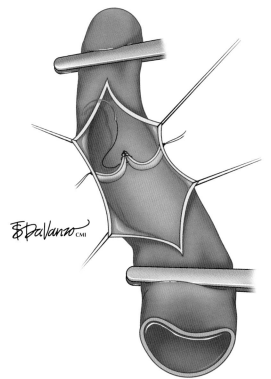

Intercommissural repair with running or interrupted sutures

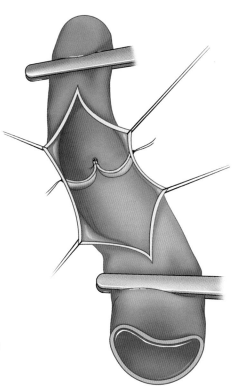

Competent valve showing good apposition of the leaflets

■ **Fig. 17.7**

External valve vein repair

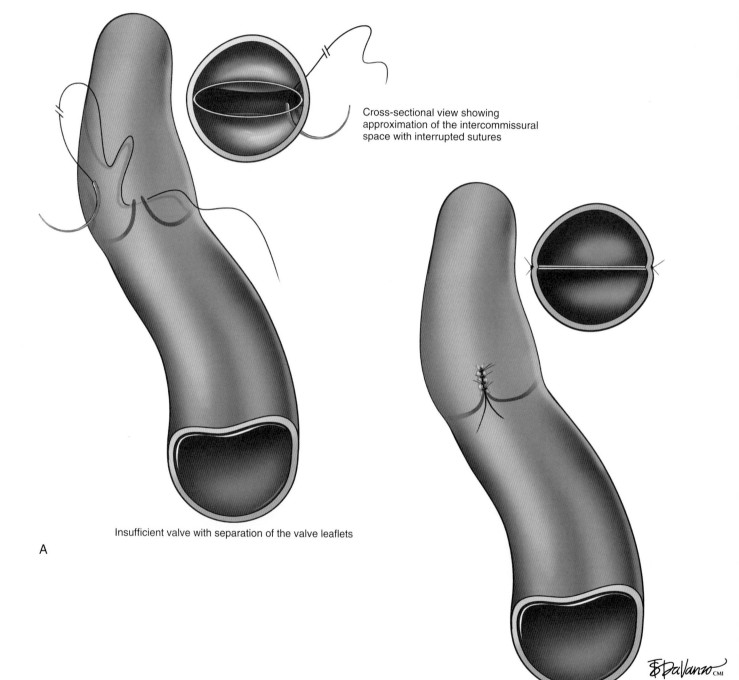

Cross-sectional view showing approximation of the intercommissural space with interrupted sutures

Insufficient valve with separation of the valve leaflets

A

Final result showing a good apposition of the valve leaflets correcting the venous reflux

B

■ **Fig. 17.8**

Axillary vein transposition

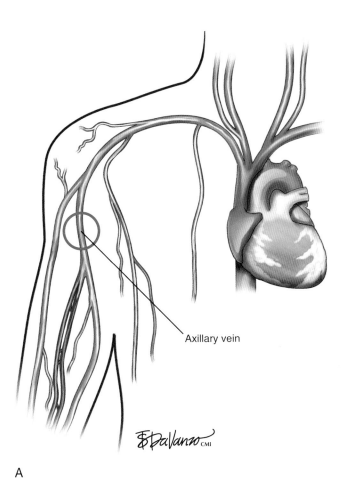

Axillary vein

A

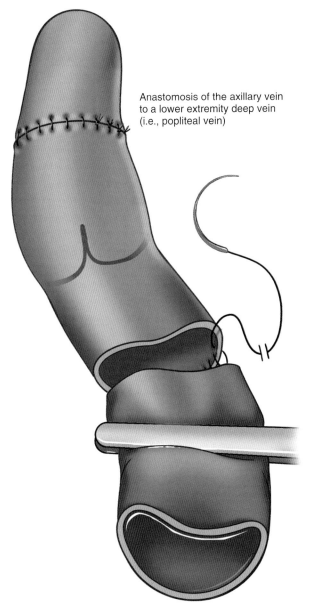

Anastomosis of the axillary vein to a lower extremity deep vein (i.e., popliteal vein)

B

■ **Fig. 17.9**

of the flow to either the femoral or profunda vein (Fig. 17.10). Contraindications of the segmental femoral vein transfer are possible dilation of the recipient vein secondary to the increased rerouted flow and, subsequently, reflux involving the femoral and the target vein.

Allied to complex surgical reconstructions or vein transfer, a temporary or long-term arteriovenous fistula (AVF) is often necessary to increase the blood flow to keep the repair patent. The drawbacks of constructing a distal AVF are the potential risk of venous dilation and valve incompetency generating venous hypertension and ultimately skin damage. In addition, anticoagulation has been advocated to improve the patency rate. Mandatory life-long anticoagulation therapy is also a concern based on risks of bleeding and its morbidity and mortality. Other disadvantages of the open procedures are low patency rates and short-term and midterm follow-up with only few long-term retrospective series, frequently with small sample size.[30]

Experimental research has been carried out including neovalve construction, cryo-preserved allograft, and prosthetic vein valve implants.[48–51] Some promising results of a multicenter phase I trial with cryopreserved allograft valves,[48] the Maleti valve,[50] and other neovalve implants[49] have been published. In preparation for neovalve reconstruction, endovenectomy of trabeculated segments is recommended. The technique consists of longitudinal incision of the vein and resection of the fibrous septa with a microsurgery scissor or ophthalmic scalpel to the level of the intima layer. Relief of the obstruction in trabeculated veins is recommended and feasible before an axillary vein segment transfer or neovalve creation.[48,49]

A neovalve creation procedure has been developed.[52] The operation encompasses endovenectomy of the venous segment and dissection of the intima layer, creating a flap that is positioned as a monocuspid or bicuspid valve with subsequent venorrhaphy in transverse fashion (Fig. 17.11). The largest experience reported is the Italian experience of 40 neovalve creations in 36 patients with recalcitrant ulcers.[49] Six valves failed in the first 19 procedures (phase I), but no failures were documented in the last 21 (phase II). No PE or major complications were reported, and overall recurrence of ulcers occurred in 8%. Mostly, the results were based on short-term and midterm follow-up (24 to 48 months for cumulative curves of competency rates).

Midterm outcomes (29-month mean follow-up) of a Russian study comprising 36 patients with both congenital avalvular deep veins ($N = 6$) or postthrombotic valve destruction, who underwent a monocuspid valve creation in the common femoral vein, showed improvement on quality of life and reduction in the severity of chronic venous disease.[53] In another case series ($N = 4$) reported by Hoshino and Hoshino from Japan, a creation of a monocuspid common femoral vein valve was responsible for ulcer healing with no recurrent symptoms at a mean follow-up of 8 months.[54]

Despite the initial good results of these series with a small number of patients from highly specialized centers based on their short to midterm outcomes, infrainguinal reconstructive deep vein reflux surgery remains incipient.

ENDOVASCULAR HORIZON

Endovenous therapy for PTS has emerged as the first option mainly for iliofemoral and IVC reconstruction because of its minimally invasive approach, lower morbidity, and promising results.[28,55] Indications and results of IVC, iliac, and femoral angioplasty and stenting are discussed in Chapter 18.

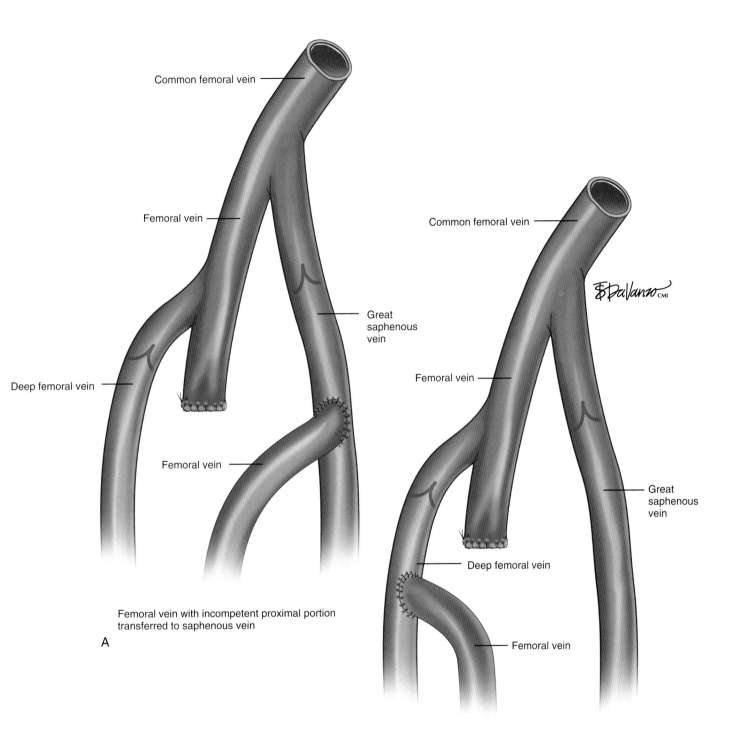

Common femoral vein

Femoral vein

Great
saphenous
vein

Deep femoral vein

Femoral vein

Femoral vein with incompetent proximal portion
transferred to saphenous vein

A

Common femoral vein

Femoral vein

Great
saphenous
vein

Deep femoral vein

Femoral vein

Femoral vein with incompetent proximal portion
transferred to deep femoral vein

B

■ Fig. 17.10

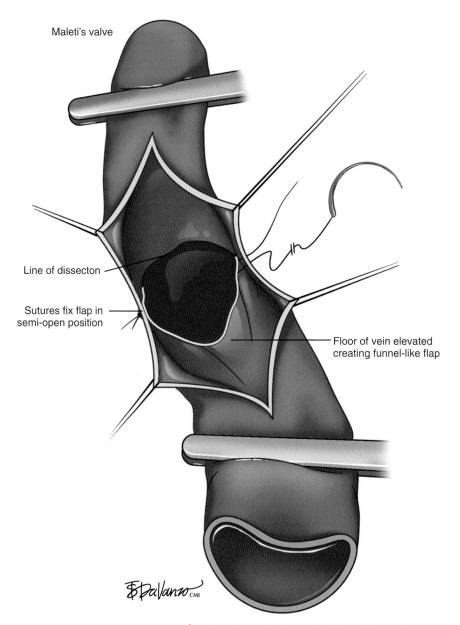

Maleti's valve

Line of dissecton

Sutures fix flap in
semi-open position

Floor of vein elevated
creating funnel-like flap

Creation of neovalve by parietal dissection and
fixing stitches to avoid readhesion

■ **Fig. 17.11** The Maleti valve.

A few experimental implantable endovascular valves have been investigated. The idea of implanting valves via the endovascular approach was first done using an external jugular vein with a competent valve mounted in a Z-stent (Cook Medical, Bloomington, IN) that was deployed in either the external ($N = 4$) or common iliac vein ($N = 1$) in dogs.[56] One of five valves implanted was patent, competent, and with minimal inflammatory surrounding reaction. Interestingly, the normal-appearing valve was deployed in the common iliac vein, which has a higher flow pattern.[56] Different valve materials, varying from glutaraldehyde-preserved bovine vein to a collagen tissue model of porcine small intestine submucosa (SIS), have been initially studied in animal models.[57,58] The former was made with thrombogenic material and leads to a higher endothelial proliferation rate and therefore carries a higher risk of early occlusion of the valve.[59] The latter, which was built with SIS, has a nonthrombogenic and nonimmunogenic surface.[58] Both prototypes are mounted on Z-stents or onto a nitinol-based stent.[57–61]

There were only two phase I trials reported, with a total of five patients in the United States. The first enrolled two patients who underwent percutaneous insertion of a glutaraldehyde-fixed bovine venous valve via right internal jugular access.[62] Both patients were anticoagulated postprocedure, but the second patient had postimplant valve thrombosis. Despite catheter direct thrombolysis, the valve was incompetent but patent. The first patient had a patent and competent valve at 12-months follow-up. Clinical improvement was achieved in both patients, although aggressive compressing therapy and other superficial vein ablation or stripping procedures were required during the follow-up.[62]

The second phase I trial comprised three patients and was performed using the SIS bioprosthetic venous valve model.[63] The patients had percutaneous implantable valves in the proximal ($N = 2$) and distal ($N = 1$) portions of the femoral vein and were anticoagulated. All three implanted SIS valves were patent but with either some degree of valve leak in the first two cases or valve tilting in the third. At 12-month follow-up, all patients but one had clinical improvement.[63] A second generation of the SIS percutaneous venous valve stents with more precise spatial configuration to prevent tilting was already tested in an animal model.[53]

Endovascular, implantable, bioprosthetic venous valves for agenesis or incompetent venous valve segments are feasible. However, further research is still warranted to improve patency and long-term valve competency.

Improvement on patients with PTS signs and symptoms has been shown after relief of chronic venous obstruction. This subject is addressed in detail in Chapter 18.

PEARLS AND PITFALLS

Compression Therapy

Compression therapy following an episode of proximal deep vein thrombosis has been advocated for decades by vascular specialists. However, the body of literature on this particular topic has not been considerably strong to make its recommendation evidence based.

Recently, a randomized controlled trial (SOX trial) was performed to gauge the PTS preventative role of compression stockings after an episode of DVT. Based on the SOX trial findings, its investigators recommended against elastic compression stockings to prevent PTS after a first proximal DVT.[24] An updated version of the last antithrombotic guidelines, published by the American College of Chest Physicians (ACCP), has also outlined that a trial of compression stockings should not be routinely prescribed to prevent chronic complication of PTS. However, this was a weak recommendation based on low-quality literature available by the time the guideline literature search was concluded in July 2014. The same ACCP updated guidelines report that a trial of graduated compression stockings, with the sole purpose of mitigating symptoms in patients with acute or chronic lower extremity deep vein thrombosis, is often justified.[64]

A recent meta-analysis of six randomized controlled trials (RCTs) including 1462 patients, which aimed to study the effect of compression stockings on PTS, concluded that the use of elastic compression stockings does not significantly reduce the development of PTS. Nonetheless, the authors did outline that the body of evidence available is still limited and that there is equipoise. From a molecular-basis standpoint, compression therapy has been shown to reduce inflammation in a study of 30 limbs with venous ulcers. Proinflammatory cytokine levels were reduced after 4 weeks of compression therapy.[65] The impact of compression therapy on inflammation remains to be elucidated and how it can modulate molecular changes after an episode of DVT in regard to prevention of PTS.

Two multicenter RCTs have been proposed to establish the role of compression stockings in PTS prevention. A Dutch trial named IDEAL (individually tailored elastic compression against long-term therapy) is designed to be a multicenter, single-blinded, allocation concealed, randomized, noninferiority trial.[66] This trial aims to enroll 864 adults with an acute, properly documented, proximal DVT of the leg, who are adequately treated with anticoagulation, with initial compression therapy started within 2 to 6 weeks. The duration of the follow-up after randomization will be 24 months. The goals of this trial are to demonstrate which patient benefits from compression therapy and to identify the optimal individual treatment duration. Another Dutch trial (DVT and postthrombotic syndrome [PTS] Bridging the Gap Study) will investigate the use of compression stockings in patients with DVT to prevent PTS in a primary-care, medical setting.[67] The study will have four arms, in which post-DVT patients will be placed, based on absence or presence of venous reflux and/or obstruction and PTS symptoms. Some arms of the study will be followed for 4 years.

Based on the aforementioned, and until strong literature to support or reject the effects of compression stockings on PTS becomes available, the use of compression stockings should still be based on a fair discussion between physician and patient.[68]

FIVE SALIENT REFERENCES

1. Comerota AJ, Oostra C, Fayad Z, et al. A histological and functional description of the tissue causing chronic postthrombotic venous obstruction. *Thromb Res.* 2015;135:882–887.
2. Kahn SR, Shrier I, Julian JA, et al. Determinants and time course of the postthrombotic syndrome after acute deep venous thrombosis. *Ann Intern Med.* 2008;18:698–707.
3. Kahn SR, Kearon C, Julian JA, et al. Predictors of the post-thrombotic syndrome during long-term treatment of proximal deep vein thrombosis. *J Thromb Haemost.* 2005;3:718–723.
4. Prandoni P, Villalta S, Polistena P, et al. Symptomatic deep-vein thrombosis and the post-thrombotic syndrome. *Haematologica.* 1995;80(suppl 2):42–48.
5. Raju S, Fredericks RK, Neglen PN, et al. Durability of venous valve reconstruction techniques for "primary" and postthrombotic reflux. *J Vasc Surg.* 1996;23:357–366, discussion 366–367.

REFERENCES

1. Heit JA, Rooke TW, Silverstein MD, et al. Trends in the incidence of venous stasis syndrome and venous ulcer: a 25-year population-based study. *J Vasc Surg.* 2001;33(5):1022–1027.
2. Ashrani AA, Heit JA. Incidence and cost burden of post-thrombotic syndrome. *J Thromb Thrombolysis.* 2009;28(4):465–476.
3. Ginsberg JS, Turkstra F, Buller HR, et al. Postthrombotic syndrome after hip or knee arthroplasty: a cross-sectional study. *Arch Intern Med.* 2000;160(5):669–672.
4. Prandoni P, Villalta S, Polistena P, et al. Symptomatic deep-vein thrombosis and the postthrombotic syndrome. *Haematologica.* 1995;80(suppl 2):42–48.
5. Widmer LK, Zemp E, Widmer MT, et al. Late results in deep vein thrombosis of the lower extremity. *VASA.* 1985;14(3):264–268.
6. Labropoulos N, Manalo D, Patel NP, et al. Uncommon leg ulcers in the lower extremity. *J Vasc Surg.* 2007;45(3):568–573.
7. Mekkes JR, Loots MA, Van Der Wal AC, et al. Causes, investigation and treatment of leg ulceration. *Br J Dermatol.* 2003;148(3):388–401.
8. Tran NT, Meissner MH. The epidemiology, pathophysiology, and natural history of chronic venous disease. *Semin Vasc Surg.* 2002;15(1):5–12.
9. Douketis JD, Foster GA, Crowther MA, et al. Clinical risk factors and timing of recurrent venous thromboembolism during the initial 3 months of anticoagulant therapy. *Arch Intern Med.* 2000;160(22):3431–3436.
10. Labropoulos N, Spentzouris G, Gasparis AP, et al. Impact and clinical significance of recurrent venous thromboembolism. *Br J Surg.* 2010;97(7):989–999.
11. Kahn SR, Shrier I, Julian JA, et al. Determinants and time course of the postthrombotic syndrome after acute deep venous thrombosis. *Ann Intern Med.* 2008;149(10):698–707.
12. Labropoulos N, Gasparis AP, Tassiopoulos AK. Prospective evaluation of the clinical deterioration in post-thrombotic limbs. *J Vasc Surg.* 2009;50(4):826–830.
13. Kahn SR, Kearon C, Julian JA, et al. Predictors of the post-thrombotic syndrome during long-term treatment of proximal deep vein thrombosis. *J Thromb Haemost.* 2005;3(4):718–723.
14. Labropoulos N, Jen J, Jen H, et al. Recurrent deep vein thrombosis: long-term incidence and natural history. *Ann Surg.* 2010;251(4):749–753.
15. Prandoni P, Lensing AW, Cogo A, et al. The long-term clinical course of acute deep venous thrombosis. *Ann Intern Med.* 1996;125(1):1–7.
16. Fink AM, Mayer W, Steiner A. Extent of thrombus evaluated in patients with recurrent and first deep vein thrombosis. *J Vasc Surg.* 2002;36(2):357–360.
17. Prandoni P, Frulla M, Sartor D, et al. Vein abnormalities and the post-thrombotic syndrome. *J Thromb Haemost.* 2005;3(2):401–402.
18. Latella J, Desmarais S, Miron MJ, et al. Relationship between D-Dimer level, venous valvular reflux, and development of the post-thrombotic syndrome after deep vein thrombosis. *J Thromb Haemost.* 2010.
19. Comerota AJ, Oostra C, Fayad Z, et al. A histological and functional description of the tissue causing chronic postthrombotic venous obstruction. *Thromb Res.* 2015;135(5):882–887.
20. Spiezia L, Campello E, Giolo E, et al. Thrombophilia and the risk of post-thrombotic syndrome: retrospective cohort observation. *J Thromb Haemost.* 2010;8(1):211–213.
21. Kearon C, Kahn SR, Agnelli G, et al. Antithrombotic therapy for venous thromboembolic disease: American College of Chest Physicians Evidence-Based Clinical Practice Guidelines (8th Edition). *Chest.* 2008;133(suppl 6):454S–545S.
22. Brandjes DP, Buller HR, Heijboer H, et al. Randomised trial of effect of compression stockings in patients with symptomatic proximal-vein thrombosis. *Lancet.* 1997;349(9054):759–762.

23. Prandoni P, Lensing AW, Prins MH, et al. Below-knee elastic compression stockings to prevent the post-thrombotic syndrome: a randomized, controlled trial. *Ann Intern Med.* 2004;141(4): 249–256.

24. Kahn SR, Shapiro S, Wells PS, et al. Compression stockings to prevent post-thrombotic syndrome: a randomised placebo-controlled trial. *Lancet.* 2014;383(9920):880–888.

25. Giannoukas AD, Labropoulos N, Michaels JA. Compression with or without early ambulation in the prevention of post-thrombotic syndrome: a systematic review. *Eur J Vasc Endovasc Surg.* 2006;32(2):217–221.

26. Kakkos SK, Daskalopoulou SS, Daskalopoulos ME, et al. Review on the value of graduated elastic compression stockings after deep vein thrombosis. *Thromb Haemost.* 2006;96(4):441–445.

27. O'Meara S, Cullum NA, Nelson EA. Compression for venous leg ulcers. *Cochrane Database Syst Rev.* 2009;(1):CD000265.

28. Meissner MH, Eklof B, Smith PC, et al. Secondary chronic venous disorders. *J Vasc Surg.* 2007;46(suppl S):68S–83S.

29. Kahn SR, Shrier I, Shapiro S, et al. Six-month exercise training program to treat post-thrombotic syndrome: a randomized controlled two-centre trial. *CMAJ.* 2010.

30. Jost CJ, Gloviczki P, Cherry KJ Jr, et al. Surgical reconstruction of iliofemoral veins and the inferior vena cava for nonmalignant occlusive disease. *J Vasc Surg.* 2001;33(2):320–327, discussion 327–328.

31. Harris JP, Kidd J, Burnett A, et al. Patency of femorofemoral venous crossover grafts assessed by duplex scanning and phlebography. *J Vasc Surg.* 1988;8(6):679–682.

32. Garg N, Gloviczki P, Karimi KM, et al. Factors affecting outcome of open and hybrid reconstructions for nonmalignant obstruction of iliofemoral veins and inferior vena cava. *J Vasc Surg.* 2011;53(2):383–393.

33. Neglen P, Raju S. Venous reflux repair with cryopreserved vein valves. *J Vasc Surg.* 2003;37(3):552–557.

34. Taheri SA, Elias SM, Yacobucci GN, et al. Indications and results of vein valve transplant. *J Cardiovasc Surg (Torino).* 1986;27(2):163–168.

35. Cheatle TR, Perrin M. Venous valve repair: early results in fifty-two cases. *J Vasc Surg.* 1994;19(3):404–413.

36. Masuda EM, Kistner RL. Long-term results of venous valve reconstruction: a four- to twenty-one-year follow-up. *J Vasc Surg.* 1994;19(3):391–403.

37. Raju S, Berry MA, Neglen P. Transcommissural valvuloplasty: technique and results. *J Vasc Surg.* 2000;32(5):969–976.

38. Raju S, Fredericks RK, Neglen PN, et al. Durability of venous valve reconstruction techniques for "primary" and postthrombotic reflux. *J Vasc Surg.* 1996;23(2):357–366, discussion 366–357.

39. Eklof BG, Kistner RL, Masuda EM. Venous bypass and valve reconstruction: long-term efficacy. *Vasc Med.* 1998;3(2):157–164.

40. Jessup G, Lane RJ. Repair of incompetent venous valves: a new technique. *J Vasc Surg.* 1988;8(5):569–575.

41. Raju S, Fredericks R. Valve reconstruction procedures for nonobstructive venous insufficiency: rationale, techniques, and results in 107 procedures with two- to eight-year follow-up. *J Vasc Surg.* 1988;7(2):301–310.

42. Cardon JM, Cardon A, Joyeux A, et al. Use of ipsilateral greater saphenous vein as a valved transplant in management of post-thrombotic deep venous insufficiency: long-term results. *Ann Vasc Surg.* 1999;13(3):284–289.

43. Eriksson I, Almgren B. Surgical reconstruction of incompetent deep vein valves. *Ups J Med Sci.* 1988;93(2):139–143.

44. Kistner RL, Ferris EB 3rd, Randhawa G, et al. The evolving management of varicose veins. Straub Clinic experience. *Postgrad Med.* 1986;80(4):51–53, 56–59.

45. Nash T. Long term results of vein valve transplants placed in the popliteal vein for intractable post-phlebitic venous ulcers and pre-ulcer skin changes. *J Cardiovasc Surg (Torino).* 1988;29(6):712–716.

46. Sottiurai VS. Surgical correction of recurrent venous ulcer. *J Cardiovasc Surg (Torino).* 1991;32(1):104–109.

47. Ferris EB, Kistner RL. Femoral vein reconstruction in the management of chronic venous insufficiency. A 14-year experience. *Arch Surg.* 1982;117(12):1571–1579.
48. Dalsing MC, Raju S, Wakefield TW, et al. A multicenter, phase I evaluation of cryopreserved venous valve allografts for the treatment of chronic deep venous insufficiency. *J Vasc Surg.* 1999;30(5):854–864.
49. Lugli M, Guerzoni S, Garofalo M, et al. Neovalve construction in deep venous incompetence. *J Vasc Surg.* 2009;49(1):156–162, 162.e151–162.e152; discussion 162.
50. Maleti O, Lugli M. Neovalve construction in postthrombotic syndrome. *J Vasc Surg.* 2006;43(4):794–799.
51. Taheri SA, Schultz RO. Experimental prosthetic vein valve. Long-term results. *Angiology.* 1995;46(4):299–303.
52. Maleti O. Venous valvular reconstruction in post-thrombotic syndrome. A new technique. *J Mal Vasc.* 2002;27(4):218–221.
53. Ignatyev IM, Akhmetzyanov RV. Long-term results of the monocusp valve formation in the common femoral vein in patients presenting with avalvular deep veins of the lower extremities. *Int Angiol.* 2016.
54. Hoshino Y, Hoshino S. The Short-term Outcomes of Neovalve Deep Venous Reconstructive Surgery. *J Vasc Surg Venous Lymphat Disord.* 2015;3(1):129.
55. Raju S, Neglen P. Percutaneous recanalization of total occlusions of the iliac vein. *J Vasc Surg.* 2009;50(2):360–368.
56. Dalsing MC, Sawchuk AP, Lalka SG, et al. An early experience with endovascular venous valve transplantation. *J Vasc Surg.* 1996;24(5):903–905.
57. Gomez-Jorge J, Venbrux AC, Magee C. Percutaneous deployment of a valved bovine jugular vein in the swine venous system: a potential treatment for venous insufficiency. *J Vasc Interv Radiol.* 2000;11(7):931–936.
58. Pavcnik D, Kaufman J, Uchida B, et al. Second-generation percutaneous bioprosthetic valve: a short-term study in sheep. *J Vasc Surg.* 2004;40(6):1223–1227.
59. de Borst GJ, Teijink JA, Patterson M, et al. A percutaneous approach to deep venous valve insufficiency with a new self-expanding venous frame valve. *J Endovasc Ther.* 2003;10(2):341–349.
60. Pavcnik D, Uchida B, Timmermans H, et al. Square stent: a new self-expandable endoluminal device and its applications. *Cardiovasc Intervent Radiol.* 2001;24(4):207–217.
61. Pavcnik D, Uchida BT, Timmermans HA, et al. Percutaneous bioprosthetic venous valve: a long-term study in sheep. *J Vasc Surg.* 2002;35(3):598–602.
62. Gale SS, Shuman S, Beebe HG, et al. Percutaneous venous valve bioprosthesis: initial observations. *Vasc Endovascular Surg.* 2004;38(3):221–224.
63. Pavcnik D, Machan L, Uchida B, et al. Percutaneous prosthetic venous valves: current state and possible applications. *Tech Vasc Interv Radiol.* 2003;6(3):137–142.
64. Kearon C, Akl EA, Ornelas J, et al. Antithrombotic Therapy for VTE Disease: CHEST Guideline and Expert Panel Report. *Chest.* 2016;149(2):315–352.
65. Beidler SK, Douillet CD, Berndt DF, et al. Inflammatory cytokine levels in chronic venous insufficiency ulcer tissue before and after compression therapy. *J Vasc Surg.* 2009;49(4):1013–1020.
66. Ten Cate-Hoek AJ, Bouman AC, Joore MA, et al. The IDEAL DVT study, individualised duration elastic compression therapy against long-term duration of therapy for the prevention of post-thrombotic syndrome: protocol of a randomised controlled trial. *BMJ Open.* 2014;4(9):e005265.
67. Michiels JJ, Michiels JM, Moossdorff W, et al. Diagnosis of deep vein thrombosis, and prevention of deep vein thrombosis recurrence and the post-thrombotic syndrome in the primary care medicine setting anno 2014. *World J Crit Care Med.* 2015;4(1):29–39.
68. Subbiah R, Aggarwal V, Zhao H, et al. Effect of compression stockings on post thrombotic syndrome in patients with deep vein thrombosis: a meta-analysis of randomised controlled trials. *Lancet Haematol.* 2016;3(6):e293–e300.

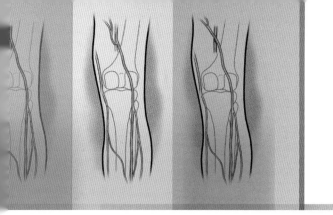

CHAPTER 18

Iliocaval and Femoral Venous Occlusive Disease

Priscila Gisselle Sanchez Aguirre, Andrew M. Abi-Chaker, and Jose I. Almeida

HISTORICAL BACKGROUND

In contrast with the right common iliac vein, which ascends almost vertically to the inferior vena cava (IVC), the left common iliac vein takes a more transverse course beneath the right common iliac artery, which may compress it against the lumbar spine before entering the vena cava. This compression causes stasis of the blood, which is one element of Virchow's triad that may precipitate deep venous thrombosis (DVT).

In approximately 40% of patients, the precursor to iliac vein obstruction is not thrombosis, but rather, a nonthrombotic iliac vein lesion (NIVL). Also known as May-Thurner syndrome[1] or iliac vein compression syndrome,[2] it is caused by web formation[3] and obstruction. A nonthrombotic blockage is defined as an absent clinical history of DVT coupled with absent findings on imaging studies, such as contrast venography and ultrasound. This lesion is classically found in the left common iliac vein of younger females; but, it is not uncommon in males or in elderly patients, and may involve the right limb. At least 15% of the limbs with primary disease have been shown to have stenosis of both common and external iliac veins.[4]

As depicted in Fig. 18.1, the right common iliac artery always crosses the left common iliac vein at the confluence of the IVC and is where classic proximal left NIVL occurs. In 75% (majority pattern), the right iliac artery continues its course to cross near the external iliac vein level, in which case, it may induce right distal NIVL. In the minority pattern (22%), the right, common iliac artery crosses the right, common iliac vein, and then down over a longer length of the external iliac vein and can thus induce either a proximal or distal right NIVL. The left distal lesion may be related to the crossing of the vein by the left hypogastric artery. These anatomic variations may explain why proximal NIVLs occur much more frequently on the left side than on the right side, why the left

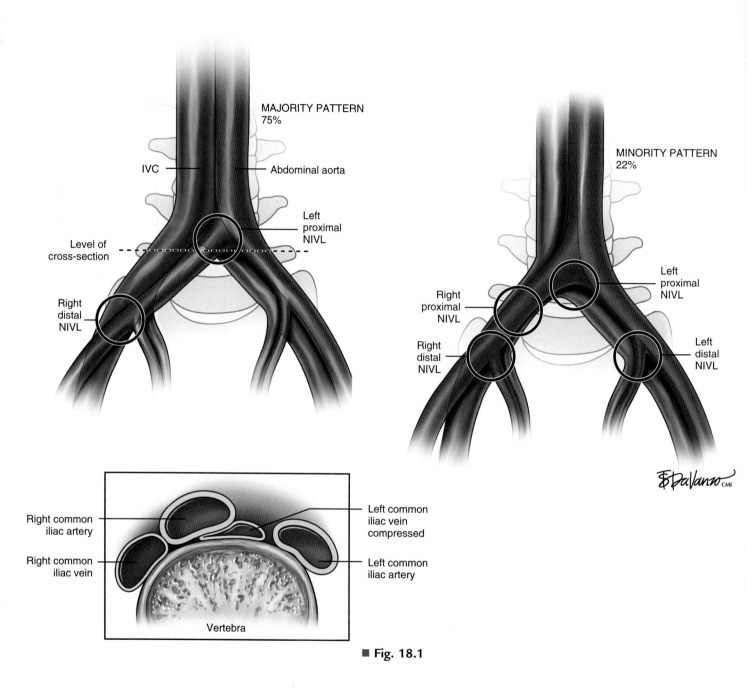

MAJORITY PATTERN
75%

IVC — Abdominal aorta

Left proximal NIVL

Level of cross-section

Right distal NIVL

MINORITY PATTERN
22%

Left proximal NIVL

Right proximal NIVL

Right distal NIVL

Left distal NIVL

Right common iliac artery

Right common iliac vein

Left common iliac vein compressed

Left common iliac artery

Vertebra

■ **Fig. 18.1**

lesion is focal and the right less so, and why the distal NIVL occurs equally on either side.[5]

Although traditional venous corrective surgery concentrated on the correction of superficial and deep venous reflux below the inguinal ligament, the introduction of minimally invasive venous stenting using venography and intravascular ultrasonography (IVUS) provides the ability to treat the "obstructive" component of the disease above the inguinal ligament. The emphasis on IVUS as the key diagnostic tool was promulgated by Raju and Neglén who have shown that iliac venous stenting alone is sufficient to control symptoms in most patients with combined outflow obstruction and deep reflux.[6]

ETIOLOGY AND NATURAL HISTORY OF DISEASE

The iliac vein is the common outflow tract of the lower extremity, and chronic obstruction of this segment can result in severe symptoms. The most frequent precursor to chronic pelvic venous outflow obstruction is iliofemoral DVT. Only 20% to 30% of iliac veins completely recanalize spontaneously after thrombosis, whereas the remaining veins recanalize partially and develop varying degrees of collaterals. This may result in significant residual obstruction to the venous outflow of the lower extremity. In the iliofemoral segment, collateral vein formation is relatively poor, and thus results in more severe symptoms than lower segmental blockage. Distal obstructions are more readily compensated for because of robust femoral-popliteal collaterals, profunda-popliteal vein connections, deep muscular tributaries in the thigh, and saphenosaphenous venous connections.[7]

Kibbe et al.[8] performed a retrospective analysis of medical records and helical abdominal computed tomography scans conducted on 50 consecutive patients evaluated in the emergency department because of abdominal pain. It was surprising that 24% ($N = 12$) of patients had greater than 50% compression and 66% ($N = 33$) had greater than 25% compression. Mean compression of the left common iliac vein was 35.5% (range, 5.6%–74.8%). The structure most often compressing the left common iliac vein against the vertebral body was the right common iliac artery (84%).

The high prevalence and pathologic role of NIVLs in symptomatic chronic venous disease (CVD) patients must be balanced with the frequent prevalence of NIVLs in the asymptomatic general population. These apparent contradictions can be resolved if the NIVL is viewed as a permissive condition predisposing to the development of CVD. Permissive conditions are pathologies that may remain silent until additional insult or pathology is superimposed. Symptom expression in many NIVL obstructions remain asymptomatic, because it probably is a slowly progressive condition. Additional insult or pathology such as trauma, cellulitis, distal thrombosis, secondary lymphatic exhaustion, or reflux, may render the extremity symptomatic.[9] The general principle in these complex pathologies is to treat the permissive condition first, which alone may provide relief, and to prevent recurrence. Correction of secondary pathology may be required only in recalcitrant and advanced cases.

In Raju's series,[9] 75% of limbs with NIVLs and concurrent reflux experienced a good or excellent outcome with stent placement alone, even when the reflux component, severe in many, was uncorrected. These results support the concept that the NIVL plays a permissive role in the genesis of CVD symptoms. NIVLs are ubiquitous in CVD with severe symptoms, and use of IVUS and stent correction when detected is recommended. Even patients with significant distal reflux benefit, thus avoiding or postponing open, reflux-corrective procedures, which are not precluded if the stents were to fail later. An alternative explanation for the observations presented here is to consider NIVLs and distal reflux as a continuum in progressive hemodynamic deterioration of the venous system; symptomatic decompensation occurs when the hemodynamics cross a certain critical threshold. However, no connection between NIVLs and distal reflux has yet been established. It should be emphasized that the hemodynamics of obstructive and reflux pathologies are poorly understood, and their measurement even less so.

Of particular interest is the subset with NIVLs with reflux that became symptom free with stent correction of the NIVL alone, even when the reflux component remained uncorrected. Notably, 67% of stasis ulcers in this subset also healed and remained healed at 2.5 years. CVD symptoms, including stasis ulcers, are not caused by reflux alone; the

NIVL plays a role in ways yet to be understood. Ulcers also occur in NIVLs without reflux, although the incidence is higher with reflux.[6]

When symptoms recur after initial remission following stent placement, often stent malfunction is found. Distal migration of the stent with recurrence of the lesion at the iliocaval junction, missed or incomplete treatment of the distal lesion, or, less commonly, in-stent restenoses were found in Raju's series.[9] When corrected, the patient is usually returned to the status of symptom remission.

PATIENT SELECTION

When planning an invasive procedure on a patient, a surgeon preferably enters the operating room with an imaging study demonstrating a pathologic lesion. In the case of iliac vein occlusive disease, this is often not possible. The group out of Mississippi has one of the largest experiences in the world with iliac vein occlusive disease, and they have emphasized the value of intraoperative IVUS for diagnosis and treatment. Their vascular laboratory runs a battery of preoperative noninvasive tests on patients with signs and symptoms of venous disease, and their data demonstrate the insensitivity of these examinations to identify lesions (Table 18.1). Magnetic resonance venography is very operator dependent, and its routine use has not elevated this technique as the

TABLE 18.1 Demographics, Intravascular Ultrasound Findings and Preinterventional Hemodynamics in Stented Limbs With Nonthrombotic Iliac Vein Lesions With and Without Venous Reflux[9]

Parameter	NIVLs With Reflux (N = 151)	NIVLs Without Reflux (N = 181)
Age, years	56 (20–85)	51 (18–90)[a]
Female-male ratio	110:36 (3.1:1)	146:31 (4.7:1)[b]
Left-right limb ratio	105:46 (2.3:1)	136/45 (3:1)[b]
IVUS degree of stenosis (%)	70 (0–95)	70 (0–100)[b]
Stenotic area (cm²)	0.66 (0.15–2.00)	0.53 (0.02–1.65)[a]
Ambulatory venous pressure		
% drop	77 (0–97)	77 (0–99)[b]
venous filling time (s)	23 (2–132)	44 (0–165)[c]
APG:VFI$_{90}$ (mL/s)	2 (0–12.3)	0.9 (0.0–6.0)[c]
Hand-foot pressure differential (mm Hg)	1 (0–8)	1 (0–10)[b]
Dorsal foot hyperemia pressure differential (mm Hg)	6 (0–26)	5 (0–23)[b]

[a]$P = .01$
[b]Not significant.
[c]$P < .001$.
APG, Air plethysmograph; *IVUS,* intravascular ultrasound; *NIVL,* nonthrombotic iliac vein lesions.
Data are presented as ratios or median (range).
(Reprinted with permission from Raju R, Neglén P. High prevalence of nonthrombotic iliac vein lesions in chronic venous disease: a permissive role in pathogenicity. *J Vasc Surg.* 2006;44:136–144.)

gold standard for diagnosis. Perhaps the most interesting phenomenon is the insensitivity of intravenous contrast venography. Although anterior-posterior and oblique views may suggest some "pancaking" of the proximal iliac vein (Fig. 18.2), oftentimes, the common iliac vein appears normal. The poor diagnostic sensitivity of venography was well documented by Negus et al.[3] Of practical importance is that up to half of the cases can be missed if frontal projection venograms alone are relied on for diagnosis.

IVUS has become the diagnostic imaging modality of choice. This coaxial technique allows the operator to examine the target lesion as sound waves are emitted from the catheter tip transducer, usually in the 10-MHz to 20-MHz range. A real-time ultrasound image of a thin section of the blood vessel is generated without radiation or nephrotoxic contrast. IVUS has also been used for placement of IVC filters; it is a more accurate method than contrast venography of localizing the renal veins and measuring vena cava diameter.

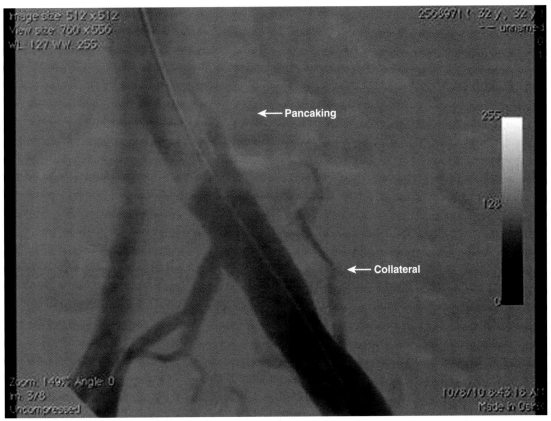

■ **Fig. 18.2** Left iliocaval contrast venography with oblique views. "Pancaking" seen at iliocaval confluence.

OPERATIVE STEPS

The patient is taken to the endovascular suite and prepped and draped in the usual manner (Fig. 18.3A). The preferred access site is the femoral vein at the upper third of the thigh with the thigh slightly externally rotated and the knee slightly bent. The femoral vein lies inferior to the superficial femoral artery and slightly lateral in most cases. If access is planned via a popliteal approach, then the prone position is preferable, but for the jugular of femoral vein access, the supine position is ideal.

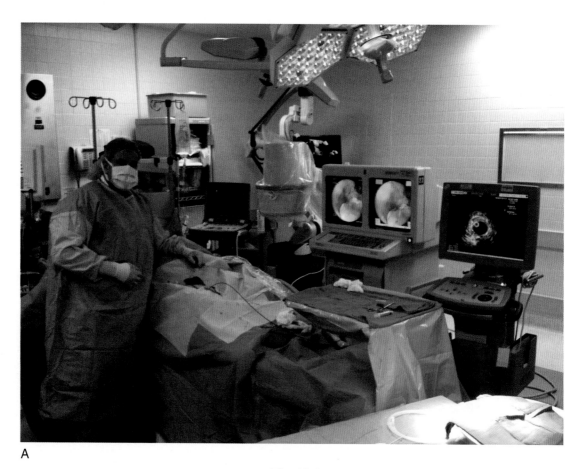

A

■ **Fig. 18.3**

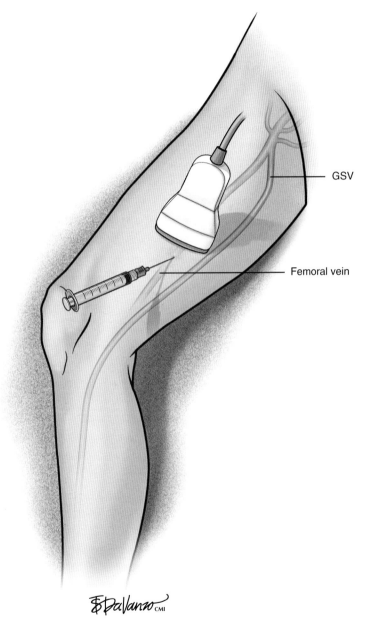

GSV

Femoral vein

B

■ Fig. 18.3, cont'd

Continued

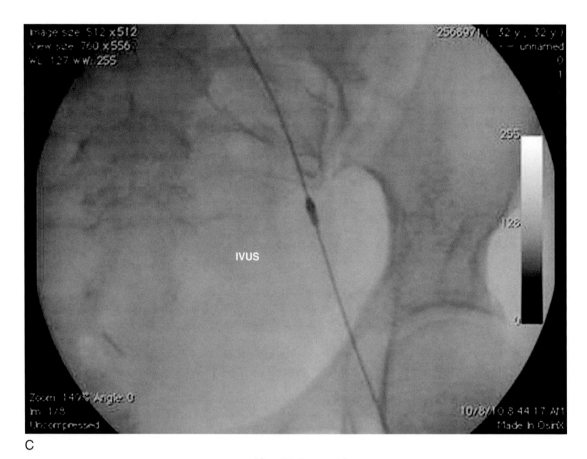

C

■ **Fig. 18.3, cont'd**

Using ultrasound, a 21-gauge needle is inserted into the femoral vein and an 0.018-inch (0.045-cm) wire placed with Seldinger technique (see Fig. 18.3B). The 4-Fr microintroducer sheath is placed and used to exchange for a 0.035-inch (0.088-cm) guidewire. Using fluoroscopy, the 0.035-inch (0.088-cm) wire is navigated into the IVC. If the 0.035-inch (0.088-cm) wire meets resistance and has difficulty entering the IVC, an intravenous contrast injection is performed to generate an anatomic roadmap. Most obstructive lesions can be crossed with a 0.035-inch (0.088-cm) glide wire.

To perform contrast venography, a larger sheath (8 Fr, 11 cm in length) is ideal. The power injector is prepared, and a digital subtraction contrast run is prepared by connecting high-pressure tubing from the injector to the side arm of the sheath. Eight mL per second for a total of 20 mL of nonionic intravenous contrast is injected. The resulting image is examined for areas of stenosis, obstruction, and/or the presence of collaterals.

NONTHROMBOTIC ILIAC VEIN LESIONS

The most common lesion encountered for these cases is a stenosis at the confluence of the left common iliac vein with the IVC. Usually a standard 0.035-inch (0.088-cm) J-tipped guidewire will cross the lesion easily. In cases where the wire does not cross, a 0.035-inch (0.088-cm), hydrophilic, angled-glide wire is selected. Hydrophilic glide wires are slippery by design; thus they are not ideal as working wires for tracking balloons, IVUS catheters, and stents. Therefore the lesion is crossed; a 5-Fr guide catheter is used to exchange the glide wire for a 0.035-inch (0.088-cm) Amplatz super-stiff wire. The super-stiff wire is parked into the subclavian or jugular vein. This maneuver is in anticipation of stent placement and will be explained later.

The IVUS catheter is brought into the field and mounted onto the 0.035-inch (0.088-cm) super-stiff guidewire (see Fig. 18.3C). IVUS imaging of the entire iliofemoral and caval outflow tract is performed. Particular attention is paid to the caliber of the veins as demonstrated by IVUS. The classic May-Thurner lesion is located at the left, common iliac vein–IVC junction. This is the location where the right, common iliac artery can be visualized as it crosses the left common iliac vein (Fig. 18.4A–D). As mentioned earlier, distal NIVLs can be seen where the hypogastric artery crosses the external iliac vein, on either the right or left sides (see Fig. 18.4E and F). Using the IVUS computerized, planimetry software, the percent area reduction of the stenosis can be calculated by comparing with a normal, adjacent, reference vessel (see Fig. 18.4G); however, this is not our current practice.

Optimum caliber values described by Raju for the entire iliac-femoral segments are shown in Chapter 2, Table 2.2. In current practice, the optimal caliber should be used as a reference in calculating common iliac vein stenosis. There are no validated criteria to determine what percent area reduction constitutes a hemodynamically significant lesion; however, as a rule of thumb, a 50% area reduction is the treatment threshold (see Table 18.2).

Once the decision to treat is made, a larger sheath, usually 11 Fr, must be placed to accommodate the larger stent delivery systems. In addition, stent delivery systems track easier over 0.035-inch (0.088-cm) stiff wires; therefore, if needed, an exchange must be performed if a stiff wire is not in place. It is critical not to lose access once a lesion has been crossed with a wire and an intermediate step is useful. A 5-Fr guide catheter will track over a glide wire into the IVC and through the heart into the innominate venous system; it can then be subsequently used for 0.035-inch (0.088-cm) stiff-wire placement. After the 0.035-inch (0.088-cm) stiff wire of exchange length is parked in the subclavian or jugular vein, the 5-Fr guide catheter is removed, and a balloon is brought into the field. Iliac veins are quite compliant and fairly resistant to rupture. A 16- to 20-mm-diameter Atlas balloon is usually chosen to dilate the lesion (Fig. 18.5). The balloon is dilated to profile until the waist is obliterated. Sequential dilatations with larger balloons may be required to completely dilate the lesion. Because venous lesions almost always recoil after dilatation, stent deployment is required. Stent diameters of 16 to 20 mm are preferred because oversized stents are necessary. The most common stents used for iliac vein work are self-expanding, braided, Elgiloy Wallstents (Boston Scientific, Nantucket, Mass) (Fig. 18.6–18.9). Gianturco Z-stents (Boston Scientific, Nantucket, Mass) are also used when projecting into the vena cava.[10]

Text continued on p. 446

TABLE 18.2 Optimal Caliber of the Iliac-Femoral Vein Segments

Vessel Segment	Diameter	Area
CIV	16 mm	200 mm^2
EIV	14 mm	150 mm^2
CFV	12 mm	110 mm^2

CIV, Common iliac vein; *CVF,* common femoral vein; *EIV,* external iliac vein.
(From Raju S, Buck WJ, Crim W, et al. Optimal sizing of iliac vein stents. *Phlebology.* 2017:268355517718763. [Epub ahead of print])[23]

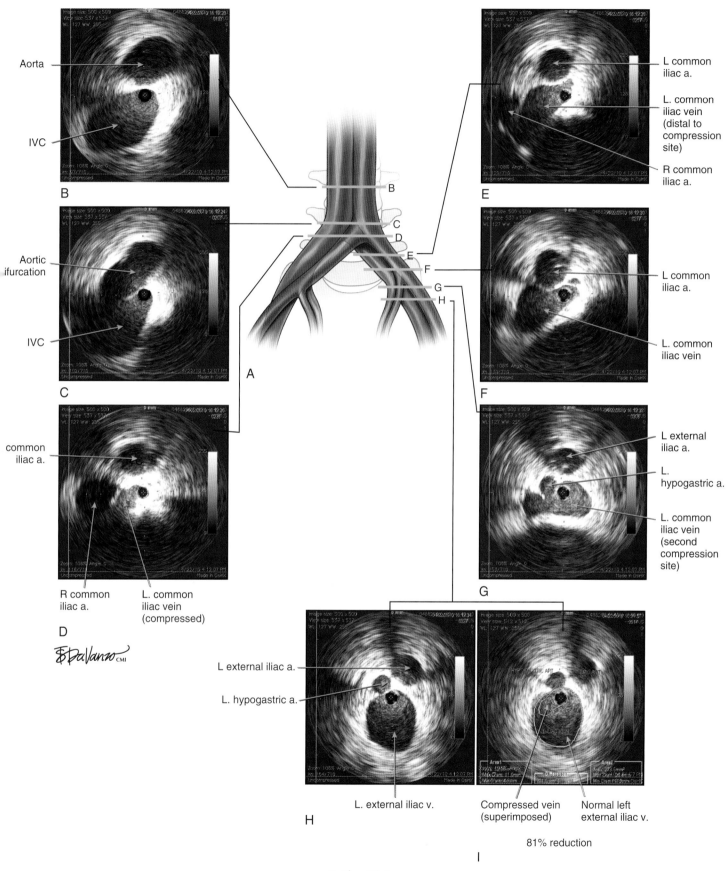

Aorta

IVC

B

Aortic bifurcation

IVC

C

common iliac a.

R common iliac a.   L. common iliac vein (compressed)

D

L common iliac a.

L. common iliac vein (distal to compression site)

R common iliac a.

E

L common iliac a.

L. common iliac vein

F

L external iliac a.

L. hypogastric a.

L. common iliac vein (second compression site)

G

L external iliac a.

L. hypogastric a.

L. external iliac v.

H

Compressed vein (superimposed)   Normal left external iliac v.

81% reduction

I

■ Fig. 18.4

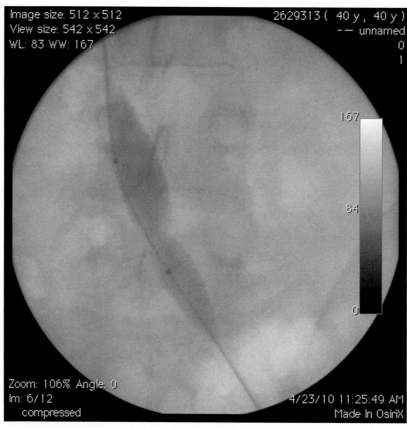

■ **Fig. 18.5**

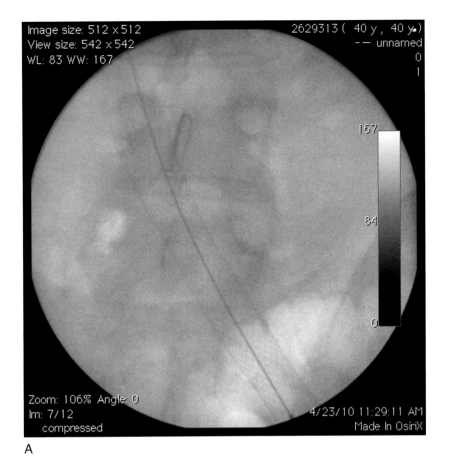

A

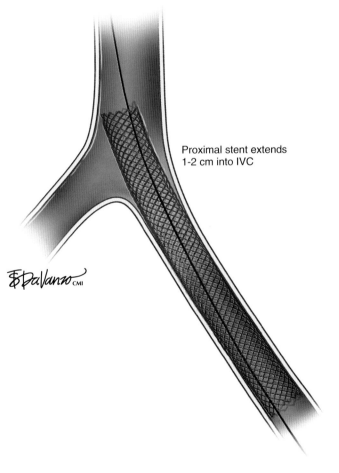

Proximal stent extends
1-2 cm into IVC

■ **Fig. 18.6** (B) After deployment of
proximal 18-mm × 9-cm Wallstent. Proximal
stent extends 1 to 2 cm into inferior vena
cava.

B

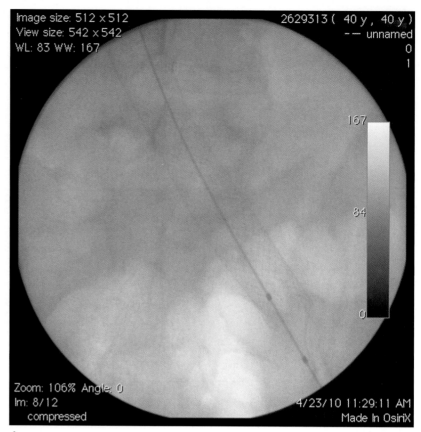

A

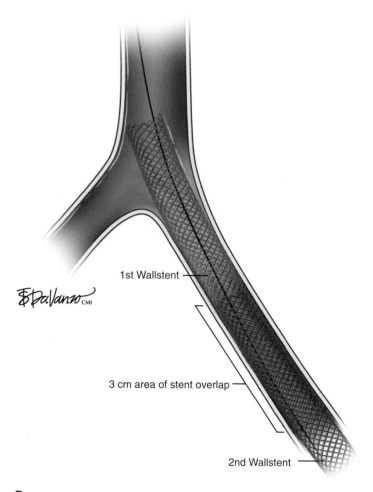

■ **Fig. 18.7** (B) After deployment of
second Wallstent (18 mm × 9 cm).
Distal aspect of stent extends below
inguinal ligament. There is a 3-cm area
of stent overlap.

1st Wallstent

3 cm area of stent overlap

2nd Wallstent

B

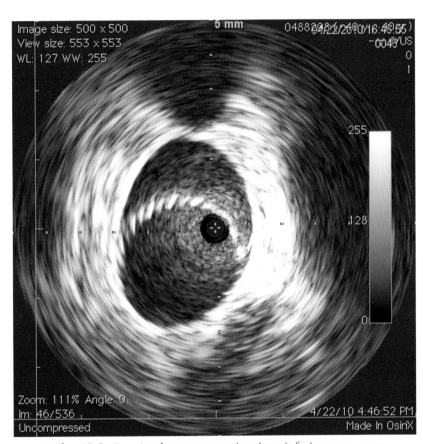

■ **Fig. 18.8** Proximal stent extension into inferior vena cava.

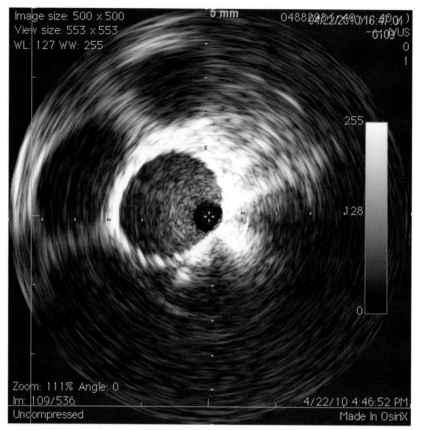

■ **Fig. 18.9** Deployed stent with complete apposition to left common iliac vein wall. Complete obliteration of the stenosis at right common iliac artery compression site.

Intravascular Ultrasonography Findings

Raju et al.[9] reported that the proximal NIVL was three times more frequently observed on the left side, whereas the distal NIVL was equally distributed bilaterally. The proximal NIVL was typically very focal on the left side and was located at the iliocaval junction; the right proximal NIVL was less focal and was located 1 to 2 cm distal to the iliocaval junction. The median area of the more severe stenosis (proximal or distal), as measured by IVUS, was 0.58 cm^2 (normal, 1.5 cm^2) representing approximately 70% stenosis. Most NIVLs were "soft" compared with postthrombotic syndrome (PTS) or arterial lesions, with waisting of the balloon often relieved at less than 2 atm.

Stent Deployment

The most dreaded complication is losing a stent and finding it in the heart. The phenomenon results when stents "jump" during deployment. Stents are packaged tightly in delivery sheaths where their potential energy is stored. During deployment, the potential energy converts to kinetic energy as it expands and finds its resting place. The stent will then apply its outward radial force to the vessel wall and maintain an open vessel.

If the stent has the opportunity to find an open area to quickly release its energy, it will. Iliocaval stent deployment for NIVL routinely deploys across a tight iliocaval stenosis into the IVC. The IVC represents a large space where a stent may quickly, and uncontrollably, convert its potential energy into kinetic energy. Thus the stent could jump into the IVC and float into the right ventricle if the operator is not careful.

Aside from careful deployment and stent oversizing, an important maneuver is parking the distal guidewire into the innominate, subclavian, or jugular vein before stent deployment. This technique will keep the stent "on a rail," or not allow migration into the right atrium, the tricuspid valve, or worse, into the right ventricle. Stent retrieval with a snare, or capturing it with a balloon, and redeploying it in another vessel is much easier when the stent is on a wire.

Scientific Evidence Nonthrombotic Iliac Vein Lesion Treatment

In four studies, with a total of 1000 lower extremities, NIVL was specifically assessed.[11–14] Technical success was achieved in 96% to 100% of cases, with a follow-up of 59 months (6–72 months). Primary patency (where the vein is open without any additional intervention) was 85% (79%–99%), and assisted primary (where the vein is patent, but an additional intervention is needed to keep it so) and secondary patencies (where the vein is patent after one or more additional interventions were required to treat an occlusion of the vein) were 100%. Rates of ulcer healing ranged from 82% to 85%,[17,19] with 5% to 8% recurrence.[17,18] There was statistically significant improvement at all points of the Chronic Venous Insufficiency Questionnaire (CIVIQ)[18] and in the Visual Analogue Scale and Quality of Life scores.[18,19] Edema decreased in 32% to 89% of cases,[17,18] and hyperpigmentation improved in 87%.[17]

POSTTHROMBOTIC ILIOCAVAL AND FEMORAL VENOUS OCCLUSIVE DISEASE

Because of the considerable incidence of iliocaval thrombosis in patients with known DVT, clinical examination should include evaluating pelvic and abdominal components to ensure that more proximal vessels are not involved and contributing to the lower extremity complaints. Duplex ultrasound (US) allows for good visualization of lower extremity veins; however, for iliocaval disease, computed tomographic venography or magnetic resonance venography may help define the landscape and aid planning venography, IVUS, with or without intervention. For patients with iliocaval disease, the goal of therapy is to improve symptoms; curing the disease is not realistic. In these patients, always remember to document clinical severity with an appropriate index such as the revised Venous Clinical Severity Score (VCSS), Villalta score, and Comprehensive Classification System for Chronic Venous Disorders (CEAP) scores.

It has been shown that in two-thirds of patients with postthrombotic disease, it is necessary to implant stents down to the groin below the inguinal ligament to improve inflow into the reconstructed iliac veins. In a report by Raju,[15] the common femoral vein was stented to the lower landing zone in 22 cases (56%). When the common femoral vein was occluded or stenosed, inflow from the profunda femoris vein was enough to maintain stent patency. When both the profunda and femoral veins have obstructive lesions, stents can be extended into them, but in this situation, there is a high risk of stent thrombosis because of poor inflow. If the popliteal vein is occluded, it may require tibial vein access to recanalize the popliteal and femoral veins to obtain inline flow.

Interventions distal to the groin, including endovenectomy or stenting further down into the femoral vein or profunda femoral vein, are also under investigation in select cases.

Once operative planning has begun, it is important to properly choose an access site. If the femoral vein is patent, it can be used for access to larger vessels. If the femoral vein is occluded, then venous drainage from the popliteal and profunda femoris veins should be evaluated. If the popliteal and profunda femoris veins are patent, the most proximal segment of an occluded femoral vein may often still be accessed. On occasion, it may be necessary to access the proximal profunda femoris vein, which may be challenging because of its depth.

Patients presenting with iliac vein occlusive disease secondary to thrombosis are much more difficult to deal with technically, and stent patency is inferior to that of NIVL cases. Recanalization techniques are required (Fig. 18.10). General endotracheal anesthesia is preferred for management of the airway in pain. A Foley catheter is placed for urinary drainage because these procedures can become lengthy.

Femoral vein access under US guidance is preferred at the midthigh level. The femoral vein is found posterolateral to the artery at midthigh. Midthigh access facilitates shorter-length instrumentation with superior pushability compared with popliteal or internal jugular access sites. We prefer an 11-Fr sheath of 11-cm length to allow space cephalad to the sheath and below the inguinal ligament to land a stent into the common femoral vein when necessary. The profunda femoris vein is usually open if the femoral vein is occluded and can be accessed 2 to 3 cm below the lesser trochanter; stent extension into the profunda femoris vein is performed without impeding inflow from an occluded femoral vein. If the femoral vein is occluded, access is often possible through the upper 3 to 5 cm of the vein, which tends to remain open.

To cross a chronic total occlusion (CTO), an antegrade venogram is performed via the sidearm of the sheath to define venous anatomy at the groin and pelvis. A 0.035-inch

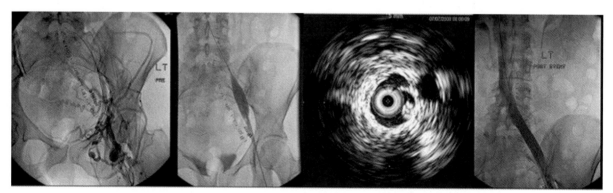

■ **Fig. 18.10** Recanalization of an occluded iliac vein. *Left panel,* initial venogram. *Second panel,* aggressive dilatation of the occluded vein and deployment of a slightly oversized stent is required to achieve a recanalized lumen approximating normal anatomy. This poses no bleeding risk. *Third panel,* intravascular ultrasound examination of the recanalized channel after maximal balloon dilatation invariably shows the glide wire in the middle of the venous channel with intact thick walls. *Right panel,* completion venogram shows a stented channel of adequate lumen without residual stenoses, good flow, and absence of previously visualized collaterals.[15]

(0.088-cm) soft-glide or stiff-glide wire (Terumo Inc, Ann Arbor, Mich) is navigated up to the occlusion. Further progress into the occlusion is made with vigorous rotation of the glide-wire tip with a torque device; the enhanced kinetic energy at the wire tip facilitates wire passage into microchannels present in the organizing fibrous tissue within the vein. Usually a straight or angled support catheter (Quick-Cross support catheter; Spectranetics, Colorado Springs, CO, or CXI support catheter; Cook, Bloomington, IN) is required to facilitate progress. If added support is required, we prefer the Triforce system (Cook Medical, Bloomington, IN). This 5-Fr braided sheath with tungsten tip adds columnar strength to the inner 4-Fr CXI support catheter and a nice transition between the two devices placed coaxially.

Glide wire passage must be guided by knowledge of topographic course of the vein. In the frontal projection, the left femoral vein overlies the medial third of the femoral head, coursing up to the lower pelvic brim across the sacroiliac joint joining the IVC variably between the fourth and fifth lumbar vertebral bodies. The right femoral and iliac veins course in a straighter line (frontal projection) to their junction with the IVC. It is useful to view progress of the recanalization intermittently by rotating the C-arm gantry into 45-degrees or 60-degrees oblique projections to ensure that the glide wire initially follows the curve of the sacrum and then turns anteriorly towards the promontorium and anterior to the spine. It is critical to recognize that the glide wire may enter collaterals and tributaries. Interval contrast injections (puff angiograms) will help aid progress into the correct anatomy. An angled-tip catheter is useful in redirecting the glide wire in the proper direction when it seems to veer off course.

Passage of the glide wire away from the expected course of the vein with sudden ease denotes perforation. The glide wire can be withdrawn and usually manipulated in the proper direction without sequelae. Withdrawal of blood through the catheter may or may not be possible during the recanalization process and has no particular significance as long as the glide wire tracks approximate to normal anatomy. Entry into the IVC should be confirmed by fluoroscopy, contrast injection through a catheter placed in the IVC, and IVUS.

From this stage of the recanalization procedure, the use of IVUS becomes crucial to assure integrity of the recanalized channel, to select optimal proximal and distal landing sites preferably free of postthrombotic disease, to ensure proper deployment and expansion of the stents, and to minimize radiation exposure.[15] The recanalized channel may be dilated, starting with smaller-sized (3-mm) balloons to allow passage of an 8-Fr IVUS catheter and large-caliber balloons. It is useful to use high-pressure balloons (16–18 atm) expanded at maximum level for at least a minute until the balloon pressure stabilizes at this level. Overdilatation and oversizing of the stent diameter by 2 to 4 mm for the anatomic location is recommended to compensate for the variable recoil of the recanalized channel. Optimal stent diameters after recoil are 18 mm for the common iliac vein, 16 mm for the external iliac vein, and 14 mm for the common femoral vein in normally sized adults. Self-expanding woven braided Elgiloy stents (Wallstent, Boston Scientific, Nantucket, Mass) in series with 3-cm to 4-cm overlap to minimize shelving along the complex course of the iliac vein are used. Because multiple stents are typically required, the maximum manufactured length for the various diameter sizes (typically 7-cm to 9-cm length) should be used, restricting shorter lengths for use at either end of the stack to tailor length. A completion IVUS examination and venogram terminate the procedure after noted defects are corrected by repeat ballooning. Patients are discharged home the same day.

Bilateral Stenting and Advanced Techniques

Patients may require stenting of both limbs. Several techniques have been described by Neglén,[16] but most noteworthy is the fenestration technique (Fig. 18.11).

Occasionally, one may encounter very recalcitrant lesions where sharp recanalization techniques should be considered (i.e., stiff wire, Rosch-Uchida needle). In addition, access from above and below may be required to snare a wire to get through-and-access across the lesion ("body floss" technique). More advanced techniques and details of the endovascular instrumentation required will be discussed at the end of this chapter.

Previously placed IVC filters incorporated in the occluded caval segment or present above the occlusion in a patent segment pose a special technical problem. In the former instance, the filter must be displaced sideways or remodeled/fractured by repeated high-pressure balloon dilation to allow stent placement. In the latter case, the filter implantation site must be assessed for significant associated stenosis. If present, the IVC filter should be disrupted or displaced for placement of the stent across the stenosis; otherwise, it is left alone.

Anticoagulation

Intraoperatively, unfractionated heparin (5000–10,000 U) is administered and allowed to circulate before balloon dilatation. In patients with stents implanted for the treatment of NIVL, usually a daily dose of 81 mg of aspirin is sufficient to maintain stent patency. However, in postthrombotic cases, we have learned that "when in doubt, anticoagulate." In patients who undergo difficult recanalizations and lengthy procedures, low-molecular-weight heparin (enoxaparin 1 mg/kg twice daily subcutaneously) is administered afterwards in the recovery room, and daily thereafter for 3 months. At this point, we will convert them to an oral agent for long-term anticoagulation. In many, especially those patients with inherited or acquired thrombophilias, lifelong oral anticoagulation is indicated to maintain stent patency.

Scientific Evidence Postthrombotic Treatment

In six studies with a total of 921 legs, secondary (postthrombotic) obstruction was specifically examined.[17-22] Technical success was achieved in 93% to 100% of cases, with a mean follow-up of 46 months (2–72 months). Primary patency (where the vein is open without any additional intervention) was 57% (50%–80%), assisted primary patency (where the vein is patent, but an additional intervention was needed to keep the vein patent) 80% (76%–82%), and secondary patency (where the vein is patent after one or more additional interventions were required to treat an occlusion of the vein) 86% (82%–90%). Ulcer healing ranged from 63% to 67%,[23] with 0% to 8% recurrence.[20,24] There was statistically significant improvement at all points of the CIVIQ[24] and VCSS[21] scores. Edema decreased in 32% to 51% of cases.[22-24]

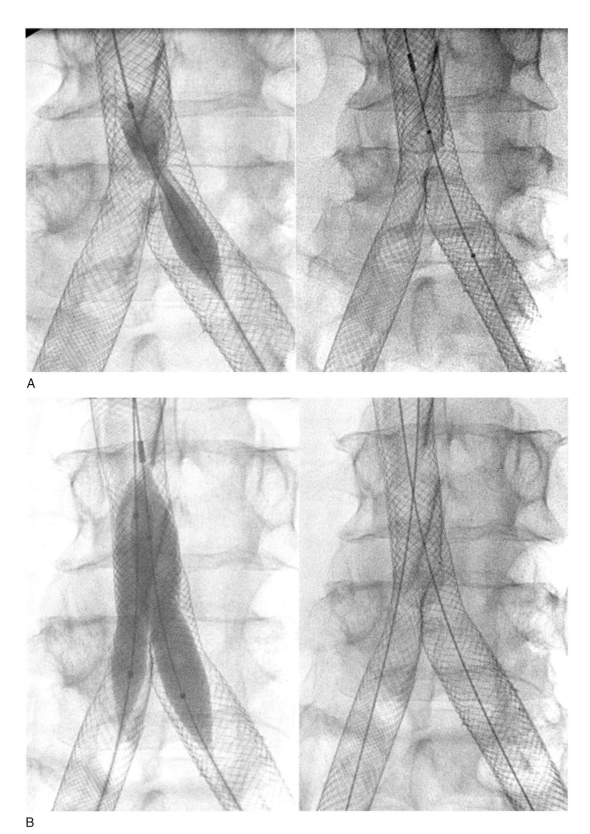

A

B

■ **Fig. 18.11** (A) Fenestration of a stent, which is placed across the outflow of one stented limb after an inverted Y fenestration. *Left,* a balloon is placed through the side of the stent and dilated, *(right)* creating a fenestra allowing unimpeded outflow. (B) The unilateral dilation may sometimes infringe on the previous created window and result in stenosis. *Left,* it may be useful to perform balloon dilation at the stent confluence by kissing balloon technique to *(right)* ensure an uninterrupted outflow from both iliac veins.[16]

Comparative Effectiveness of Existing Treatments

Historically, the venous femoral-femoral bypass using great saphenous vein as a bypass conduit (Palma procedure) was the procedure of choice for iliac vein occlusions. Direct iliac vein surgery, such as iliac vein bypass using prosthetic grafts, never gained much popularity because of the high failure rate. Anticoagulation, with or without adjunctive arteriovenous fistula support, was the norm to maintain primary patency of all venous reconstructions, and despite these efforts, the procedures performed poorly in general.

CASES AND INNOVATIVE TECHNIQUES

Case 1: Recanalization of Left Iliac Chronic Total Occlusion, Endovascular Reconstruction With Wallstent/Z-Stent Stack (Figs. 18.12–18.20)

Lesions that involve the iliac confluence have been previously treated with Wallstents, with proximal extension further into the vena cava to prevent stent retraction into the common iliac vein. These have the risk of partially or totally jailing the contralateral side. As mentioned earlier, the Gianturco Z stent has large interstrut spaces and provides good support to the upper end of Wallstents to avoid their compression/migration. A technical modification in which a Gianturco Z stent tops the Wallstent stack at the upper end appears to contribute greater radial strength to withstand the tight constricting lesion at the iliac caval junction, reduces the chance of "jailing" contralateral iliac vein, and greatly improves the technical ease of simultaneous or sequential bilateral iliac vein stenting.

Text continued on p. 460

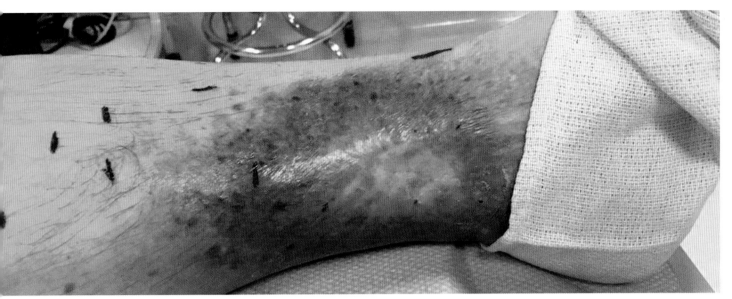

■ **Fig. 18.12** 45 yo WM presented to us with worsening signs and symptoms of LLE postthrombotic syndrome. At age 18 he suffered an accident requiring three abdominal operations for a testicular injury. He developed pain and swelling of the left lower extremity after the third procedure and was treated for lymphangitis with antibiotics. Patient with no knowledge of any previous thromboembolic event. Duplex imaging in our office demonstrated postthrombotic changes in the common femoral vein, femoral vein, and popliteal vein.

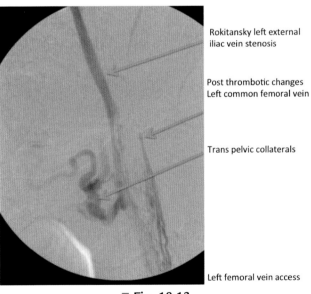

Rokitansky left external iliac vein stenosis

Post thrombotic changes Left common femoral vein

Trans pelvic collaterals

Left femoral vein access

■ **Fig. 18.13**

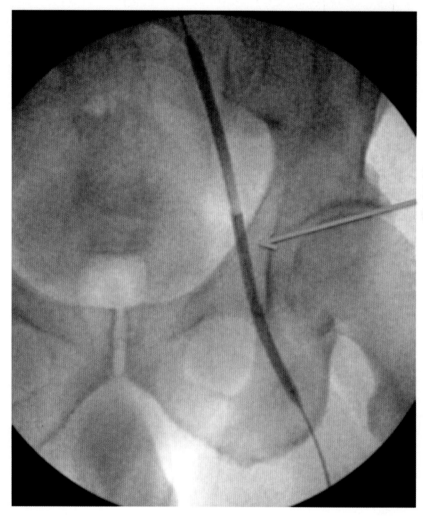

Serial balloon angioplasty
begun with long length
8 mm Mustang balloon

■ Fig. 18.14

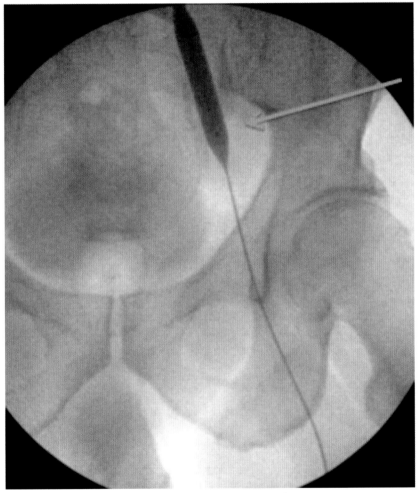

Serial balloon angioplasty upsizing to 14 mm Atlas balloon

■ Fig. 18.15

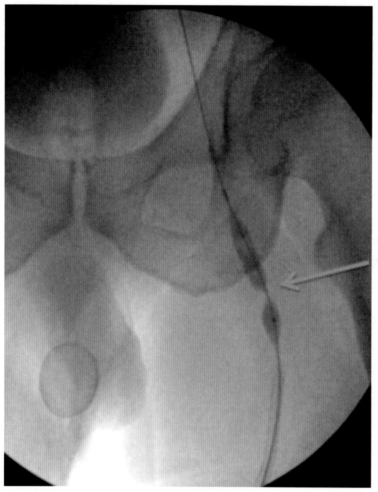

Tight waist at lesser trochanter (femoral vein confluence)

■ Fig. 18.16

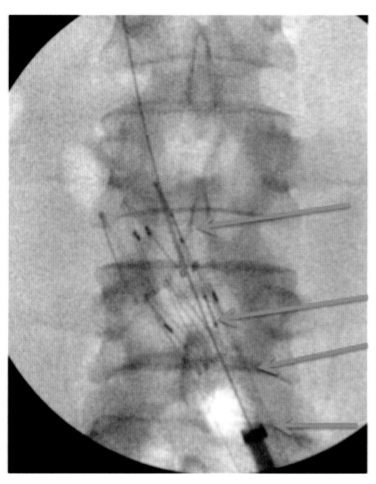

Z stent deployment-
caudad Z-stent component deployed
within Wallstent; cranial component
deployed in vena cava

20 mm Cook Z-stent
(cranial component)

20 mm Cook Z-stent
(caudad component)

18 mm BSCI Wallstent

16 FR Cook Z-stent
delivery system

■ Fig. 18.17

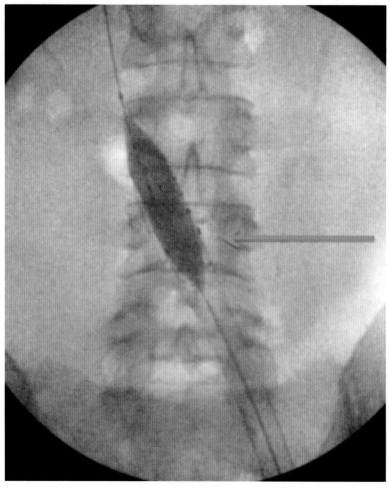

Post-Z-stent balloon dilatation with 18 mm Atlas balloon to 16 atm

■ Fig. 18.18

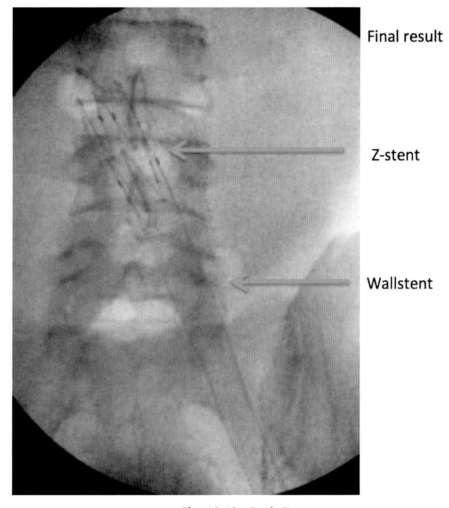

Final result

Z-stent

Wallstent

■ **Fig. 18.19** Cook Z-stent.

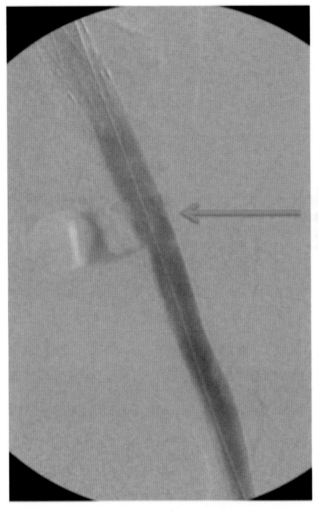

Final run:
notice luminal gain
post stenting

■ Fig. 18.20

Case 2: IVC Filter Induced Vena Cava Occlusion, Extract Filter and Stent Cava (Figs. 18.21–18.30)

Remove the Inferior Vena Cava Filter and Attempt to Traverse the Lesions

It is important to remove, if possible, any filters present because they may migrate and erode through the vein and/or stent. IVC filters are supposed to be temporary and recommendations are to remove them as soon as they are no longer indicated. If a filter is not removable, then crushing the filter can be an option (see Case 3).

Text continued on p. 468

65-year-old white male with 10 year history of bilateral femoro-iliocaval chronic total occlusions secondary to inferior vena cava filter thrombosis. Severe post-thrombotic syndrome of bilateral lower extremities with edema, advanced lipodermatosclerosis, and recurrent venous ulcerations. On lifelong anticoagulation.

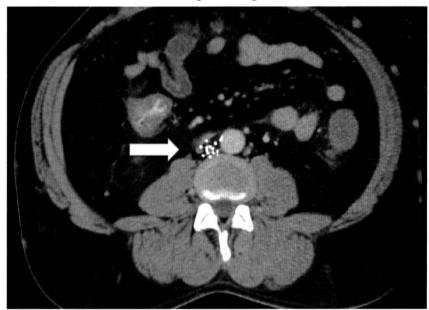

■ Fig. 18.21

Inferior vena cava obstruction produces abdominal collateral veins to bypass the blocked inferior vena cava and permit venous return from the legs.

How to differentiate portal hypertension (caput medusae) from caval occlusion?

Determine the direction of flow in the veins below the umbilicus by compressing a prominent vein:
if flow toward the legs -> caput medusae
if flow toward the head-> inferior vena cava obstruction

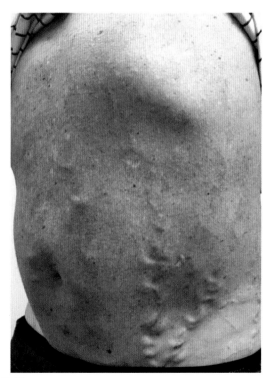

■ Fig. 18.22

CT scan demonstrates embedded
Bard G2 filter with distal IVC
occlusion.
Large collateral vein enters vena
cava above filter from the right
side.
Filter legs embedded in a aorta
and lumbar spine.

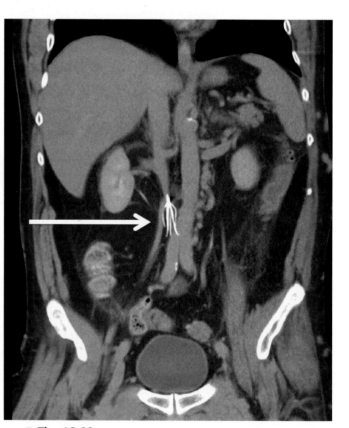

■ Fig. 18.23

Caval venogram, jugular
approach, shows
occlusion of IVC filter

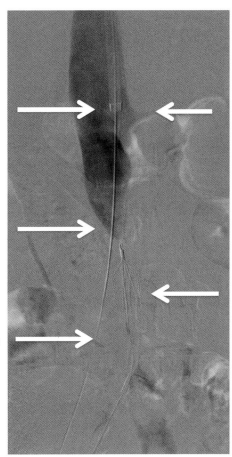

guide sheath

left renal vein

birds beak
caval occlusion

thrombosed
IVC filter

guidewire in collateral vein

■ Fig. 18.24

Right internal jugular vein
accessed using ultrasound
16 FR, 45 cm length sheath
placed to support Cook
clover snare

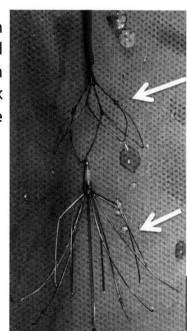

Cook
clover snare

Bard G2
filter

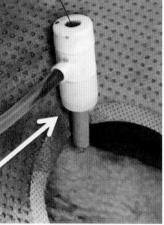

16 FR, 45 cm length
guide sheath

■ Fig. 18.25

Right internal jugular vein
accessed using ultrasound.
16 FR, 45 cm length sheath
placed to support Cook
clover snare
Using aggressive traction, IVC
filter retrieved in its entirety
after 10 years

Localized extravasation of
contrast visualized after
extraction. Patient remained
hemodynamically stable

guidewire in collateral
vein right side

Triforce catheter for
left iliac vein
recanalization

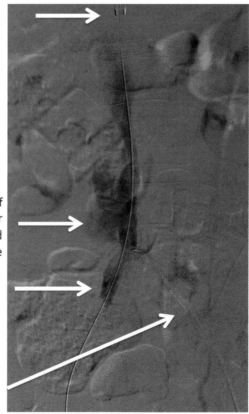

■ Fig. 18.26

Initial venogram demonstrates bilateral iliac vein occlusion
with large pelvic collaterals

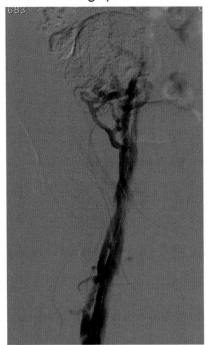

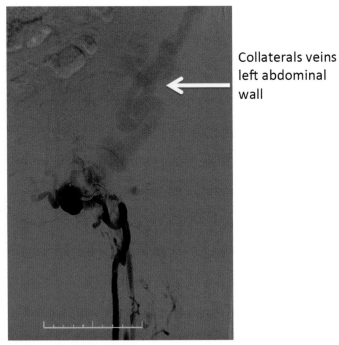

Collaterals veins
left abdominal
wall

RLE venogram

LLE venogram

■ Fig. 18.27

5 Fr Cook Tri-force system
provides good columnar
support
.035 angled stiff glidewire for
recanalization of left iliac vein

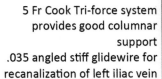

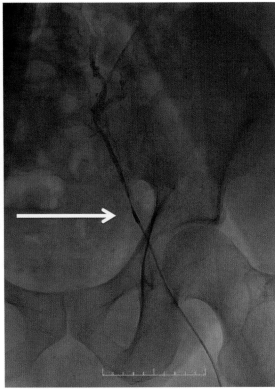

■ Fig. 18.28

Post-stent dilatation with 16 mm
Bard Atlas balloons to 16 atm
Double-barrel
16 mm Wallstents
placed in IVC extending
into iliac veins

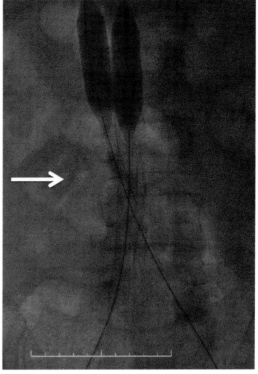

■ Fig. 18.29

Final bilateral iliocaval
endovascular reconstruction
and completion venogram
demonstrating excellent venous
flow

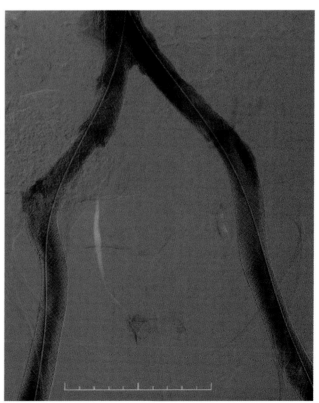

■ Fig. 18.30

Using a Cloversnare, the IVC filter was controlled and able to be safely removed in its entirety by withdrawing it into a 16-Fr sheath. Once removed, the left femoral vein was able to be recanalized using an 0.035-inch (0.088-cm) angled glide wire supported by the 5-Fr TriForce system, gaining access to the left common iliac vein. Similarly, the right common iliac vein was able to be accessed.

Access and Bilateral Lower Extremity Venograms

The patient had patent femoral veins bilaterally and the left femoral vein was accessed first using the micropuncture system under US guidance. Left lower extremity (LLE) venography was performed showing proximal femoral vein obstruction and occlusion of the proximal iliofemoral veins. Next, the same procedure was carried out on the right side with similar findings. Then the right internal jugular (RIJ) was accessed with US-guided micropuncture system and exchanged for an 0.035-inch (0.088-cm) angled glide wire, which was placed into the distal IVC followed by a 16-Fr sheath for support.

Intravascular Ultrasonography, Venography, and Percutaneous Transluminal Angioplasty/Stenting

Once the lesions were traversed and the wires safely advanced to the right subclavian vein, systemic anticoagulation was administered with 10,000 units of intravenous (IV) heparin. Serial balloon dilations were performed with 6-mm and 10-mm Mustang balloons followed by 16-mm Atlas balloons inflated to 16 atm throughout the IVC to common femoral veins. IVUS was then performed and demonstrated a stenotic IVC inferior to the renal veins down to the level of the femoral confluences. Wallstents were deployed using an 18-mm Wallstent for the IVC, 16-mm Wallstents for the iliac veins, and 14-mm Wallstents in the bilateral common femoral veins using a generous telescoping technique.

Poststent Dilation and Completion Venography

Following stenting, a 16-mm Atlas balloon at 16 atm was used throughout the stented regions bilaterally. Completion IVUS and venography showed good apposition of the stents to the venous wall and brisk contrast emptying suggesting widely patent iliocaval system. Compression dressings were applied, and the patient was discharged with follow-up in 4 days.

Case 3: IVC Filter Induced Vena Cava Occlusion, Crush Filter and Stent Cava (Figs. 18.31–18.39)

Preoperative diagnosis includes postthrombotic syndrome with bilateral venous ulcers, iliac vein occlusion, and IVC filter occlusion in the presence of thrombophilia.

Text continued on p. 474

The major collateral pathways seen with IVC obstruction are the azygos-hemiazygos and vertebral pathways

guide sheath

birds beak caval occlusion

thrombosed IVC filter

collateral vein

Triforce catheter for left iliac vein recanalization

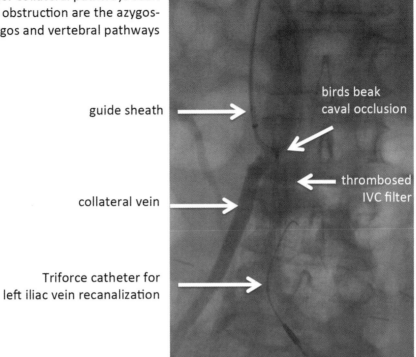

■ Fig. 18.31

Occluded permant IVC filter (Braun) traversed with sharp end of an .035 Amplatz super-stiff wire supported with 45cm 16 FR Cook sheath and 5 FR 55 cm Triforce system

Amplatz Superstiff Guidewire (back end – sharp)

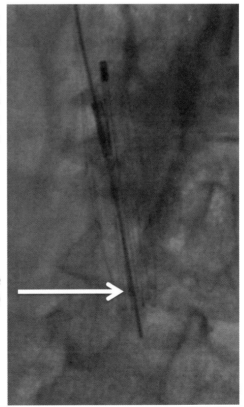

■ Fig. 18.32

Channel created
between IVC
and left common iliac
vein to allowed passage
of an .014 floppy tip wire
from below without
having to snare from
above

Amplatz Superstiff Guidewire
(back end – sharp)

Triforce for
left iliac vein recanalization
the 4 FR CXI Support
catheter used to deliver the
.014 floppy tip wire into IVC

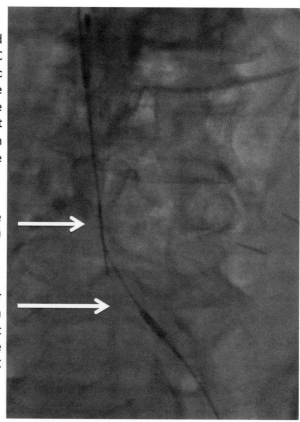

■ Fig. 18.33

With through-and-though access from left femoral vein to right internal jugular vein serial balloon dilatation begun

Here we "endosmash" the IVC filter using a 16 mm Bard Atlas balloon

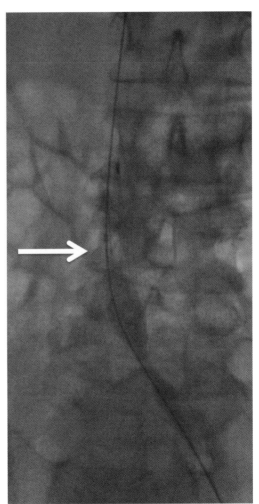

■ Fig. 18.34

Filter "endotrashed" to the caval sidewall by stenting across it, 24 mm Wallstent

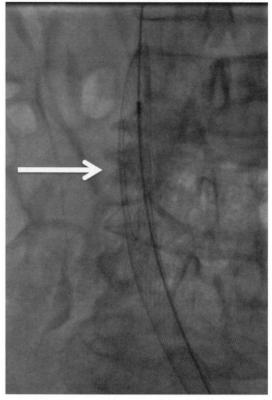

■ Fig. 18.35

Post-stent dilatation of IVC with 20 mm Bard Atlas balloon, inflations to 16 atm

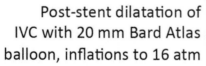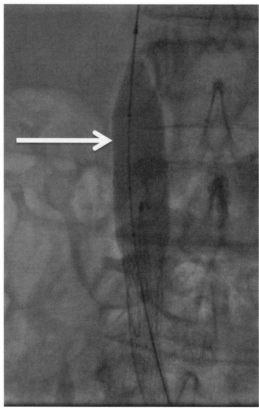

■ Fig. 18.36

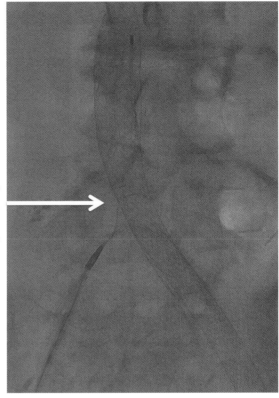

Stent fenestration initiated
by traversing stent struts
right iliac vein recanalized with
.035 angled glidewire supported
by Triforce system

■ Fig. 18.37

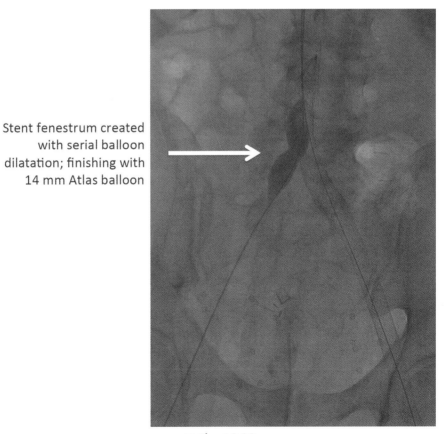

Stent fenestrum created
with serial balloon
dilatation; finishing with
14 mm Atlas balloon

■ Fig. 18.38

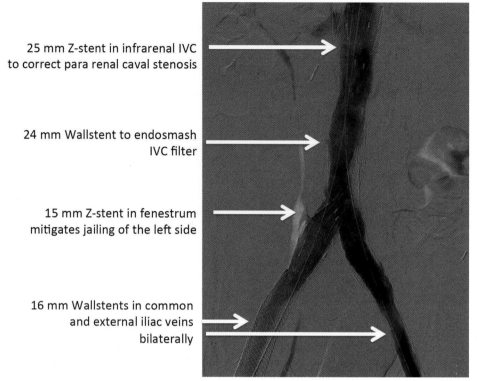

25 mm Z-stent in infrarenal IVC
to correct para renal caval stenosis

24 mm Wallstent to endosmash
IVC filter

15 mm Z-stent in fenestrum
mitigates jailing of the left side

16 mm Wallstents in common
and external iliac veins
bilaterally

■ **Fig. 18.39** Radiographic image after recanalization of occluded IVC secondary to chronic filter thrombosis. The filter was compacted by balloon dilation and then stented across. The stent stack extends into the common femoral vein bilaterally crossing the groin crease. Extensive metal load is well tolerated, but missed lesions often lead to stent thrombosis because of poor inflow/outflow.

Access and Initial Bilateral Lower Extremity Venography

In the supine position, the right neck and both groins were prepped. A Foley was placed, and the right femoral vein was accessed first using US-guided micropuncture system followed by an 0.035-inch (0.088-cm) glide wire. Contrast venography was performed showing a chronic occlusion of the proximal femoral vein and common femoral vein. An 11-Fr sheath was placed, and the Triforce system was used to attempt right iliac vein recanalization. Once further progress appeared stunted, attention was turned to the left side. There was a similar presentation with the exception of the proximal femoral vein remaining patent.

The TriForce system was used on the left side as well and was able to recanalize the left external iliac and obtain access to the left external iliac. Attempts were further tried with an 0.035-inch (0.088-cm) roadrunner glide wire supported by the TriForce system. Again, progress was stunted and so the decision was to access from the RIJ.

Using US-guided micropuncture followed by an 11-Fr sheath, a 0.035-inch (0.088-CM) glide wire was advanced through the heart into the IVC. The TriForce system was used through the RIJ access, and contrast venography revealed an occluded IVC filter.

Attempts were made to traverse the occluded IVC filter with the TriForce system from above (RIJ access). Ultimately it required the additional support of a 14-Fr sheath and the back end of an Amplatz super-stiff guidewire to pierce and traverse the occluded Braun permanent filter.

Using an 0.014-inch (0.035-cm) floppy coronary wire from below, the filter was traversed via the small 0.035-inch (0.088-cm) channel created by the back end of the Amplatz super-stiff wire. The 0.014-inch (0.035-cm) coronary wire was exchanged for an 0.035-inch (0.088-cm) Amplatz super-stiff guidewire using a CXI support catheter from below and advanced cephalad into the RIJ.

The patient was given systemic anticoagulation with 10,000 U of IV heparin, and balloon dilations of the femoral veins, iliac veins, IVC, and IVC filter were performed beginning with a 5-mm balloon followed by a 10-mm, 14-mm, 16-mm, 18-mm, and 20-mm Atlas balloons inflated to 16 atm. IVUS was performed followed by placement of 24-mm Wallstents in the IVC through the IVC filter, displacing the filter towards the wall followed by telescoped 18-mm Wallstents in the common iliac vein, and 16-mm Wallstents in the external iliac vein and common femoral vein. Completion venography was performed, and the procedure was terminated with the right side planned for a separate date because of length of surgery.

Stage II Contralateral (Right) Side

Two months following the first procedure, the patient returned for right-sided symptoms and recurrent left-sided symptoms. Access was achieved again using US-guided micro-puncture system and exchanged an 11-Fr sheath with a 7-Fr pinnacle sheath and the 5-Fr TriForce system with an 0.035-inch (0.088-cm) glide wire. The right external and common iliac veins were able to be recanalized this time.

RIJ access was obtained and an 11-Fr sheath was placed through which a 9-Fr sheath was used to steer a guidewire through the stenotic IVC stent followed by balloon dilation with 20-mm Atlas balloon at 16 atm. A new 25-mm Z stent was placed using access from the left femoral access. Completion venography was performed and showed good iliofemoral flow bilaterally with some persistent chronic disease within the IVC. Compression dressings were placed, and the patient was sent to the recovery room with follow-up in 2 to 4 days.

Using a glide wire, the left iliac stent was able to be traversed and a fenestration was created within the left iliocaval stent with serial high-pressure balloon angioplasty using 5-mm, 10-mm, and 18-mm balloons.

Intravascular Ultrasonography and Percutaneous Transluminal Angioplasty/Stenting of the Right Side

IVUS was performed and confirmed intraluminal placement and right-sided disease. Systemic anticoagulation was given, and balloon angioplasty of the right iliofemoral veins were performed up to 18 mm using Atlas balloons with 16 atm. The right iliac vein was then stented with a 20-mm Z stent into the fenestration of the left iliocaval stent into the IVC in a T configuration. This is telescoped to an 18-mm Wallstent in the external iliac on the right side and 16-mm Wallstent in the common femoral vein. Poststenting balloon dilation is the performed with an 18-mm Atlas balloon at 16 atm.

Bilateral iliofemoral vein recanalizations are performed at the same session or staged, depending on the duration and difficulty of the initial procedure. The right and left stent assemblies are connected through a fenestration.

Case 4: Caval Agenesis and Recurrent VTE-Treated With Staged Complex Reconstruction (Figs. 18.40–18.48)

This 59-year-old Caucasian male had been followed conservatively in our practice for 10 years. He had a history of right iliac vein injury during pelvic tumor resection as a child. He also came with a history of vena cava agenesis. He had been managed lifelong with bilateral thigh high compression hose (30–40 mm Hg) and oral anticoagulation with a vitamin K antagonist. He had developed hepatitis B after blood transfusion but had good hepatic function. Throughout his life, he had suffered multiple bilateral episodes of DVT and multiple bilateral venous ulcers.

He had a brother and sister, each of whom were surgeons, who asked if we could offer an endovascular solution. Venography demonstrated bilateral chronic femoroiliocaval occlusions.

The left side was successfully recanalized, dilated, and stented. The stent stack consisted of a 24-mm Wallstent extending into the intrahepatic vena cava superiorly, with additional Wallstents placed in continuity, gradually tapering in size, terminating with a 16-mm Wallstent at the lesser trochanter.

We usually allow 2 to 3 months for the skin to recover from radiation dosages, and the kidneys to recover from contrast boluses, before operating the other limb. The right femoral vein had extensive synechiae from previous recurrent thromboembolism; it was accessed with a micropuncture system and an 8-Fr sheath was placed. Venography showed chronic total occlusion of the right iliofemoral venous outflow tract with significant formation of pelvic collaterals; drainage into the thoracic cavity was via the azygous vein. Multiple attempts were made to find and recanalize the native right iliac system using a variety of different wires (0.035-inch [0.088-cm] angled stiff and soft glide wires and 0.018-inch [0.045-cm] CTO wires) supported with 2.6-Fr and 4-Fr CXI support catheters

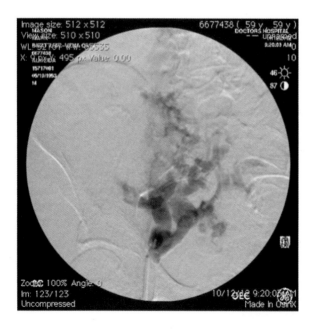 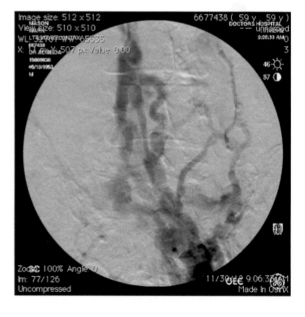

right iliac   left iliac

■ **Fig. 18.40**

post- thrombotic LLE
with iliac vein occlusion and
caval outflow lesions

supra and infrarenal
vena cava post-thrombotic
intraluminal fibrosis

left renal vein

caval occlusion with
left sided pelvic collaterals

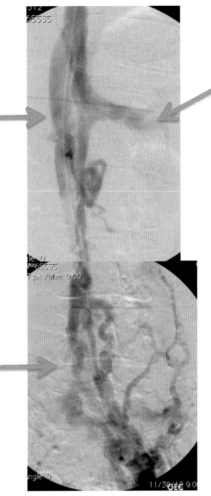

■ Fig. 18.41

and 6-Fr braided guide sheaths. The iliac system could not be identified; instead, a robust retroperitoneal collateral system had developed draining toward the paravertebral azygous system.

Access of the RIJ allowed placement of a 0.035-inch (0.088-cm) Bentson wire through the right atrium and into the intrahepatic portion of the IVC. A Kumpe catheter was then used to navigate the wire down into the left iliac stent. Through this, venography was performed and an attempt to visualize the caval entry of the right iliac system. However, no remnant right iliac system could be found.

The azygous vein appeared to be patent and rather robust with direct runoff into the superior vena cava (SVC), but there were several areas of stenosis. The right femoral 8-Fr sheath was exchanged for an 11-Fr sheath and the glide wire (supported by 5-Fr multipurpose A curve [MPA] catheter) was advanced through the azygous system into the SVC. The angled glide wire was exchanged for an Amplatz super-stiff wire over the MPA catheter.

s/p recanalization & serial dilatation of visceral cava
intra-hepatic IVC with post-thrombotic intraluminal scar (webs)

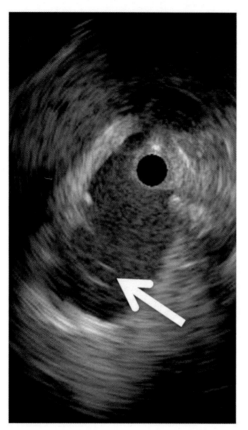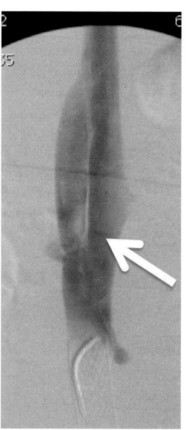

■ **Fig. 18.42**

IVUS was performed showing multiple lesions and the patient was anticoagulated with 10,000 units of heparin before balloon dilatation. Serial balloon dilatation was performed commencing with 5-mm balloons followed by 10-mm, and 14-mm. Venous recoil was observed, and the decision was made to stent with 14-mm Wallstents, connecting the femoral system through collaterals to the azygous. Following stenting, completion venography was performed and showed some areas of persistent stenosis. These were treated with 16-mm balloon angioplasty. Finally, completion venography showed obliteration of many, but not all, collateral vessels implying significantly improved outflow.

Text continued on p. 484

left iliocaval stent terminates at infrahepatic cava

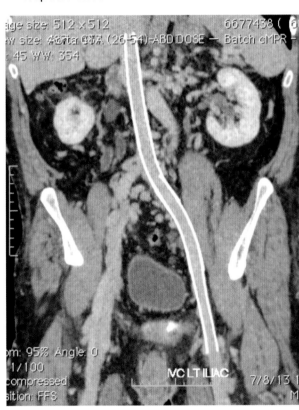
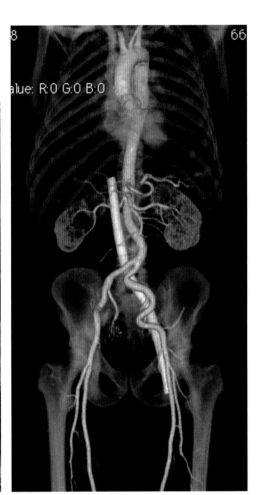

■ Fig. 18.43

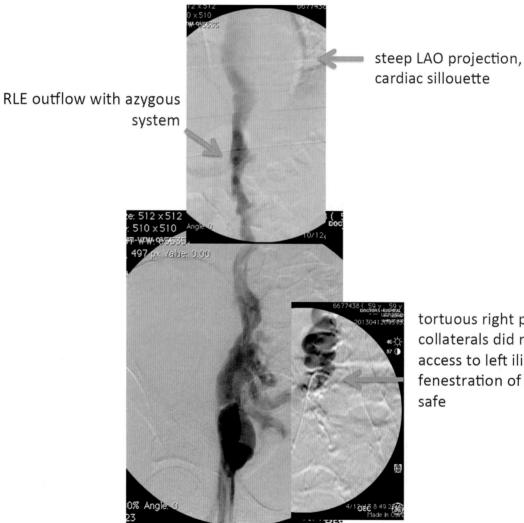

RLE outflow with azygous system

steep LAO projection, cardiac sillouette

tortuous right pelvic collaterals did not provide access to left iliac stent; fenestration of stent not safe

■ Fig. 18.44

Steep RAO view

5 FR Davis catheter
in SVC

Azygous Vein is outflow
source for RLE

Superimposed
left iliocaval stent

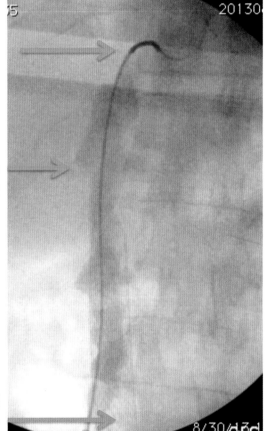

■ Fig. 18.45

Serial balloon
angioplasty of
azygous vein
(14 mm Atlas)

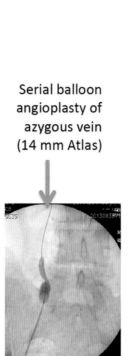

level of pelvis

Left iliocaval stent

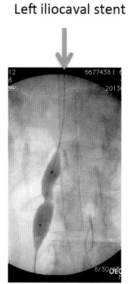

level of abdomen

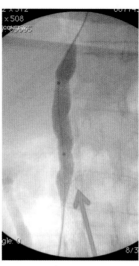

level of thorax
14 mm Atlas balloon
angioplasty of azygous
vein

■ Fig. 18.46

14 mm Atlas balloon
angioplasty of azygous-
SVC confluence

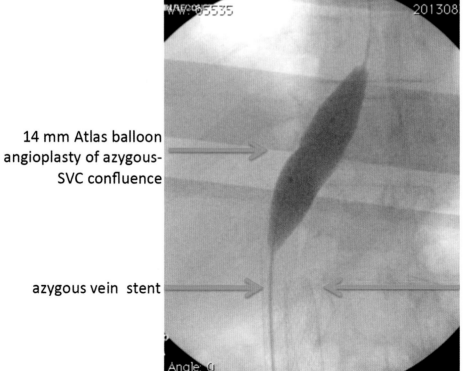

azygous vein stent   left iliocaval stent

■ Fig. 18.47

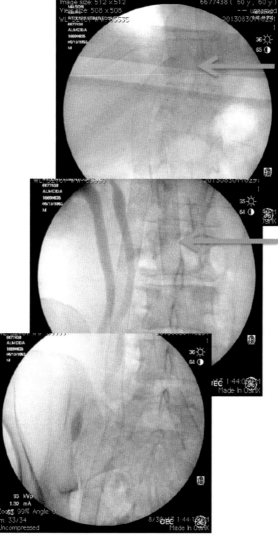

RLE venous system
drains into SVC

LLE venous system
drains into IVC

■ Fig. 18.48

Case 5: Femoral Vein Stenting to Add Inflow Support to Iliocaval Endovascular Reconstruction (Figs. 18.49–18.56)

A 52-year-old woman with multiple episodes of deep venous thrombosis had an iliocaval stent placed for worsening postthrombotic syndrome 2 years earlier. Warfarin was discontinued by primary care physician (PCP) and the patient developed stent thrombosis and recurrent of the femoral and popliteal veins.

The stent was reopened using phamacomechanical thrombolysis (Angiojet; Boston Scientific, Marlborough, MA) and the patient anticoagulation with rivaroxaban.

Femoral Vein Intervention steps:

Anesthesia: Monitored anesthesia care in the office-based laboratory

Step 1: Access the small saphenous vein (SSV) and perform low-extremity venography

Patient is placed in the prone position for easy access to the SSV with a micropuncture system under US guidance. Using an 0.035-inch (0.088-cm) guidewire, a 10-Fr sheath is placed and lower extremity venography is performed.

Step 2: Vena cava catheterization and venography

LLE diseased veins are noted and a 5-Fr Kumpe catheter is placed for selective vena cava catheterization and venography. The Kumpe catheter is then advanced beyond the heart and into the right subclavian vein. An 0.035-inch (0.088-cm) Amplatz super-stiff wire is then placed via the catheter.

Step 3: IVUS

Using a volcano intravascular ultrasound catheter, IVUS is performed from the femoral vein to the heart. Significant findings are recorded.

Step 4: Venous angioplasty

Systemic anticoagulation is given. We typically give 10,000 units of IV heparin. For femoral popliteal disease, a 10-mm balloon is used to angioplasty the diseased area, which may encompass the entire femoral popliteal tract.

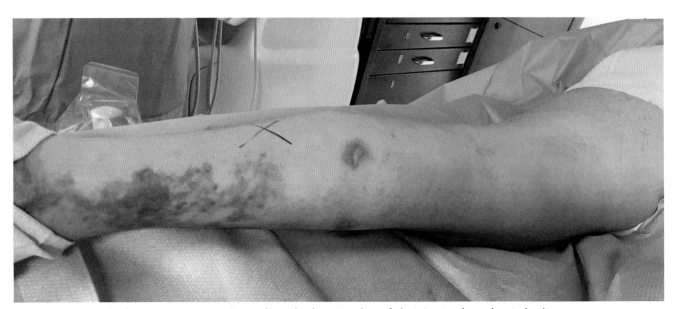

■ **Fig. 18.49** 52 yo WM with multiple episodes of deep vein thrombosis had iliocaval stent placed for worsening postthrombotic syndrome. Warfarin discontinued by PCP and patient developed recurrent LLE iliofemoral and popliteal deep vein thrombosis.

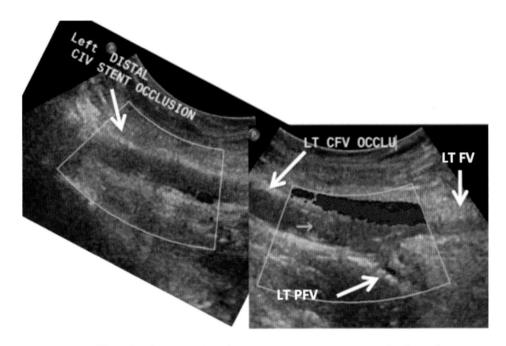

An office duplex imaging demonstrates an acute occlusion of stent extending from left common iliac vein to common femoral vein. native femoral vein and profunda femoris vein also occluded.

■ Fig. 18.50

Left iliofemoral re-intervention restores stent patency patient symptoms improved. Notice inflow to stent via profunda femoris vein. Femoral vein recanalized with intraluminal fibrosis.

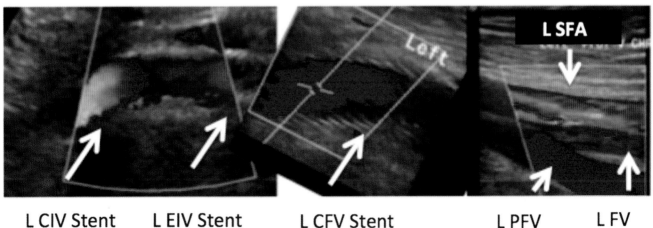

■ Fig. 18.51

2 years later, left femoral vein with chronic obstruction and reflux
patient wanted intervention to improve venous claudication in calf
L SFA
L SFA
Short Axis
L FV
Long Axis
L FV

■ Fig. 18.52

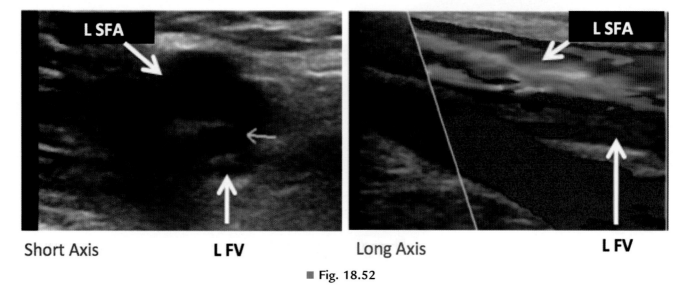

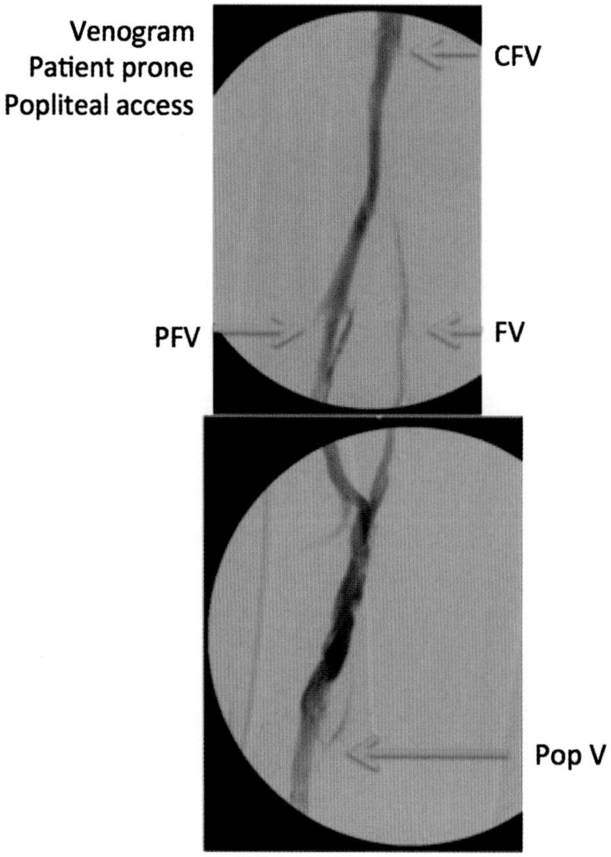

Venogram
Patient prone
Popliteal access
CFV
PFV
FV
Pop V

■ Fig. 18.53

IVUS, popliteal access

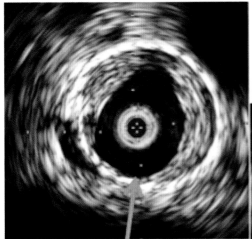

**Recanalized EIV-CFV
16 mm Wallstent
with ISR**

Sub-total occlusion FV

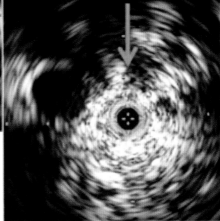

Recanalized Pop V

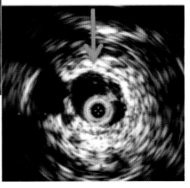

■ Fig. 18.54

Step 5: Venous stenting

For femoral-popliteal stenting, 10-mm overlapping nitinol uncovered stents should be used with 1 cm overlap from the femoral vein confluence to the proximal popliteal vein. Care should be taken to not jail off the profunda proximally or distally. Poststent balloon angioplasty is then performed with a 10-mm balloon up to 16 atm (or the appropriate rating per the manufacturer).

Step 6: Completion venography

Completion venography is then performed to ensure proper positioning and stent expansion with resolution of stenosis.

Step 7: Catheter removal and completion

The Amplatz wire and sheath are then removed and a circumferential compression dressing is applied on the calf at the puncture site. The patient is sent to the recovery room and discharged home with pain medications for the following 2 to 4 days. A follow-up visit is scheduled for 4 days postprocedure for in-clinic assessment of the stent with US.

Venogram
Patient prone
Popliteal access
s/p FV stent

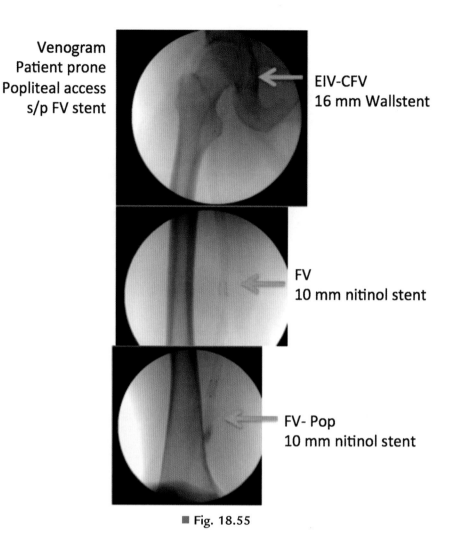

EIV-CFV
16 mm Wallstent

FV
10 mm nitinol stent

FV- Pop
10 mm nitinol stent

■ Fig. 18.55

Duplex at 6-months shows patent femoral vein stent,
patent popliteal vein. Patient anti-coagulated on rivaroxaban

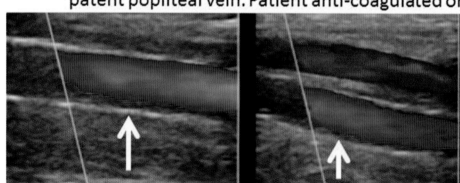
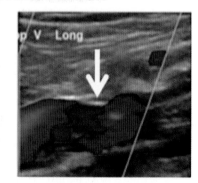

proximal FV   mid-thigh FV   popliteal vein

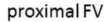

■ Fig. 18.56

Case 6: Infrarenal Caval Occlusion With Dissection. Treatment With Sharp Recanalization, Through-and-Through (Body Floss) Access and Endovascular Stent Reconstruction

See Figs. 18.57–18.65.

Text continued on p. 496

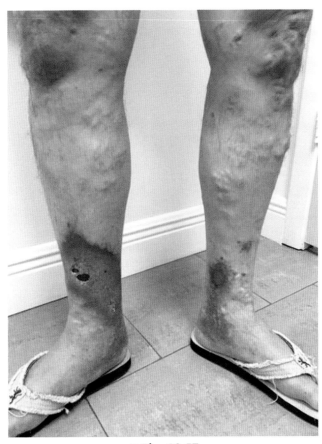

■ **Fig. 18.57**

Caval venogram
jugular approach
shows infrarenal occlusion

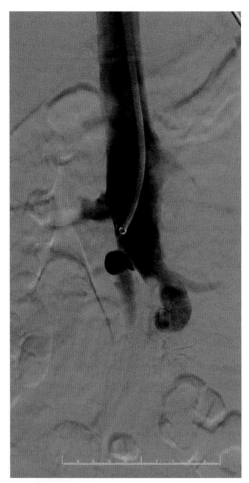

■ Fig. 18.58

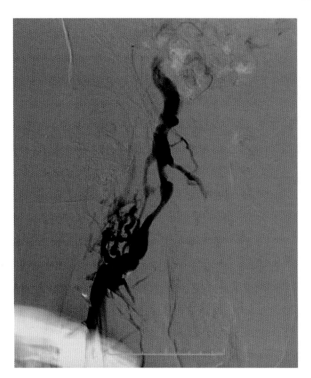

R iliac CTO

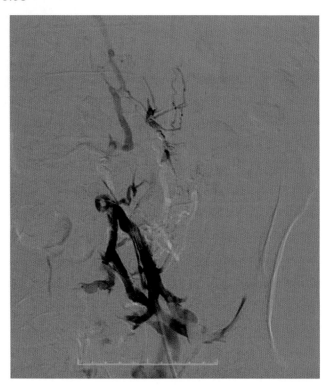

L iliac CTO

■ Fig. 18.59

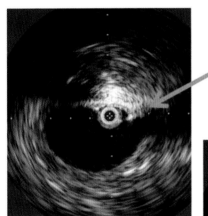

Dissection flap of IVC originating at level of the left renal vein

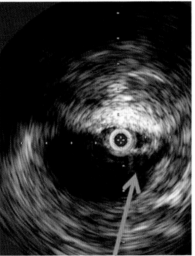

Caval dissection with true and false lumen depicted

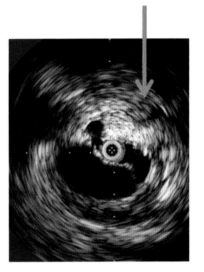

Dissection flap of IVC progressing caudad towards iliocaval confluence

▪ Fig. 18.60

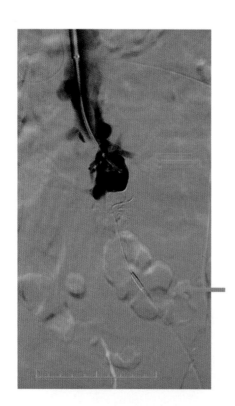 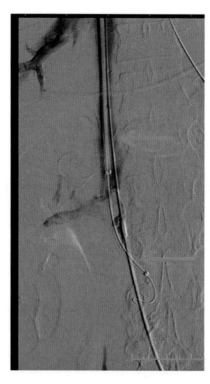

successful recanalization from above and below gives through-and-through access

.035 stiff angled glidewire supported with 5FR Triforce system from below

.035 stiff angled glidewire supported with 5FR Triforce system and 9 FR Performer sheath from above

■ Fig. 18.61

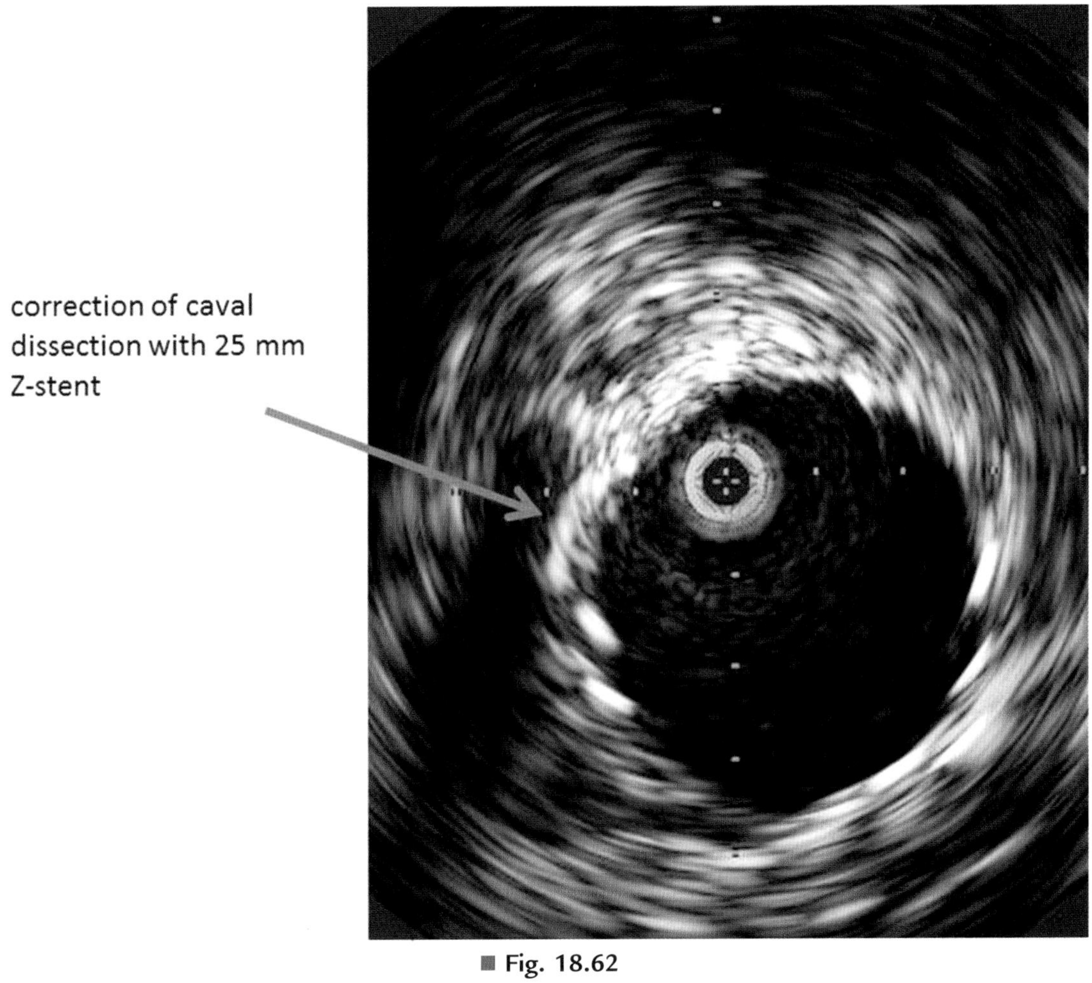

correction of caval
dissection with 25 mm
Z-stent

■ Fig. 18.62

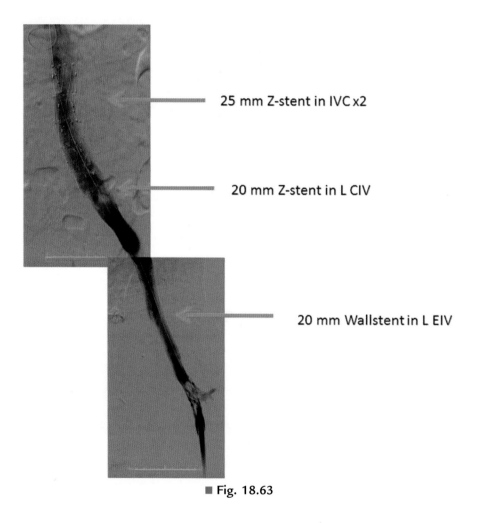

25 mm Z-stent in IVC x2

20 mm Z-stent in L CIV

20 mm Wallstent in L EIV

■ Fig. 18.63

Rösch-Uchida Needle

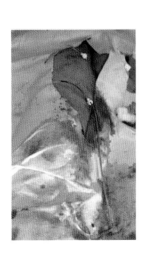

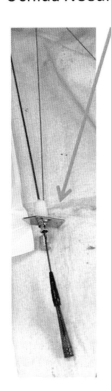

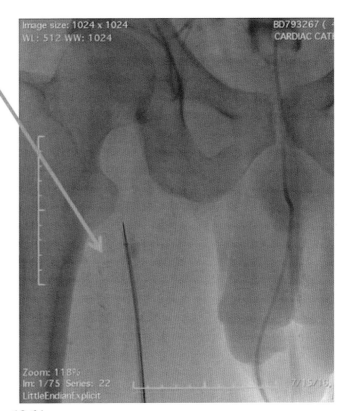

■ Fig. 18.64

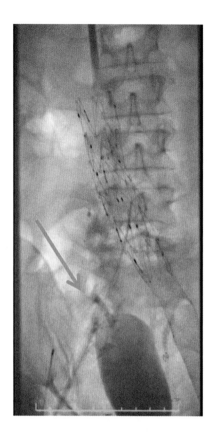

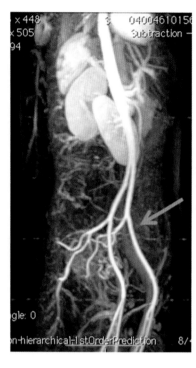

Always keep in mind,
the curvatures of the pelvis.
Multiple oblique views required when
traversing occluded vessels in the pelvis.

■ **Fig. 18.65**

Case 7: Biconical IVC Filter Caval Extraction With Loop Snare and Rigid Bronchial Forceps (Figs. 18.66–18.70)

A 65-year-old woman with history of deep venous thrombosis 10 years earlier had placement of biconical IVC filter for unclear reasons.

Presented to us with chronic BLE edema and lipodermatosclerosis; found caval occlusion secondary to filter on cross-sectional imaging.

16 FR Braided Sheath
Will Allow Wire & Snare (2 devices)
via one RIJ Access

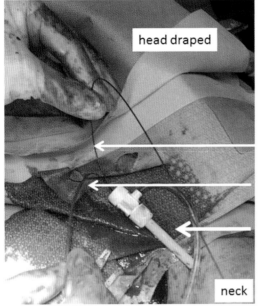

head draped

wire

clover snare

16 FR RIJ
Sheath

neck

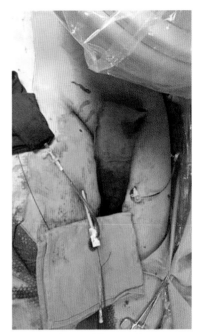

Bilateral femoral access

■ Fig. 18.66

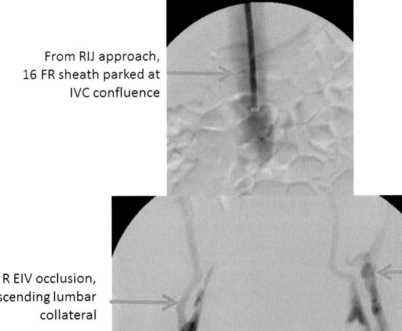

From RIJ approach,
16 FR sheath parked at
IVC confluence

R EIV occlusion,
ascending lumbar
collateral

L EIV occlusion,
ascending lumbar
collateral

■ Fig. 18.67

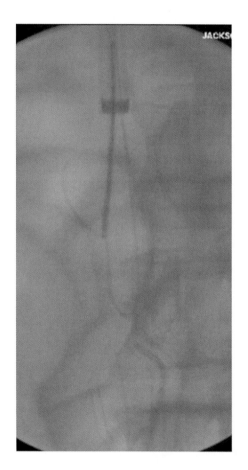 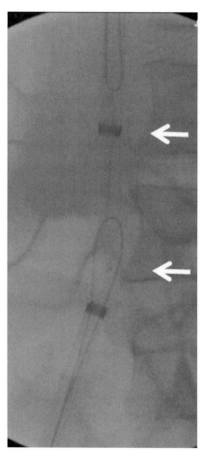

Loop snares from above and below allow counter traction to "cinch down" the filter

■ Fig. 18.68

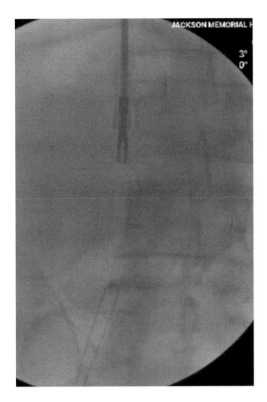
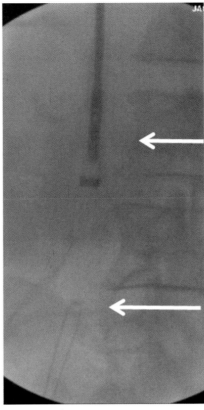

Rigid bronchoscopy forceps allow firm grasp of filter. Then slide sheath downward to collapse the filter and enclose with sheath for removal

Notice downward traction from below

■ **Fig. 18.69**

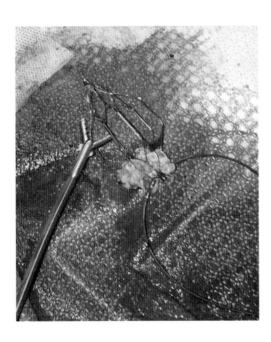
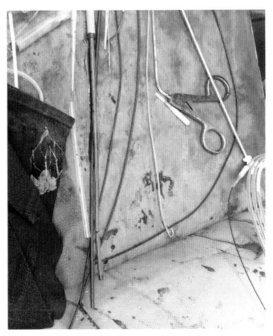

Successfully retrieved biconical IVC filter – note the adherent tissue typically seen with long dwell times, and the array of endo-tools required for retrieval.

■ **Fig. 18.70**

Case 8: Vena Cava Atresia Presented With Acute Bilateral Iliofemoral Deep Vein Thrombosis. Treated With Catheter Directed Thrombolysis Followed by Endovascular Stenting (Figs. 18.71–18.74)

A 37-year-old Caucasian female with known vena cava atresia presented with acute bilateral iliofemoral deep venous thrombosis while running a marathon.

Via bilateral popliteal access, the femoral and iliac veins were crossed and the vena cava entered. Overnight catheter-directed thrombolysis performed with tissue plasminogen activator.

Selective caval venography demonstrated absent renal vein drainage
into vena cava.
Serial balloon dilatation of infrahepatic and infrarenal vena cava performed; final inflations with 24 mm Atlas balloon to 16 atm.

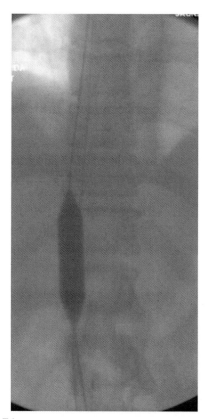

■ Fig. 18.71

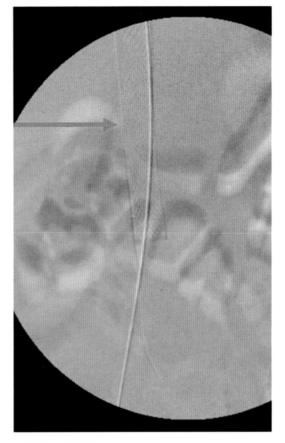

24 mm Wallstent placed in intrahepatic vena cava and extended into infrarenal vena cava; post-dilatation with 24 mm Atlas balloon to 16 atm.

■ **Fig. 18.72**

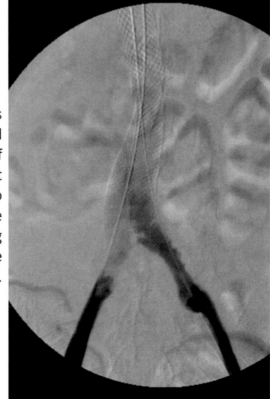

Two 16 mm Wallstents placed inside inferior aspect of caval stent and brought down into each respective common iliac vein using double barrel technique.

■ **Fig. 18.73**

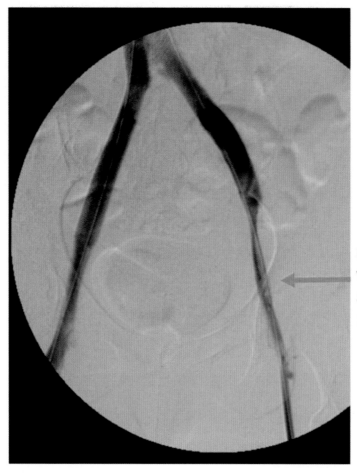

residual left external iliac
vein stenosis required an
additional
16 mm Wallstent

■ Fig. 18.74

Case 9: Severe Thromophilia, Venous Ulceration, Failed Femoral Vein Stenting

See Figs. 18.75–18.83.

Text continued on p. 508

31 yo WM s/p 5 DVT over the course of 15 years;
3 right lower extremity and
2 left lower extremity.

Thrombophilia work-up negative.
Recommended lifelong anticoagulation.

Presented with recurrent RLE venous ulcer.

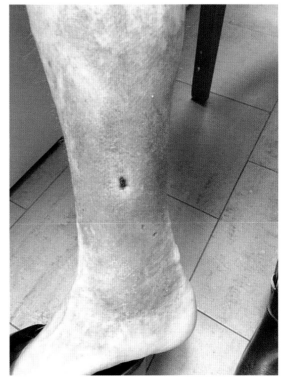

■ Fig. 18.75

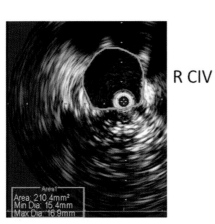

R CIV

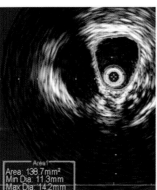

R EIV

Iliac vein evaluation with IVUS
showed a normal right common
and external iliac vein.

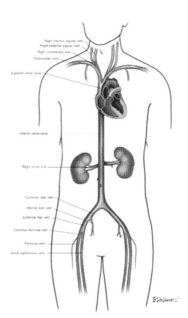

■ Fig. 18.76

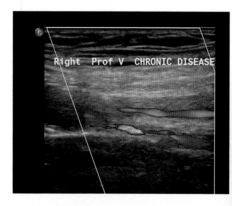

Duplex ultrasound shows severe femoral – popliteal (including profunda femoris vein) post-thrombotic obstruction

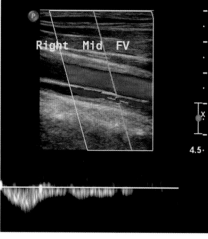

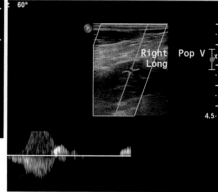

■ Fig. 18.77

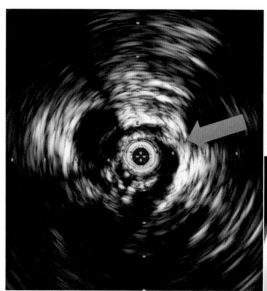

R CFV post-thrombotic webs found with IVUS imaging

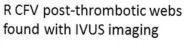

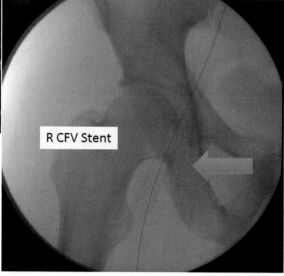

Treated with right common femoral vein stent placement

■ Fig. 18.78

1 year later patient with recurrent
RLE ulcer-
desired further intervention.
Prone venogram
left gastrocnemius
vein access

pre-stent

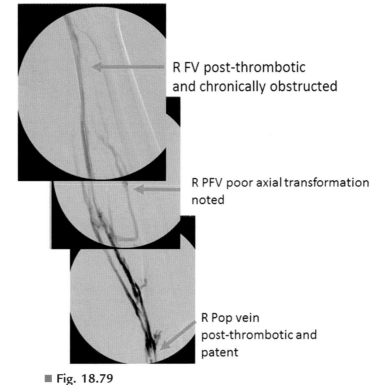

R FV post-thrombotic
and chronically obstructed

R PFV poor axial transformation
noted

R Pop vein
post-thrombotic and
patent

■ Fig. 18.79

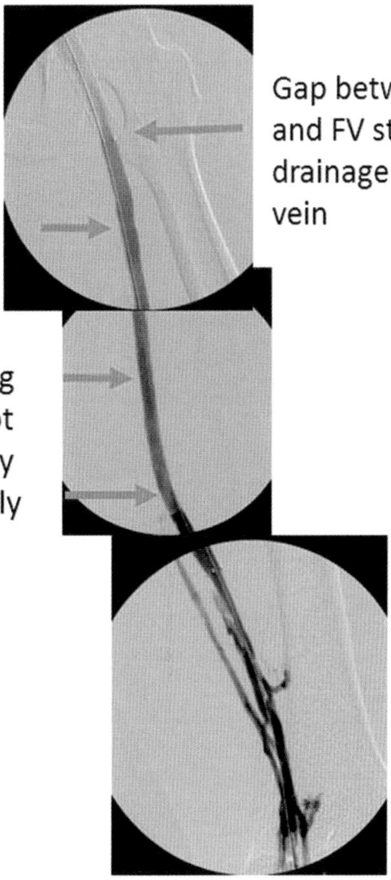

Prone venogram
left gastrocnemius
vein access, advised to continue
his warfarin INR 2-3

Gap between CFV stent
and FV stent to allow
drainage of profunda femoris
vein

Femoral vein stented using
10mm nitinol with care not
to jail profunda proximally
or distally

■ Fig. 18.80

Shows up 4 weeks later with INR 1.4
Patient supine, PT vein access, venogram shows FV stent thrombosis

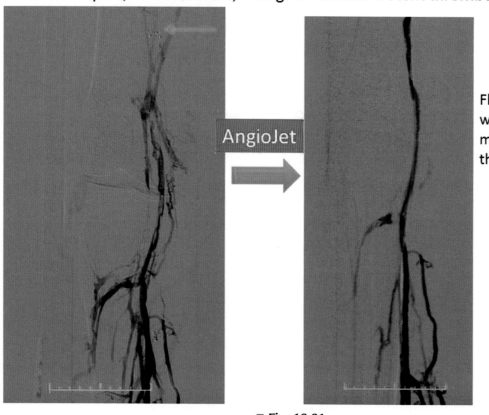

AngioJet

Flow restored
with pharmaco-
mechanical
thrombolysis

■ **Fig. 18.81**

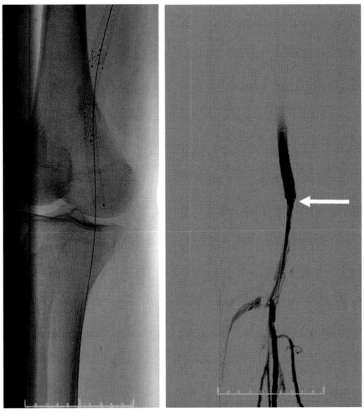

Extended FV Stent
into popliteal vein,
but did not cross
knee joint because of
concern of potential future stent
fracture

■ Fig. 18.82

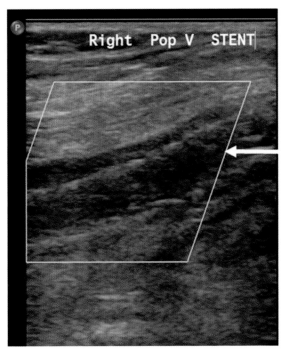

FV stent
re-occluded at
3 day f/u
Advised to continue
anti coagulation,
local wound care, and
compression

■ Fig. 18.83

Case 10: Iliac Vein Occlusion, Recanalization From Above

See Figs. 18.84–18.87.

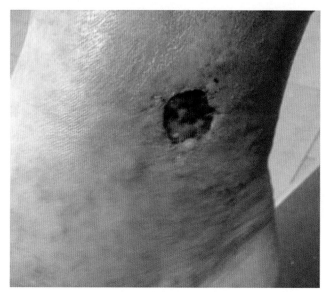

■ **Fig. 18.84** 80 yo WF recurrent postthrombotic venous ulcer. R ilio-femoral vein CTO seen on cross sectional imaging.

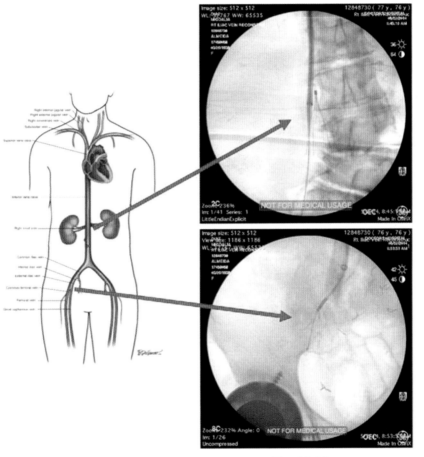

From RIJ approach,
16 FR sheath parked at
IVC confluence

5 FR Triforce system
used to cross the right
CIV from above

■ Fig. 18.85

"Body-Floss"

RIJ Access & cross R CIV from above

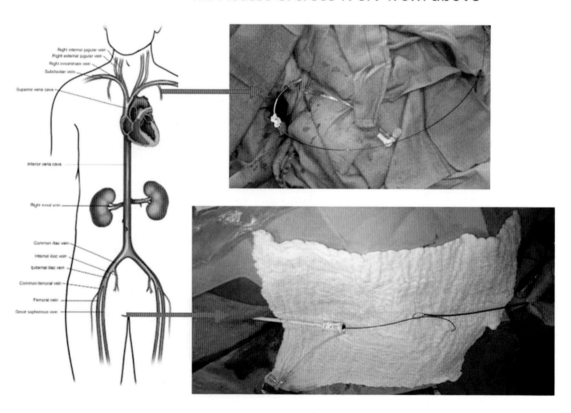

R FV Access & snare wire from below

■ Fig. 18.86

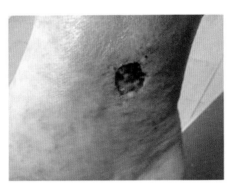

pre-stent

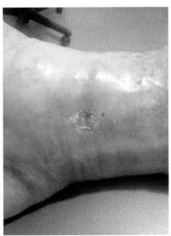

ulcer healing
post-stent

■ Fig. 18.87

Case 11: Acute DVT Treated With "One-and-Done" Rheolytic Pharmacomechanical Thrombolysis (Figs. 18.88–18.91)

A 40-year-old Caucasian female underwent left iliocaval stenting for May-Thurner syndrome 5 years earlier.

Presented 3 years ago with calf vein thrombosis; treated with anticoagulation alone for 3 months then discontinued. Now presents with right lower extremity iliofemoral deep venous thrombosis with pain and edema.

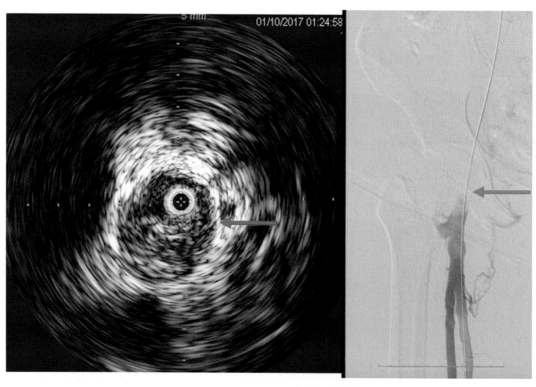

Right lower extremity venogram demonstrates patent femoral venous inflow with acute occlusion of the common femoral vein (blue arrow). IVUS shows thrombus within iliac vein system (red arrow).

■ Fig. 18.88

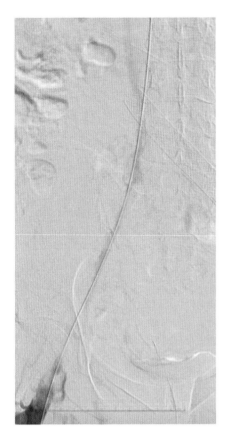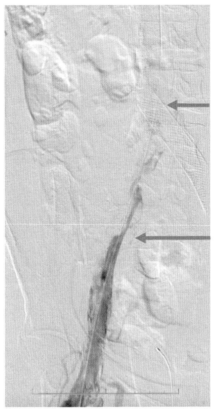

Notice right iliac vein "jailing" from previously placed left ilio-caval stent

One pass with angioJet demonstrated "acute-on-chronic" right iliofemoral venous thrombosis

■ Fig. 18.89

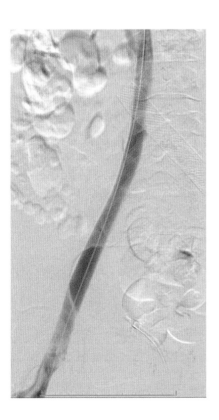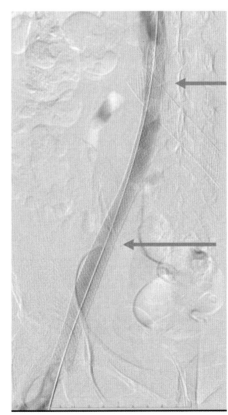

Successful restoration of flow after right side Ilio-caval stenting. Contrast leaves the Field-Of-View rapidly indicating adequate inflow and outflow.

■ Fig. 18.90

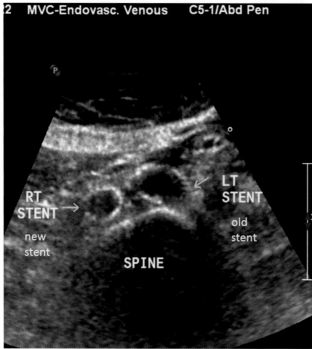

Patient seen in office 1-week post procedure. Transabdominal ultrasound imaging (transverse view) demonstrates new stent being compressed by old stent; very typical finding, because chronic stent endothelialization enhances stent rigidity. Both stents widely patent with resolution of symptoms. Patient will be maintained on lifelong anticoagulation.

■ **Fig. 18.91**

REFERENCES

1. May R, Thurner J. The cause of the predominantly sinistral occurrence of thrombosis of the pelvic veins. *Angiology.* 1957;8:419–428.
2. Cockett FB, Thomas ML. The iliac compression syndrome. *Br J Surg.* 1965;52:816–821.
3. Negus D, Fletcher EWL, Cockett FB, et al. Compression and band formation at the mouth of the left common iliac vein. *Br J Surg.* 1968;55:369–374.
4. Neglén P, Raju S. Intravascular ultrasound scan evaluation of the obstructed vein. *J Vasc Surg.* 2002;35:694–700.
5. Neglén P, Berry MA, Raju S. Endovascular surgery in the treatment of chronic primary and post-thrombotic iliac vein obstruction. *Eur J Vasc Endovasc Surg.* 2000;20:560–571.
6. Raju S, Darcey R, Neglén P. Unexpected major role for venous stenting in deep reflux disease. *J Vasc Surg.* 2010;51(2):401–408.
7. Mavor GE, Galloway JMD. Iliofemoral venous thrombosis: pathological considerations and surgical management. *Br J Surg.* 1969;56:45–59.
8. Kibbe M, Ujiki M, Lee A, et al. Iliac vein compression in an asymptomatic patient population. *J Vasc Surg.* 2004;39(5):937–943.
9. Raju R, Neglén P. High prevalence of nonthrombotic iliac vein lesions in chronic venous disease: a permissive role in pathogenicity. *J Vasc Surg.* 2006;44:136–144.
10. Raju S, Ward M Jr, Kirk O. A modification of iliac vein stent technique. *Ann Vasc Surg.* 2014;28:1485–1492.
11. Lou WS, Gu JP, He X, et al. Endovascular treatment for iliac vein compression syndrome: a comparison between the presence and absence of secondary thrombosis. *Korean J Radiol.* 2009;10:135–143.
12. Meng QY, Li XQ, Qian AM, et al. Endovascular treatment of iliac vein compression syndrome. *Chin Med J.* 2011;124:3281–3284.
13. Neglén P, Hollis KC, Olivier J, et al. Stenting of the venous outflow in chronic venous disease: long-term stent-related outcome, clinical, and hemodynamic result. *J Vasc Surg.* 2007;46:979–990.

14. Ye K, Lu X, Li W, et al. Long-term outcomes of stent placement for symptomatic nonthrombotic iliac vein compression lesions in chronic venous disease. *J Vasc Interv Radiol.* 2012;23:497–502.

15. Raju S, Neglén P. Percutaneous recanalization of total occlusions of the iliac vein. *J Vasc Surg.* 2009;50:360–368.

16. Neglén P, Darcey R, Olivier J, et al. Bilateral stenting at the iliocaval confluence. *J Vasc Surg.* 2010;51:1457–1466.

17. Raju S, Hollis K, Neglén P. Obstructive lesions of the inferior vena cava: clinical features and endovenous treatment. *J Vasc Surg.* 2006;44:820–827.

18. Rosales A, Sandbaek G, Jorgensen JJ. Stenting for chronic post-thrombotic vena cava and iliofemoral venous occlusions: mid-term patency and clinical outcome. *Eur J Vasc Endovasc Surg.* 2010;40:234–240.

19. Alhadad A, Kolbel T, Herbst A, et al. Iliocaval vein stenting: long term survey of postthrombotic symptoms and working capacity. *J Thromb Thrombolysis.* 2011;31:211–216.

20. Nayak L, Hildebolt CF, Vedantham S. Postthrombotic syndrome: feasibility of a strategy of imaging-guided endovascular intervention. *J Vasc Interv Radiol.* 2012;23:1165–1173.

21. Neglén P, Hollis KC, Olivier J, et al. Stenting of the venous outflow in chronic venous disease: long-term stent-related outcome, clinical, and hemodynamic result. *J Vasc Surg.* 2007;46:979e90.

22. Oguzkurt L, Tercan F, Ozkan U, et al. Iliac vein compression syndrome: outcome of endovascular treatment with long-term follow-up. *Eur J Radiol.* 2008;68:487–492.

23. Raju S, Buck WJ, Crim W, et al. Optimal sizing of iliac vein stents. *Phlebology.* 2017:268355517718763. [Epub ahead of print].

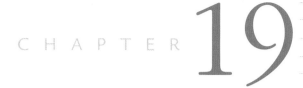

CHAPTER 19

Deep Venous Incompetence and Valve Repair

Michael C. Dalsing and Robert L. Kistner

Deep venous insufficiency and the techniques used to repair the valve damage or valve incompetence is technically challenging when compared with the treatment of superficial, perforator, and iliofemoral deep venous occlusive disease, and therefore has been relegated to a "last consideration" in the treatment of patients with advanced clinical stage disease. Whether or not this should be the case can be debated but, in practicality, this is the current state and is mainly based on consensus risk/benefit determinations.[1] If we only consider the patient with a venous ulcer as a potential candidate for deep venous valve reconstruction, approximately 2% of the 6 million US citizens with at least clinical stage 4 venous disease (C4) will progress to a venous ulcer (120,000). Medical treatment may heal 70% to 80% of venous ulcers but the recurrence rate is high and dependent on compliance.[2] My best estimate is that 50% will be recurrence free over a 3-year period, leaving about 60,000 with a venous ulcer requiring more advanced treatment.[3] The majority of patients with venous ulcers have reflux in multiple systems and treating all superficial and perforator vein insufficiency (with 89% also afflicted with deep venous insufficiency) will result in healing 80% but with a recurrence rate of 20% at 3 years.[4] This would suggest that 12,000 did not heal and that another 9600 recurred for 21,600 patients still afflicted with a chronic disabling ulcer. If we assume that 55% of these patients have associated deep venous occlusive disease amenable to iliofemoral venous stent treatment and that 60% have long-term healing,[5,6] we are left with nearly 5000 patients with deep venous insufficiency as the only uncorrected venous pathology to address. The approach to this cohort of patients must be prominent in the minds of those who care for such patients, or these patients will be deprived of a critical treatment opportunity because of sheer physician ignorance. These estimates are intentionally conservative, so it is certainly important to keep venous valve repair in our treatment toolbox. At least 20 surgeons adept at deep venous reconstruction would be required to treat these patients if each performed 250 operations yearly. If we add those with advanced C4b tissue changes and incapacitating swelling because of venous reflux to those with actual ulceration, the numbers increase significantly.

NORMAL CONDITION: EMPHASIS ON LOWER EXTREMITY DEEP VENOUS VALVES

Anatomy

The lower extremity deep venous system with consistent valve presence begins in the foot and ceases at the inguinal ligament. The deep veins lie within the investing fascia of the muscles of the leg and thigh. The anterior tibial, posterior tibial, and peroneal veins are most often dual interconnected veins and follow the like-named arteries. The anterior tibial veins are found in the anterior compartment whereas the posterior tibial and peroneal veins lie within the deep posterior compartment (Fig. 19.1). The anterior tibial veins and closely associated deep peroneal nerve lie between the tibialis anterior and extensor digitorum longus muscles in the proximal leg. The posterior tibial and peroneal veins lie within a rather-thin fascial layer between the superficial and deep posterior muscle groups and, in the upper extent, lie on the tibialis posterior muscle in close association with the tibial nerve. The posterior tibial and peroneal veins can join shortly before joining with the anterior tibial veins as it penetrates the tough interosseous membrane and becomes the popliteal vein(s) (PVs), which can be dual and reside near the popliteal artery (see Fig. 19.1). The popliteal vein(s) lie(s) behind the knee, can interconnect around the artery, and are noted anterior to the oblique popliteal ligament and popliteus muscle and is surrounded by a small fat pad. The gastrocnemius muscles are positioned laterally and medially, with the hamstrings more cephalad. The tibial nerve runs within this space whereas the common peroneal nerve lies laterally and cephalad, spiraling around the biceps insertion to reach the lateral aspect of the leg. The small saphenous vein may join the PV within this space. The popliteal vein(s) become the femoral vein(s) (FV) as the vein(s) pass(es) through the adductor magnus where it/they split(s) to form the adductor hiatus (see Fig. 19.1). The distal connection with the deep femoral vein (DFV) is a constant finding near this location. Two layers of tough fascia separate the quadriceps of the thigh from the adductors medially and hamstrings posteriorly. Superficially, there is an additional piece of fascia separating vastus medialis from adductors and above that the sartorius muscle. The vessels run within this fascial sling. The FV(s) rest in the deep fascia, deep to the sartorius muscle

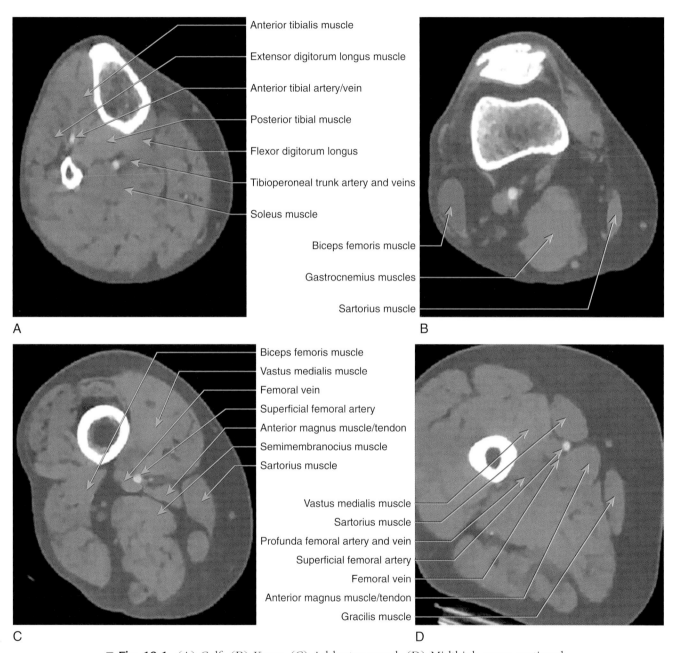

Anterior tibialis muscle

Extensor digitorum longus muscle

Anterior tibial artery/vein

Posterior tibial muscle

Flexor digitorum longus

Tibioperoneal trunk artery and veins

Soleus muscle

Biceps femoris muscle

Gastrocnemius muscles

Sartorius muscle

Biceps femoris muscle
Vastus medialis muscle
Femoral vein
Superficial femoral artery
Anterior magnus muscle/tendon
Semimembranocius muscle
Sartorius muscle

Vastus medialis muscle
Sartorius muscle
Profunda femoral artery and vein
Superficial femoral artery
Femoral vein
Anterior magnus muscle/tendon
Gracilis muscle

A

B

C

D

■ **Fig. 19.1** (A) Calf. (B) Knee. (C) Adductor canal. (D) Midthigh cross-sectional computed tomography to demonstrate anatomy.

while flanked by the vastus medialis and adductor longus muscles (Fig. 19.2). The inguinal ligament marks the transition from common femoral vein (CFV) to external iliac veins, and the vessels lie beneath the midpoint of the inguinal ligament. In the groin, the femoral vessels lie in the femoral sheath and are flanked laterally by the sartorius muscle and medially by the adductor longus muscle (see Fig. 19.2). The fascia lata forms an anterior roof over the femoral triangle and an opening in this fascia allows the lymphatics and great saphenous vein (GSV) to enter. The DFV joins the FV to form the CFV about 1 cm below the inguinal ligament.

The axillary vein lies below the lateral margin of the first rib and above the lateral edge of the teres major muscle. It lies on the subscapularis muscle with the lowest segment resting on the teres major and latissimus dorsi insertions. It resides in a cleft formed by muscles originating in the scapula with medial wall being the serratus anterior muscle. The coracoid process lies over the axillary neurovascular bundle and some of the muscle which overlay the neurovascular bundle attach to it. The pectoralis minor

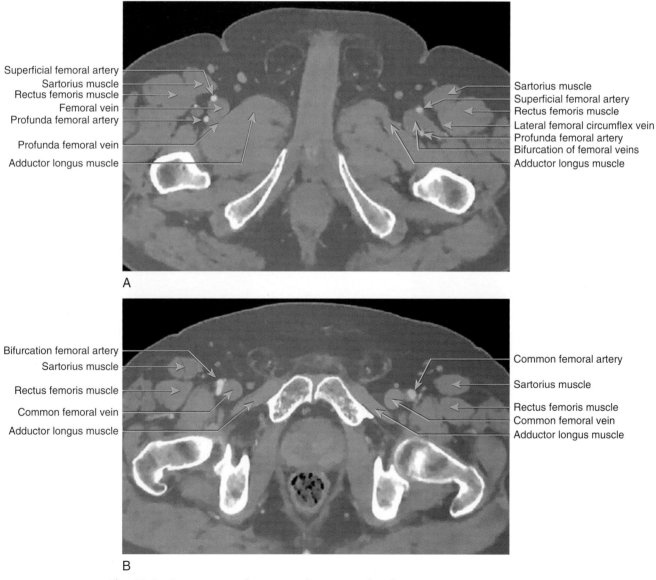

Superficial femoral artery
Sartorius muscle
Rectus femoris muscle
Femoral vein
Profunda femoral artery

Profunda femoral vein

Adductor longus muscle

Sartorius muscle
Superficial femoral artery
Rectus femoris muscle
Lateral femoral circumflex vein
Profunda femoral artery
Bifurcation of femoral veins
Adductor longus muscle

A

Bifurcation femoral artery
Sartorius muscle

Rectus femoris muscle

Common femoral vein
Adductor longus muscle

Common femoral artery

Sartorius muscle

Rectus femoris muscle
Common femoral vein
Adductor longus muscle

B

■ **Fig. 19.2** Cross-sectional computed tomography demonstrating anatomy at groin. (A) Caudal. (B) Cephalad.

muscle, which lies directly over the bundle separates the vein and artery into three parts. The pectoralis major is the most superficial covering whereas the vein parallels the cora-cobrachialis and short head of the biceps brachii. The brachial vein lies below and within a fascial sheath, which when entered allows displacement of the biceps brachii and triceps muscles exposing the vessels because the vessels run in a parallel fashion with these muscles. Same named arteries and associated nerves lie in close proximity. This anatomy is included because it becomes important when considering a venous valve transplantation operation.

Venous valves are thin but very strong connective tissue structures with minimal muscular media covered by endothelium and are generally bicuspid in nature (Fig. 19.3). The tibial and peroneal veins typically have 3 to 12 valves present in each.[7] The majority of popliteal veins have one to three valves, with a tendency to be located more caudal within the vein.[7] The FV has one to five valves, and in approximately 90% of patients, the most constant valve is located proximally within 1 to 2 cm of joining the DFV.[7–9] About 90% of DFVs will have venous valves and some have up to four present.[7] Only 30% to 50% of CFVs have a valve, but in those that do, there may be one or even two valves within a few centimeters of the inguinal ligament.[7–9] Rarely does the external iliac vein have a valve present (~25%), and the common iliac vein lacks a venous valve in most cases.[10] The GSV usually contains more than six valves (4–25), and at least one of these is within a few centimeters of the saphenofemoral junction.[11] Axillary veins have at least one valve, with about 70% having a second, and 30% or less having one-third more distally located valve.[12]

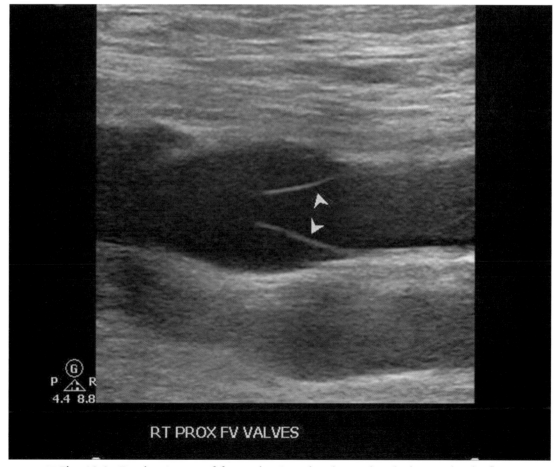

■ **Fig. 19.3** Duplex image of femoral vein valve (*arrowheads* show valve leaflets in semi-open position with valve sinuses on opposite side).

Physiology

Dynamic duplex imaging has demonstrated that the large intramuscular veins (femoral[s]/popliteal), are supported on all sides by connective tissue, and therefore, when subjected to changes in volume, expand or collapse in direct response to those changes and in a circular manner. There compliance curves mimic those of an artery in that pressure changes reflect volume changes, they act as conduits rather than compliance vessels. The vein valves are not crushed together when the vein empties as might be expected in a completely compliant vessel. The valves within the vein function on a four-phase cycle consisting of opening, equilibrium, closing, and closed.[13] After opening, the equilibrium phase demonstrates separation occurring at the valve edge on duplex imaging and the flow splits into two streams, with one directed into the valve sinus possibly to prevent stasis (clot prevention). When maximally open, the two cusps create a 35% narrowing of the outflow tract, which might aid in overall flow.[13] Most of the time, the valve is in the open position. Valve closure normally occurs rapidly in response to the loss of the forward pressure/flow gradient and less so to retrograde blood flow. In fact, in normally functioning valves, closure is likely instantaneous without reverse blood flow noted.[14] In clinical practice when evaluated by duplex imaging, the precise location of the valve is often not known and so reverse flow as an estimate of normal valve closure time is less than 500 ms for the deep femoral and tibial veins, although slightly longer for the FV and popliteal vein at 1 second.[15,16] The hemodynamic result of a normal functioning venous system, both as conduit for blood to return to the heart and with valve function to prevents reflux, is decreased venous blood pooling and prevention of sustained/consistent high venous pressures in the lower leg when in the erect position.

DISEASED CONDITION: INSUFFICIENCY IN THE LOWER LEG VENOUS SYSTEM

Etiology/Pathology

The rare patient may congenitally lack vein valves.[17] In primary venous insufficiency, the valve may be structurally normal but floppy or redundant; the vein diameter may be enlarged preventing cusp apposition; or asymmetric insertion or development may result in a malfunctioning valve.[18–21] There is no clear inciting event for the changes noted and except for developmentally defective valves, tightening of the valve leaflets can reestablish function.

In contradistinction to primary venous insufficiency described earlier, secondary venous insufficiency has an inciting event, which is often acute venous thrombosis. The associated inflammation can result in scarring following recanalization demonstrated as valve fibrosis, foreshortening, perforation, and wall adhesion in a potential environment of luminal narrowing (Fig. 19.4).[18] The valve leaflets are not repairable and other options to reestablish a lower extremity deep venous system free of reflux is required. Because acute thrombosis and recanalization is variable in extent and resolution, there are conditions in which a valve is preserved either within a normal vein segment or within a damaged shrunken vein, potentially the result of isolated wall scarring.[18,22–24]

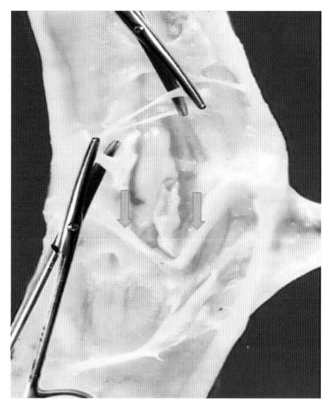

■ **Fig. 19.4** Scarring, webs (being cut), and foreshortening of the valve *(arrows)* after venous thrombosis and recanalization.

Pathophysiology

Unrelieved ambulatory venous hypertension in the lower leg (especially in the gaiter area) is a major factor causing the signs and symptoms of chronic venous disease (CVD).[1,25] Correcting free reflux into the lower leg by even one competent valve has demonstrated clinical improvement for prolonged periods as long as that valve remained competent. This has been demonstrated by the results of valve repair preformed for this condition and will be reviewed in detail later in this chapter. The anatomic fact that the popliteal vein is directly connected to both the FV and DFV establishes it in a unique position as "gatekeeper" for reflux into the lower leg. This is clearly demonstrated by the fact that an isolated FV valve repair may clinically fail if the deep femoral system is also incompetent (free reflux into the popliteal and then the lower leg), although isolated femoral repair will be successful when the deep femoral valve(s) is/are competent.[26,27] FV occlusion may result in significant DFV dilation, such that correction of reflux in the DFV will dramatically improve venous hemodynamics.[28] Alternatively, preventing reflux through the DFV (gatekeeper) can correct significant axial insufficiency into the lower leg and has been associated with delayed healing when not addressed.[29–32] Repairing multiple tibial vein valves can have a similar effect.[33]

THE CLINICAL EVALUATION: CLINICAL; ETIOLOGIC; ANATOMIC; PATHOPHYSIOLOGIC

Typical Diagnostic Evaluation

A history and physical examination with handheld Doppler examination of lower leg veins (level of investigation 1) can provide an idea of the etiology of the patient's condition[34] and rule out other causes of the patient's symptoms. Patients considered for venous valve surgery should have symptomatic advanced disease: C3 (unrelenting edema), C4 (skin damage), C5 (healed venous ulcer), or C6 (active venous ulcer).

When considering a deep venous valve repair, a more in-depth evaluation is essential for clarifying your patient's precise anatomic situation and planning the appropriate operation. A complete noninvasive venous duplex evaluation that typically includes plethysmography (level of investigation 2) is essential in determining the location of reflux, which specific veins are involved, and provides some indication of overall lower extremity hemodynamic effects attributable to the insufficiency present.[1,15,34] Assuming that other venous systems in the lower extremity are functionally normal or have been corrected by intervention before considering a valve repair, this investigation specifically defines the deep venous system. Prolonged reflux time (valve closure time), after a provocative test (compression distal to the femoral junction) conducted in the standing position and throughout the deep venous system, is standard protocol for determining reflux.[35,36] Although some studies have demonstrated that 1 second or more should be the cut-off abnormal value for the FV and popliteal vein, current consensus suggests that a valve closure time 0.5 second or more is best considered abnormal for all vein segments.[37] Venous duplex imaging is variably capable of valve visualization to determine cusp presence and its function or lack thereof (see Fig. 19.3). Venous plethysmography is not a routine study in standard clinical practice but adds some insight into differentiation between hemodynamic reflux and obstruction when considering a deep venous valve repair. It also provides the potential to demonstrate quantitative improvement after repair.[38,39] It may help to establish the effect an abnormal calf pump function may have on the patient's condition.[40,41] The ejection volume and residual volume fraction are good indicators of calf muscle pump function and are abnormal when the ejection volume is less than 60% and the residual volume fraction is greater than 35%. The residual volume fraction reflects the ambulatory venous pressure quite well.[42,43]

Advancement to the third level of investigation includes invasive venography and is recommended before valve repair.[34] Descending venography provides detail of valve anatomy and the degree of reflux within the deep system.[44] Kistner used a four-grade system with grade 4 (the most severe) involving reflux down the entire lower leg venous system, whereas grade 3 reflux went through the popliteal vein during descending venographic evaluation. Both are considered for valve repair. Visualization and interrogation of the DFV is an important component of this investigation as a potential alternate source of axial reflux and an indication for valve repair within the DFV itself or placement of the valve in the popliteal vein rather than the upper FV. The success of FV valve repair depends upon elimination of axial reflux by all axial routes, including femoral-popliteal, deep femoral-popliteal, and other random anatomic pathways. Descending venography is not perfect,[18] but when paired with duplex imaging and ascending venography is the best available preoperative diagnostic combination to define repairable, deep venous reflux. Ascending venography provides some anatomic detail of segmental obstructions and the opportunity to measure ambulatory venous pressure as an estimate of venous insufficiency.[45] Computed tomographic imaging and magnetic resonance imaging are performed in the supine position, which renders the study unreliable for valve anatomy and function, although such can be useful to rule out other cause of venous pathology.

These anatomic and functional investigations lead to a precise determination of your patient's current venous pathologic state to be compared with a complete clinical application of CEAP (clinical, etiologic, anatomic, pathophysiologic) including full determination of clinical presentation (with or without symptoms), etiology, anatomy involved, and pathophysiology by anatomic segment.[34,46] Included in the classification is the level of investigation (potentially 3) and the date of investigation. Integral to demonstrating success after an intervention, it is helpful to have a baseline physician determined disease severity score (Venous Clinical Severity Score) and a patient-estimated impact on life and functional status score (Quality of Life survey[s]).[47,48] Measurement of clinical and pathologic status using current assessment tools (for planned venous interventions) can be given a grade 1 recommendation.[1,15]

OPERATIVE INTERVENTION

Routine Operative Considerations

General anesthesia is generally required for these open procedures, which can be technically challenging and therefore lengthy. Confirmation of respiratory and cardiac stability for a safe operative intervention and the elimination of arterial occlusive disease as a confounding issue, especially in a patient with an ulcer, are highly recommended.[1] A patient with diabetes, renal failure, or collagen vascular disorders requires optimal medical treatment before operative intervention. Perioperative antibiotics are frequently used (first-generation cephalosporin) and heparin is recommended for open vein procedures, so allergies must be considered.

Operative Exposure

The exposure of the lower extremity veins mimics that used for exposure of the associated artery. If reconstruction of the proximal FV or DFV is planned, a generous groin incision (Fig. 19.5A) is made in the direction of the vessels to expose the first and second femoral valves. Extending the dissection distally through the fascia will allow lateral displacement of the sartorius muscle and exposure of a longer length of either vein as needed (Fig. 19.5B). Ligate any apparent lymphatic chains to prevent postoperative lymphocele or lymph leak. To determine if valve cusps are present and to allow later valve repair, dissection of the vein's adventitial layer is critical (Fig. 19.6). It will allow confirmation of a valve (which may have been missed on primary imaging) or determine the lack of a valve in cases where one was thought present. A lack of clear valve attachment lines signifies high likelihood of significant postthrombotic valve damage and suggests that

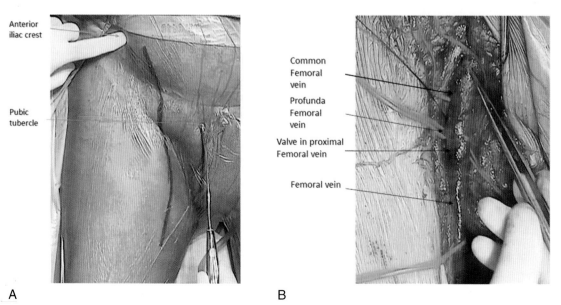

A   B

■ **Fig. 19.5** (A) Incision for femoral vein exposure. (B) Femoral vein exposed and branches controlled.

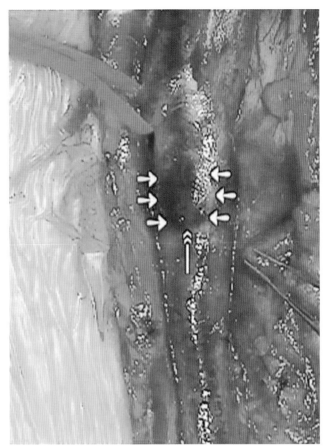

■ **Fig. 19.6** Adventitial dissection allows clear outline of white line of valve attachment to vein wall dissected before vein opening (note *double-headed arrow* is bottom of valve attachment; other *arrows* outline valve attachment from outside vein).

techniques other than in situ repair will be required for success. This incision also provides exposure of the lower CFV, proximal FV, and DFV as needed for valve transposition, transplantation, or other less-conventional valve reconstructions. The GSV insertion into the FV is also within this field and medial dissection in the subcutaneous tissues will quickly expose its proximal extent and associated branches.

Distal femoral, proximal popliteal, or even tibial veins can be exposed through medial incisions as one would use to expose the associated artery. Detailed descriptions of these exposures are available for review.[49] The best exposure to the popliteal vein is a posterior S-shaped incision with the transverse incision made in the posterior knee crease to decrease the chance of scar contraction.[49] Bear in mind the associated nerves (as noted in the anatomy section), which are prone to iatrogenic injury in this confined area of dissection.

Following the generous dissection of the target vein with valve within, the "strip test" is used to determine valve incompetence. The strip test is performed by occluding antegrade venous blood flow (finger compression or instrument) distal to the valve and pushing the trapped blood into the vein above the valve. If flow into the empty vein below the valve is observed upon applying pressure on the vein above the valve, valve incompetence is confirmed. If the valve is totally competent, the segment above the valve balloons out and the segment below the valve remains collapsed.

Treatment Option 1

When valve cusps are structurally intact within the incompetent venous system of interest, the specific operative technique to use in any given case is determined by the degree of valve prolapse, surgeon preference/experience, and expected long-term success. Intraoperative vasospasm resulting in a competent valve at the time of open surgical exposure (potential wall dilation as the underlying issue) may suggest change of the surgical technique to an external valve repair or external banding as a reasonable option.[50] With more prominent wall dilation, external valvuloplasty may provide the less-invasive, yet functional, outcome. For severe valve leaflet prolapse or as the "go to" procedure (based on best outcome as discussed later), internal valvuloplasty may be the appropriate option.

External Banding

An exoskeleton of synthetic (e.g., dacron, polytetrafluoroethylene) is wrapped circumferentially around the vein at the valve site and then tightened to reduce the diameter of the vein lumen, thereby realizing valve competence.[31,51,52] To avoid sleeve slippage, the synthetic is anchored in place to the adventitia. One investigator used a spiral device screwed around the outside of the vein, which decreased the diameter until valve competence was determined by endoscopic inspection.[53]

External Valvuloplasty

The technique of external valvuloplasty, pioneered by Kistner in the late 1980s, is demonstrated in Fig. 19.7A and B.[54] The advantage is valve repair without venotomy, the latter risks cusp damage on opening. External valvuloplasty is performed with an interrupted or a running transmurally placed, fine Prolene suture through the valve attachment lines and, when tied causing a decreased vein diameter, decreased commissural angle, and ultimately a competent valve. Both anterior and/or posterior plications can result in clinical success, and the same is true when performed with or without angioscopic guidance.[55–57] Raju and colleagues' method of transcommissural valvuloplasty stresses the need for identifying the valve cusp attachment lines and full thickness suture placement placed less obliquely as the repair proceeds caudally and directed by the line of cusp demarcation.[58] A continuous suture can also be used to accomplish this repair.[59] A limited anterior plication involves anterior vein dissection only and placement of a running mattress suture at the anterior commissure, which runs from a point 3 to 4 mm proximal to the angle of the valve cusp insertion lines up to the angle of the valve cusp insertion and incorporates about 3 mm of the vein wall.[60] The last option has been most studied in association with a simultaneously performed saphenous vein stripping and limited to the FV valve.

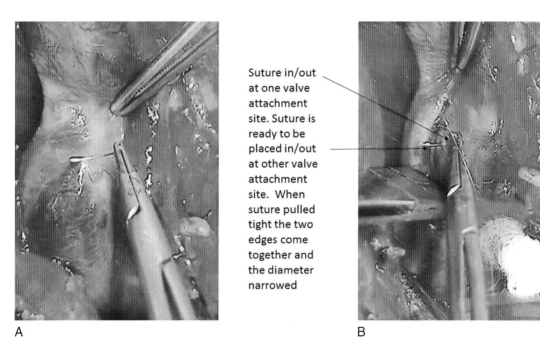

A   B

■ **Fig. 19.7** External valvuloplasty. (A) Start suture in and out at proximal most attachment site (tie). (B) Approximate in caudal manner by placing suture at valve attachment site (in/out) on side and same on other to narrow the vein diameter and close the valve cusp gap.

Internal Valvuloplasty

The open method of direct valve cusp tightening (reefing) involves a venotomy (Figs. 19.8A–C and 19.9A) to expose the incompetent valve (Fig. 19.9B). Fig. 19.8A depicts a marking suture placed to mark precisely where the two leaflets meet and is placed before opening the vein. This suture is a marking suture to guide the venotomy between the valve cusps because the venotomy must be precise to avoid damage to the delicate valve leaflets (see Fig. 19.8B and C). The reefing sutures to shorten the valve cusps consist of interrupted 6 or 7 polypropylene suture, which penetrate the external vein at the commissural attachment; when inside the vein, the suture penetrates the valve leaflet (full thickness), and then exits the vein near the site of initial insertion. Figs. 19.10 and 19.11 demonstrate the steps used to reef the anterior valve leaflet on one end. This can be accomplished on both sides at the site of vein opening with similar sutures placed until the cusps are tightened appropriately. Fig. 19.11 demonstrates the steps required to tighten the valve leaflets (both sides simultaneously because the vein wall is closed)

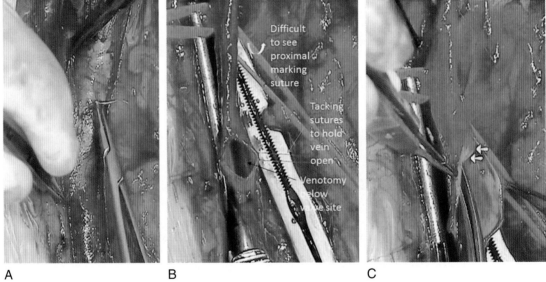

A   B   C

■ **Fig. 19.8** Internal valvuloplasty. (A) Suture placement to mark proximal edge where two valve leaflets meet. (B) Vein opened and tacking sutured placed to hold open. (C) Extending incision proximally along commissure (*arrows* show valve just coming to view).

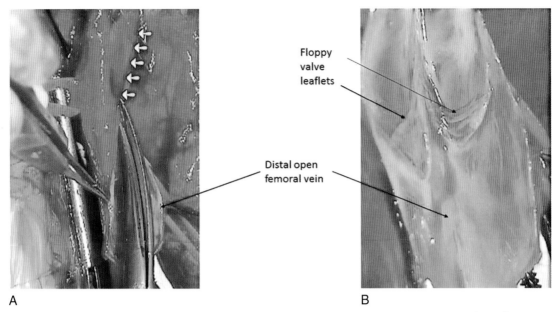

■ **Fig. 19.9** Internal valvuloplasty. (A) Open vein to mark suture where edge of both valves meet proximally. (B) Floppy valve leaflets, intact on both sides.

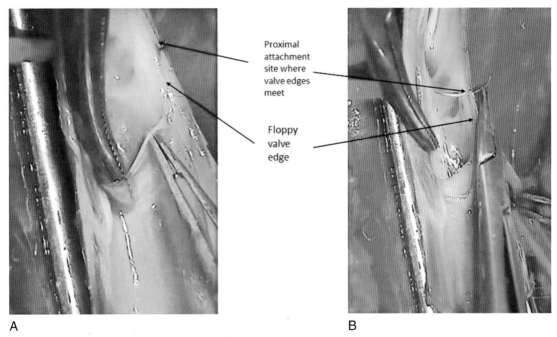

■ **Fig. 19.10** Internal valvuloplasty. (A) Floppy valve, thin, edge well defined and intact. (B) Initial suture to reef valve, suture needle placed outside in at proximal attachment site.

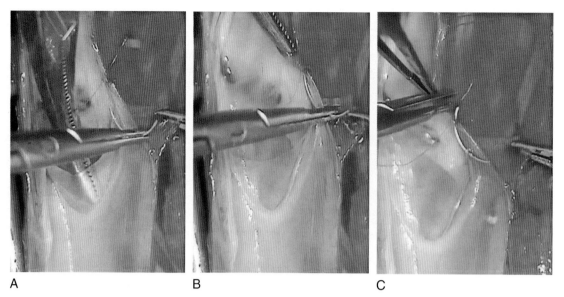

A   B   C

■ **Fig. 19.11** Internal valvuloplasty. (A) Suture into the valve leaflet slightly away from wall. (B) Inside out at original suture placement. (C) Pull needle through and tie to tighten cusp.

on the posterior wall. Figs. 19.8 to 19.12 show the original method of Kistner (circa 1968) as performed by him through a longitudinal venotomy extending through and past the valve commissure.[61]

Alternative valve repair techniques have been described and reported in large series. Raju used a transverse venotomy performed at least 2.5 cm above the valve, providing a view down into the valve, with suture(s) placed to tighten the valve leaflets (Fig. 19.13).[62] Sottiurai used a combination T-shaped venotomy with transverse incision above the valve and distal extension into the valve sinus.[63] Creating an incision above and below the valve with transverse incision through the site of common origin of the cusps, a "trap door" approach, has been reported by Tripathi and Ktenidis.[64]

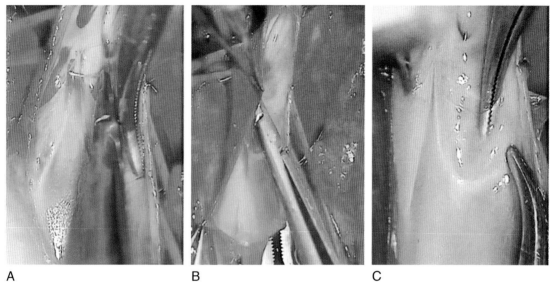

■ **Fig. 19.12** Internal valvuloplasty. Reefing of valve, posterior vein (A) suture placed outside in at proximal attachment site, take individual edge of each valve slightly away from vein wall (separate bites). (B) Place suture inside out at original site of suture placement and tie (valves tight and flat on wall). (C) Operative picture of completed valve reefing with nonfloppy valve leaflet present and held open by hemostat.

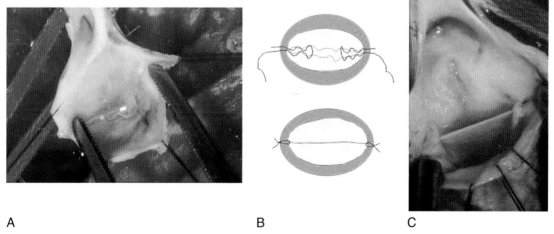

■ **Fig. 19.13** Internal valvuloplasty (Raju method). (A) Transverse opening, viewing floppy valve in depth (operative photo). (B) Running suture of about one-fifth of valve length on both sides (top), tied to tighten valve. (C) Reefed valve (operative photo).

Regardless of the exposure, the ultimate goal of suture placement is to tighten the valve and produce competent valve function. A running suture can be used to reef the valve (see Fig. 19.13) rather than an interrupted approach, or a combination thereof may be required to obtain the desired result. Reefing approximately 20% of the length of the valve leaflet can restore valve competency in most cases.[65] At the completion of the procedure and with vein closed, a repeat strip test demonstrates valve competency (Fig. 19.14).

Treatment Option 2

When there is no in situ valve available for repair, alternative approaches have been designed to obtain the goal of preventing free reflux of blood from heart to calf without interruption when ambulating. Rerouting of the incompetent axial systems distal to a competent valve, transplanting a functional venous valve containing segment from the upper extremity into the incompetent system, or fashioning an autogenous valve substitute have been the alternatives reported to be successful.

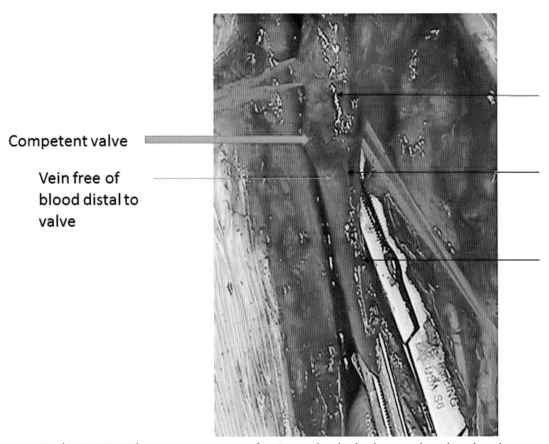

Competent valve

Vein free of blood distal to valve

■ **Fig. 19.14** Valve now competent after internal valvuloplasty, valve closed and strip test preformed (*black arrows* show suture line closure of vein).

Valve Transposition

The presence of a single competent proximal leg valve provides the opportunity to perform a valve transposition procedure, which positions the incompetent axial venous system distal to that competent valve. The most common clinical scenario is a femoral system devoid of competent valves while a deep femoral valve remains competent. The incompetent FV can be transected and implanted distal to the competent DFV valve in an end-to-end or end-to-side fashion (Fig. 19.15). A competent valve in the GSV can serve as a similar surrogate valve. Alternatively, incompetency of the deep femoral system can be compensated for by placing it below a competent valve in the FV or the GSV. The size discrepancy of the GSV and FV has been addressed by using an end-to-side reconstruction of femoral to saphenous vein with ligation of the proximal FV below the deep femoral orifice to allow maximal outflow and prevent reflux in the FV.[66]

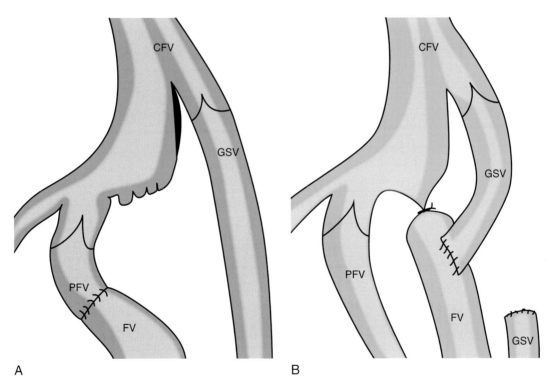

■ **Fig. 19.15** Valve transposition. (A) Incompetent femoral vein (FV) transposed below a competent profunda femoral vein, (B) Great saphenous vein (GSV) anastomosis end-to-side to incompetent FV and proximal ligation to prevent reflux into FV with protection by GSV valve. *CFV,* Common femoral vein; *PFV,* profunda femoral vein.

Valve Transplantation

When no available valves are present in the incompetent lower leg venous system(s), using a competent valved vein segment from the upper extremity, which can be transplanted into the lower leg incompetent axial system is a viable option (Fig. 19.16A and B) first described by Taheri and his group.[67] A 2-cm-long to 3-cm-long axillary or brachial vein with competent valve is first removed as the donor valve. In some cases, a contralateral GSV or small saphenous vein segment containing a competent valve can be used.[68] In general, a damaged-free segment of incompetent FV is exposed below the takeoff of the DFV, and the donor valve sewn in place with fine interrupted Prolene sutures after removal of a corresponding length of FV to allow accommodation for the donor vein length.[65] This last step prevents redundancy and kinking. By performing the proximal anastomosis first, release of the proximal clamp will confirm donor valve competency while distending and lengthening of the vein to facilitate completion of the distal anastomosis. In trabeculated, postthrombotic veins, excision of intraluminal synechiae to create a single lumen and more suitable recipient bed has been described with success.[69] Following repair, some surgeons have placed an external band to prevent later dilation and valve failure.[56,65,70] If the donor valve is found to be incompetent after transplantation as determined by proximal clamp release or postimplantation strip test, valvuloplasty may be required and can be performed as a bench repair if known before implantation.[56,65,71] The best valve available should be sought and harvested before resorting to this extra step in the repair.

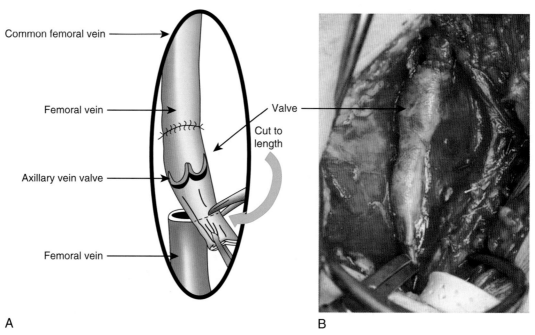

A   B

■ **Fig. 19.16** Valve transplant. (A) Artist depiction of valve transplant. (B) Operative photo. *(Courtesy Dr. Raju).*

Valve Substitutes

Autogenous valve replacement has been made by using a piece of autogenous vein wall to make a semilunar cusp(s) sewn into the recipient vein. They have functioned successfully in one small series. Valve cusps are made by trimming the adventitia and part of the media from the vein wall and then suturing the tissue into a leaflet design with nonendothelial surface directed toward the lumen.[56] Plagnol and associates used the stump of the GSV invaginated into the FV to fashion a bicuspid valve generally in conjunction with saphenous vein stripping.[72] To date, neither study has been repeated for confirmation of the technique.

Maleti and colleagues use an ophthalmic knife to make a cut into the media (half or nearly circumferential) and, with elevation of flaps, fashion one or two cusps after opening the incompetent and postphlebitic vein.[73,74] Recent experience demonstrating valve collapse with failure resulted in adding the placement of two sutures to hold the valve in the semi-open position and improve neovalve competence in the long term (Fig. 19.17). Very informative illustrations and images can be found in a recent review by the inventor.[75,76] This work has been verified.[77]

A hybrid approach, invented by Opie, invaginates a cuboidal cut piece of the vein wall attached at its caudal edge into the vein lumen with two sutures attached to the cephalad edge to prevent complete reflux of the flap into the distal vein on standing. The defect in the vein is repaired with a flexible specially designed polytetrafluoroethylene patch, thereby forming a monocusp valve.[78] It is difficult to explain how the valve can prevent all reflux, because it is open on both sides, but its effects are reported to be sufficient to have a clinical result. Investigators from Russia have used the technique with some success.[79]

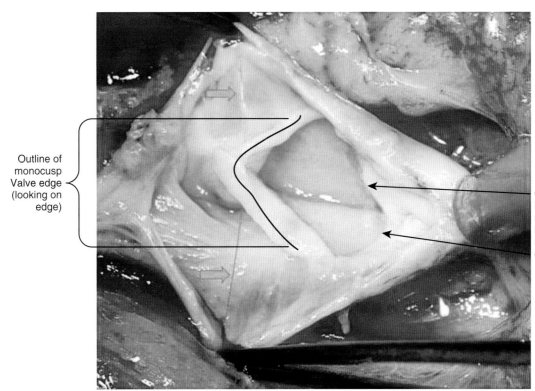

Outline of monocusp Valve edge (looking on edge)

Ophthalmic knife used to make a flap into the media and elevate a flap

■ **Fig. 19.17** Neovalve. Monocusp design with sutures to hold valve in semi-open position *(arrows)*. *(Courtesy Dr. Oscar Maleti).*

POSTOPERATIVE CARE

Pneumatic compression devices can aid in decreasing swelling, the risk of deep venous thrombosis (DVT), and increase the flow in the sedentary patient across the valve repair.[58,70,80–82] Therapeutic or low-dose heparin is generally administered postoperatively, and therefore some surgeons place a drain to control postoperative drainage, which could result in a hematoma or seroma formation. The use of therapeutic anticoagulation post valve repair is quite variable and for some surgeons is only provided after open valvuloplasty.[60,81] When therapeutic anticoagulation is deemed appropriate, one investigator starts warfarin on postoperative day 1 with an initial target international normalized ratio (INR) of 2 to 2.5 for the first 6 weeks, then subsequently decreased to a target INR of 1.7 to 2 for an additional 4 months at which point it is stopped.[58] Some surgeons use "minidose" warfarin, 1 to 2.5 mg per day, for long-term anticoagulation.[56] Others use warfarin at therapeutic levels for 3[70,80,82–84] or 6 months.[85] One investigator uses therapeutic low-molecular-weight heparin for 3 months.[59] None of these alternatives have been tested with comparative studies. Most surgeons encourage the use of compressive support after venous valve surgery, but many patients do not comply and yet experience good clinical outcomes.[18,86]

Routine Follow-Up

Typical clinical follow-up includes a history and physical examination at 2 to 6 weeks, 3 to 9 months, and then annually. During each visit, venous duplex ultrasonography determines valve site patency and valve competence as well as any changes in other components of the venous system since the last evaluation. Noninvasive testing has generally replaced descending venography, which was often used in earlier series.[81,86] Surgeons have often included some type of hemodynamic assessment.[51,52,58,80,82–85] If pain and swelling are symptom components, some have used a visual analogue score or assessment to determine success.[58,60,70] Reclassification by the CEAP criteria, venous severity scoring, and use of quality of life assessment tools are encouraged to provide quantifiable parameters of clinical success.

RESULTS

Early Results

Valve repair series of all varieties have reported no mortality and a low, associated morbidity.[56,58,60,70,83,85,87,88] Although somewhat higher in series reporting the use of more intense anticoagulation, hematoma and seroma formation has been noted in 15% or less of cases.[58,65,70,80,82,83,86,89] Although of great concern, most investigators have observed a clinical DVT rate of less than 10%.[51,56,58,65,70,80,86,89] In one report, the venographic rate of DVT studied 2 days after valve repair was quoted to be about 20% but the thrombus noted was often nonocclusive, not extensive and had no reported clinical sequelae.[82] The etiologic basis of the underlying venous insufficiency is associated with the risk of postoperative DVT in one in-depth study being observed in only 6.7% of those with primary disease and 25.4% in patients treated for the postthrombotic disease.[83] Catheter-directed thrombolysis resulted in complete thrombus clearing in 60% of these cases and resulted in a functioning valve in 50% (one of two cases).[58] Pulmonary embolism is rarely reported but, in one series, one of 129 patients did experience this complication.[58] Wound infections have been reported in 1% to 7% of cases.[56,58,65,70,83,86] The overall 30-day postoperative vein patency for all types of repairs is excellent, with some isolated events of early failure, but even when reported was overall less than 1% of all cases.[56,58] Valve leaflet trauma can occur especially when venotomy is a component of the operation, seven cases were reported by one investigator.[83] Repair with fine Prolene suture resulted in four of seven valves competent at 2 years.

Late Results: Option 1

External Banding

The prosthetic sleeve method of valve repair has achieved acceptable results in selected patients with less advanced disease or even when venospasm does not necessarily result in competence.[31,51] If even one wrapped, valved vein segment remains competent, 86% of those with a venous ulcer will obtain long-term healing at 7 years.[51] Another group confined banding to the proximal FV valve in patients with grade 3 or grade 4 reflux and only in those in whom the DFV was competent. They reported a 78% competency rate and symptom relief at 4 years.[52]

External Valvuloplasty

External valvuloplasty may be a less durable repair than open valvuloplasty.[31] Much of the current reports involving external valvuloplasty have involved the repair of multiple valves in the same patient, which can confuse interpretation per valve repair. As an example, transcommissural valve repair of 179 valves in 141 limbs demonstrated a competence rate of 63%, with clinical improvement in about 70% of cases at 3 years.[58] Another series reported a 3-year and 5-year competency rate of 64% and 52% respectively in 17 patients, but many patients had multistation or multilevel repairs.[59]

Internal Valvuloplasty

Kistner and colleagues have monitored their patients who required internal valvuloplasty for decades and have reported a symptom relief rate of greater than 81% by life-table analysis. Of the 22 patients for which actual valve competence was determined long-term, 73% were competent.[86] Valves are competent in 60% to 70% of patients at 5 years in most series, and fortunately, there are many such experiences. This is, by far, the best studied of the venous valve repairs and has demonstrated consistent findings from multiple investigators. In general, a patent and competent valve translates into clinical improvement, whereas the reverse results in recurrent symptoms.[26,31,62,64,80,82–84,88,90–92]

Late Results: Option 2

Valve Transposition

Some 40% to 50% of those patients amenable to valve transposition have experienced good clinical results at 5 years of follow-up.[27,66,86,90,92,93] A recent review, specifically addressing those with venous ulcers as the indication for surgery, summarizes the current experience.[1] The method of placing a large femoral system below a competent great saphenous valve with ligation to offset the size discrepancy has resulted in 55% of patients being free of ulcers at 10 years in one series.[66]

Valve Transplantation

Clinical improvement is seen in about 50% of patients, even at 8 years of follow-up, and it remains a viable option in cases in which other options are not possible.[29,30,62,65,67,92–98] The use of GSV or small saphenous vein valve transplants provide a similar result at 3 and 7 years.[68]

Venous Valve Substitutes

The Plagnol type of valve has clinical results reported, with 19 of 20 reconstructions being patent and competent at a mean of 10 months in the author's experience.[72] One valve demonstrated reflux because of insufficient valve length at the time of reconstruction. Invagination of an adventitial surface into the venous lumen is of some concern but was not substantiated in this study.

The Maleti neovalve initial configuration demonstrated that early thrombosis below the valve occurred in two patients, and there was one late occlusion shortly after starting oral contraceptives. Therefore 95% of treated segments remained primarily patent and competent, with significantly improved duplex and air plethysmography results at a mean 22 months of follow-up. Ulcer healing occurred in 16 cases (88.9%) at a median of 12 weeks with no recurrences. There was no associated mortality.[74] However at a mean of 57 months, valve competence was demonstrated in 13 of 19 cases (68%). The one case added to the 2006 report included an episode of DVT, and the long-term ulcer healing rate was now 84% with two recurrences. The modification noted in the techniques section was instituted to improve these results. The second group studied (modification included) consisted of 21 operations with a mean 11 months of surveillance. All valves were competent, and there was a 95% ulcer healing rate and two recurrences (9.5%).[75,76]

Opie reported no incompetent valves in 14 operations at 4 years and excellent clinical improvement.[78]

Late Results

Multilevel Valve Reconstruction

There is increasing evidence that multilevel valve reconstruction (more than one valve repair in the same axial system) does improve maintenance of valve competence in at least one of the repaired valves and, as a consequence, improves clinical outcome. Raju and his group have been advocates of this approach for years.[33,58] At 2 years, Tripathi and colleagues found that patients with primary reflux disease undergoing single-level valvuloplasty could expect a 59.4% valve competence rate and 54.7% ulcer healing rate, which was statistically different ($P < .05$) from multilevel repair, which demonstrated rates of 79.7% and 72.9%, respectively.[83] A similar trend was noted in those requiring valve transplantation; valve competence and ulcer healing rates were 38.9% and 46.1%, respectively for single-level repairs versus 55.8% and 57% for multilevel repairs.[83] Rosales and colleagues have accumulated data on external valvuloplasty that suggest improved clinical results, especially in CEAP class 4 patients, with the use of a multilevel (different locations in the same axial system) and multistation (more than one valve in the same location) technique, but statistical significance was not obtained, and clear determination of valve competence was not provided.[59] Lane and associates found that as the number of external banding repairs per axial system increased, so did long-term ulcer healing.[51]

SUMMARY

This review demonstrates that a wide experience has accumulated in deep venous valvular reconstructions, most of which were performed for advanced CEAP class 4b to 6 CVDs. For the most part, these are cases that would have been severely lifestyle limiting and in many instances disabling without deep venous repair. The technical approaches have been widely varied; some of these have been extensively reproduced by different surgeons, and others have been isolated reports by individuals with small series.

The commonalities among these reports has been the sustained clinical success ranging from 40% to 80% over periods greater than 5 years in persons who could not have been healthy and active with conventional management. The significant element appears to be maintenance of a patent vein with a competent valve for sustained positive long-term results of healed ulceration and relief of pain and swelling. It is to be expected that the results obtained to date can be improved upon by comparative clinical studies going forward.

This experience has been performed by surgeons around the world, so it is not something that is too difficult to master. It has required careful diagnostic workup to allow selection of the proper surgical candidates to an extent not customarily devoted to venous patients. It has taught us that the chronically diseased venous system responds to surgical manipulation in a positive manner using known surgical principles of adequate inflow and outflow and delicate precise surgical techniques well within the abilities of the trained vascular surgeon.

The ultimate development of ideal patient selection and surgical technique will continue to evolve and may simplify by better understanding of venous physiology, management of the inflammatory cascade, and by comparative study of diagnostic and technical surgical techniques. The story to date is reflected in the references cited in this chapter. The authors are excited by the potential of those innovative clinicians setting their sights on the care of the venous patient.

REFERENCES

1. O'Donnell TF, Passman MA, Marston WA, et al. Management of venous leg ulcers: clinical practice guidelines of the Society for Vascular Surgery (SVS) and the American Venous Forum (AVF). *J Vasc Surg.* 2014;60(2 suppl):3S–59S.
2. Kalra M, Gloviczki P. Surgical treatment of venous ulcers: role of subfascial endoscopic vein ligation. *Surg Clin North Am.* 2003;83(3):671–705.
3. Mayberry JC, Moneta GL, Taylor LM Jr, et al. Fifteen-year results of ambulatory compression therapy for chronic venous ulcers. *Surgery.* 1991;109:575–581.
4. Kalra M, Gloviczki P, Noel A, et al. Subfascial endoscopic perforator vein surgery in patients with post-thrombotic syndrome: Is it justified? *Vasc Endovascular Surg.* 2002;36:41–50.
5. Neglen P, et al. Venous outflow obstruction: an underestimated contributor to chronic venous disease. *J Vasc Surg.* 2003;38:879–885.
6. Raju S, et al. The clinical impact of iliac venous stents in the management of chronic venous insufficiency. *J Vasc Surg.* 2002;35:8–15.

7. Sun J, et al. Anatomic and histologic studies on the valves of the venous system in lower extremities. *Vasc Surg.* 1990;24:85–90.

8. Powell T, et al. The valves of the external iliac, femoral, and upper third of the popliteal veins. *Surg Gynecol Obstet.* 1951;92:453–455.

9. Basmajian JV. The distribution of valves in the femoral, external iliac, and common iliac veins and their relationship to varicose veins. *Surg Gynecol Obstet.* 1952;95:537–542.

10. LePage PA, Villavicencio JL, Gomez ER, et al. The valvular anatomy of the iliac venous system and its clinical implications. *J Vasc Surg.* 1991;14:678–683.

11. Pang AS. Location of valves and competence of the great saphenous vein above the knee. *Ann Acad Med Singapore.* 1991;20:248–250.

12. Celepci H, Brenner E. Position of valves within the subclavian and axillary veins. *J Vasc Surg.* 2011;54(6 suppl):70S–76S.

13. Lurie F, Kistner RL, Eklof B, et al. Mechanism of venous valve closure and role of the valve in circulation: a new concept. *J Vasc Surg.* 2003;38:955–961.

14. Lurie F, Kistner RL, Eklof B. The mechanism of venous valve closure in normal physiologic conditions. *J Vasc Surg.* 2002;35:713–717.

15. Gloviczki P, Comerato AJ, Dalsing MC, et al. The care of patients with varicose veins and associated chronic venous disease: clinical practice guidelines of the Society for Vascular Surgery and the American Venous Forum. *J Vasc Surg.* 2011;53:2S–48.

16. Labropoulos N, Tiongson J, Pryor L, et al. Definition of venous reflux in lower-extremity veins. *J Vasc Surg.* 2003;38:793–798.

17. Plate G, et al. Physiologic and therapeutic aspects in congenital vein valve aplasia of the lower limb. *Ann Surg.* 1983;198:229–233.

18. Raju S, et al. Venous valve station changes in "primary" and post-thrombotic reflux: an analysis of 149 cases. *Ann Vasc Surg.* 2000;14:193–199.

19. Budd TW, et al. Histopathology of veins and venous valves of patients with venous insufficiency syndrome: ultrastructure. *J Med.* 1990;21:181–199.

20. Sandri JL, et al. Diameter-reflux relationship in perforating veins of patients with varicose veins. *J Vasc Surg.* 1999;30:867–875.

21. Clarke H, et al. Role of venous elasticity in the development of varicose veins. *Br J Surg.* 1989;76:577–580.

22. Killewich LA, et al. Spontaneous lysis of deep venous thrombi: rate and outcome. *J Vasc Surg.* 1989;9:89–97.

23. Masuda EM, et al. The natural history of calf vein thrombosis: lysis of thrombi and development of reflux. *J Vasc Surg.* 1998;28:67–73.

24. McLafferty RB, et al. Late clinical and hemodynamic sequelae of isolated calf vein thrombosis. *J Vasc Surg.* 1998;27:50–56.

25. Eberhardt RT, Raffetto JD. Chronic venous insufficiency. *Circulation.* 2005;111:2398–2409.

26. Eriksson I, et al. Influence of the profunda femoris vein on venous hemodynamics of the limb: experience from thirty-one deep vein valve reconstructions. *J Vasc Surg.* 1986;4:390–395.

27. Queral LA, et al. Surgical correction of chronic deep venous insufficiency by valvular transposition. *Surgery.* 1980;87:688–695.

28. Raju S, et al. Axial transformation of the profunda femoris vein. *J Vasc Surg.* 1998;27:651–659.

29. O'Donnell TF, et al. Clinical, hemodynamic, and anatomic follow-up of direct venous reconstruction. *Arch Surg.* 1987;122:474–482.

30. Bry JD, et al. The clinical and hemodynamic results after axillary-to-popliteal vein valve transplantation. *J Vasc Surg.* 1995;21:110–119.

31. Raju S, et al. Durability of venous valve reconstruction techniques for "primary" and post-thrombotic reflux. *J Vasc Surg.* 1996;23:357–367.

32. Brittenden J, Bradbury AW, Allan PL, et al. Popliteal vein reflux reduces healing of chronic venous ulcers. *Br J Surg.* 1998;85:60–62.

33. Raju S. Multiple-valve reconstruction for venous insufficiency: indications, optimal technique, and results. In: Veith FJ, ed. Current Critical Problems in Vascular Surgery. 4th ed. St. Louis: Quality Medical Publishing; 1992:122–125.

34. Eklof B, Rutherford RB, Bergan JJ, et al. Revision of the CEAP classification for chronic venous disorders: consensus statement. *J Vasc Surg.* 2004;40:1248–1252.

35. Masuda EM, Kistner RL, Eklof B. Prospective study of duplex scanning for venous reflux: comparison of Valsalva and pneumatic cuff techniques in the reverse Trendelenburg and standing positions. *J Vasc Surg.* 1994;20:711–720.

36. Markel A, Meissner MH, Manzo RA, et al. A comparison of the cuff deflation method with Valsalva's maneuver and limb compression in detecting venous valvular reflux. *Arch Surg.* 1994;129:701–705.

37. Lurie F, Comerota A, Eklof B, et al. Multicenter assessment of venous reflux by duplex ultrasound. *J Vasc Surg.* 2012;55:437–445.

38. Owens LV, Farber MA, Young ML, et al. The value of air plethysmography in predicting clinical outcome after surgical treatment of chronic venous insufficiency. *J Vasc Surg.* 2000;32:961–968.

39. Weingarten MS, Czeredarczuk M, Scovell S, et al. A correlation of air plethysmography and color flow-assisted duplex scanning in the quantification of chronic venous insufficiency. *J Vasc Surg.* 1996;24:750–754.

40. Labropoulos N, Giannoukas AD, Nicolaides AN, et al. The role of venous reflux and calf muscle pump function in nonthrombotic chronic venous insufficiency. Correlation with severity of signs and symptoms. *Arch Surg.* 1996;131:403–406.

41. Araki CT, Back TL, Padberg FT, et al. The significance of calf muscle pump function in venous ulceration. *J Vasc Surg.* 1994;20:872–877.

42. Nicholaides AN. Investigation of chronic venous insufficiency: a consensus statement. *Circulation.* 2000;102:E126–E163.

43. Criado E, Farber MA, Marston WA, et al. The role of air plethysmography in the diagnosis of chronic venous insufficiency. *J Vasc Surg.* 1998;27:660–670.

44. Kistner RL, et al. A method of performing descending venography. *J Vasc Surg.* 1986;4:464–468.

45. Nicolaides AN, Hussein MK, Szendro G, et al. The relationship of venous ulceration with ambulatory venous pressure measurements. *J Vasc Surg.* 1993;17:414–419.

46. Kistner RL, Eklof B. Classification and etiology of chronic venous disease. In: Gloviczki P, ed. Handbook of Venous Disorders. 3rd ed. London, UK: Hodder Arnold; © 2009:37–46.

47. Vasquez MA, et al. Revision of the venous clinical severity score: venous outcomes consensus statement: special communication of the American Venous Forum Ad Hoc Outcomes Working Group. *J Vasc Surg.* 2010;52:1387–1396.

48. Rutherford RB, et al. Outcome assessment in chronic venous disease. In: Gloviczki P, ed. Handbook of Venous Disorders: Guidelines of the American Venous Forum. 3rd ed. London: Hodder Arnold; 2009:684–693.

49. Valentine RJ, et al. Vessels of the leg. In: Valentine RJ, Wind GG, eds. Anatomic Exposures in Vascular Surgery. 2nd ed. Philadelphia: Lippincott Williams & Wilkins; 2003:467–522.

50. Camilli S, et al. External banding valvuloplasty of the superficial femoral vein in the treatment of primary deep valvular incompetence. *Int Angiol.* 1994;13:218–222.

51. Lanc JL, et al. Intermediate to long-term results of repairing incompetent multiple deep venous valves using external valvular stenting. *Aust N Z J Surg.* 2003;73:267–274.

52. Guarnera G, et al. External banding of the superficial femoral vein in the treatment of recurrent varicose veins. *Int Angiol.* 1998;17:268–271.

53. Makhatilov G, et al. Endoscopically directed external support of femoral vein valves. *J Vasc Surg.* 2009;49:676–680.

54. Kistner RL. Surgical technique of external venous valve repair. *Straub Found Proc.* 1990;55:15–16.

55. Nishibe T, et al. Intermediate-term results of angioscopy-assisted anterior valve sinus plication for primary deep venous insufficiency. *J Cardiovasc Surg (Torino).* 2007;48:21–25.

56. Raju S, et al. Technical options in venous valve reconstruction. *Am J Surg.* 1997;173:301–307.

57. Gloviczki P, et al. Femoral vein valve repair under direct vision without venotomy: a modified technique with use of angioscopy. *J Vasc Surg.* 1991;14:645–648.

58. Raju S, et al. Transcommissural valvuloplasty: technique and results. *J Vasc Surg.* 2000;32:969–976.

59. Rosales A, et al. External venous valve plasty (EVVP) in patients with primary chronic venous insufficiency (PCVI). *Eur J Vasc Endovasc Surg.* 2006;32:570–576.

60. Belcaro G, et al. External femoral vein valvuloplasty with limited anterior plication (LAP): a 10-year randomized, follow-up study. *Angiology.* 1999;50:531–536.

61. Kistner RL. Surgical repair of a venous valve. *Straub Clin Proc.* 1968;24:41–43.

62. Raju S. Venous insufficiency of the lower limb and stasis ulceration: changing concepts and management. *Ann Surg.* 1983;197:688–697.

63. Sottiurai VS. Technique in direct venous valvuloplasty. *J Vasc Surg.* 1988;8:646–648.

64. Tripathi R, Ktenidis KD. Trapdoor internal valvuloplasty: a new technique for primary deep vein valvular incompetence. *Eur J Vasc Endovasc Surg.* 2001;22:86–89.

65. Raju S, et al. Valve reconstruction procedures for nonobstructive venous insufficiency: rationale, techniques, and results in 107 procedures with two- to eight-year follow-up. *J Vasc Surg.* 1988;7:301–310.

66. Cardon JM, et al. Use of ipsilateral greater saphenous vein as a valved transplant in management of post-thrombotic deep venous insufficiency: long-term results. *Ann Vasc Surg.* 1999;13:284–289.

67. Taheri SA, et al. Vein valve transplant. *Surgery.* 1982;91:28–33.

68. Rosales A, Jorgensen JJ, Slagsvold CE, et al. Venous valve reconstruction in patients with secondary chronic venous insufficiency. *Eur J Vasc Endovasc Surg.* 2008;36:466–472.

69. Raju S, et al. Axillary vein transfer in trabeculated post-thrombotic veins. *J Vasc Surg.* 1999;29:1050–1064.

70. Jamieson WG, et al. Clinical results of deep venous valvular repair for chronic venous insufficiency. *Can J Surg.* 1997;40:294–299.

71. Sottiurai VS. Supravalvular incision for valve repair in primary valvular insufficiency. In: Bergan JJ, Kistner RL, eds. Atlas of Venous Surgery. Philadelphia: WB Saunders; 1992:137–138.

72. Plagnol P, et al. Autogenous valve reconstruction technique for post-thrombotic reflux. *Ann Vasc Surg.* 1999;13:339–342.

73. Maleti O. Venous valvular reconstruction in post-thrombotic syndrome. A new technique. *J Mal Vasc.* 2002;27:218–221.

74. Maleti O, et al. Neovalve construction in postthrombotic syndrome. *J Vasc Surg.* 2006;43:794–799.

75. Lugli M, et al. Neovalve construction in deep venous incompetence. *J Vasc Surg.* 2009;49:156–163.

76. Maleti O, et al. Reconstructive surgery for deep vein reflux in the lower limbs: techniques, results and indications. *Eur J Vasc Surg.* 2011;41:837–848.

77. Corcos L, et al. A new autologous venous valve by intimal flap. One case report. *Minerva Cardioangiol.* 2003;51:395–404.

78. Opie JC, et al. Monocusp—novel common femoral vein monocusp surgery uncorrectable chronic venous insufficiency with aplastic/dysplastic valves. *Phlebology.* 2008;23:158–171.

79. Ignat'ev IM, et al. First experience in forming a multi-flap valve of the common femoral vein in avalvulation of the deep veins of lower extremities. *Angiol Sosud Khir.* 2010;16:77–79.

80. Cheatle TR, et al. Venous valve repair: early results in fifty-two cases. *J Vasc Surg.* 1994;19:404–413.

81. Nishibe T, et al. Femoral vein valve repair with angioscopy-assisted anterior valve sinus plication. Early results. *J Cardiovasc Surg (Torino).* 2001;42:529–535.

82. Perrin M. Reconstructive surgery for deep venous reflux: a report on 144 cases. *Cardiovasc Surg.* 2000;8:246–255.

83. Tripathi R, et al. Deep venous valve reconstruction for non-healing leg ulcers: techniques and results. *Aust N Z J Surg.* 2004;74:34–39.

84. Perrin M, et al. Results of valvuloplasty in patients presenting with deep venous insufficiency and recurring ulceration. *Ann Vasc Surg.* 1999;13:524–532.

85. Us M, et al. The use of external banding increases the durability of transcommissural external deep venous valve repair. *Eur J Vasc Endovasc Surg.* 2007;33:494–501.

86. Masuda EM, et al. Long-term results of venous valve reconstruction: a four to twenty-one year follow-up. *J Vasc Surg.* 1994;19:391–403.

87. Wang S, et al. Effect of external valvuloplasty of the deep vein in the treatment of chronic venous insufficiency of the lower extremity. *J Vasc Surg.* 2006;44:1296–1300.

88. Kistner RL. Surgical repair of the incompetent femoral vein valve. *Arch Surg.* 1975;110:1336–1342.

89. Welch H, et al. Femoral vein valvuloplasty: intraoperative angioscopic evaluation and hemodynamic improvement. *J Vasc Surg.* 1992;16:694–700.

90. Ferris EB, et al. Femoral vein reconstruction in the management of chronic venous insufficiency: a 14-year experience. *Arch Surg.* 1982;117:1571–1579.
91. Lurie F, et al. Results of deep-vein reconstruction. *Vasc Surg.* 1997;31:275–276.
92. Perrin MR. Results of deep-vein reconstruction. *Vasc Surg.* 1997;31:273–275.
93. Johnson ND, et al. Late objective assessment of venous valve surgery. *Arch Surg.* 1981;116:1461–1466.
94. O'Donnell TF. Chronic venous insufficiency: an overview of epidemiology, classification, and anatomic considerations. *Semin Vasc Surg.* 1988;1:60–65.
95. Sottiurai VS. Results of deep-vein reconstruction. *Vasc Surg.* 1997;31:276–278.
96. Nash T. Long-term results of vein valve transplants placed in the popliteal vein for intractable post-phlebitic venous ulcers and pre-ulcer skin changes. *J Cardiovasc Surg (Torino).* 1988;29:712–716.
97. Rai DB, et al. Chronic venous insufficiency disease: its etiology: a new technique for vein valve transplantation. *Int Surg.* 1991;76:174–178.
98. Taheri SA, et al. Indications and results of vein valve transplant. *J Cardiovasc Surg.* 1986;27:163–168.

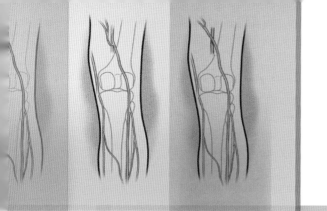

Venous Ulcers

William Marston

Venous leg ulcers (VLUs) are an important medical problem. The chronic and recurrent nature of VLUs causes morbidity, severely reduces patient quality of life, and increases costs placed on health care systems. Standard care supported by evidence includes compression therapy and the use of adjunctive agents, which have been shown to accelerate healing, improve patient quality of life, and likely reduce health care costs.

The American Venous Forum and Society for Vascular Surgery published treatment guidelines for venous leg ulcers in 2014.[1] These comprehensive practice guidelines include recommendations on therapy to prevent ulceration, therapies to heal VLUs, and to prevent recurrent ulceration. Nonhealing venous ulcers are typically characterized by uncontrolled inflammation generated by venous hypertension, bacterial colonization of the wound, and excessive wound exudate, containing high concentrations of proteases and inflammatory cytokines. Elimination of this inflammation, control of bacterial load and exudate must all be achieved to initiate healing of the chronic ulcer. Control of underlying venous hypertension can be achieved with either sustained, high-strength compression or intervention to eliminate venous insufficiency. The other components of venous ulcer care must be continued after achieving control of venous hypertension to achieve reliable ulcer healing.

CONTROL OF VENOUS HYPERTENSION

Compression

Sustained high-strength compression of the limb remains the basis of treatment for venous leg ulcers. Compression must be initiated before other therapies and throughout the treatment course to attain healing. Adjuvant therapies will uniformly fail if limb compression is not maintained during treatment in an ambulatory patient. It is important to understand that multiple methods of compression may be necessary to treat patients of varying types. Multilayered compression bandaging, Unna's boot, compression stockings, inelastic compression garments, and intermittent pneumatic compression are all useful methods for achieving compression and should be used when they are the best option for the patient. Multilayer compression systems, incorporating absorptive padding layers and 2 to 3 layers of compression, are able to absorb excess wound exudate and eliminate edema and are a good choice for large wounds with heavy exudative drainage (Fig. 20.1).

Using high-strength sustained compression, 60% to 70% of venous ulcers will heal in 3 to 4 months of treatment.[2] Larger wounds, those of long duration before treatment, and wounds in men are slower to heal. Those responding slowly to compression therapy should be considered for venous intervention.

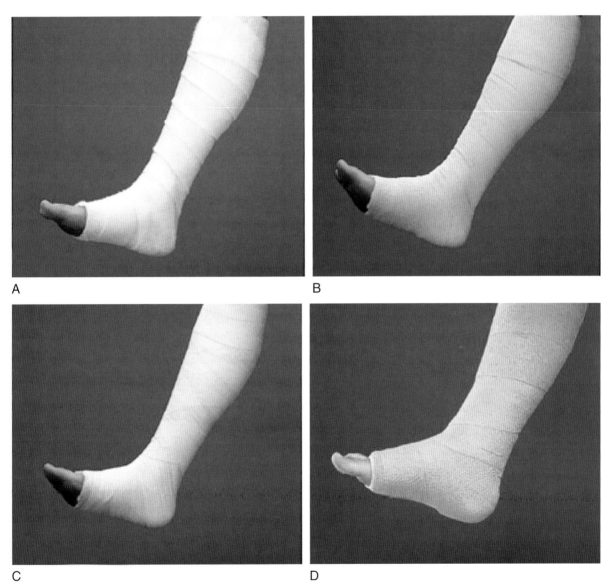

A

B

C

D

■ **Fig. 20.1** Multilayer elastic compression. (A) Layer 1: orthopedic wool padding. (B) Layer 2: Light long-stretch elastic compression. (C) Layer 3: figure 8 wrapped elastic compression. (D) Layer 4: self-retaining elastic wrap.

INTERVENTION TO CORRECT VENOUS HYPERTENSION

Indications for Intervention

Based on a review of the literature, there is significant support for performing intervention to control saphenous reflux in patients with venous ulcers, particularly to prevent recurrent ulceration. Barwell et al.[3] performed a randomized study comparing the efficacy of saphenous stripping plus compression with compression alone for the healing and prevention of venous leg ulcers in patients with superficial venous reflux. Although there was no difference in the healing rate between the two groups, significantly fewer patients in the surgery group experienced recurrent ulceration (15%) compared with the compression-only group (34%) at 1-year follow-up.

Superficial Venous Ablation

When performing ablation of the great or small saphenous vein for ulceration, several key principles should be considered. The saphenous vein should be mapped with ultrasound before ablation to follow the venous path bringing venous hypertension to the ulcer bed, with the goal of eliminating this entire pathway. In some cases, the great saphenous vein will be enlarged all the way down to and under the ulcer bed. In this case, the saphenous vein should be accessed as low as possible in the leg, close to the area of ulceration rather than performing access higher in the leg (Fig. 20.2). If the enlarged saphenous vein gives off large branches to varicosities in the upper calf and then is normal below the large branches, it should be accessed at the location where the large branches come off to ablate from the saphenofemoral to this location. The large varicose channels down to the ulcer bed should also be eliminated. In a study of ulcer healing and recurrence after endovenous thermal ablation (EVTA) in C6 patients, limbs in which phlebectomy of varicose veins was performed along with EVTA experienced significantly lower ulcer recurrence than those treated with EVTA alone. There is also limited evidence supporting the removal of varicose channels extending into the ulcer bed to eliminate the final channel of venous hypertension extending into the area of ulceration.[4] This may be done surgically or with sclerotherapy.

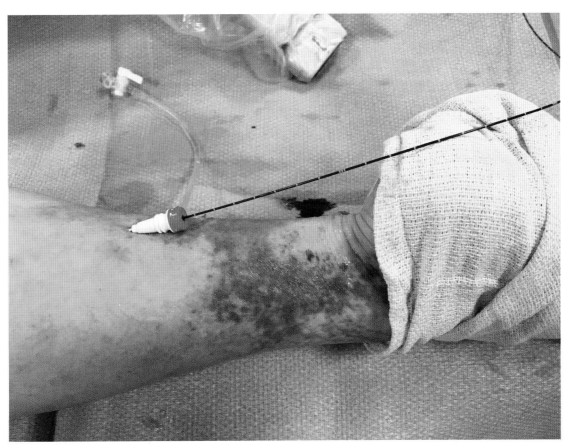

■ **Fig. 20.2** Illustration of access of great saphenous vein in lower calf just above ulcer in medial ankle.

Methods of saphenous ablation in retrograde fashion have been reported using the mechanochemical method (MOCA), allowing catheter passage under the ulcer bed to ablate the incompetent vein all the way to the wound while avoiding access in compromised, scarred periulcer skin[5] (Fig. 20.3).

Perforator Insufficiency

The contribution of incompetent perforators to global venous insufficiency remains controversial. When refluxing perforators are identified along with saphenous reflux, many perforators will no longer reflux after saphenous and varicosity ablation. However, infrequently, leg ulcers are associated with large incompetent perforators alone or with associated deep venous reflux. Based on a series of studies by Lawrence et al., it appears that ablation of perforators in these situations promotes venous ulcer healing.[6,7] The technical details of perforator ablation are outlined in Chapter 9.

Based on this information, we advocate an approach to eliminate the pathway of reflux bringing venous hypertension to the area of ulceration. This involves detailed duplex imaging to evaluate the deep and superficial venous systems to identify obstruction or axial reflux patterns as well as any saphenous branches, perforators, or chains of varicosities extending from the primary area of reflux to the ulcer bed itself. This process identifies any abnormal reflux or obstruction between the heart and the ulcer bed, and identifies a set of therapies designed to eliminate the pathway and each of its components. The potential causes of venous hypertension are listed in Table 20.1 along with their reported frequency in venous ulcer patients. A significant majority of patients with venous ulcers have correctible venous pathology that can reduce or eliminate the venous hypertension leading to ulceration.

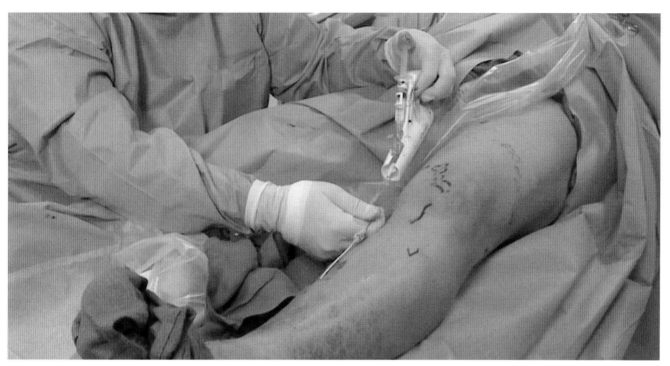

■ Fig. 20.3 Illustration of the mechanochemical method using retrograde access in great saphenous vein.

TABLE 20.1 Venous Pathology in Patients With Venous Ulceration[2]

Proximal venous obstruction > 70% (May-Thurner)	23%
Isolated great or small saphenous reflux	18%
Isolated perforator reflux	6%
Superficial and perforator reflux	11%
Deep and superficial reflux	21%
Deep venous reflux	43%

TERMINAL INTERRUPTION OF REFLUX SOURCE

All the potential venous interventions for the venous pathology listed in Table 20.1 have been described in detail in other chapters, except for methods to interrupt the terminal reflux source to the venous ulcer (terminal interruption of the reflux source [TIRS]). This technique is designed to eliminate the final pathway linking deep, superficial, or perforator incompetence to the ulcer bed itself. This method may be particularly useful when the more proximal source cannot be eliminated, most commonly in patients with uncorrected deep venous reflux. In these patients, compression therapy may not be able to adequately control venous hypertension and the resultant inflammation inhibiting healing. Interrupting the venous channels at the wound bed may protect the periulcer tissue, resulting in reduced venous hypertension to support healing. Although recurrence of these channels will likely occur over time, the healed ulcer may not recur with compression and avoidance of mechanical trauma to the skin.

Bush reported a series of 20 patients treated with the TIRS technique; healing occurred in 90% of patients within 8 weeks. All patients had been treated with compression for 18 to 24 months before treatment.[8]

The TIRS technique requires good interpretive ultrasound skills and the ability to safely deliver the foamed sclerotherapy with the aid of ultrasound guidance. Only the most distal venous branches draining the area of the ulcer are identified. In some patients, especially those with anterior calf ulcers, a perforator leading directly to the ulcer bed may be identified, the proximal source of reflux, if correctible, should be performed before or concurrent with TIRS (Fig. 20.4).

The sites of injection when performing TIRS are illustrated for a variety of ulcer locations in Figs. 20.5 to 20.7. Using ultrasound guidance, the target periwound vessels are identified for injection (Fig. 20.8). The target vein is then accessed with needle penetration through normal skin, or the ulcerated skin if necessary. Using a 3-mL syringe and a 25-gauge needle, the foam is slowly injected as the operator observes sonographic venous filling (Fig. 20.9A and B). A variety of sclerosants can be used including physician-compounded, foam sclerosants and Varithena polidocanol foam (BTG International, London).

In the series reported by Bush, the authors prepared a 4:1 mixture of sodium tetradecyl sulfate (Sotradecol) and carbon dioxide.[8] After injection of the foamed solution, compression was applied, and local wound care was performed. The patients were rescanned at weekly intervals and foam injections were repeated if necessary. A 1% concentration was used for most patients. A 3% foamed solution of sodium tetradecyl sulfate was used for patients on anticoagulation or where unusually high-flow was found in the target veins.

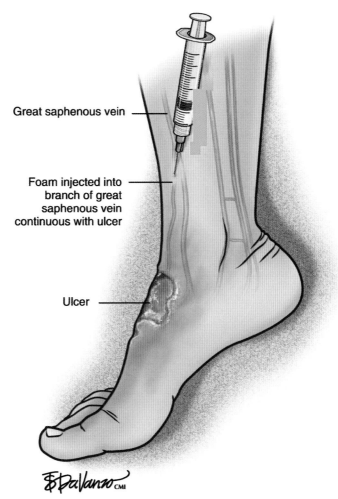

Great saphenous vein

Foam injected into
branch of great
saphenous vein
continuous with ulcer

Ulcer

■ **Fig. 20.4** Schematic drawing of anterior ulcer secondary to incompetent branch of the saphenous vein with associated greater saphenous insufficiency.

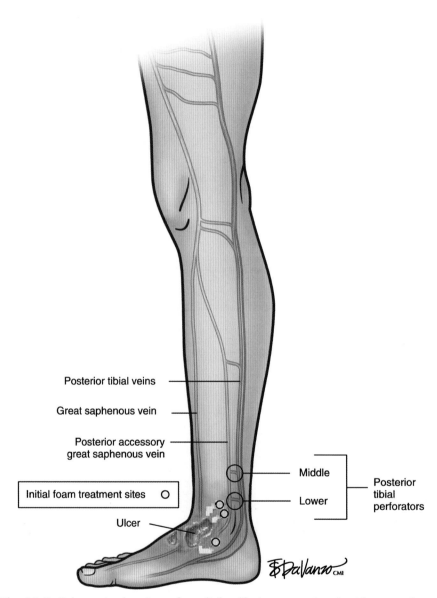

Posterior tibial veins

Great saphenous vein

Posterior accessory great saphenous vein

Initial foam treatment sites   O

Middle

Lower

Posterior tibial perforators

Ulcer

■ **Fig. 20.5** Schematic drawing of medial calf ulcer associated with posterior calf perforator.

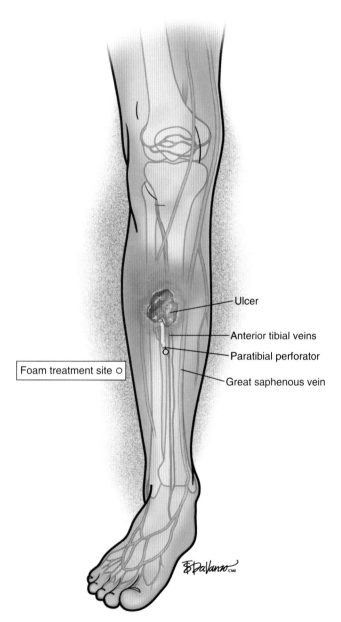

Ulcer

Anterior tibial veins

Paratibial perforator

Foam treatment site ○

Great saphenous vein

■ **Fig. 20.6** Schematic drawing of anterior ulcer secondary to perforator associated with deep venous insufficiency.

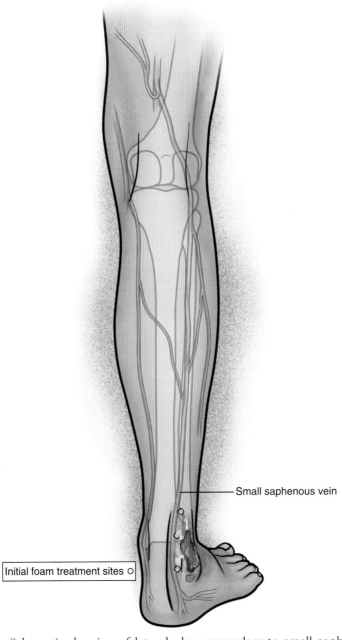

Small saphenous vein

Initial foam treatment sites ○

■ **Fig. 20.7** Schematic drawing of lateral ulcer secondary to small saphenous vein insufficiency.

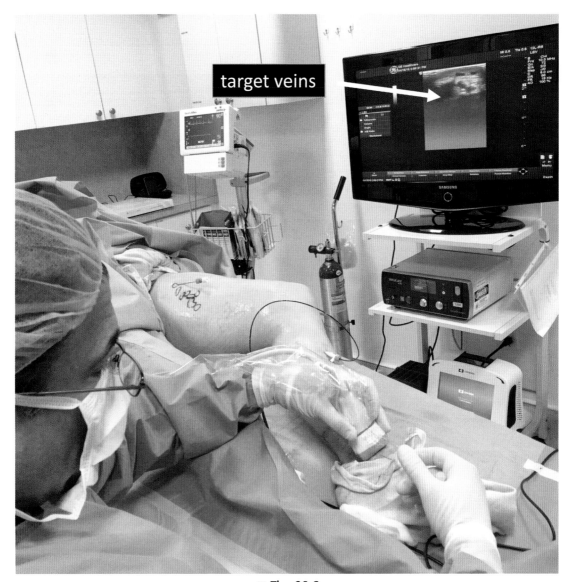

■ Fig. 20.8

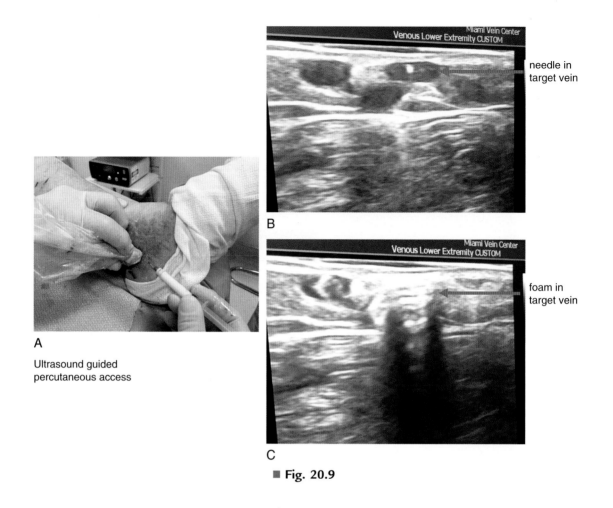

needle in
target vein

foam in
target vein

A

Ultrasound guided
percutaneous access

B

C

■ Fig. 20.9

MANAGEMENT OF THE VENOUS ULCER TO FACILITATE HEALING

Once control over the venous hypertension is achieved, either by compression methods or venous intervention, reduction of the inflammatory process inhibiting healing occurs. However, many ulcers will still not heal without careful attention to the wound itself. Wounds of long duration often have developed senescent fibroblasts and significant bacterial colonization that will inhibit normal healing mechanisms despite elimination of venous hypertension. Wound bed preparation describes the process of eliminating other barriers to healing allowing normal epithelial growth and migration to occur.

Wound Bed Preparation

The components of this process include debridement of nonviable tissue, identification and correction of bacterial involvement, control of chronic inflammation, elimination of limb edema, and control of wound exudate.

Debridement

Debridement is required to excise nonviable tissue and should be aggressive, particularly at the initial evaluation. Cellular senescence has been identified in wound tissue around chronic venous ulcers of long duration, indicating the need for wound excision to remove all surrounding tissue in these cases.[9,10]

Numerous alternatives to surgical debridement have evolved, including chemical debridement, ultrasound debridement, hydrodebridement (Fig. 20.10), and larval therapy. In general, there are two situations in which alternatives to surgical debridement may be desirable: patients in long-term nursing facilities, and those who have difficulty traveling to wound or surgical clinics for surgical debridement when required. These patients may benefit from chemical debridement or some other method.

Larval

Larval therapy using medical maggots has been studied as an alternative to conventional therapy in several nonrandomized studies. A randomized study of larval therapy compared with hydrogel for the management of chronic leg ulcers was reported in 2009.[11] All other wound therapies were similar for each group. The study found that larval-treated wounds experienced significantly faster debridement than the hydrogel-treated group, but at the expense of significantly higher ulcer-related pain scores. No difference in ulcer healing or patient quality of life was demonstrated.

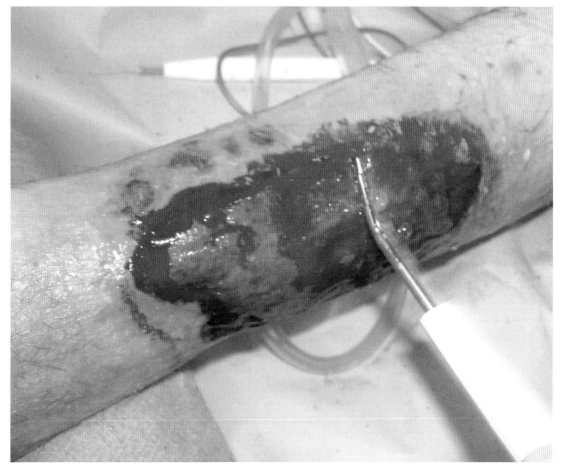

■ **Fig. 20.10** Hydrodebridement.

Bacterial Colonization

Bacterial colonization is a common complication in chronic wounds. Bacteria form biofilms in wounds that appear to multiply to the point at which they inhibit healing by stimulating chronic inflammation, inactivating growth factors critical to the healing process, and preventing orderly angiogenesis required for healing (Fig. 20.11).[12] If untreated, it is believed that biofilms will continue to inhibit wound healing or may lead to more significant systemic infection.

Given the emergence of this clinical problem, wounds with poor progress and those demonstrating any evidence of enlargement or infection, should be evaluated with quantitative cultures. If cultures demonstrate greater than 10^5 bacterial counts per cubic millimeter, the patient should receive systemic therapy guided by bacteria-specific sensitivities.[13]

Properties and Categories of Wound Dressings

In general, the selection of a wound dressing should be based on wound characteristics, including location, inflammation and amount of exudate. Moisture balance is important, and the dressing should maintain a moist environment conducive to tissue growth and epithelial migration. Based on the high concentration of inflammatory cytokines and proteases in chronic wound fluid, excessive fluid should be wicked away from the ulcer and the skin surface to prevent further tissue inflammation and damage from prolonged contact. For this reason, foam and alginate dressings with high absorptive capacities are good choices for primary dressings on exudative venous ulcers underneath the chosen method of compression.

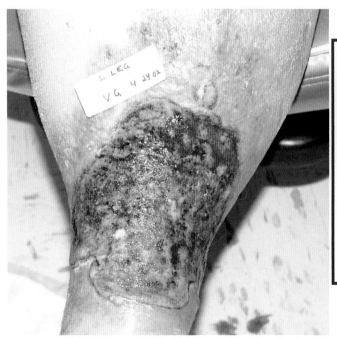
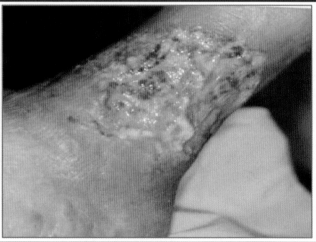

■ Fig. 20.11

Adjunctive Therapies to Accelerate Healing

Numerous adjunctive methods have been studied in an attempt to accelerate the healing process, including skin grafting, growth factors, living human skin equivalents, collagen matrices, platelet releasates, topical therapies, ultrasound, electrical stimulation, and other modalities. The majority of these therapeutic strategies have limited data supporting their efficacy.

Human Skin Equivalents

Apligraf (Organogenesis, Canton, Mass) is a cultured bilayer cellular construct (BLCC) originating from neonatal foreskin. A bovine collagen lattice is used as a base to support the organization of dermal fibroblasts and epithelial cells. A layer of allogeneic keratinocytes is cultured over the fibroblast layer to form a stratified epidermis. The bilayer has a structure similar to human skin, with the absence of hair follicles or sweat glands (Fig. 20.12). The growth factors and cytokines secreted by the cellular components of BLCC include fibroblast growth factor (GF), vascular endothelial GF, platelet-derived GF, transforming GF-β, and multiple interleukins, paralleling those secreted by healthy human skin.[14] The product requires a well-granulated wound bed in which exudate and bacterial levels have been controlled to yield positive results. The BLCC is easily applied in a clinic or operating room setting after aggressive wound debridement and hemostasis. Standard compression bandaging is then applied to maintain control of venous hypertension.

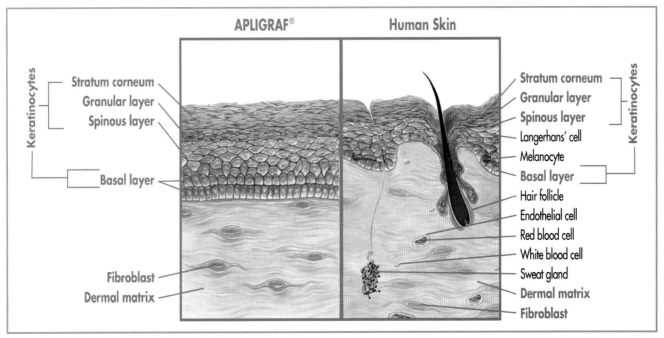

■ **Fig. 20.12**

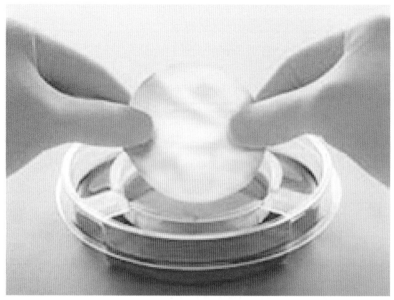

■ **Fig. 20.13**

Apligraf (Fig. 20.13) was studied in a prospective randomized multicenter trial of 240 patients with nonhealing venous leg ulcers present for more than 1 month.[15] Patients were randomized to a standard compression bandaging regimen or compression bandaging plus BLCC. The primary study outcome measure was complete healing at 24 weeks of treatment. In the BLCC-treated group, 57% of venous leg ulcers closed at 24 weeks, compared with 40% in the control group (P = .02). For ulcers that had been present for more than 1 year, 47% healed at 24 weeks, compared with 19% in the control group (P = .002).

Porcine small intestine submucosa (OASIS wound matrix, Healthpoint Ltd, Fort Worth, Texas) has also been shown in a prospective randomized controlled trial to accelerate healing of VLUs.[16] In a study by Mostow et al., in 2005, a total of 120 patients with VLUs were randomized to receive either weekly topical treatment of small intestine submucosa (SIS) plus compression or compression therapy alone. After 12 weeks of treatment, 55% of wounds treated with SIS healed versus 34% in the control group (P = .0196).

SUMMARY

Reliable and durable healing of venous leg ulcers requires control of numerous factors, which coalesce to create an environment that prevents healing and places the patient at risk for recurrent ulceration. Venous hypertension must be controlled consistently. This can be achieved in many patients through the consistent use of compression garments, but must be performed daily to be effective. In many patients, better control can be achieved by intervention to eliminate the venous pathology leading to venous hypertension. Intervention has also been proven to reduce the risk of recurrent ulceration, likely because of the difficulty in maintaining effective compression for years after ulcer healing. After control of venous hypertension, the wound itself must be managed effectively to remove nonviable tissue and excess bacteria, control exudate and edema to facilitate rapid ulcer healing. Adjunctive therapies may be useful in recalcitrant wounds to accelerate healing.

REFERENCES

1. O'Donnell TF Jr, Passman MA, Marston WA, et al. Management of venous leg ulcers: clinical practice guidelines of the Society for Vascular Surgery and the American Venous Forum. *J Vasc Surg*. 2014;60(2 suppl):3S–59S.
2. Marston WA, Carlin RE, Passman MA, et al. Healing rates and cost efficacy of outpatient compression treatment for leg ulcers associated with venous insufficiency. *J Vasc Surg*. 1999;30:491–498.
3. Barwell J, Davies C, Deacon J, et al. Comparison of surgery and compression with compression alone in chronic venous ulceration (ESCHAR STUDY): randomized controlled trial. *Lancet*. 2008;363:1854–1859.
4. Marston WA, Crowner J, Kouri A, et al. Incidence of venous leg ulcer healing and recurrence after treatment with endovenous laser ablation. J Vasc Surg. In press.
5. Sullivan LP, Quach G, Chapman T. Retrograde mechanic-chemical endovenous ablation of infrageniculate great saphenous vein for persistent venous stasis ulcers. *Phlebology*. 2014;29:654–657.
6. Lawrence PF, Alktaifi A, Rigberg D, et al. Endovenous ablation of incompetent perforating veins is effective treatment for recalcitrant venous ulcers. *J Vasc Surg*. 2011;54:737–742.
7. Harlander-Locke M, Lawrence PF, Alktaifi A, et al. The impact of ablation of incompetent superficial and perforator veins on ulcer healing. *J Vasc Surg*. 2012;55:458–464.
8. Bush R. New technique to heal venous ulcers: terminal interruption of the reflux source (TIRS). *Perspect Vasc Surg Endovasc Ther*. 2010;22:194–199.
9. Stanley AC, Fernandez NN, Lounsbury KM, et al. Pressure-induced cellular senescence: a mechanism linking venous hypertension to venous ulcers. *J Surg Res*. 2005;124:112–117.
10. Cardinal M, Eisenbud DE, Armstrong DG, et al. Serial surgical debridement: a retrospective study on clinical outcomes in chronic lower extremity wounds. *Wound Repair Regen*. 2009;17:306–311.
11. Dumville JC, Worthy G, Bland JM, et al. Larval therapy for leg ulcers (VenUS II): randomized controlled trial. *BMJ*. 2009;338:b773.
12. James GA, Swogger E, Wolcott R, et al. Biofilms in chronic wounds. *Wound Repair Regen*. 2008;16:37–44.
13. Robson MC, Heggers JP. Bacterial quantification of open wounds. *Mil Med*. 1969;134:19–24.
14. Streit M, Braathen LR. Apligraf—a living human skin equivalent for the treatment of chronic wounds. *Int J Artif Organs*. 2000;23:831.
15. Falanga V, et al. A bilayered living skin construct (APIGRAF) accelerates complete closure of hard-to-heal venous ulcers. *Wound Repair Regen*. 1999;7:201–207.
16. Mostow EN, Haraway GD, Dalsing M, et al. Effectiveness of an extracellular matrix graft (OASIS Wound Matrix) in the treatment of chronic leg ulcers: a randomized clinical trial. *J Vasc Surg*. 2005;41:837–843.

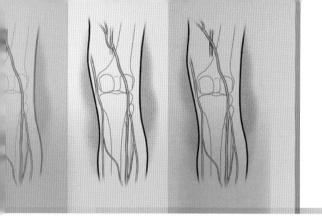

CHAPTER 21

Pelvic Venous Disorders

Mark H. Meissner and Peter Gloviczki

Venous disorders of the abdomen and pelvis are often referred to as a number of syndromes, including pelvic congestion, May-Thurner, and nutcracker syndrome (NCS), which are of historical significance, but inadequately reflect the underlying pathophysiology of these disorders. For example, May and Thurner described anatomic "spurs" of the left common iliac vein (CIV) beneath the right common iliac sarterial crossing in 24% of 342 cadavers. Although one-third of these were associated with distal thrombosis, the relationship to other symptoms of chronic venous disease is unknown. Similarly, in 1949, Lo described a spectrum of chronic pelvic symptoms and attributed them to pelvic congestion, arising from a combination of obesity and tight-fitting corsets. Classification of symptomatic patients into these syndromes has, unfortunately, impeded real understanding of the underlying pathophysiology and may lead to inappropriate treatment.

There have been tremendous advances in our understanding and treatment of chronic venous disorders of the lower extremity over the past century. As the pathophysiology of chronic venous disorders has become better understood, there have been corresponding advances in the classification and treatment of lower extremity venous disease. Unfortunately, although venous disorders of the abdomen and pelvis are part of the spectrum of chronic venous disease and often play a role in lower extremity disease, the anatomy, pathophysiology, and treatment of pelvic venous disease is only beginning to be understood. Rather than being a disparate group of syndromes (e.g., May-Thurner, pelvic congestion, and nutcrackers syndromes), it is becoming clear that, although much more complex, the abdominal and pelvic venous systems should be approached in a systematic way similar to the lower extremities. Reflux and/or obstruction in various components of the abdominal and pelvic veins often results in similar clinical symptoms, posing complex diagnostic and therapeutic questions. In the lower extremities, pelvic venous disease, particularly obstruction, may be primary or secondary to a previous episode of deep venous thrombosis; however, this chapter will focus on primary abdominal and pelvic venous disorders. Although our understanding remains incomplete, it is only through an appreciation of the complex anatomy and physiology that appropriate therapeutic decisions can be made.

ABDOMINAL AND PELVIC VENOUS ANATOMY

It is useful to consider that the venous circulation of the pelvis consists of three multiply-interconnected venous systems: the left renal and ovarian veins, the iliac veins (common, external and internal), and the lower extremity veins. In addition to communications between these three systems, there is frequently crossover from one side to the other within the pelvis. In the female, the ovarian veins drain the venous territories of the parametrium, cervix, mesosalpinx, and pampiniform plexus, which may also drain through the internal iliac veins as a collateral pathway. These plexuses form the ovarian vein, which may have two to three trunks before becoming a single trunk at the level of L4. The ovarian vein has a mean diameter of approximately 3 mm, which increases with pregnancy, and usually has two to three valves, which are incompetent in about half of women. Although variations may occur, the right ovarian vein usually drains directly into the inferior vena cava (IVC), whereas the left drains into the left renal vein. In males, the gonadal veins do not primarily drain the pelvis but rather pass through the inguinal canal as the testicular vein. A similar tributary in females, the round ligament vein, may bypass the pelvis and pass through the inguinal canal to the labia.

The left renal vein most commonly follows a course between the superior mesenteric artery (SMA) anteriorly and the aorta posteriorly, although it may also pass posterior to the aorta (retroaortic or circumaortic renal vein). The SMA normally arises from the aorta at a near 90-degree angle and courses ventrally for 4 to 5 mm to form a rectangular tunnel through which the left renal vein passes. Both the third portion of the duodenum and retroperitoneal fat are postulated to be of importance in maintaining a wide aorto-mesenteric angle. Important tributaries that may function to drain the kidney include the left adrenal, gonadal, ascending lumbar, hemiazygous, periureteric, and capsular veins.

Compression of the left renal vein over the abdominal aorta has variously been termed *nutcracker phenomenon, aortomesenteric compression of the left renal vein,* or *left renal vein entrapment.* This has most commonly been attributed to compression of the left renal vein between the SMA and abdominal aorta (anterior nutcracker phenomenon), and the SMA does indeed arise at a much more acute angle in many patients with NCS. However, there is wide variability in both the distance between the aorta and SMA and the aortomesenteric angle, and it remains unclear if either of these measurements are predictive of hemodynamically significant renal vein compression. The aortomesenteric angle has also noted to be position dependent, decreasing substantially when upright. Anterior nutcracker phenomenon has been attributed to a variety of anatomic variants including an acute or lateral origin of the SMA, fibrosis surrounding the origin of the SMA, a high trajectory of the left renal vein, and posterior ptosis of the left kidney. In at least some patients, compression may be more related to the steep posterior to anterior course of the renal vein in the retroperitoneum with direct posterior compression by the aorta alone. The relative importance of compression by the SMA versus stretching of the renal vein over the aorta in patients with a paucity of retroperitoneal fat is unclear but may have important anatomic implications for treatment (Fig. 21.1). The left renal vein may also course posterior to the abdominal aorta (retroaortic or circumaortic renal

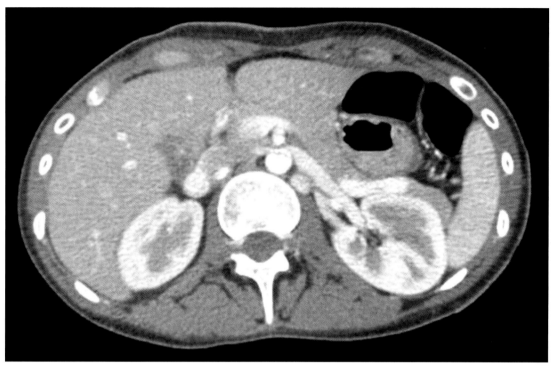

■ **Fig. 21.1** Computed tomography of the abdomen demonstrating compression of the left renal vein. Note the paucity of retroperitoneal fat and steep posterior to anterior course of the left renal vein. The relative importance of compression of the left renal vein by the overlying superior mesenteric artery versus stretching of the vein over the abdominal aorta is unknown.

vein), allowing compression between the aorta and vertebral column (posterior nutcracker). The development of symptoms is likely related to the adequacy of collateral pathways and the development of renal venous hypertension. Inadequate drainage may lead to left flank pain, orthostatic hematuria, and proteinuria. In contrast, decompression through the gonadal veins may lead to pelvic symptoms in women and varicocele in men.

The CIV is formed by the confluence of the external iliac vein, draining the lower extremity, and the internal iliac vein, which provides drainage of the pelvis. Nonthrombotic compression of the CIV most commonly arises from compression of the central left CIV by the overlying right common iliac artery and is often associated with secondary intraluminal band or web formation (May-Thurner syndrome). However, approximately 15% of limbs with primary disease will have involvement of both the common and external iliac veins. It is also now clear that compressive lesions can occur elsewhere, specifically at the crossing of the right common iliac artery over the right CIV, the crossings of the internal iliac arteries, and at the inguinal ligament. However, left-sided lesions are at least 3 times more common than right-sided lesions. Compressive lesions of the CIVs may cause lower extremity symptoms or, in the presence of collateral drainage into a refluxing internal iliac vein, pelvic symptoms.[1]

The internal iliac vein is formed by the confluence of the obturator, branches of the internal pudendal, and gluteal veins, which originate in the thigh, perineum, and buttock respectively. They function as important collaterals for the venous territories drained by the ovarian veins and may also communicate with the lower extremity veins through "escape points" in the pelvic floor. In this manner, the caudal tributaries of the internal iliac veins function much as perforating veins, connecting the deep veins of the pelvis with the superficial veins of the lower extremity. Four escape points from the pelvic veins are commonly identified: the P, I, G, and O points.[2] The perineal or "P" point connects the internal and external pudendal systems and communicates with the veins of the medial thigh and further with the saphenofemoral junction (Fig. 21.2). The inguinal or "I" point connects the ovarian vein, through the round ligament vein and inguinal canal, with the labial veins and saphenofemoral junction (Fig. 21.3). The obturator or

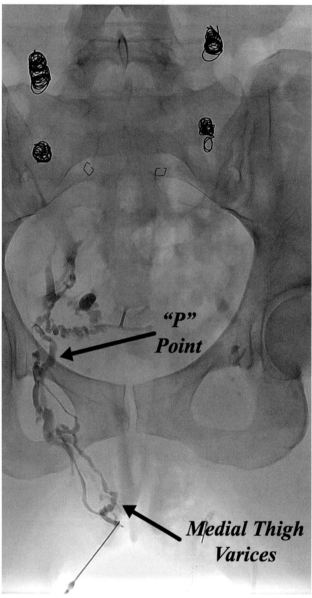

◼ **Fig. 21.2** Retrograde venography of medial thigh varices demonstrating the perineal "P" with filling of internal pudendal tributaries of the internal iliac vein.

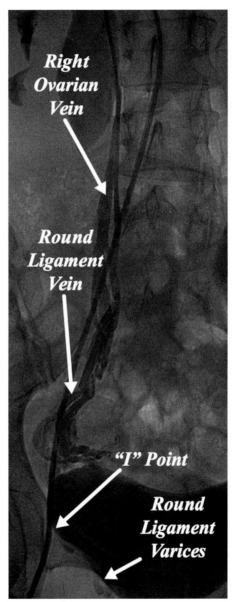

■ **Fig. 21.3** Right ovarian venography demonstrating the vein of the round ligament arising from the ovarian vein and passing through the inguinal canal (inguinal "I" point) to communicate with labial varices.

"O" point connects the obturator vein with the veins of the medial thigh (Fig. 21.4), and the gluteal or "G" point connects the gluteal veins with the sciatic and posterior thigh veins Fig. 21.5). The drainage of the female vulva is particularly complex and includes the internal pudendal, obturator, and round ligament veins from the pelvis as well as the superficial and deep external pudendal veins.

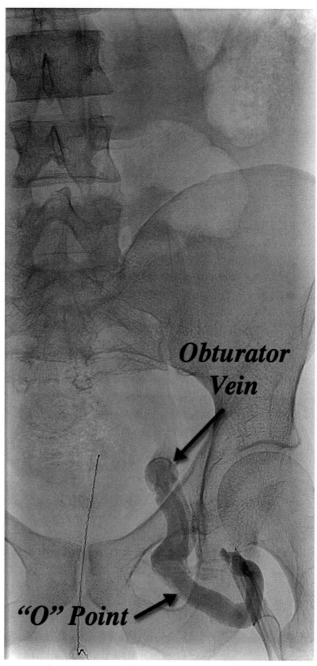

■ **Fig. 21.4** Retrograde venogram demonstrating communication of the great saphenous vein with the obturator tributary of the internal iliac vein through the "O" point.

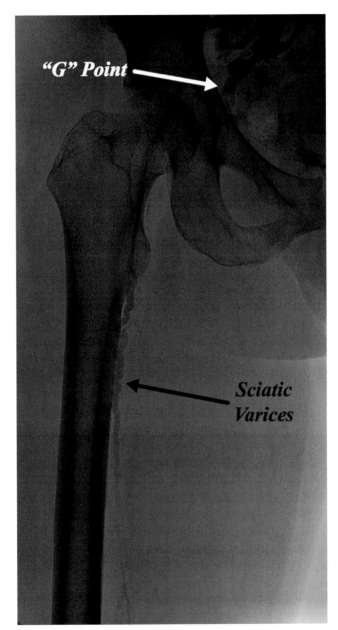

■ **Fig. 21.5** Balloon occlusion venography demonstrating communication of the internal iliac gluteal tributaries with sciatic varices through the gluteal ("G") escape point.

All three venous systems, the renal/ovarian, common/internal iliac, and lower extremity veins can be thought of as terminating in venous "reservoirs" (Fig. 21.6A–C). In general terms, venous symptoms can be considered to arise from distention of one of these three venous reservoirs: those of the left renal hilum (NCS), the pelvis (pelvic congestion syndrome), and the lower extremities (pelvic congestion and May-Thurner syndromes).

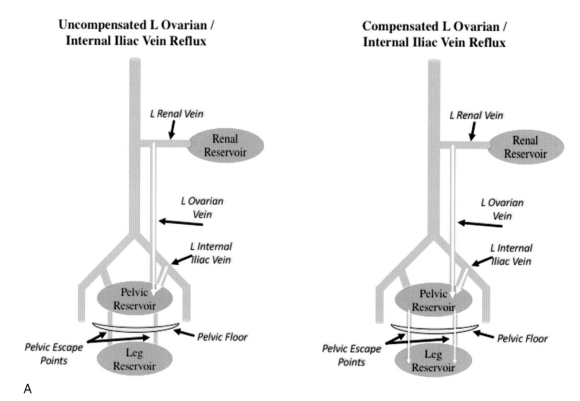

Uncompensated L Ovarian / Internal Iliac Vein Reflux

Compensated L Ovarian / Internal Iliac Vein Reflux

A

■ **Fig. 21.6** The venous reservoirs of the abdomen and pelvic. Depending on whether pressure is transmitted directly to the distal reservoir or is decompressed via collaterals, individual pathologies (reflux or obstruction) can be classified as "uncompensated" or "compensated." (A) Primary ovarian/internal iliac reflux. An uncompensated pattern is associated with distension of the pelvic venous reservoir and predominant pelvic symptoms in women. In contrast, decompression via the pelvic escape points is associated with typical or atypical lower-varices, often with few pelvic symptoms.

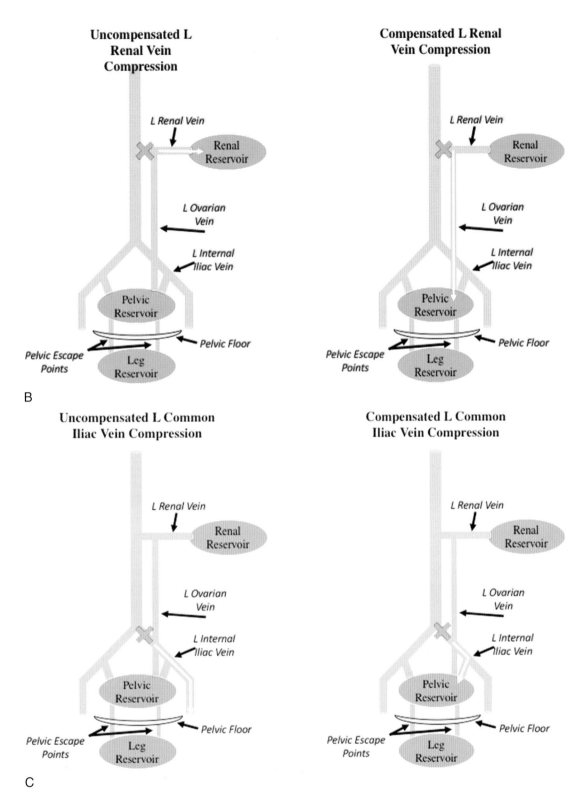

Uncompensated L Renal Vein Compression

Compensated L Renal Vein Compression

Uncompensated L Common Iliac Vein Compression

Compensated L Common Iliac Vein Compression

■ **Fig. 21.6, cont'd** (B) Left renal vein compression. An uncompensated pattern is associated with pressure transmission directly to the renal hilum with the development of hilar varices and symptoms of flank pain and hematuria. If collateral drainage via the left gonadal vein is adequate, a compensated pattern of disease may lead pelvic symptoms in women or a varicocele in men. (C) Left common iliac vein compression. In an uncompensated pattern, elevated upstream pressure is transmitted directly to the leg resulting in pain and edema. In compensated disease, decompression via an incompetent internal iliac vein may be associated with pelvic symptoms.

The pelvic venous reservoir, consisting of the plexus of veins associated with the pelvic viscera and broad ligament is central to the clinical manifestations of pelvic venous disorders. Although normally draining via the ovarian veins and tributaries of the internal iliac vein, under pathologic conditions, the plexus may serve as the primary reservoir for drainage of an obstructed left renal vein (NCS); refluxing ovarian or internal iliac veins (pelvic congestion syndrome); or an obstructed left CIV (May-Thurner syndrome). Similarly, the pelvic venous plexus may decompress into the lower extremity reservoir via tributaries of the internal iliac veins. A thorough knowledge of these venous interconnections is critical in understanding the pathophysiology, diagnosis, and management of pelvic venous disorders.

CLINICAL MANIFESTATIONS OF PELVIC VENOUS DISORDERS

The spectrum of pelvic venous disorders includes four clinical presentations: chronic pelvic pain, pelvic source varices of the leg, symptoms related to renal venous hypertension, and leg swelling. These in turn result from two patterns of reflux; reflux in the ovarian and internal iliac veins, and two patterns of obstruction associated with compression of the left renal and left CIVs. Left renal and common iliac obstruction may in turn cause reflux in the ovarian and internal iliac veins respectively.

Each of the four individual pathologies can be regarded as being either compensated or uncompensated, depending on whether venous pressure is transmitted directly to the distal venous reservoir (renal hilar, pelvic, or leg) or decompressed via collaterals into more caudal veins. For example, uncompensated primary ovarian or internal iliac vein reflux leads to distension of the pelvic venous reservoir and predominant pelvic symptoms in women, whereas decompression via the pelvic escape points in compensated disease leads to typical or atypical lower extremity varices with fewer pressure-related symptoms in the pelvis (see Fig. 21.6A). In a similar fashion, uncompensated compression of the left renal vein is associated with venous hypertension transmitted to the renal hilar reservoir and symptoms of flank pain and hematuria, whereas collateral drainage via the left gonadal vein in a compensated pattern results in either pelvic symptoms in women or varicocele in men (see Fig. 21.6B). Finally, elevated upstream venous pressure associated with CIV compression may result in either lower extremity symptoms in uncompensated disease or pelvic symptoms related to decompression via an incompetent internal iliac vein in the compensated state (see Fig. 21.6C).

Chronic pelvic pain is defined as intermittent or constant pelvic pain persisting for at least 6 months, unassociated with pregnancy, and not occurring exclusively with intercourse or menstruation.[3] Pain is typically noncyclic, that is, background symptoms are often present throughout the month, but typically worsens with menstruation as well as intercourse and prolonged standing. Associated symptoms may include dyspareunia, dysuria, and dysmenorrhea. Postcoital pain is often described as a bursting or aching sensation that may take several hours to resolve. These symptoms are frequently accompanied by depression (25%–50%), anxiety (10%–20%), and somatic complaints (10%–20%).

Pelvic pain of venous origin is presumably related to venous hypertension with dilation and distension of the pelvic venous reservoir, either caused by primary reflux in the ovarian and/or internal iliac veins (uncompensated reflux, Fig. 21.7), or secondary

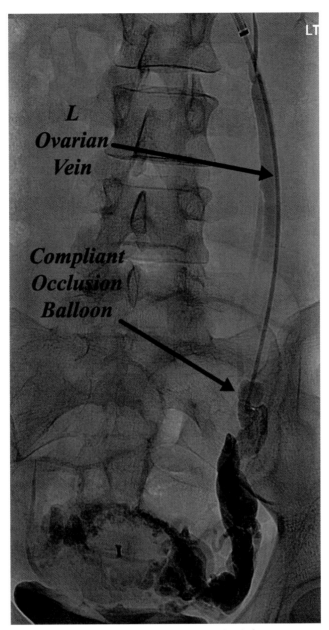

■ **Fig. 21.7** Primary ovarian vein incompetence. The left ovarian vein is markedly dilated and refluxing resulting in periuterine varicosities and pelvic symptoms.

reflux because of compression of the left renal or CIVs (compensated obstruction, Fig. 21.8). Given the nonspecific and historical nature of the term, pelvic congestion syndrome, it should be replaced by more specific terms, such as chronic pelvic pain, because of primary ovarian or internal iliac venous incompetence, left renal vein compression, or left CIV compression.

Lower extremity varicose veins, occurring either alone or in combination with chronic pelvic pain, are also a manifestation of pelvic venous disorders. The leg reservoir is the most distal of the three venous reservoirs and pelvic source varices may represent a compensated pattern of primary ovarian or internal iliac venous incompetence or of common iliac or left renal compression. These may develop in atypical locations (vulva, perineum, or buttocks) or, by way of communication with the superficial and deep external pudendal veins, in a great saphenous distribution. Great saphenous varices of pelvic origin may be particularly associated with an incompetent preterminal valve in

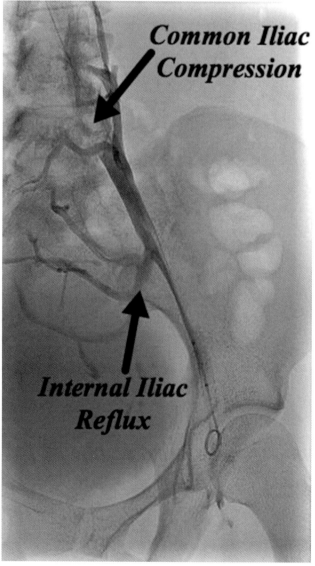

■ **Fig. 21.8** Left common iliac venous compression (May-Thurner syndrome). Elevated pressure upstream from the venous compression is compensated by drainage through the refluxing internal iliac vein and the ascending lumbar vein.

the presence of a competent terminal valve. An overlooked pelvic origin of lower extremity varices is also a common cause of recurrent varicose veins in women.

Compression of the left renal vein may be associated with either renal (uncompensated pattern) or pelvic (compensated pattern) symptoms. If collateral outflow from the kidney is inadequate, compression of the left renal vein may lead to renal venous hypertension and hilar varices associated with clinical symptoms of left flank pain, orthostatic proteinuria, and hematuria, which may be either gross or microscopic[4] (Fig. 21.9). However, if there is adequate decompression of an obstructed renal vein via collaterals, renal symptoms may be minimal and symptoms related to the more caudal pelvic reservoir may predominate. The gonadal veins are among the most important collateral pathways draining the left renal vein, and differences in anatomy account for the gender differences in the manifestations of compensated disease. In women, the ovarian vein communicates with the pelvic venous plexus, and compensated left renal vein obstruction may be associated with

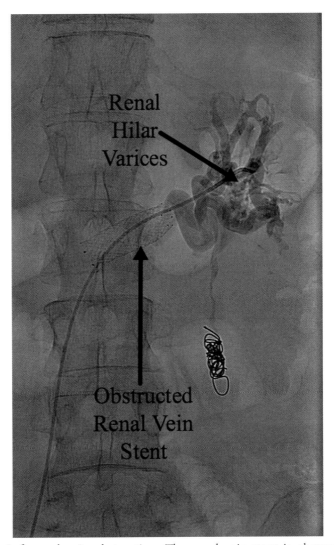

■ **Fig. 21.9** Left renal vein obstruction. The renal vein stent is obstructed with limited collateral outflow from previous left ovarian embolization. There is direct pressure transmission to the renal hilum with the formation of varices and symptoms of flank pain and hematuria. A similar pattern may occur in uncompensated left renal vein compression (nutcracker syndrome).

pelvic pain, dysuria and dyspareunia as well as pelvic origin lower extremity varices. In contrast, there is no collateral flow through the pelvis in men, and secondary gonadal vein reflux may lead to a left-sided varicocele (Fig. 21.10). Symptoms are usually more prominent when standing, a finding attributed to visceral proptosis and narrowing of the aortomesenteric angle in the upright position.

Finally, lower extremity symptoms, including pain spelling and varices, caused by compression of the iliac veins, most commonly on the left side, should be included in the spectrum of pelvic venous disorders. In the event of adequate decompression of increased venous pressure through an incompetent internal iliac vein, primary pelvic symptoms may predominate in women. In contrast, lack of collateralization via the internal iliac vein may lead to primary lower extremity pain and swelling.

EPIDEMIOLOGY

As discussed earlier, the clinical manifestations of pelvic venous disease are varied. The precise presentation depends not only on the pattern and distributions of reflux and

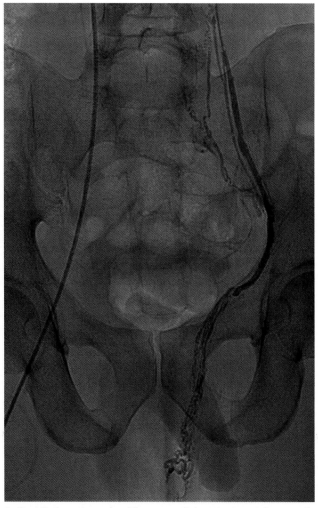

■ **Fig. 21.10** Left-sided varicocele. The gonadal vein in males rarely communicates with tributaries of the internal iliac vein.

obstruction, but also on a number of demographic factors including gender, age, parity, and body habitus.

Chronic pelvic pain accounts for approximately 10% of gynecologic visits, with a prevalence estimated to vary from 5.7% in Austria to 26.6% in Egypt.[3] Underlying causes of chronic pelvic pain include endometriosis, pelvic venous disorders, adhesions, uterine leiomyomata, adenomyosis, malignancy, uterine prolapse, and inflammatory bowel disease. Pelvic venous disorders are responsible for approximately one-third of cases and are second only to endometriosis as a cause of chronic pelvic pain. Pelvic symptoms related to underlying pelvic venous disease most commonly occur in premenopausal, multiparous women. Among 57 patients evaluated by Scultetus, the mean age of patients presenting with pelvic venous disorders was 34 years (range 24–48 years) and the mean number of pregnancies was 3.1 (range 2–5). However, note that pelvic varicosities do not uniformly lead to disabling symptoms and asymptomatic varicosities have been reported in 38% to 47% of women patients undergoing cross-sectional computed tomographic (CT) or magnetic resonance (MR) imaging.

Pelvic origin, lower extremity varices may occur either in isolation or in association with typical pelvic symptoms. Vulvar varicosities are reported to account for 4% of women presenting with varicose veins. They complicate 8% and 10% of pregnancies, risk increasing with parity, and usually resolve within 6 weeks of delivery. Approximately one-third of women with pelvic venous disorders have vulvovaginal varices and up to 90% may have lower-limb varices. Conversely, approximately 5% of women presenting with lower extremity varicose veins will have concurrent pelvic symptoms.

Asymptomatic radiographic evidence of left renal vein compression (nutcracker "phenomenon") is common and must be distinguished from compression associated with clinical symptoms (NCS). The incidence of 50% or more left renal vein compression in patients undergoing routine imaging has varied from 10.9% to 72%. Among patients with CT findings of left renal vein compression, Poyraz found that only 8.8% had hematuria or proteinuria whereas 5.5% had either a varicocele or pelvic congestion. Symptoms have been reported to be more common in asthenic patients, presumably caused by a paucity of retroperitoneal fat, and those with an aortomesenteric angle of less than 16 degrees (normal 35–40 degrees). Symptoms also appear to have a predominance in women and have peak onset in the second or third decade of life. Some have suggested a bimodal age distribution with one peak in adolescents and young adults and a second in middle-aged women. It has been suggested that spontaneous resolution of symptoms may be more common in children and adolescents, presumably caused by either the development of collaterals or changes in anthropomorphic proportions. Spontaneous resolution of hematuria has been reported in up to 75% of adolescents. Left renal vein compression may also present as a varicocele in men, particularly in adolescents, in whom up to one-quarter of patients may have anatomic evidence of left renal vein compression.

As for left renal vein compression, asymptomatic CIV compression is far more common than symptomatic lesions. Nonthrombotic iliac vein lesions are more common in women with a female-to-male ratio of 4:1. The original autopsy studies of May and Thurner found spurs at the arterial crossing in 24% of 342 adult cadavers. These spurs were associated with distal thrombosis in one-third of cases. Similarly, Kibbe identified more than 50% compression of the left CIVs in almost one-quarter of patients undergoing CT scanning for abdominal pain, with greater mean compression in females. Marston found the prevalence of such lesions to be higher in patients with advanced venous disease, reaching up to 37% in patients with healed or active venous ulcers. Patients at highest risk for an underlying iliac vein lesion are those with a history of deep venous thrombosis or with axial deep venous reflux.

DIAGNOSIS OF PELVIC VENOUS DISORDERS

Venography has historically been the gold standard for the diagnosis of pelvic venous disorders. Diagnostic criteria for primary ovarian vein incompetence, initially proposed by Beard, included an ovarian vein diameter 6 mm or greater, contrast retention in the pelvic venous plexus of more than 20 seconds, congestion of the pelvic venous plexus and/or opacification of the ipsilateral (or contralateral) internal iliac vein, and/or filling of vulvovaginal and thigh varicosities (Fig. 21.11). Each variable was assigned a value of 1 to 3, depending on the degree of abnormality, with a score greater than 5 indicating pelvic congestion syndrome. Fortunately, contrast venography is now largely used to guide intervention and has been replaced by a variety of noninvasive modalities.

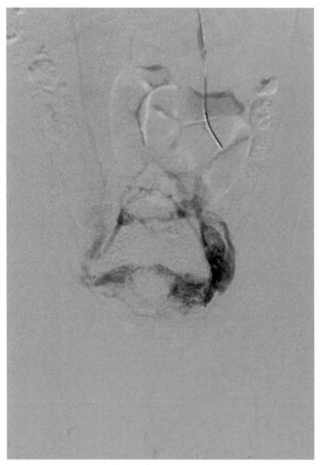

■ **Fig. 21.11** Digital subtraction left ovarian venogram. Note diagnostic criteria (see text) including congestion of the pelvic venous plexus, prolonged contrast retention in the pelvic venous plexus, and opacification of the contralateral internal iliac vein.

Cross-sectional imaging with CT or MR venography is commonly used to establish the etiology of pelvic venous disorders in symptomatic patients. Both modalities are sensitive for pelvic varices, ovarian vein dilation, and compression of the left common iliac and renal veins. Pelvic varices appear as dilated and tortuous parauterine tubular structures, which may extend laterally in the broad ligament and reach the pelvic side wall or extend inferiorly to communicate with the paravaginal venous plexus. Coakley has proposed cross-sectional diagnostic criteria for pelvic varices including at least four ipsilateral tortuous parauterine veins, at least one of which measures over 4 mm in diameter, or an ovarian vein diameter greater than 8 mm. Unfortunately, CT requires radiation, and neither modality provides hemodynamic information, a clear benefit of duplex ultrasonography.

Duplex ultrasound has become the diagnostic test of choice in most venous centers. Although transvaginal ultrasound can clearly demonstrate pelvic varices, routine trans-abdominal ultrasound often provides more complete interrogation of the entire abdominal, pelvic, lower extremity venous circulation. The patient, fasting and with a full bladder, is positioned in reverse Trendelenburg position and the fundus of the uterus and periuterine crossing veins are first evaluated. The number of periuterine crossing veins are estimated, and vein diameters are measured (Fig. 21.12). The patient then empties their bladder and in reverse Trendelenburg position, renal vein compression is evaluated using a

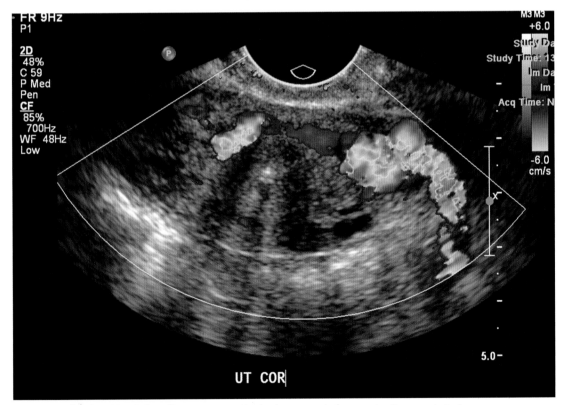

■ **Fig. 21.12** Color flow transvaginal ultrasound demonstrating periuterine varicosities.

combination of renal vein diameter and velocity ratios (Fig. 21.13). In comparison with the main renal vein, a diameter ratio of 5 (main renal vein to point maximal compression diameter) and a velocity ratio of 5 (maximal point of compression to main renal vein velocity) at the point of maximal compression are suggestive of significant renal vein compression. The sensitivity and specificity of duplex ultrasound for the detection of left renal vein compression have been reported to be between 69% to 90% and 89% to 100% respectively.[4] The left and right ovarian veins are then identified on the anterior surface of the psoas muscle and their respective diameters and flow direction (antegrade or retrograde) determined (Fig. 21.14). The IVC and bilateral CIV and external iliac vein are next examined. The presence of left common iliac compression is evaluated using a combination of planimetric diameter measurements and velocity ratios (Fig. 21.15). Labropoulos has suggested a velocity ratio greater than 2.5 across the stenosis as a criterion for hemodynamically significant venous stenosis. The presence of reflux is then evaluated in both internal iliac veins. A combination of an elevated venous velocity ratio and ipsilateral internal iliac reflux have been reported to be reliable diagnostic criteria for hemodynamically significant iliac venous compression.[1]

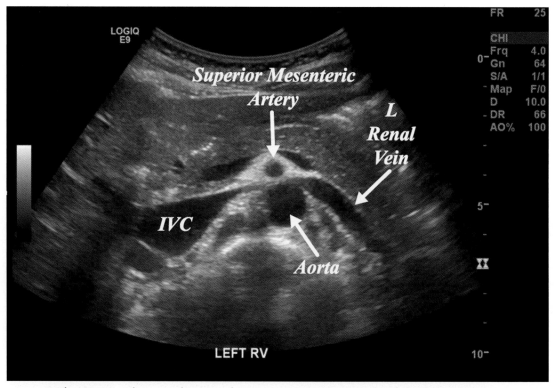

■ **Fig. 21.13** Ultrasound image demonstrating compression of the left renal vein between the superior mesenteric artery and abdominal aorta. *IVC,* Inferior vena cava; *RV,* renal vein.

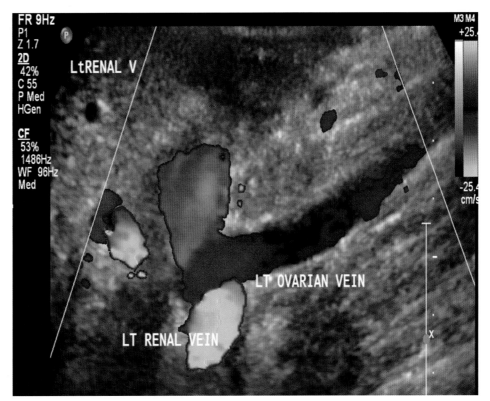

■ **Fig. 21.14** Color flow duplex image demonstrating the origin of the left ovarian directly overlying the psoas muscle, an important landmark in identifying the ovarian veins.

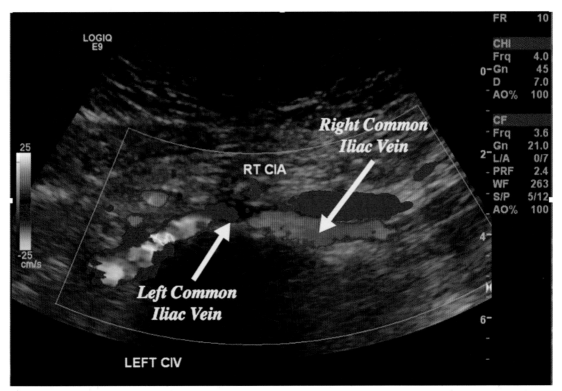

■ **Fig. 21.15** Color flow duplex imaging demonstrating compression of the left common iliac vein beneath the right common iliac artery. The degree of stenosis is estimated by comparing the diameter at the point of maximal compression with that of the normal caliber caudal common iliac vein, as well as by determination of a velocity ratio in comparison to the normal caudal vein. *CIA,* Common iliac artery; *CIV,* common iliac vein.

Invasive diagnostic measures including venography, intravascular ultrasound (IVUS), and pullback pressure measurements are currently used primarily as a guide to intervention. A tilting fluoroscopy table capable of placing the patient in reverse Trendelenburg position is valuable in demonstrating spontaneous reflux. Depending on the operator's preference, either a right internal jugular or a common femoral vein approach can be used. The evaluation begins with contrast venography of the left renal vein (Fig. 21.16).

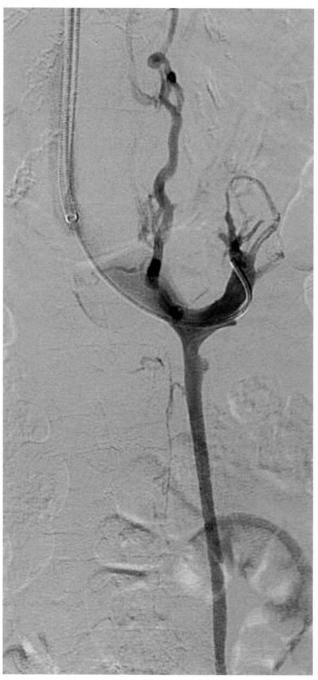

■ **Fig. 21.16** Left renal vein compression. Digital subtraction venography demonstrates contrast attenuation over the abdominal aorta with distal stagnation and the presence of prominent collaterals, particularly the left ovarian vein.

Contrast attenuation over the abdominal aorta, stagnation in the proximal renal vein, and the presence of collaterals may suggest left renal vein compression. In addition, in contrast to the pelvic contrast stagnation seen in patients with primary ovarian incompetence, rapid pelvic drainage via either an antegrade right ovarian vein or the ipsilateral or contralateral internal iliac vein is frequently observed in patients with significant left renal vein compression. However, despite these findings, accurate estimation of the degree of renal vein obstruction may be precluded both by the course of the renal vein in the retroperitoneum and the anteroposterior nature of the compression. A combination of three-dimensional rotational venography (Fig. 21.17A and B), IVUS, and pullback pressures are therefore often helpful if left renal vein compression is suspected on preoperative imaging studies. The normal gradient between the left renal vein and IVC is approximately 1 mm Hg and, although lacking consensus, a pressure gradient of 3 mm Hg or greater is often cited as diagnostic of NCS.[4] In a large series of patients with largely left flank symptoms, a mean gradient of 13 ± 4.5 mm Hg was reported.[5] However, although a gradient may be diagnostic in patients with uncompensated compression and flank pain, it may be absent in women with pelvic symptoms or men with a varicocele who are well decompressed through the left gonadal vein.

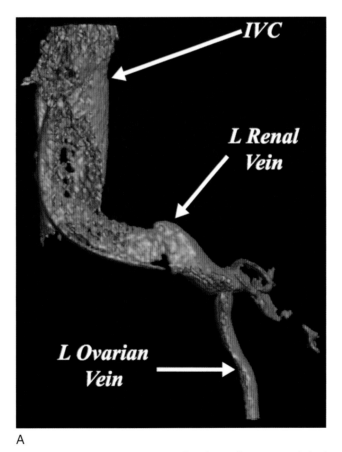

A

■ **Fig. 21.17** Workstation reconstruction of a three-dimensional (3D), rotational venogram of the left renal vein. Software allows creation of a 3D image that can be rotated 360 degrees in all directions. (A) Anteroposterior view of the left renal vein demonstrating no significant stenosis.

Continued

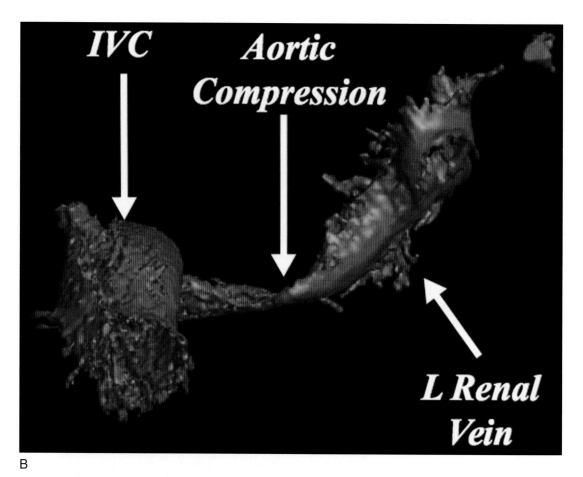

B

■ **Fig. 21.17, cont'd** (B) The left renal vein image is rotated 90 degrees as if observing from the patient's head. Marked compression of the left renal vein is seen overlying the abdominal aorta. *IVC,* Inferior vena cava.

The left ovarian vein is next selected, and the fluoroscopy table moved to a steep reverse Trendelenburg position. Contrast venography is then performed with the catheter positioned both centrally and just above the pelvis. The diagnostic catheter is then exchanged for a compliant occlusion balloon, which is positioned just above the confluence of the ovarian vein tributaries in the pelvis. Balloon occlusion venography (Fig. 21.18) can assist in identifying escape points from the pelvis, as well as in performing balloon occlusion foam sclerotherapy in patients with primary ovarian vein incompetence. If sclerotherapy and coil embolization of the pelvic venous plexus and left ovarian vein are performed, it is important to insure adequate left renal drainage with selective left renal venography on completion. The catheter is then withdrawn into the IVC, the right ovarian vein selected and evaluated in a similar fashion.

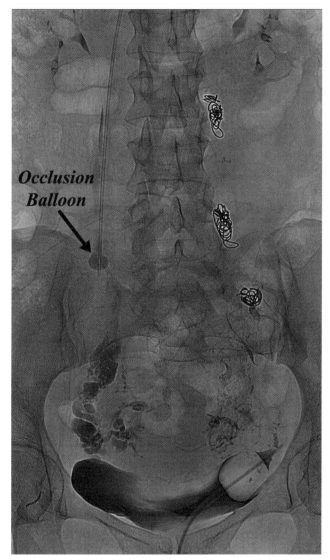

■ **Fig. 21.18** Balloon occlusion venography of the right ovarian vein. A compliant occlusion balloon is inflated above the confluences of the ovarian vein tributaries in the pelvis. Both foam sclerotherapy and coil embolization can be performed through the wire lumen of the occluding balloon.

Both internal iliac veins are then evaluated with balloon occlusion venography (Fig. 21.19). Even in the presence of internal iliac reflux, antegrade flow may preclude adequate visualization of caudal varices and escape points. A compliant occlusion balloon is therefore initially inflated in the internal iliac vein just proximal to the confluence with the external iliac vein and progressively advanced over a glide wire into selected distal varicose tributaries. Balloon occlusion sclerotherapy of more distal tributaries and escape points can then be performed based upon the findings. Finally, if suggested by the patient's symptoms and preoperative imaging, the left CIV is evaluated using a combination of contrast venography and IVUS.

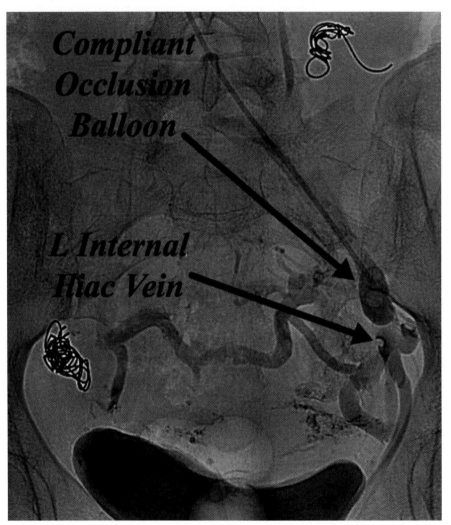

■ **Fig. 21.19** Balloon occlusion venography of the left internal iliac vein.

THE MANAGEMENT OF PELVIC VENOUS DISORDERS

Patients are often referred for management of a primary venous disorder after an extensive evaluation ultimately demonstrates pelvic varices on laparoscopy, ultrasound, or cross-sectional imaging studies. Despite an initial diagnosis based on the finding of pelvic varices, effective treatment is critically dependent on an accurate diagnosis of the precise underlying pathology. A generic approach to treatment, as implied by the term pelvic congestion syndrome, is destined to lead to suboptimal results. Unfortunately, because more than one pathology may coexist, such as concurrent left renal vein and common iliac compression, an understanding of the underlying pathophysiology, careful attention to the diagnostic imaging studies, and clinical judgement are often required in selecting among treatment options. The specific treatment options for each specific pelvic venous disorder will be considered subsequently.

Primary Ovarian/Internal Iliac Venous Incompetence

A variety of medical, surgical, and endovascular approaches have been proposed for the treatment of primary ovarian and internal iliac venous incompetence. Primary ovarian vein incompetence is thought to be related to both mechanical factors, primarily a 60-fold increase in pelvic blood flow during pregnancy, and endocrine factors. Because the ovarian veins may be particularly sensitive to estrogen-mediated vasodilation, pharmacologic suppression of ovarian function would seem logical and treatment with medroxyprogesterone acetate or the gonadotropin-releasing hormone analogue, goserelin, may provide short-term relief of symptoms.[6] Unfortunately, many women fail to attain adequate pain relief and beneficial effects are often not sustained. Furthermore, the side effects of pharmacotherapy, weight gain and bloating with medroxyprogesterone acetate and pseudomenopausal symptoms including hot flashes and bone loss with goserelin, may be unacceptable in the long term.

Surgical approaches to pelvic congestion syndrome have included hysterectomy, with or without oophorectomy, and ovarian vein resection. Hysterectomy fails to directly address the underlying pathophysiology and, in addition to potential morbidity and fertility concerns, has been associated with residual and recurrent symptoms in 33% and 20% of patients respectively. Hysterectomy with bilateral oophorectomy appears more effective than hysterectomy alone.[7] Ovarian vein ligation and/or excision has also been used to eliminate ovarian vein reflux. Because there are frequently multiple venous trunks, Hobbs has emphasized the importance of resecting the ovarian vein from the confluence with the left renal vein or IVC past the confluence of the ovarian tributaries in the pelvis. At least some evidence suggests that bilateral ovarian vein resection may be more effective than unilateral approaches.

Endovascular approaches to primary ovarian and internal iliac venous reflux have largely supplanted medical and surgical approaches. A variety of percutaneous embolization approaches have been reported including simple coil embolization of the refluxing trunks, glue embolization, and a combination of sclerotherapy and coil embolization. Compared with hysterectomy with unilateral or bilateral oophorectomy, the only randomized trial comparing modalities for the management of primary pelvic reflux found a greater 12-month reduction in visual analog pain scores among those undergoing ovarian vein embolization.[7] However, most of the data supporting ovarian and internal iliac embolization comes from case series (Table 21.1). Such series have reported complete or partial symptom resolution in 68.2% to 100% of patients with improvement in mean visual analog pain scores from 7.3 to 7.6 preoperatively to 0.5 to 3.2 postoperatively. However, note that improvement may continue for months after the initial procedure.

These series have reported wide variation in both the technique and extent of embolization. Although an argument can perhaps be made for treating only those veins with clearly documented reflux, reported variability in the extent of ovarian and internal iliac involvement is clearly far greater than can be attributed solely to anatomic variability and be more likely related to the operator's treatment biases and endovascular skills. A thorough search for all refluxing pathways, including both ovarian and internal iliac veins, using balloon occlusion venography should be made in all patients. There does appear to be a tendency toward recurrence in veins that are not embolized and improved results have been reported with bilateral embolization.

Unfortunately, no studies have directly compared glue, coils, and sclerosants either alone or in combination. Although glue embolization does appear to be associated with more treatment failures, the remaining approaches do not appear to differ substantially and there is little solid data to recommend one approach over another (see Table 21.1). However, given the central role of the pelvic venous reservoir in both pelvic and lower extremity manifestations, the addition of sclerosants has theoretical advantages over simple mechanical occlusion of the ovarian and internal iliac veins. Sclerotherapy of the pelvic venous plexus below the confluence of the ovarian and internal iliac trunks might better address the robust anastomoses in the uteroovarian arcade and treat the distal pelvic venous reservoir.

We typically prefer a sandwich technique for embolization of the ovarian veins, alternating sclerosant with clusters of coils (Fig. 21.20). Foam sclerosants, which displace

TABLE 21.1 Outcomes of Pelvic Venous Embolization

Author	N	Treatment	Symptoms Resolved	Symptoms Improved	No Improvement/ Worse	VAS Pre[a]	VAS Post[a]	P
Chung	52	Coils only	—	—	—	7.8 (± 1.2)	3.2 (± 0.9)	<.05
Asciutto	71	Coils only	—	—	53%	—	—	—
Laborda	179	Coils only	—	—	6.2%	7.34 (± 0.7)	0.78 (± 1.2)	.0001
Nasser	100	Coils only	53%	47%	0	7.34 (± .07)	0.47 (± .05)	<.001
Kim	97	Sclerosant + coils	—	—	17%	7.6 (± 1.8)	2.9 (± 2.8)	<.000001
Monedero	100	Sclerosant + coils	64%	29%	7%	—	—	—
Hocquelet	33	Sclerosant + coils	61%	33%	6%	7.37 (± .99)	1.36 (± 1.7)	<.0001
Capasso		Glue and/or coils	57.9%	15.8%	26.3%	—	—	—
Maleux	41	Glue	58.5%	9.7%	31.8%	—	—	—
Van der Vleuren	21	Glue	14.3%	61.9%	23.8%	—	—	—
Pieri	33	Sclerosant only	61%	—	—	—	—	—

[a]*VAS*, 10-point visual analogue pain score before (pre-) and after (post-) embolization.
(Reprinted with permission from Meissner MH, Gibson K. Clinical outcomes after treatment of pelvic congestion syndrome: sense and nonsense. *Phlebology.* 2015;30:73–80.)

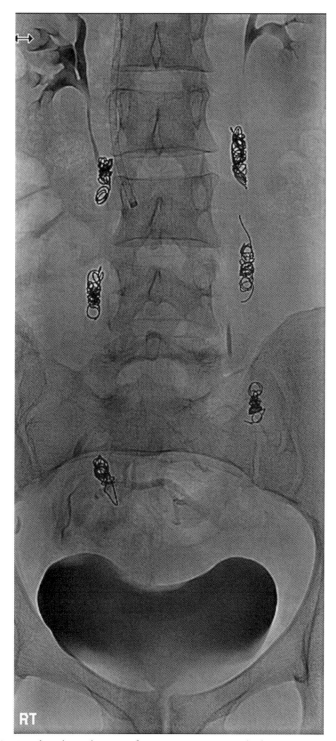

■ **Fig. 21.20** Sandwich technique for ovarian vein embolization. Treatment is performed through a compliant occlusion balloon, and the pelvic venous plexus is initially treated with foamed sclerosant mixed with radiographic contrast under fluoroscopic guidance. Approximately three clusters of coils are then deployed, through the occlusion balloon, along the course of the ovarian vein. Coil clusters are alternated with the installation of foamed sclerosant.

blood and prolong contact with the venous endothelium, have been demonstrated to be more efficacious than liquid sclerotherapy in a variety of other circumstances and are preferred. A compliant occlusion balloon is deployed just above the confluence of the ovarian vein tributaries at L4-L5 and after calibration of the pelvic venous volume with balloon occlusion venography, a similar volume of foam sclerosant diluted with contrast is injected through the occlusion balloon. While allowing the sclerosant to dwell below the occlusion balloon, a cluster of appropriately sized coils is then deployed through the catheter lumen. The balloon is then deflated, the catheter withdrawn several centimeters, after which the balloon is reinflated and additional sclerosant injected followed by the deployment of additional coils. Three clusters of coils, alternated with sclerosant, are typically deployed along the course of the ovarian vein. Such an approach may better address the multiple ovarian trunks and communicating collateral tributaries that are frequently observed.

A similar approach is followed for embolization of the internal iliac veins, although because of the risk of coil migration in these veins, we commonly use foam sclerosants without coil deployment. Coils are occasionally used as an adjuvant if dictated by the specific anatomy. A compliant occlusion balloon is initially inflated just below the confluence of the external and internal iliac veins. After identification of more peripheral varices with balloon occlusion venography, abnormal tributaries are individually selected and treated in a similar fashion with balloon occlusion sclerotherapy.

PELVIC ORIGIN LOWER EXTREMITY VARICES

The optimal management of pelvic-origin, lower extremity varices remains poorly defined and often guided more by the clinician's skills and site of practice (office vs. hospital or outpatient imaging facility) than by clinical evidence. Management options include treating proximal reflux first with pelvic venous embolization, blind treatment of the leg varices with ultrasound-guided sclerotherapy or phlebectomy, and ultrasound and fluoroscopically guided sclerotherapy with the intent of refluxing sclerosant into the pelvic venous reservoir in a controlled fashion.

Initial embolic treatment of any proximal pelvic venous reflux is consistent with the fundamental tenets of lower extremity venous disease but likely represents overtreatment in many patients without pelvic symptoms and has some limitations. Patients with pelvic source varices appear to respond less well to proximal embolization than do those with isolated pelvic symptoms. Such findings are consistent with clinical experience that a single procedure (either pelvic embolization or sclerotherapy of leg varices) rarely addresses all symptoms in patients with concurrent pelvic symptoms and external varices.

Sclerotherapy of external varices, either visual or ultrasound guided, may in contrast fail to suppress reflux from the pelvic venous reservoir, and although results may initially be satisfactory, recurrence rates are likely higher. Despite anecdotal reports of good outcomes,[8] there is little long-term follow-up of patients treated in this fashion.

Although also not supported by long-term data, fluoroscopically guided sclerotherapy (foam or liquid) via direct puncture of the leg varices may allow both control of the pelvic venous reservoir and treatment of external varices (Fig. 21.21). After initial ultrasound-guided puncture of the varices, the escape points and associated pelvic venous anatomy are defined with volume calibrated retrograde direct puncture venography. A similar volume of contrast diluted foam or liquid sclerosant is then slowly injected, following its course centrally into the pelvis with fluoroscopy. Because this approach often requires only a single treatment and may effectively control the pelvic venous plexus as a source

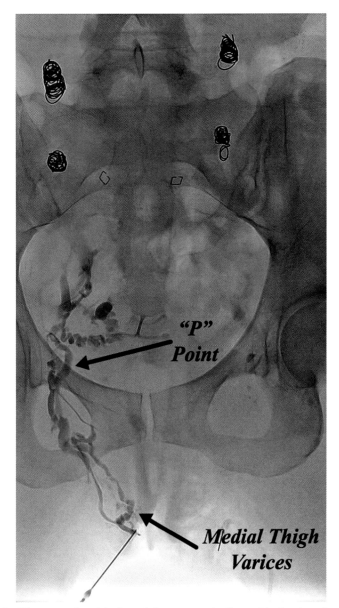

■ **Fig. 21.21** Ultrasound-guided and fluoroscopically guided sclerotherapy of pelvic-origin medial thigh varices. The perineal or "P" point connects the internal and external pudendal systems and communicates with the veins of the medial thigh and further with the saphenofemoral junction.

of recurrence, it is our procedure of choice for pelvic-source, lower extremity, and labial varices.

Primary Left Renal Vein Compression (Nutcracker Syndrome)

Not all patients with compression identified on noninvasive imaging will have symptoms, and among those with trivial symptoms, most can be managed conservatively. However, for adults with disabling symptoms, both surgical and endovascular approaches have been proposed. Surgical approaches have included nephropexy, external renal vein stenting, aortomesenteric transposition, renal autotransplantation, gonadal vein transposition, and left renal vein transposition. However, except for left renal and gonadal vein transposition, most procedures have been described in case reports with little long-term follow-up. Although laparoscopic approaches have been described, left renal vein transposition is generally approached through a small midline incision with mobilization of the left renal vein and IVC, division of the left renal vein at its confluence with the IVC, oversewing of the IVC, and reimplantation of the renal vein inferiorly on the vena cava (Fig. 21.22A–C). Unfortunately, the renal vein may continue to be compressed over the abdominal aorta in a number of cases, again raising questions as to the true underlying etiology of this lesion. Erben and Gloviczki[9] have described a variety of modifications to overcome this limitation, including the use of cuffs, patches, and adjuvant stents. Among 31 patients undergoing renal vein transposition, such adjunctive procedures were required in 14 patients. Unfortunately, despite these modifications, two patients required early reintervention within 30 days whereas 8 patients required late reintervention.

Left ovarian vein transposition may also be an option in patients with pelvic symptoms, although the presence of flank symptoms despite decompression into the pelvis suggests that this may be a less reliable option in these patients. Ovarian transposition to the IVC is performed laparoscopically or through a small, left, lower-quadrant or midline incision, mobilizing and dividing the ovarian vein just above the pelvis, and transposing it medially onto the distal IVC or external iliac vein. The distal ovarian vein can also be cannulated after its division and foam sclerotherapy of the pelvic venous plexus performed under fluoroscopic guidance (Fig. 21.23).

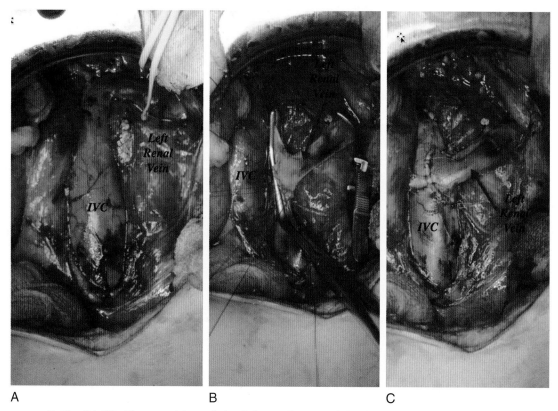

A   B   C

■ **Fig. 21.22** Transposition of the left renal veins. (A) The left renal vein and inferior vena cava (IVC) are mobilized through a small midline incision. (B) The left renal vein is transected including a small cuff of IVC. The IVC defect is oversewn and the renal vein transposed several centimeters distally. (C) An end-renal vein to side IVC anastomosis is constructed, insuring that the renal vein is not stretched over the abdominal aorta.

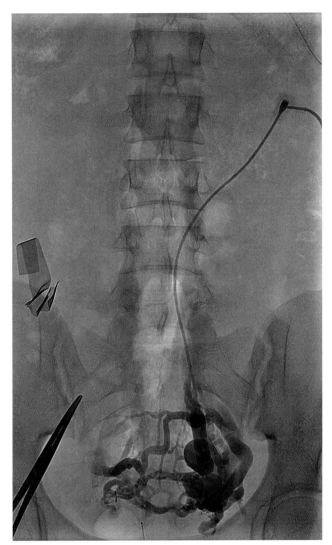

■ **Fig. 21.23** Intraoperative fluoroscopically guided foam sclerotherapy of the pelvic venous plexus performed at the time of left ovarian transposition. A long 5-Fr sheath is brought through the abdominal wall and used to cannulate the distal ovarian vein after its division. Intraoperative venography and foam sclerotherapy are performed after completion of the ovarian vein to inferior vena cava anastomosis.

Endovascular treatment of the left renal vein compression has also been described. Both stainless steel Wallstents (Boston Scientific-Schneider, Minneapolis, MN) and self-expanding nitinol stents have been used. Stent sizing should be based upon the patient's anatomy. Because renal vein diameter may increase 50% to 58% with Valsalva, some have suggested calibrated IVUS measurements be made during such a maneuver. Approximately 20% oversizing is often suggested, commonly resulting in selection of 14-mm to 16-mm stents. Insuring adequate purchase on both sides of the compressive lesion is important and the stent should be partially extended into the IVC. Although short-term results suggest good resolution of symptoms with renal vein stenting, the long-term consequences are unknown. Unfortunately, stent migration, either into the distal renal vein or the heart, remains a significant complication after stenting. A migration rate of

6.7% (5/75) has been reported in one large series, which included two patients requiring surgical extraction for migration to the heart.[5] It is also clear that stent migration is not purely an early phenomenon, with several cases being reported months after initial deployment.

SYMPTOMATIC INTERNAL ILIAC REFLUX CAUSED BY COMMON ILIAC VEIN COMPRESSION (MAY-THURNER SYNDROME)

Endovascular management of lower extremity symptoms caused by iliac compression is covered in more detail elsewhere in this book. However, as discussed previously, pelvic symptoms may also arise from iliac venous compression, and limited data suggests that endovascular stenting of the left CIV is also effective in these patients. Among 19 patients reported by Daugherty, endovascular stenting improved pelvic pain and dyspareunia in 79% and 82% patients respectively.

PITFALLS IN THE MANAGEMENT OF PELVIC VENOUS DISORDERS

Despite the favorable results reported in the literature, not all interventions for pelvic venous disorders benefit all patients. For example, 6% to 31.8% of patients do not get substantial relief following ovarian embolization. At least some of these may represent a failure to correctly diagnose the underlying pathophysiology with subsequent ineffective treatment. Other explanations for an inadequate response to treatment include patient variability, procedural variability, and inadequate outcome measures.

Relevant patient factors may include a differential response of individual symptoms to treatment, underlying psychosocial issues, and issues related to the processing of chronic pain. Certain symptoms, including dyspareunia, urinary frequency, and concurrent pelvic pain and lower extremity varices, may portend a less favorable outcome. In addition, concurrent psychosocial issues, such as anxiety and depression, are frequently present and may also be associated with a poor response to treatment. Finally, at least some evidence suggests that women with chronic pelvic pain may have some disordered pain processing, with a heightened response to noxious stimuli.

In addition to diagnostic uncertainty, procedural variability and the lack of robust data to guide interventions may also lead to poor outcomes. As discussed earlier for ovarian embolization, there is wide variation both in the techniques used and the extent of embolization.

Finally, there is a lack of adequate, disease-specific, outcome measures to assess the response to treatment. Most studies have used either a subjective assessment of degree of improvement or visual analog pain scales. However, such measures fail to account for improvement in psychosocial distress and sexual functioning, both of which have been shown to improve after embolotherapy for primary ovarian vein incompetence. There is a clear need for a disease-specific quality of life instrument that includes both the physical and psychosocial components of pelvic venous disease.

SUMMARY

Although the pathophysiology, diagnosis, and management of lower extremity venous disorders is well understood, our understanding of the complexities of pelvic venous disorders is evolving. Rather than being a disconnected set of syndromes, it is becoming clear that the manifestations of pelvic venous disorders arise from the complex interconnections of three venous systems: those of the left renal and ovarian veins, the internal iliac veins, and the superficial veins of the lower extremity. These are associated with two patterns of reflux affecting the ovarian and internal iliac veins and two patterns of obstruction related to compression of the common iliac or renal veins. Symptoms are often determined by whether or not rises in pressure are directly transmitted to the distal venous reservoir (uncompensated reflux or obstruction) or decompressed into more caudal reservoirs by associated collaterals (compensated reflux or obstruction). Treatment of these disorders is critically dependent on appropriate identification of the underlying pathophysiology. Unfortunately, appropriate diagnosis is often confounded by concurrence of multiple lesions, and treatment must often be guided by the results of small case series rather than rigorous randomized trials. Improving the care of women with these disorders will require a better understanding of abdominal and pelvic venous anatomy, as well as the connections to the lower extremity veins, improved comprehension of the relative importance of pelvic venous reflux and obstruction in individuals patients, validation of diagnostic protocols, particularly with respect to ultrasound, robust clinical trials evaluating the management of pelvic venous reflux and obstruction, and validated patient-centered outcome measures.

REFERENCES

1. Daugherty SF, Gillespie DL. Venous angioplasty and stenting improve pelvic congestion syndrome caused by venous outflow obstruction. *J Vasc Surg Venous Lymphat Disord.* 2015;3:283–289.
2. Kachlik D, Pechacek V, Musil V, et al. The venous system of the pelvis: new nomenclature. *Phlebology.* 2010;25:162–173.
3. Meissner MH, Gibson K. Clinical outcome after treatment of pelvic congestion syndrome: sense and nonsense. *Phlebology.* 2015;30:73–80.
4. Kurklinsky AK, Rooke TW. Nutcracker phenomenon and nutcracker syndrome. *Mayo Clin Proc.* 2010;85:552–559.
5. Wu Z, Zheng X, He Y, et al. Stent migration after endovascular stenting in patients with nutcracker syndrome. *J Vasc Surg Venous Lymphat Disord.* 2016;4:193–199.
6. Soysal ME, Soysal S, Vicdan K, et al. A randomized controlled trial of goserelin and medroxyprogesterone acetate in the treatment of pelvic congestion. *Hum Reprod.* 2001;16:931–939.
7. Chung MH, Huh CY. Comparison of treatments for pelvic congestion syndrome. *Tohoku J Exp Med.* 2003;201:131–138.
8. Scultetus AH, Villavicencio JL, Gillespie DL, et al. The pelvic venous syndromes: analysis of our experience with 57 patients. *J Vasc Surg.* 2002;36:881–888.
9. Erben Y, Gloviczki P, Kalra M, et al. Treatment of nutcracker syndrome with open and endovascular interventions. *J Vasc Surg Venous Lymphat Disord.* 2015;3:389–396.

CHAPTER 22

Nutcracker Syndrome

Manju Kalra and Peter Gloviczki

Compression of the left renal vein (LRV) between the superior mesenteric artery (SMA) and the abdominal aorta was first described by Grant in 1937, who found the anatomic relationship analogous to a nut in a nutcracker.[1] The first clinical report was by El-Sadr in 1950, although the compression was documented by venography only 2 decades later by Chait.[2] The term *nutcracker* phenomenon was coined by de Schepper in 1972. The importance of retroperitoneal fat in maintaining a wide aortomesenteric angle was suggested by Stavros et al., and classically an asthenic body habitus has since been associated with nutcracker syndrome (NCS) or symptoms secondary to the nutcracker phenomenon (Fig. 22.1). Stretching the LRV secondary to a posteriorly ptotic left kidney, excess fibrous tissue aortomesenteric angle and wasted paraspinal muscles have also been incriminated. The LRV may also be compressed between the aorta and the vertebral body, leading to a description of a posterior NCS by Lau et al. in 1986.

The most common symptoms of LRV compression include flank pain and hematuria secondary to the increased venous pressure and development of varices in the renal pelvis that rupture into the urinary collecting system. Other reported symptoms include left-sided varicocele in males, pelvic congestion syndrome in females, orthostatic proteinuria, and chronic fatigue. Diagnosis is difficult, often delayed and made only after ruling out all other causes of hematuria and flank pain. It is established by a combination of cystoscopy, ultrasonography, computed tomography (CT) scan and venography with measurement of pressure gradients between the LRV and the inferior vena cava (IVC).[3,4]

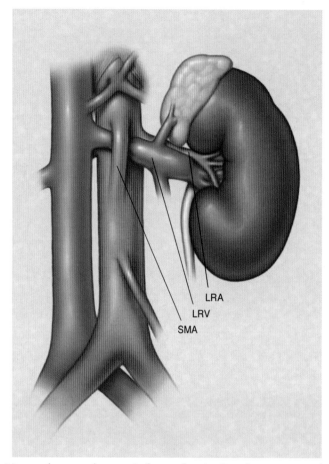

■ Fig. 22.1 Nutcracker syndrome. Left renal vein (LRV) compressed as it passes between the aorta and the superior mesenteric artery (SMA). *LRA*, Left renal artery. *(From Said SM, Gloviczki P, Kalra M, et al. Renal nutcracker syndrome: surgical options.* Semin Vasc Surg. *2013;26(1):35–42.)*

DIAGNOSIS

Cystoscopy is indicated in all patients with hematuria to rule out other causes and localize the source to the left ureteric orifice. It, however, may be normal or noncontributory in patients with intermittent or no hematuria.

Duplex Ultrasonography

Color duplex ultrasound (DUS) is a good screening study to confirm the presence of anatomic LRV compression and has been used for the diagnosis of LRV compression syndrome since 1986.[3,5–7] This should be the initial test if the diagnosis is suspected. However, it has the drawbacks of poor visualization on occasion and operator dependence. A variety of diagnostic criteria have been described. The major ultrasound features are the aortomesenteric angle, aortomesenteric and hilar renal vein anteroposterior (AP) diameter, and peak systolic velocity (PSV) ratios with a ratio greater than 4:5 being acceptable to consider the diagnosis (Fig. 22.2).

Arima demonstrated symptomatic compression of the LRV when the aortomesenteric angle was less than 6 to 16 degrees (normal around 40 degrees). Other criteria include an AP diameter ratio of 4 and a mean PSV ratio of greater than 5 in patients with symptomatic NCS. However, these vary widely; in a study by Park et al., only 49% of patients had a PSV and AP diameter ratio greater than 4.[8] Kim reported a mean PSV ratio of 7.9 ± 2.7 in patients with clinical NCS and 2.8 ± 1.5 in asymptomatic controls.[9] They reported 90% sensitivity and 100% specificity to diagnose NCS when the mean of the two ratios (AP diameter and PSV) was greater than 5. Park et al., in a similar study, designated an AP diameter to PSV ratio of 4 to be diagnostic.[8] Takebayashi et al. compared DUS with conventional left renal venography and reported sensitivity and specificity of DUS to diagnose NCS of 78% and 100%, respectively, when the color flow in the collateral veins is included in the diagnostic criteria.[7]

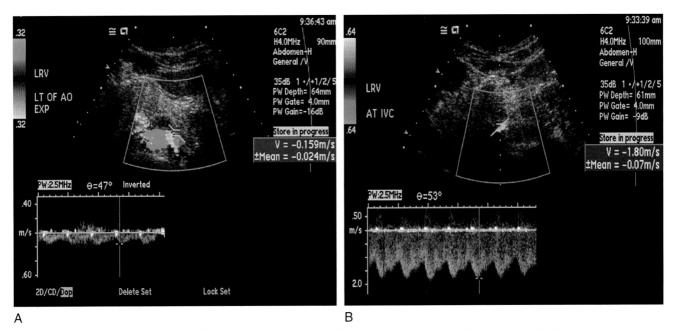

■ **Fig. 22.2** Duplex ultrasound images showing the peak systolic velocity (PSV) (A) at the hilar segment of the left renal vein and (B) in the aortomesenteric angle; PSV ratio = 11.3.

Computed Tomography/Magnetic Resonance Imaging/Intravascular Ultrasound

CT venography and magnetic resonance imaging (MRI) scans can also demonstrate the nature and degree of LRV narrowing, retroperitoneal, and renal hilar collaterals (Fig. 22.3). A "beak sign" (triangular shape of LRV caused by severe aortomesenteric narrowing) is described. Similar to DUS features, an LRV (hilar-aortomesenteric) diameter ratio cut-off of 4.9 and an angle of less than 41 degrees between the SMA and the aorta are considered diagnostic.[10] However, it is imperative that the CT scan be performed specifically to capture the venous phase with maximal distention of the LRV because a CT scan done for other purposes may demonstrate a false-positive compression of the LRV (Fig. 22.4). MRI, although less commonly used, has findings similar to those seen on CT venography. Intravascular ultrasound (IVUS) has also been used to measure the degree of venous stenosis.[11] Positive imaging findings of nutcracker phenomenon must always be correlated with the clinical situation.

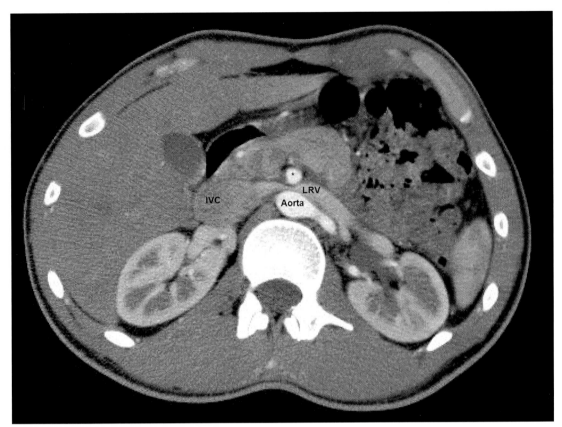

■ **Fig. 22.3** Computed tomography venography showing the left renal vein being (LRV) compressed as it passes between the aorta and the superior mesenteric artery (*). *IVC,* Inferior vena cava. *(From Reed NR, Kalra M, Bower TC, et.al. Left renal vein transposition for nutcracker syndrome.* J Vasc Surg. *2009;49(2):386–393.)*

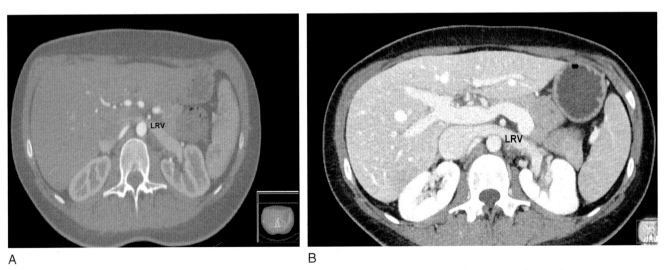

A   B

■ **Fig. 22.4** (A) Computed tomography (CT) imaging of the abdomen performed at outside institution reported as nutcracker syndrome, and (B) repeat CT venography to specifically evaluate left renal vein demonstrating no compression. *LRV,* Left renal vein.

Venography

A venous pressure gradient of 2 to 14 mm Hg between the hilar LRV and the IVC during venography has been considered the gold standard for diagnosis, the normal being 0 to 1 mm Hg. Venography also demonstrates narrowing, collaterals, and the nature of venous reflux in the left gonadal vein, as well as direction of flow across the narrowed segment of LRV (Fig. 22.5). However, interpretation of pressure gradients may be fallacious because of high variability in healthy subjects; variation with position, hydration, degree of collateralization, and overlap in values between normal and symptomatic patients. Conversely, postoperative symptom resolution has been reported with no change in pressure gradients.[12] Thus radiographic evidence alone is not sufficient to prompt invasive treatment because imaging criteria do not necessarily correlate with symptomatology.[12]

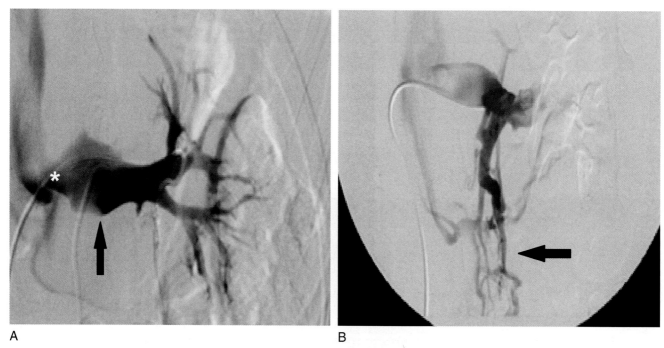

A   B

■ **Fig. 22.5** Contrast venography showing (A) narrowing of the left renal vein as it crosses the aorta underneath the superior mesenteric artery (*), dilatation of the peripheral left renal vein (*arrow*) and (B) opacification of gonadal, ascending lumbar, adrenal and other collateral veins (*arrow*).

PATIENT SELECTION CRITERIA

The aim of intervention for NCS is to reduce LRV hypertension. The lack of correlation of symptoms with radiologic features makes prediction of operative outcomes difficult. Imaging is necessary to confirm significant, anatomic LRV compression, but the indications for intervention remain clinical. Our protocol is guided by patient symptoms (Fig. 22.6). Most operative or endovascular procedures are reserved for severe hematuria and/or debilitating flank pain. For those presenting with a varicocele and flank pain, operative treatment resulted in resolution of the pain, but the varicocele recurred in the majority. Hence in patients presenting with a varicocele alone, we advise traditional treatments (gonadal vein coil occlusion or local ligation). Those with mild or atypical symptoms are offered medical/pain management as the first line of treatment. We compared radiologic criteria in patients we treated surgically with those who were managed conservatively based upon clinical presentation and severity of symptoms and found a significant overlap (Table 22.1).[12]

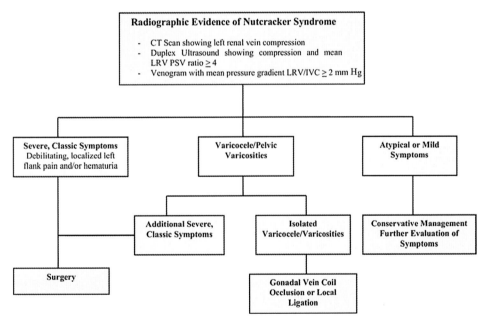

■ **Fig. 22.6** Nutcracker syndrome: proposed diagnostic and management protocol. *CT,* Computed tomography; *IVC,* inferior vena cava; *LRV,* left renal vein; *PSV,* peak systolic velocity. *(From Reed NR, Kalra M, Bower TC, et.al. Left renal vein transposition for nutcracker syndrome.* J Vasc Surg. *2009;49(2):386–393.)*

TABLE 22.1 Patient Demographics in 23 Patients With Nutcracker Syndrome

	Surgical Management (N = 11)	Conservative Management (N = 12)
Median age (years)	23 (16–43)	18 (14–67)
Male/female	4/7	6/6
Left flank pain	10	3
Hematuria	7	5
Pelvic varicosities/varicocele	3	6
Atypical symptoms	1[a]	5[a]
Mean LRV PSV ratio	6.6 (2.5–10)[b]	8.4 (4–12)[b]
Mean pressure gradient LRV/IVC (mm Hg)	4 (2–6)[c]	4 (4–5)[c]

[a]Atypical symptoms include bilateral flank pain, postural tachycardia, orthostatic hypotension, painless hematuria, back pain, renal stones, urinary incontinence, weight loss, vomiting, and diarrhea.
[b]Ultrasounds performed in 7 of 11 surgically managed patients; 8 of 12 conservatively managed patients.
[c]Venography performed in 10 of 11 surgically managed patients; 4 of 12 conservatively managed patients.
IVC, Inferior vena cava; *LRV,* left renal vein; *PSV,* peak systolic velocity.
(From Reed NR, Kalra M, Bower TC, et.al. Left renal vein transposition for nutcracker syndrome. *J Vasc Surg.* 2009;49(2):386–393.)

TREATMENT

Open, endovascular, and hybrid treatment options are described albeit with limited concentration of experience because of rarity of the disorder.

Open Reconstruction

Left Renal Vein Transposition

Left renal vein transposition: Because the basic pathology responsible for NCSs is compression of the renal vein, direct procedures on the LRV are likely to be most efficacious with least risk to other structures. This is the most common and most effective procedure in which the LRV is transposed distally onto the IVC at an area where the aortomesenteric space is wider (Fig. 22.7). Through a transabdominal, transperitoneal minilaparotomy, the small bowel is retracted to the right and in part toward the distal abdomen. The retroperitoneum is opened between the fourth part of the duodenum and the inferior mesenteric vein, in front of the infrarenal abdominal aorta. The LRV is mobilized, and the left adrenal and descending left lumbar vein are ligated and divided to facilitate adequate mobilization. The left gonadal vein is preferably preserved for subsequent coiling to treat unresolved pelvic congestion or as a conduit for bailout secondary procedures. Intraoperative measurement of the pressure gradient can be performed before transecting the LRV. Following systemic heparinization, the IVC is controlled with a side-biting Satinsky clamp across the LRV confluence. The LRV is then transected and a tension-free end-to-side reanastomosis to the IVC at a more distal location is performed. The original insertion site on the IVC is oversewn. Following restoration of flow, patency may be documented with intraoperative DUS, IVUS, or venography.

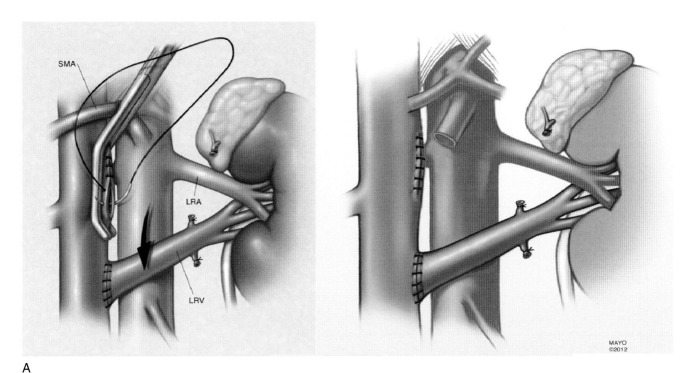

A

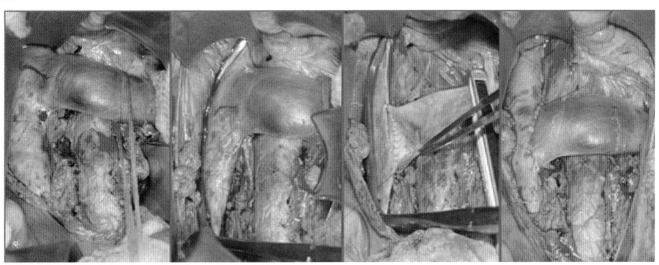

B

■ **Fig. 22.7** Left renal vein transposition. (A) Illustration showing inferior vena cava (IVC) control, transection of left renal vein, tension-free, end-to-side reanastomosis to the IVC at a distal location and oversewing of the IVC (B) Intraoperative images demonstrating the same. *LRA,* Left renal artery, *LRV,* left renal vein; *SMA,* superior mesenteric artery. *(From Said SM, Gloviczki P, Kalra M, et al. Renal nutcracker syndrome: surgical options. Semin Vasc Surg. 2013;26(1):35–42.)*

Left renal vein transposition with patch venoplasty: Permanent distortion of the vein with sclerosis and fixed narrowing of the venous lumen, akin to that seen in the subclavian vein in venous thoracic outlet syndrome, may be present with chronic compression. In patients with a stretched out LRV (ptotic kidney/lack of retroperitoneal fat), a tension-free anastomosis may not be possible once the LRV is transected. A great saphenous vein (GSV) patch across the anterior wall of the anastomosis to augment the LRV–IVC confluence after LRV transposition is a useful adjunct (Fig. 22.8).

Left renal vein transposition with saphenous vein cuff: In circumstances where the LRV length is totally inadequate to transpose to a sufficiently wide area of the aortomesenteric space, a GSV cuff extension to the LRV may be performed to ensure a

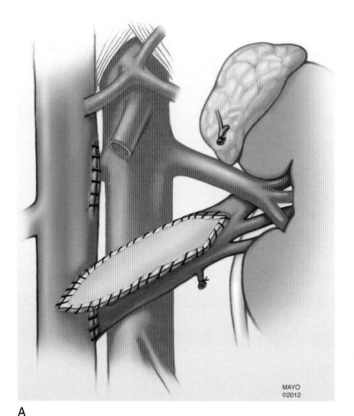

A

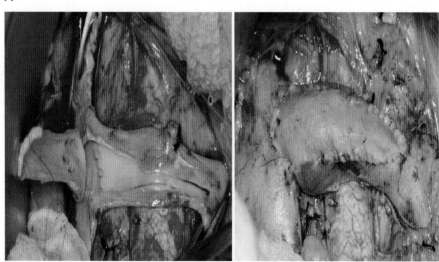

B

■ **Fig. 22.8** Left renal vein transposition with patch venoplasty. (A) Illustration showing a great saphenous vein patch across the anterior wall of the left renal vein–inferior vena cava (LRV-IVC) anastomosis to augment the LRV-IVC confluence after LRV transposition. (B) Intraoperative images demonstrating the same. *(From Said SM, Gloviczki P, Kalra M, et al. Renal nutcracker syndrome: surgical options.* Semin Vasc Surg. *2013;26(1):35–42.)*

tension-free anastomosis. The GSV cuff is created and first sutured to the IVC with a continuous polypropylene suture following which it is anastomosed end-to-end to the LRV with interrupted 5 or 6 polypropylene sutures (Fig. 22.9).

Stenosis or thrombosis of the transposed LRV can occur with recurrence of symptoms. The predisposing causes are a scarred distorted vein, especially one with previous thrombosis with inadequate length to perform a tension-free anastomosis to the IVC.[13]

Venous Bypass Procedures

In patients who have compression of a retroaortic LRV or in those with chronic LRV thrombosis, anterior transposition alone may not be sufficient, and an interposition graft or implantation of the gonadal vein to the IVC may be better alternatives.

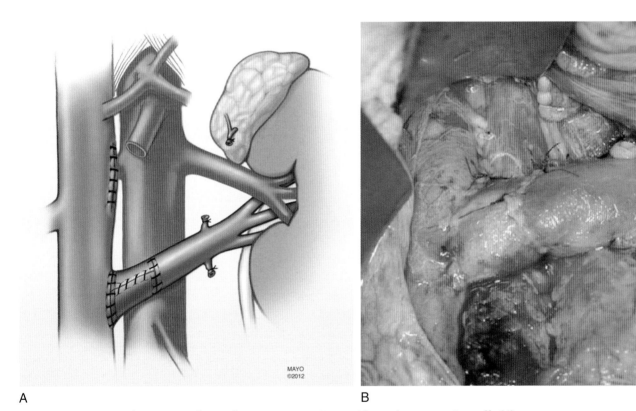

A   B

■ **Fig. 22.9** Left renal vein transposition with saphenous vein cuff. (A) Illustration showing great saphenous vein cuff extension to elongate the left renal vein. (B) Intraoperative image demonstrating the same. *(From Said SM, Gloviczki P, Kalra M, et al. Renal nutcracker syndrome: surgical options.* Semin Vasc Surg. *2013;26(1):35–42.)*

Gonadal vein transposition: In this technique, the left gonadal vein is transected and reimplanted into the IVC (Fig. 22.10). This is a particularly suitable alternative in patients with NCS and an incompetent left gonadal vein with symptomatic pelvic congestion, or in the setting of thrombosis of the LRV, either de novo or following transposition. This also serves the purpose of decompressing the LRV through the gonadal vein without actual transection and translocation of the LRV itself. The left gonadal vein is approached through the transverse mesocolon similar to the exposure used for LRV transposition. The side branches of the gonadal vein are ligated and divided. The gonadal vein is ligated distally, divided and tunneled under the inferior mesenteric vessels over the abdominal aorta toward the IVC. Following systemic heparinization, the IVC is controlled with a side-biting Satinsky clamp and an end-to-side anastomosis using interrupted 6 polypropylene sutures is performed.

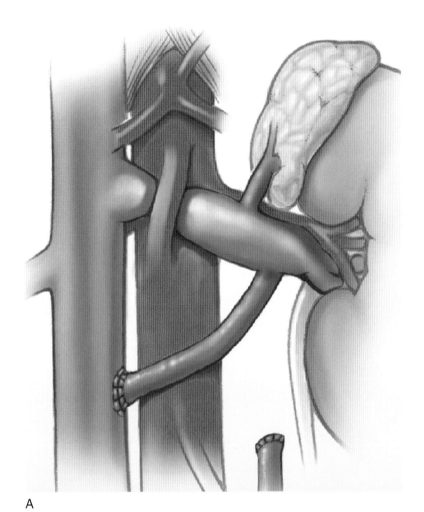

A

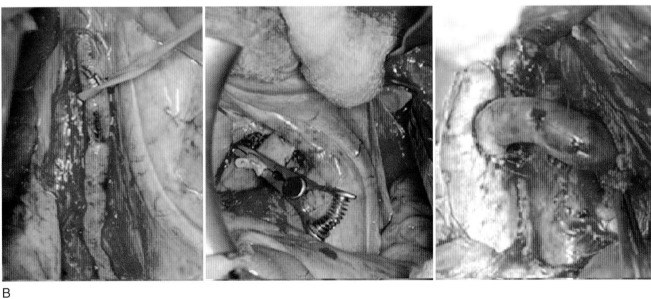

B

■ **Fig. 22.10** Left gonadal vein transposition. (A) Illustration. (B) Intraoperative images showing the vein isolation, distal transection, tunneled under the inferior mesenteric vessels and reimplantation into the inferior vena cava. *(From Said SM, Gloviczki P, Kalra M, et al. Renal nutcracker syndrome: surgical options. Semin Vasc Surg. 2013;26(1):35–42.)*

Renocaval great saphenous vein bypass: In the absence of a large-caliber, refluxing gonadal vein, a GSV conduit can be used to bypass the compressed segment of the LRV without the need for transection and transposition (Fig. 22.11). This is an excellent option especially when the compressed segment of LRV has suffered thrombosis as well.

Renal autotransplantation: This is a potentially more complete procedure but has the advantage of correcting concomitant posterior ptosis. It involves a much more extensive dissection, longer period of renal ischemia, and additional renal artery and ureteric anastomoses with their attendant risk of complications. It is, however, worth considering as a bailout in the setting of failed prior operative procedures before resorting to nephrectomy in these young patients.

Other Procedures

In patients who have fibrous or fibrolymphatic tissue in the etiology of renal vein compression, excision of this tissue may provide immediate relief.[14] Anterior or anteromedial

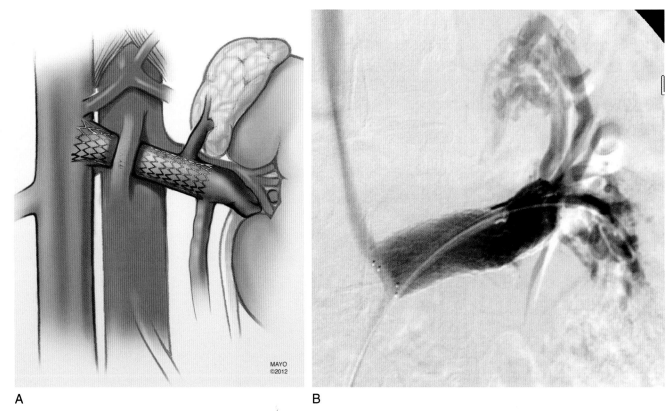

A   B

■ **Fig. 22.11** Left renal vein stent. (A) Illustration. (B) Intraoperative images, stent placed from the first division of the renal vein. *(From Erben Y, Gloviczki P, Kalra M, et.al. Treatment of nutcracker syndrome with open and endovascular interventions. J Vasc Surg Venous Lymphat Disord. 2015;3(4),389–396.)*

nephroplexy has been used successfully in patients with posterior ptosis.[15,16] Other open operative procedures reported include transposition or bypass of the SMA,[17] external stenting of the LRV using ringed polytetrafluoroethylene (PTFE),[11,18] and placement of a wedge of Dacron to increase the mesoaortic angle.[14] SMA transposition, rarely performed now, incurs the added risks of bowel ischemia and has been reported only rarely. Both the external stent and the wedge have the potential to cause kinking of the SMA in thin patients and risks possible erosion of the Dacron into the bowel.

Posterior Nutcracker Syndrome

Anterior transposition of the left renal vein: The posterior NCS can be repaired by transposing the retroaortic LRV from its original course to be anterior to the aorta and reimplanting it onto the IVC. The operative technique is similar to that used for the anterior NCS. A retroaortic LRV is more friable and frequently has multiple small tributaries. It may be associated with larger lymph vessels, which require careful ligation to avoid lymphatic leak. The vein is then translocated anterior and cephalad for a tension-free reimplantation into the IVC. The anastomosis can be performed in a continuous fashion to the posterior wall and with interrupted sutures for the anterior wall. If further widening of the LRV is indicated, an incision is made in the anterior wall of the LRV and the anterior wall of the IVC. A vein (GSV) patch is sewn in with a continuous 6 polypropylene suture. GSV patches or cuffs will be frequently required to provide adequate length for successful anterior transposition.

Endovascular Treatment

Following work published by Neste et al. in 1996, endovascular options have emerged as an alternative treatment option for NCS. Stents with high radial strength, good conformability, and minimal shortening with deployment systems that allow accurate placement are ideal. In the absence of availability of dedicated venous stents, self-expanding stents (Wallstent, SMART stent) are commonly used. Oversizing is recommended and a 6-cm or longer stent is placed, extending from the first division of the renal vein centrally to the IVC to minimize the risk of migration, the most common complication (see Fig. 22.11). Embolization of the stent to the lung has been reported. Stent protrusion into the IVC is a common observation, but it does not seem to cause any complication. Factors affecting stent migration may include a shorter distance between the ostium and the first large branch of the LRV, the increase in the LRV intraluminal pressure, pulsatility, and proximity of the stent to the abdominal aorta. Other complications, such as stent thrombosis, in-stent restenosis, kinking, and fracture are rare; this may be caused by a high-flow rate and endogenous urokinase. Unfortunately, an ideal stent for use specifically in this anatomic situation does not exist, making the results of stenting suboptimal in the long-term in spite of excellent early relief from symptoms reported.[18–25]

This minimally invasive approach may become the treatment of choice. However, clearly the long-term fate of intrarenal stents in these young patients with the potential associated complications of stenosis, thrombosis, embolization, and erosion remains to be evaluated.

Hybrid reconstruction, combining open repair followed by stenting, is an attractive option. The stent is sewn in place to the vein to prevent migration and ensure a better postoperative result (Fig. 22.12). This procedure has been recently adopted by us and combines the advantages of transposing the LRV to a more favorable site in the aortomesenteric angle, with the radial force of the stent serving to keep the vein open

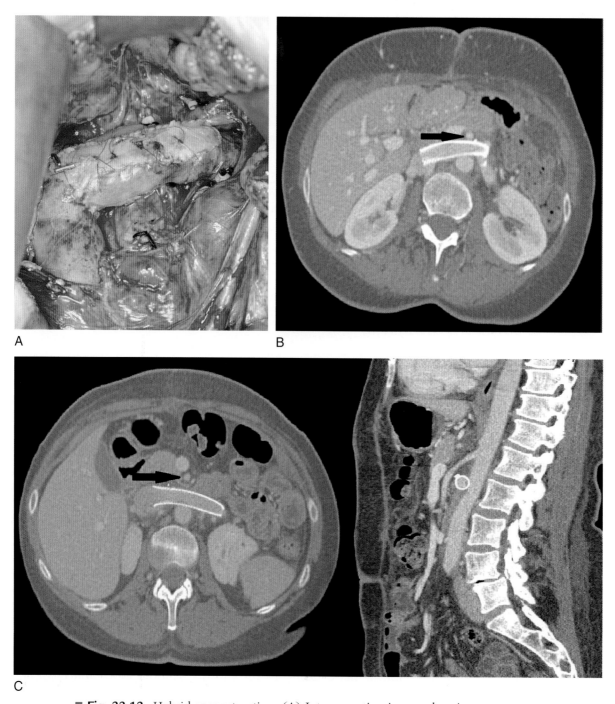

■ **Fig. 22.12** Hybrid reconstruction. (A) Intraoperative image showing open repair followed by stenting, stent is sewn in place to the vein to prevent migration. (B) Postoperative computed tomography venography following percutaneous left renal vein stenting and (C) axial and sagittal imaging following hybrid reconstruction demonstrating significant widening of aortomesenteric space *(arrow)* between (B) and (C).

at the site of anastomosis to the IVC. Durability and clinical outcome will need to be evaluated.

CONCLUSION

In patients with suspected NCS, symptom severity may not correlate with imaging parameters. Careful evaluation of clinical symptoms and thorough investigation of radiologic evidence of LRV compression is advisable before recommending surgical/endovascular intervention to obtain the best long-term outcomes. Patients with severe, classic, and chronic symptoms should be offered intervention. Renal vein transposition is safe and effective, and should be considered first-line therapy along with whatever adjuncts, including hybrid repair, needed to ensure a wide, tension-free anastomosis to the IVC. Early results of primary stenting are satisfactory, but long-term outcome results are limited. Both treatment modalities are invaluable in the event of failure of the other modality.

REFERENCES

1. Grant JCB, ed. A method of anatomy, descriptive and deductive. 3rd ed. Baltimore: The Williams and Wilkins company; 1944:822. xxiv.
2. Chait AMK, Fabian CE, Mellins HZ. Vascular impressions on the ureters. *Am J Roentgen Rad Ther.* 1971;3:729–749.
3. Stavros AT, Sickler KJ, Menter RR. Color duplex sonography of the nutcracker syndrome (aortomesenteric left renal vein compression). *J Ultrasound Med.* 1994;13(7):569–574.
4. Imamura A, Nakamura M, Maekawa N, et al. [Usefulness of renal CT scan for analysis of nutcracker phenomenon]. *Nippon Hinyokika Gakkai Zasshi.* 1992;83(11):1861–1865.
5. Wolfish NM, McLaine PN, Martin D. Renal vein entrapment syndrome: frequency and diagnosis—a lesson in conservatism. *Clin Nephrol.* 1986;26:96–100.
6. Arima MH, Hosokawa S, Ogino T. Ultrasonographically demonstrated nutcraker phenomenon: alternative to angiography. *Int Urol Nephrol.* 1990;22:3.
7. Takebayashi S, Ueki T, Ikeda N, et al. Diagnosis of the nutcracker syndrome with color Doppler sonography: correlation with flow patterns on retrograde left renal venography. *AJR Am J Roentgenol.* 1999;172(1):39–43.
8. Park SJ, Lim JW, Cho BS, et al. Nutcracker syndrome in children with orthostatic proteinuria: diagnosis on the basis of Doppler sonography. *J Ultrasound Med.* 2002;21(1):39–45, quiz 6.
9. Kim SH, Cho SW, Kim HD, et al. Nutcracker syndrome: diagnosis with Doppler US. *Radiology.* 1996;198(1):93–97.
10. Said SM, Gloviczki P, Kalra M, et al. Renal nutcracker syndrome: surgical options. *Semin Vasc Surg.* 2013;26(1):35–42.
11. Barnes RW, Fleisher HL 3rd, Redman JF, et al. Mesoaortic compression of the left renal vein (the so-called nutcracker syndrome): repair by a new stenting procedure. *J Vasc Surg.* 1988;8(4):415–421.
12. Reed NR, Kalra M, Bower TC, et al. Left renal vein transposition for nutcracker syndrome. *J Vasc Surg.* 2009;49(2):386–393, discussion 93–94.
13. Erben Y, Gloviczki P, Kalra M, et al. Treatment of nutcracker syndrome with open and endovascular interventions. *J Vasc Surg Venous Lymphat Disord.* 2015;3(4):389–396.
14. Ariyoshi A, Nagase K. Renal hematuria caused by "nutcracker" phenomenon: a more logical surgical management. *Urology.* 1990;35(2):168–170.
15. Wendel R, Crawford ED, Hehman K. The "nutcracker" phenomenon: an unusual cause for renal varicosities with hematuria. *J Urol.* 1980;123:761–763.
16. Lopatkin NA, Morozov AV, Lopatkina LN. Essential renal hemorrhages. *Eur Urol.* 1978;4:115–119.

17. Zhang H, Zhang N, Li M, et al. Treatment of six cases of left renal nutcracker phenomenon: surgery and endografting. *Chin Med J.* 2003;116(11):1782–1784.

18. Scultetus AH, Villavicencio JL, Gillespie DL. The nutcracker syndrome: its role in the pelvic venous disorders. *J Vasc Surg.* 2001;34(5):812–819.

19. Lin WQ, Huang HF, Li M, et al. [Diagnosis and therapy of the nutcracker phenomenon: long-term follow-up]. *Zhonghua Wai Ke Za Zhi.* 2003;41(12):889–892.

20. Segawa N, Azuma H, Iwamoto Y, et al. Expandable metallic stent placement for nutcracker phenomenon. *Urology.* 1999;53(3):631–633.

21. Park YB, Lim SH, Ahn JH, et al. Nutcracker syndrome: intravascular stenting approach. *Nephrol Dial Transplant.* 2000;15(1):99–101.

22. Neste MG, Narasimham DL, Belcher KK. Endovascular stent placement as a treatment for renal venous hypertension. *J Vasc Interv Radiol.* 1996;7(6):859–861.

23. Kim SJ, Kim CW, Kim S, et al. Long-term follow-up after endovascular stent placement for treatment of nutcracker syndrome. *J Vasc Interv Radiol.* 2005;16(3):428–431.

24. Hartung O, Grisoli D, Boufi M, et al. Endovascular stenting in the treatment of pelvic vein congestion caused by nutcracker syndrome: lessons learned from the first five cases. *J Vasc Surg.* 2005;42(2):275–280.

25. Zhang H, Li M, Jin W, et al. The left renal entrapment syndrome: diagnosis and treatment. *Ann Vasc Surg.* 2007;21(2):198–203.

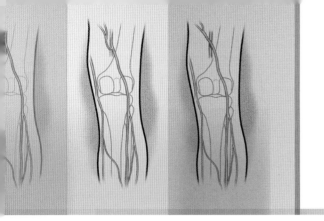

CHAPTER 23

Treatment of Spider Telangiectasias

Edward G. Mackay

HISTORICAL BACKGROUND

The treatment of telangiectasias was not seriously attempted until the 1930s, with Biegeleisen taking the credit for initially attempting an injection into the perivascular space around telangiectatic areas. Later, he implemented intravascular injections using homemade microneedles.[1] These early efforts led to disappointing results, primarily because the sclerosing solutions, such as sodium morrhuate, were very caustic. It was not until the 1970s that others attempted to treat spider telangiectasias with intravascular injection using less caustic solutions such as sodium tetradecyl sulfate (STS) (Sotradecol) and hypertonic saline. It was these agents that propelled the treatment of telangiectasias forward. The enthusiasm for these treatments increased steadily as Foley's publication, relating to this new technique, gained momentum.[2]

Etiology

Although research continues to be done in this area, there is consensus today that telangiectasias can result from many causes, alone, or more likely in combination with other etiologic factors. Telangiectatic leg veins, according to the contemporary research, arise as a result of venous hypertension secondary to a number of different causes and conditions. The etiology of varicose veins and telangiectasias, for the most part, is similar. The pathophysiology of telangiectasias is usually broadly categorized as genetic/congenital, acquired, and iatrogenic. Some of the genetic causes of telangiectasias include nevus flammeus (port-wine stains), nevus araneus (spider telangiectasia, which can also result from acquired diseases), and Klippel-Trenaunay syndrome. Congenital conditions associated with telangiectasias include Maffucci syndrome and Rothmund-Thomson syndrome (poikiloderma). Acquired causes of telangiectasias can arise from a primary cutaneous disorder, such as varicose veins and keratosis lichenoides chronica, or the result of a disorder with a secondary cutaneous component, such as lupus erythematosus, a collagen disorder, and mastocytosis (telangiectasia macularis eruptiva perstans). Hormonal influences (estrogen and progesterone) also play a role in the pathogenesis of telangiectasia. Pregnancy places the person at risk for the development of telangiectasia as early as a couple of weeks after conception. Birth control pills, menses, and the time just before ovulation are also associated with the development or worsening of telangiectasia and increased venous dispensability. Topical steroids, particularly at high doses, have also been identified as a possible causative factor. Lastly, physical insults, such as trauma (contusions) and infection, have also been implicated as causal forces. See Box 23.1 for a comprehensive listing of the many causes of lower-leg cutaneous telangiectasia.

Telangiectasia is also associated with a number of other conditions and traits. These include, but are not limited to, those listed here:

- Age (peaks during age 50 to 69 years)
- Female gender
- Occupation and lifestyle: sedentary occupations and lifestyles are associated with telangiectasia
- Diseases such as cirrhosis
- Excessive exposure to the sun
- Therapeutic radiation (Figs. 23.1–23.8).

Patient Selection

Patients with spider telangiectasias typically present with primarily cosmetic complaints. Patient selection for the treatment of spider telangiectasias, as with all medical treatments, begins with a thorough assessment, which includes not only an assessment of the person's telangiectasia, but also the medical history, chief complaint, family history, and the patient's expectations relating to their possible spider telangiectasias. Based on this assessment, the physician must determine whether or not the treatment can resolve the patient's cosmetic complaints. At times, the telangiectasia is the result of a more generalized, systemic problem such as venous insufficiency. If venous insufficiency is present, it must be treated before the treatment of spider telangiectasia; otherwise, the venous hypertension would likely thwart the desired outcome. Second, determine whether or not the patient's expectations are realistic and achievable. The patient must clearly understand that the treatment is elective and that it is not likely to produce any significant health benefits. The patient should also understand that multiple treatments are often necessary for optimal results. Some patients may not be willing to do this. As with all invasive procedures, the patient must be educated about the benefits, risks, and alternatives to treatment. They must be thoroughly aware of all potential adverse sequelae and possible complications. Last, the patient must be informed that the treatment of spider telangiectasias is not curative and that further development of telangiectatic areas is likely.

Although there are no absolute contraindications to this treatment, people taking certain medications and/or patients with some chronic illnesses, especially those that could affect the occurrence of sclerotherapy complications, should be approached with extreme caution. For example, conditions including diabetes and peripheral vascular disease may lead to serious complications, such as ulcers. Some medications, for example, minocycline or isotretinoin, can lead to adverse reactions if not discontinued before the treatment.

Text continued on p. 626

BOX 23.1 Causes of Cutaneous Telangiectasia of the Lower Extremities

Genetic/congenital factors

Vascular nevi
Nevus flammeus
Klippel-Trenaunay syndrome
Nevus araneus
Angioma serpiginosum
Bockenheimer syndrome

Congenital neuroangiopathies

Maffucci syndrome
Congenital poikiloderma (Rothmund-Thomson syndrome)
Essential progressive telangiectasia
Cutis marmorata telangiectatica congenita
Diffuse neonatal hemangiomatosis
Acquired disease with a secondary cutaneous component

Collagen vascular diseases

Lupus erythematosus
Dermatomyositis
Progressive systemic sclerosis
Cryoglobulinemia

Other

Telangiectasia macularis eruptiva perstans (mastocytosis)
Human T-lymphotrophic virus type III (HTLV-III)

Component of a primary cutaneous disease

Varicose veins
Keratosis lichenoides chronica

Other acquired/primary cutaneous diseases

Necrobiosis lipoidica diabeticorum
Capillaritis (purpura annularis telangiectodes)
Malignant atrophic papulosis (Degos disease)

Hormonal factors

Pregnancy
Estrogen therapy
Topical corticosteroid preparations

Physical factors

Actinic neovascularization and/or vascular dilation
Trauma
Contusion
Surgical incision/laceration

Infection

Generalized essential telangiectasia
Progressive ascending telangiectasia
Human T-lymphotrophic virus type III (HTLV-III)
Radiodermatitis
Erythema ab igne (heat/infrared radiation)

Modified from Goldman MP, Bennett RG. Treatment of telangiectasia: a review. *J Am Acad Dermatol.* 1987;17:167–182.

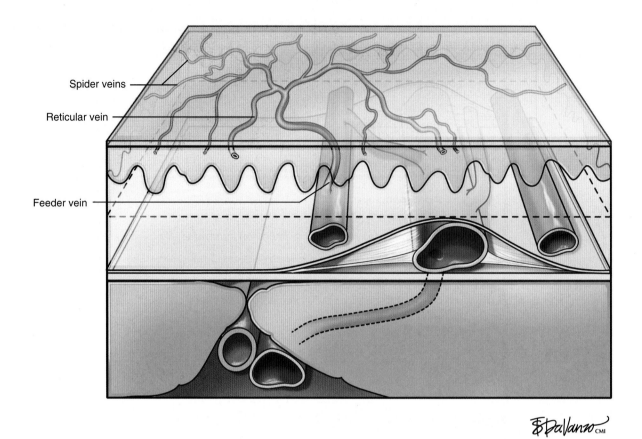

Spider veins

Reticular vein

Feeder vein

■ **Fig. 23.1** Normal subcutaneous venous anatomy.

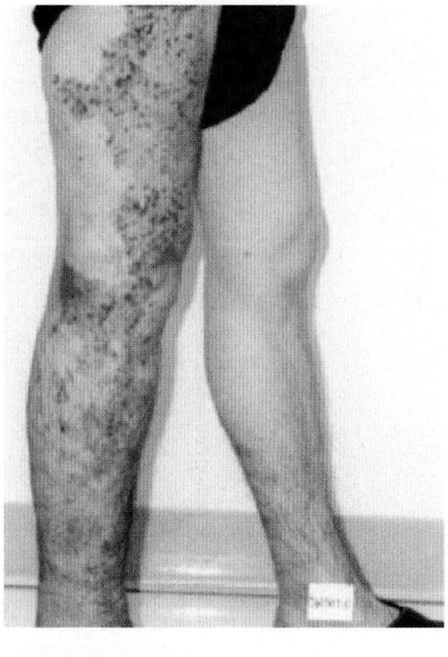

■ **Fig. 23.2** Patient with Klippel-Trenaunay syndrome.

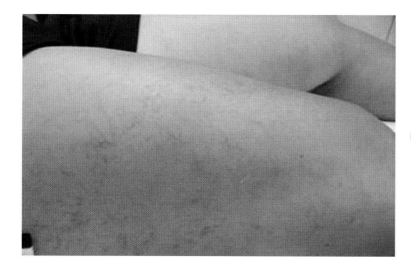

■ **Fig. 23.3** Spider vein.

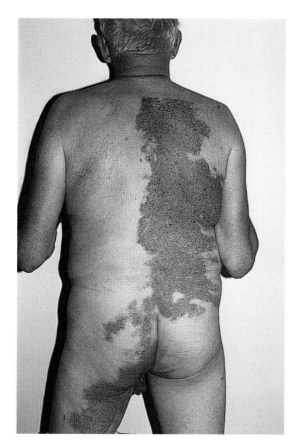

■ **Fig. 23.4** Nevus flammeus. *(From Weiss RA, Goldman MP, Bergan JJ, et al.* Sclerotherapy: Treatment of Varicose and Telangiectatic Leg Veins. *St Louis: Elsevier, 2007, Fig. 4.6, p. 76.)*

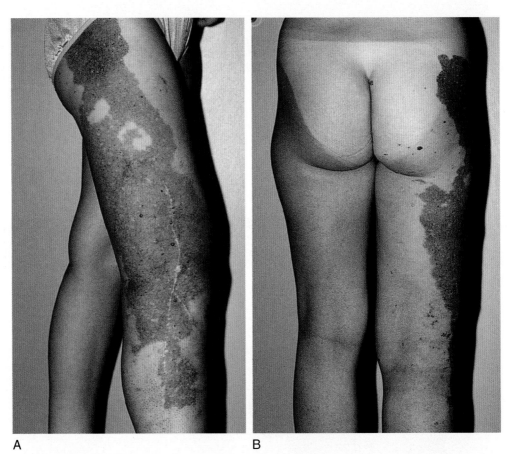

A   B

■ **Fig. 23.5** (A, B) A 16-year-old female with Klippel-Trenaunay syndrome and associated varicose veins and nevus flammeus of the right lower extremity from the toes to the buttock. *(From Weiss RA, Goldman MP, Bergan JJ, et al. Sclerotherapy: Treatment of Varicose and Telangiectatic Leg Veins. St Louis: Elsevier, 2007, Fig. 4.17, p. 84.)*

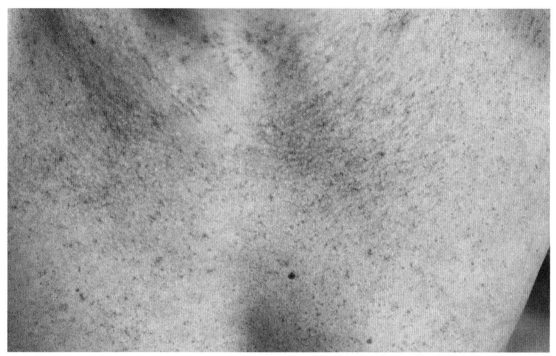

■ **Fig. 23.6** Extensive fine red telangiectasia on the chest of a severely sun-damaged 50-year-old woman. *(From Weiss RA, Goldman MP, Bergan JJ, et al. Sclerotherapy: Treatment of Varicose and Telangiectatic Leg Veins. St Louis: Elsevier, 2007, Fig. 4.19, p. 85.)*

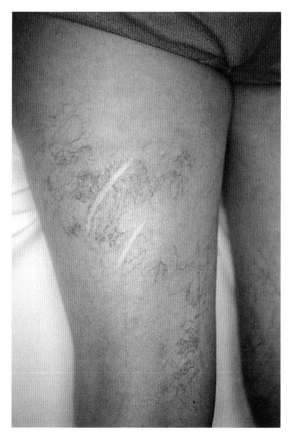

■ **Fig. 23.7** This woman underwent an extensive ligation and stripping of her varicose veins at 18 years of age. She developed extensive telangiectasia around all the surgical sites within weeks of the surgical procedure. This photograph was taken 22 years after the surgical procedure. *(From Weiss RA, Goldman MP, Bergan JJ, et al. Sclerotherapy: Treatment of Varicose and Telangiectatic Leg Veins. St Louis: Elsevier, 2007, Fig. 4.20, p. 86.)*

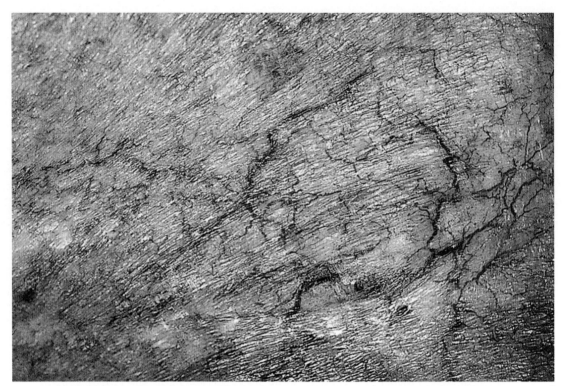

■ **Fig. 23.8** Appearance of telangiectasia occurring as a result of radiation treatment on the lateral neck for laryngeal carcinoma 20 years previously. *(From Weiss RA, Goldman MP, Bergan JJ, et al.* Sclerotherapy: Treatment of Varicose and Telangiectatic Leg Veins. *St Louis: Elsevier, 2007.)*

Endovascular Instrumentation

The basic endovascular instrumentation used for the treatment of spider telangiectasias includes needles for access and syringes to deliver the sclerosant to the affected areas. The needles used for telangiectasia are typically 30-gauge, although a 27-gauge butterfly needle may be used sometimes for larger reticular veins. Smaller needles, as small as a 33 gauge, can also be used, but they tend to bend too easily when they are penetrating the skin (Fig. 23.9).

The syringes that are typically used vary from a 1-mL tuberculin syringe to a 3-mL syringe. Most prefer a 3-mL syringe because it exerts the lowest pressures during injection, and it is also manually manipulated more precisely by the practitioner than a 1-mL syringe, especially if it is only filled to 2 mL.

The environment of care for sclerotherapy should include a comfortable table for the patient, a comfortable room temperature, and ample lighting. The treatment table height should permit the physician to sit comfortably on a stool with their legs under the table, without having to lean over the table and the patient for access. Environmental lighting should be bright and capable of providing adequate indirect illumination without any glare on the patient's skin (Fig. 23.10).

General supplies would include alcohol swabs, cotton balls, tape, and compression supplies such as ACE wraps or Coban. Patients can supply their own stockings, or they can be provided by the practice, which would require keeping a fairly large inventory (Figs. 23.11 and 23.12).

Last, but also most important, is emergency equipment. Fortunately, life-threatening complications are very rare; however, they are always possible. Basic emergency equipment must minimally include oxygen, airway equipment, epinephrine, steroids, and antihistamines (Fig. 23.13).

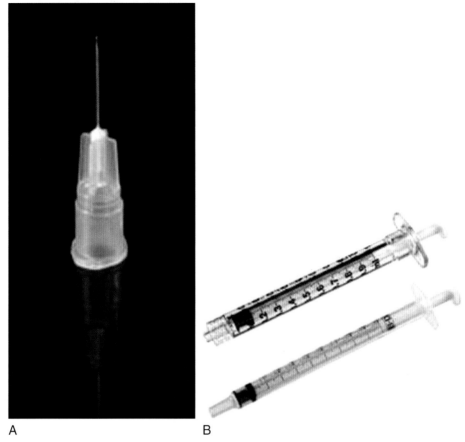

A   B

■ **Fig. 23.9** (A, B) Needles and syringes. *(Courtesy Dr. M. Nerney.)*

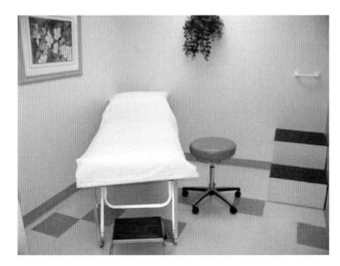

■ **Fig. 23.10** Table and chair.

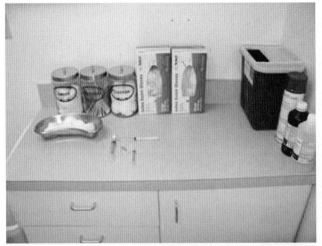

A

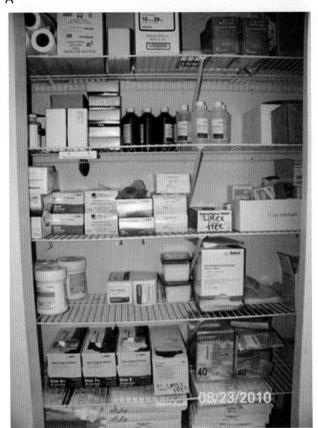

B

■ **Fig. 23.11** (A, B) Surgical supplies.

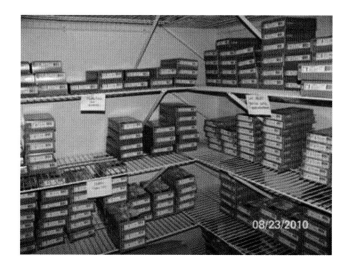

■ **Fig. 23.12** Compression stockings.

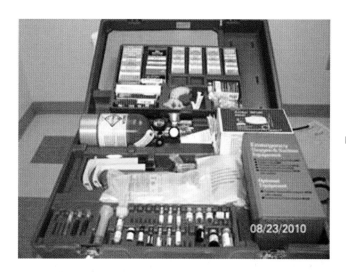

■ **Fig. 23.13** Emergency equipment.

Imaging

Spider telangiectasias are primarily a cosmetic, aesthetic concern for the patient; therefore they are primarily treated visually. Several things can be used to aid in the visualization.

First and foremost are magnifying glasses or loupes. These aids help to visualize the insertion of the needle into the smaller veins, particularly those that are less than 1 mm in diameter. Because loupes typically have 2.5 times the magnification, they facilitate good visualization while the needle pierces the skin and enters the vein (Fig. 23.14).

A number of lighting systems are used for visualization of veins to be treated. Vein lights provide visualization of vessels just under the skin that are sometimes too deep for normal visualization. These lights create a "shadow" from the absorption of the blood in the vein. Polarized lights are also used to provide better visualization through the skin (Fig. 23.15).

Syris polarized lights with magnification (Syris, Gray, ME) also provide better visualization through the skin (Fig. 23.16).

Infrared visualization is also done. Infrared lights allow the practitioner to see veins a few millimeters under the skin because these lights provide infrared images of the hemoglobin contained within the red cells circulating in the vessel, which is then projected back onto the skin using the VeinViewer or a camera. This is particularly helpful for identifying "feeding" reticular veins that could be causing the telangiectasias (Fig. 23.17).

Duplex imaging is also an invaluable tool. This imaging is primarily used for the diagnostic workup of venous insufficiency. It is also used for directing that treatment, including varicose veins. New high-frequency probes, in the 15-MHz to 17-MHz range, can identify very small veins, as small as 1 to 2 mm, such as reticular, feeding veins. These reticular, feeding veins may demonstrate reflux that may contribute to spider telangiectasias.

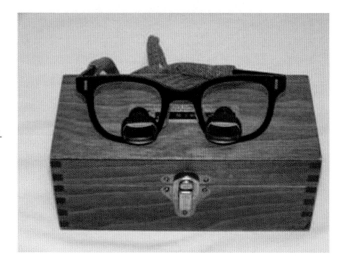

◾ **Fig. 23.14** Loupes.

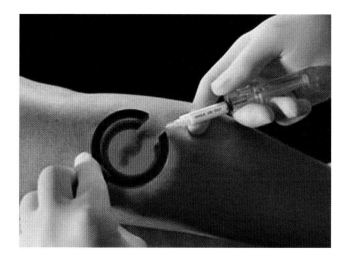

■ **Fig. 23.15** Vein light. *(Courtesy Dr. M. Nerney.)*

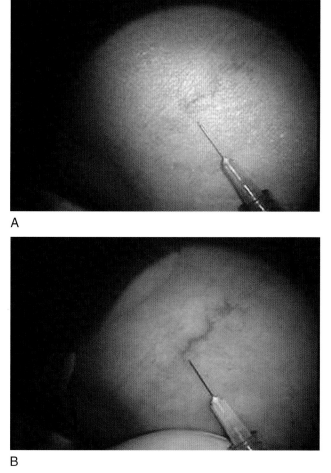

A

B

■ **Fig. 23.16** (A, B) Syris polarized light. *(Courtesy Dr. M. Nerney.)*

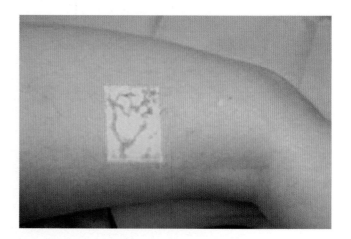

■ **Fig. 23.17** Vein viewer. *(Courtesy Dr. M. Nerney.)*

Sclerosants

Sclerosants used for the treatment of spider telangiectasias can be divided into three main groups: detergents, hyperosmolar, and chemical irritants. This section will cover the most frequently used sclerosants for treatment of telangiectasias in the United States.

The detergent solutions are primarily STS (Sotradecol) and polidocanol (POL). These solutions work by attacking the endothelial cells at their cell surface lipids. STS has been around since 1946. It is manufactured in the United States by BionichePharma. STS is used for the treatment of spider telangiectasias in various concentrations from 0.05% to 0.5%. It can be foamed if desired. POL, used for the treatment of spider telangiectasias, comes in concentrations of 0.25% to 1% and it, too, can be used as a foam. POL just recently became approved by the US Food and Drug Administration (FDA), so experience with it is not nearly as extensive as it is in Europe.

The hyperosmolar, or hypertonic, sclerosant group consists primarily of hypertonic saline (HS), hypertonic dextrose, sodium salicylate, and a combination of HS and hypertonic dextrose. These agents work by dehydrating the endothelial cells. HS is used in concentrations of 11.7% to 23.4%. Hypertonic dextrose comes in a concentration of 75% that can be diluted. The combination of 10% saline and 25% dextrose is sold as Sclerodex and manufactured by Omega laboratories in Canada.

Chemical irritant sclerosants that are currently used in the United States are primarily limited to glycerin 72%. It works as a caustic agent on the vessel wall. Glycerin can be diluted, most frequently with lidocaine 1% with or without epinephrine (Fig. 23.18).

ACCESS AND CLOSURE

As previously stated, access is primarily done through visualization with aspiration for the larger vessels. Smaller vessels are located by palpation alone because these veins are too small for aspiration. These smaller vessels are accessed by direct visualization while maintaining slight pressure on the plunger. Access is then confirmed when the sclerosing solution is seen going through the vein. Pressure should be light so as not to cause a bleb under the skin. The injection should be stopped, and a different site used if a bleb is seen. Larger veins, such as reticular veins, can be aspirated before being injected. This aspiration and injection should be effortless and without any resistance. The injection should be stopped if any resistance is met because this may indicate that

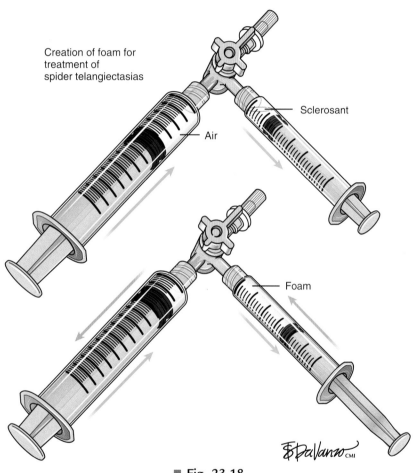

Creation of foam for treatment of spider telangiectasias

Air

Sclerosant

Foam

■ Fig. 23.18

the needle has come out of the vein. Closure, or hemostasis, is accomplished with digital pressure after the removal of the needle. A cotton ball can be applied with atraumatic tape, such as paper tape, over the puncture site for additional compression.

OPERATIVE STEPS

After appropriate informed consent is obtained and patient education is complete, the next step is to obtain photographic documentation of the areas being treated to establish a baseline for later posttreatment comparison. This comparison is useful for both the physician and the patient. Minimally, four views should be obtained with additional close-up views as indicated.

After this photographic documentation, the patient is then placed in the supine position, preferably with the head slightly lower than the legs. As previously mentioned, the height of the table itself should be comfortable for the person performing the injections. Good, indirect lighting, without glare on the skin, is also necessary. The skin should be cleansed with alcohol, not only for asepsis but also to remove the outermost dead layer of skin to make the veins more visible to the practitioner.

Treatment should begin at the source of reflux, if the source has been determined, or proximal to it if the precise location is not known. In the latter case, the larger veins are treated before the smaller ones. It can be assumed that the source of reflux is the perigeniculate perforators, located usually just above the knee, for the lateral venous plexus area (Fig. 23.19).

Complete treatment of the reticular, feeding veins is performed in a given area, before moving to the treatment of the smaller spider telangiectasias in the same area. Sclerosant injected into the feeder vein often travels into the spider veins, thus effectively treating both the feeding veins and the spider veins. Access with the needle, as described earlier, is done with aspiration to confirm placement into the larger reticular feeder veins. The method of injection should be smooth and with very little pressure on the plunger. The volume of the injection solution depends on the size of the reticular vein. By definition, reticular veins range from 1 to 3 mm in diameter. Using 2 mm as an average, the volume of a 5-cm segment is 0.16 mL. Therefore a 15-cm segment would require 0.5 mL of sclerosant. Imaging with vein lights, a vein viewer, and polarized lights is sometimes very helpful (Figs. 23.20–23.22).

The practitioner has a choice of sclerosant and concentration for reticular veins. Typically chosen is 0.5% to 1% STS liquid or 0.25% to 0.5% foamed STS. When POL is chosen, it is generally 0.75% to 1% liquid or 0.5% to 0.75% foam. Other choices may include 23.4% HS or 66% dextrose.

Following the reticular, feeding vein treatment, the spider telangiectasia can immediately be treated during the same visit or postponed for a later date. When the spider veins are ready for treatment, these veins are accessed with visual cues or with the tactile feel of the needle and plunger. As the needle enters the vein, there is a lessening of resistance and, with a light touch on the plunger, the sclerosant will clear the vessel. If there is any evidence of extravasation, the injection must be stopped immediately.

The volume of injection is dependent on the size of the vein being treated. It is important to keep in mind that a 1-mm vein has only 0.1 mL of volume for every 13 cm of length. The injection of the appropriate volume of the solution is often ascertained by a visual determination by the experienced practitioner. Gentle positive pressure on the plunger and the injection of the sclerosing solution continue until the segment of vein fills with approximately 0.1 mL.

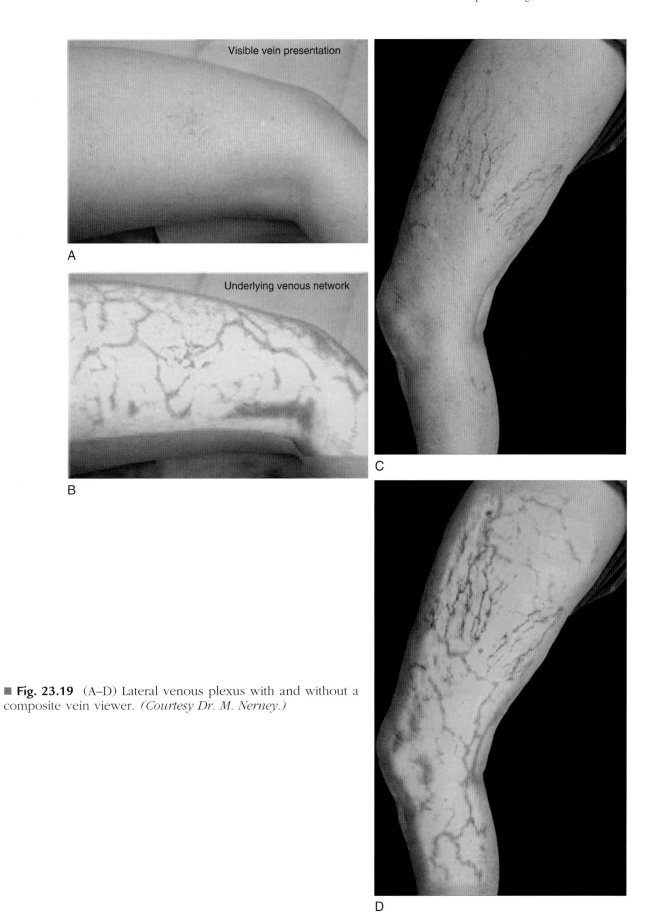

Fig. 23.19 (A–D) Lateral venous plexus with and without a composite vein viewer. *(Courtesy Dr. M. Nerney.)*

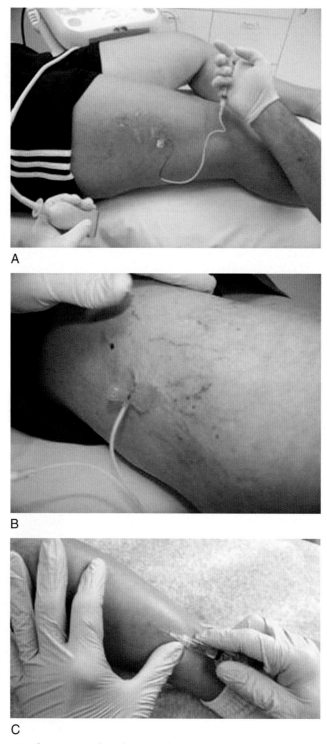

■ **Fig. 23.20** (A–C) Lateral venous plexus injection.

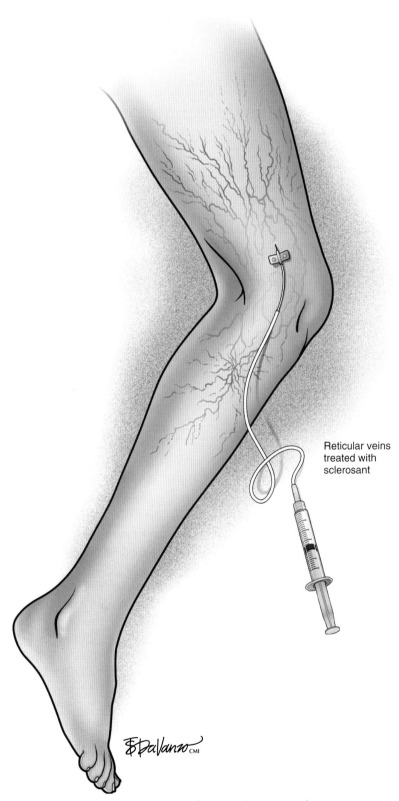

Reticular veins
treated with
sclerosant

■ **Fig. 23.21** Illustration of a lateral venous plexus injection.

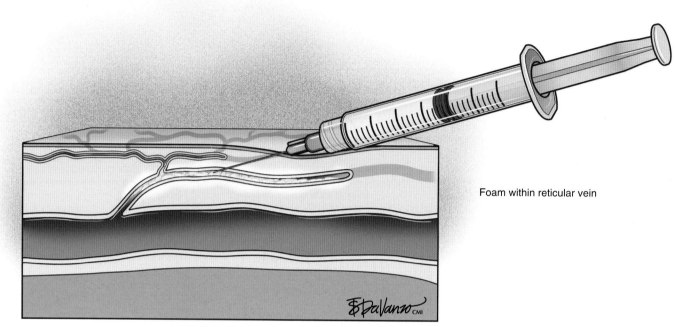

Foam within reticular vein

■ **Fig. 23.22** Illustration of a lateral venous plexus injection.

After the injection is stopped, the needle is then held in position for several seconds, up to 30 seconds. This increases the contact time of the sclerosant with the vein wall. The choice and concentration of sclerosant for spider veins are based on the size of the spider vein and practitioner preference, with ranges from 0.05% to 0.25% for STS and from 0.25% to 0.5% for POL, 11.7% HS, and 48% glycerin diluted with lidocaine. The total volume of the injection depends on which type and concentration of sclerosant are being used. For example, the maximum dose for STS is 10 mL of 3%, so if one is injecting a 0.25% solution, the total volume would be 120 mL (Figs. 23.23 and 23.24).

Many recommend placing a cotton ball over the injection site immediately after each injection to achieve hemostasis, to compress the vein walls together, and to prevent the filling of the vein with blood, which would lead to a clot. Atraumatic tape, such as paper tape, is used to hold the cotton ball in place when it is used. Further compression may be accomplished with foam pads, ACE wraps, or compression stockings. There is some data to suggest that compression stockings worn for several weeks after treatment can decrease adverse events, such as staining, but there are no data to suggest that compression stockings enhance the effectiveness of the treatment.[3]

Many practitioners recommend that patients elevate their legs, ambulate frequently, and avoid hot showers after treatment to decrease venous pressure or to avoid vasodilatation, although there is no research to support these posttreatment recommendations.

Follow-up treatments can be scheduled from a few days to several months later. There is concern that frequent treatments within a few weeks to the same area can increase the risk of inflammation in the area and possibly increase adverse effects. Again, there are no data that statistically support this concern.

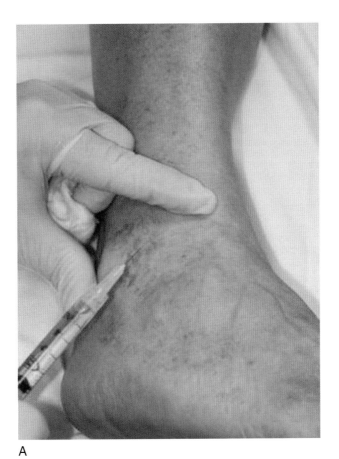

A

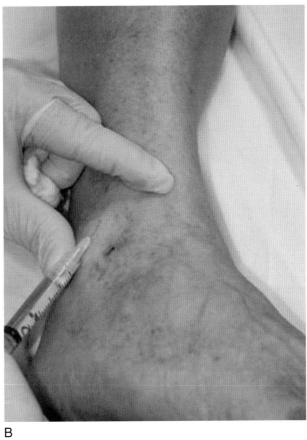

B

■ **Fig. 23.23** (A, B) Injections.

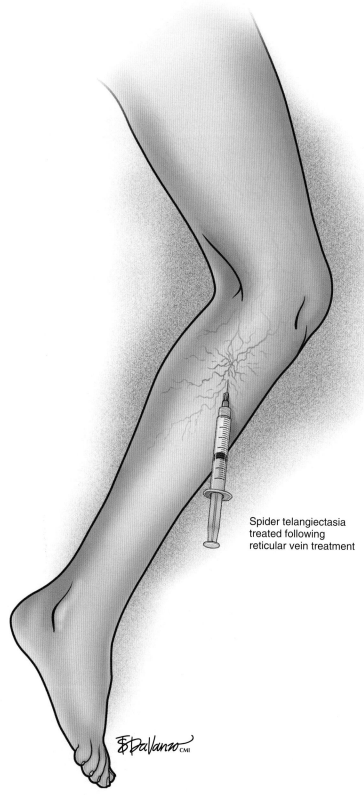

Spider telangiectasia
treated following
reticular vein treatment

■ **Fig. 23.24**

PEARLS AND PITFALLS

Foam sclerotherapy has greatly improved the outcome of varicose vein sclerotherapy.[4] However, its merits in terms of the treatment of spider telangiectasias are less clear. The foam actually increases the surface area of contact by displacing the blood as opposed to injecting the sclerosing agent only, which is diluted by the blood. The foam then thickens the blood vessel wall, causing less blood to pass through. The same effect of foaming can be achieved with the use of only the sclerosing agent by keeping the needle within the vein after injection and maintaining slight pressure on the plunger. The reticular feeding veins may benefit from foam because they are larger and more difficult to visualize.

Foam sclerotherapy is also associated with greater risk in terms of potential complications because air is added to the vascular system. Several reports of neurologic events have been noted. These risks may be reduced by using carbon dioxide (CO_2) as the gas rather than air. CO_2 rapidly dissolves in blood, whereas the nitrogen in air does not.[5]

Sclerotherapy may not improve spider telangiectasias if matting develops in the vasculature. Matting is the formation of new, fine spider veins in an area previously injected. This area may improve with additional treatments or may need further evaluation. Various imaging devices may be used to assess for venous hypertension caused by an incompetent saphenous or perforator vein. Ultrasound may show an underlying refluxing vein that should be treated. Vein lights and infrared imaging, such as the vein viewer and polarized light, may help to identify the reticular vein feeding the spider complex (Fig. 23.25).

Pain is one of the most common complaints during the procedure, and several methods have been used in an attempt to allay and reduce the pain. Adding lidocaine to the solution or pretreating the area with a topical anesthetic, such as topical lidocaine or EMLA, can reduce the pain from the needle stick but these measures do not typically reduce the pain from the sclerosing solution itself. Alternative pain minimization procedures are consistently being investigated. One method, popular in South America, uses hypertonic solutions that are cooled to −30°C while cold air is blown onto the area being injected with this cold solution. The cold solution acts not only as an anesthetic but also increases contact time with the vein walls because it is more viscous than solutions at room temperature. Advocates of this method believe that these colder solutions improve the outcomes of the procedure as well.

If, after several weeks posttreatment there is no significant improvement of the affected area(s), a different, stronger, and/or higher concentration of the sclerosant can be attempted for better results. Before this is done, however, it must be determined if there is some overlooked, underlying problem, such as venous insufficiency, that must be addressed. In addition, the feeder veins must be assessed to determine whether they were adequately treated. A repeat ultrasound may reveal an underlying problem that was missed on the initial assessment and examination. The imaging techniques previously described may also reveal feeder veins that must be addressed before the spider veins can be successfully treated.

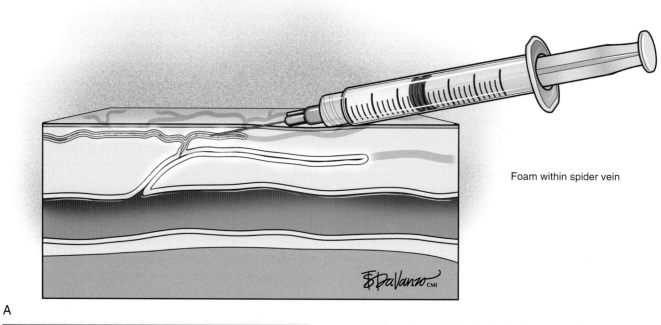

Foam within spider vein

A

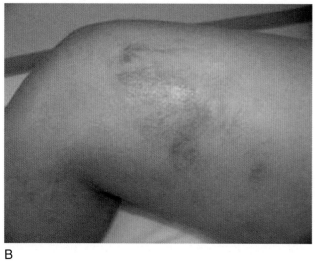

B

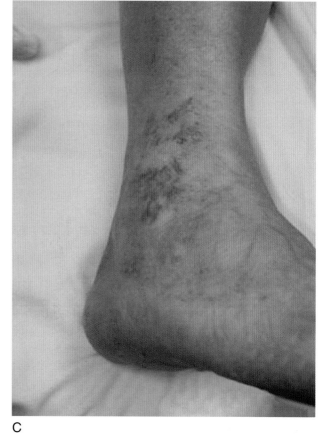

C

■ **Fig. 23.25** (A–C) Matting.

COMPLICATIONS AND ADVERSE SEQUELAE

The potential complications of sclerotherapy for telangiectatic veins and varicosities are numerous and varied, but most often, they are temporary in nature and not serious. Some of the most commonly occurring, and less-severe, complications and adverse sequelae of these treatments include the following:

- Injection site pain
- Edema
- Urticaria localized over the injection site
- Tape compression blisters and folliculitis
- Hyperpigmentation
- Recurrence of treated vessels
- Other conditions such as staining and matting

Included among the more serious and less commonly occurring complications and adverse sequelae associated with these procedures are the following:

- Nerve damage
- Superficial thrombophlebitis
- Pulmonary emboli and deep venous thrombosis (DVT)
- Air emboli
- Distal necrosis resulting from an inadvertent injection of a sclerosing agent into an artery
- Allergic reactions
- Cutaneous necrosis

Pain

Pain and soreness are sometimes experienced. However, there are a number of interventions that can be used to minimize and eliminate this discomfort. The pain and discomfort are a function of several variables including the treatment site, the injection technique, the sclerosing agent, and the needle itself. The level of discomfort is typically greatest when the feet, ankles, medial knees, and/or medial upper thighs are treated. Pain and discomfort can be prevented or diminished with the use of the smallest-possible gauge, bevelled needle that is silicone coated, sclerosing agents with a lidocaine additive, and slow infusion followed immediately by massage.

The hypertonic solutions used for sclerotherapy are synonymous with pain and discomfort. However, the pain can be decreased without any compromise in terms of desired outcome when a 2% solution of nonacidified lidocaine is added to the sclerosing agent and no more than 0.1 mL is slowly injected into each site followed by massage. Although the effectiveness of the treatment is not compromised, the addition of lidocaine may increase the risk of an allergic response. The addition of 1% lidocaine and a limitation of no more than 0.1 mL per site are recommended for glycerin sclerosing solutions to prevent pain and cramping. STS and POL are virtually painless with proper technique; however, STS can lead to pain when it is accidentally injected into perivascular areas.

Any transient pain or discomfort can be effectively treated with properly fitting graduated compression stockings for a week or two after the treatment. The presence of severe and/or unrelieved pain signals the need to assess the patient for venous thrombosis and inflammation.

Edema

Temporary swelling can result from a number of factors, including the nature of the treated site, perivascular and intravascular space differentials, endothelial permeability, the strength of the sclerosing solution, the volume of the sclerosing solution, and the lack of proper graduated compression after the treatment (tourniquet effect).

Posttelangiectasia treatment edema is most often associated with treatment areas below the ankle; however, edema can be present in other areas as well. Limiting volume to no more than 1 mL for each ankle can prevent or minimize swelling in this area. The extent of inflammation and resulting edema in the perivascular area is affected by the strength of the sclerosing agent and the client's unique status in terms of mast cells (sensitivity), medication profile (e.g., nonsteroidal antiinflammatory drugs [NSAIDs], corticosteroids), and a history of sclerosing agent sensitivity. The application of graduated compression stockings for up to 3 weeks posttreatment may be helpful for some patients, as is the application of a topical corticosteroid to enhance the antiinflammatory response. Patients must be educated about the proper application of their graduated compression stockings and about the signs of edema that can occur as a result of their poor application.

Urticaria

Localized urticaria, typically occurring over the injection site and lasting only a few minutes, is a result of transient irritation and the release of histamine. This transient complication, however, must be scrupulously differentiated from sensitivity and the onset of a systemic allergic response, which can be very serious.

The intensity of the localized itching tends to be positively correlated with the strength of the sclerosing agent. The incidence of urticaria is most often associated with the use of POL and STS as well as a failure to limit the volume of the agent. Prevention and treatment consist of the application of a topical corticosteroid to the injection sites immediately after treatment and limiting the volume of the solution for each injection site.

Blisters and Folliculitis

Blisters and folliculitis usually occur as the result of tape used to secure dressing pads. Blisters most commonly occur:
- During the summer months (perspiration and moisture)
- Among those who are thin
- Among the elderly and other people who have fragile skin
- On areas behind the knee, the interior aspect of the thigh, and other areas where there is tissue movement

Tapes with the greatest adhesiveness place patients at more risk for blisters than less-adhesive tapes like paper tape. Although blisters are relatively harmless, they must be assessed to determine whether these lesions are an allergic response, infection, or a sign of early cutaneous necrosis. Blisters can be prevented with the use of a tubular support bandage, rather than tape, over the pad for stability as the compression stocking is applied. An occlusive hydroactive dressing can be placed over the blister if it does not resolve on its own.

Folliculitis, like a blister, most commonly occurs during the summer months and as a result of a tape dressing. The treatment consists of the application of a topical antibiotic, such as clindamycin or erythromycin, and/or an antibacterial cleanser, such as Hibiclens. This complication is often self-limiting or effectively treated with topical antimicrobials. Folliculitis rarely requires the use of a systemic antimicrobial drug.

Hyperpigmentation

Hyperpigmentation, or cutaneous pigmentation, is a relatively common occurrence after treatment, regardless of the sclerosing agent used (Fig. 23.26). Hyperpigmentation is often very temporary in nature; however, rare persistence can occur for a small number of patients 1 year posttreatment. Most areas of pigmentation occur along the linear aspect of the treated vein. These areas indicate that the vein is no longer functioning. Less commonly encountered occurrences, such as those found at the injection site(s), can also occur as the result of the sclerosing agent's endothelial damage, inflammation, and red blood cell extravasation into the area. Areas below the knee and vessels from 0.6 to 1.2 mm in diameter are at greatest risk. Affected areas usually resolve within 6 to 12 months after sclerotherapy.

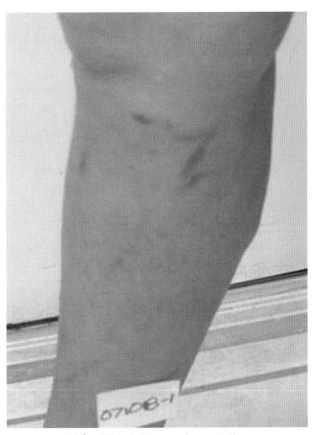

■ **Fig. 23.26** Hyperpigmentation.

Hyperpigmentation results from a number of factors, including the type of sclerosing agent, the concentration of the agent, the technique used, the postprocedure treatment(s), the diameter of the vessel, and pressures (gravitational and intravascular). In addition, the risk of hyperpigmentation increases with some unique patient characteristics, including an innate predisposition for hyperpigmentation, and medication(s), particularly minocycline (Dynacin, Minocin), taken at the time of the treatment.

Prevention aims to minimize necrosis and to avoid total endothelial destruction as well as accompanying red blood cell extravasation. The incidence of hyperpigmentation can be decreased with a number of preventive measures including, but not limited to, those listed next.

Use sclerosing agents that have been scientifically associated with the least incidence of hyperpigmentation and inflammation. These solutions include sodium salicylate, glycerin, and chromated glycerin (CG).

Keep the concentration of the sclerosing agent to the minimum necessary for effectiveness. Liquid agents are less potent than foams, so when a foam is used, it is necessary to modify the concentration, particularly when spider veins are treated.

Inject the agent with a 3-mL syringe, rather than a smaller one, because injection pressure increases proportionately with smaller piston diameters. Red blood cell extravasation and vessel rupture are more apt to occur with increased injection pressures.

Remove posttreatment coagulation using a gentle rocking expression of the clot via a small incision made with a 21-gauge needle (Fig. 23.27).

Although a number of hyperpigmentation treatments have been used, it appears that many have limited and/or questionable effectiveness, other than treatment with a Q-switched laser.

Recurrence of Treated Vessels

The recurrence of treated veins is common but also troublesome, particularly for the patient who has undergone the treatment. The practitioner may be able to rule out suspected recurrence with a thorough examination 1 year posttreatment that identifies the area(s) as new or previously untreated telangiectasia, rather than a recurrence of the treated vessels.

When it is present, the degree and extent of recurrence are positively correlated with the degree of intravascular thrombosis; therefore the most important preventive measures aim to limit intravascular thromboses. Adequate compression for an adequate duration of time is necessary to prevent recurrence.

Other Minor Conditions

Other complications and adverse sequelae include harmless suntan fading, telangiectatic matting (as discussed earlier), staining, vasovagal reflex (stress related), localized hypertrichosis, and transient urticaria, which warrants attention because it may signal a systemic allergy.

Nerve Damage

Temporary paresthesia and permanent nerve damage can occur because of the proximity of some nerves to the sclerotherapy injection sites. Temporary paresthesia, most often

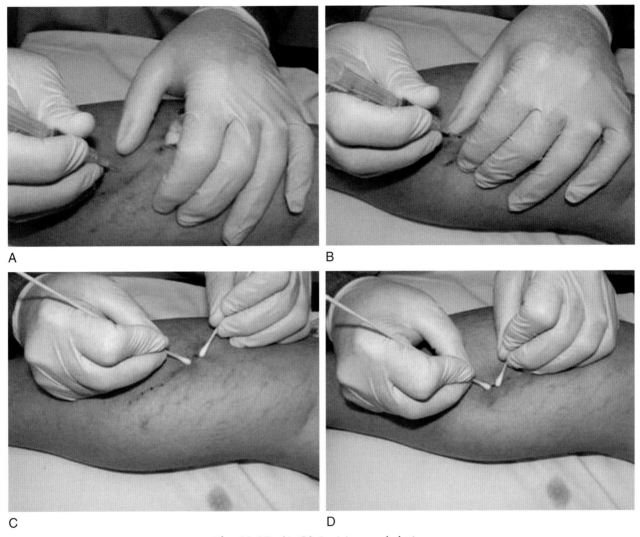

■ **Fig. 23.27** (A–D) Incision and drainage.

lasting less than 6 months, can occur when the local inflammatory process affects superficial sensory nerves. Treatment consists of the administration of NSAIDs. Major nerve damage, although very rare, can occur. This damage occurs from poor technique and malformations or anomalies of the patient's venous system.

In a systematic search by two independent reviewers, a total of 10,819 patients undergoing sclerotherapy were reviewed. There were 12 case reports of cerebrovascular accident (CVA) with confirmatory brain imaging and 9 reports of transient ischemic attack (TIA). There were 97 (0.90%) reports of neurologic events overall, including TIA, visual and speech disturbances, and 29 cases of reported migraine (0.27%). Symptoms occurred at times ranging from minutes to several days following sclerotherapy. Eleven patients with TIA or CVA were found to have a right-to-left cardiac shunt, usually a patent foramen ovale. Thus neurologic side effects following sclerotherapy are a rare occurrence; however, CVA associated with the use of sclerotherapy is clearly documented. The pathologic mechanisms resulting in CVA are likely to be different to those leading to migraine and visual disturbances; however, care should be exercised in patient selection, particularly in those with known cardiac defects.[6]

Superficial Thrombophlebitis

The advent of posttreatment graduated compression has greatly diminished the incidence and prevalence of thrombophlebitis; however, it does occur on some occasions for a variety of reasons. Some patients are at risk for thrombophlebitis because they are predisposed to it as a result of an innate state of hypercoagulopathy. Other examples of predisposition are conditions and disorders such as pregnancy, genetic excesses of coagulation factor VII, and a protein C deficiency.

Superficial thrombophlebitis presents as an induration that is tender and reddened or an area of hyperpigmentation along the vein, usually from 1 to 3 weeks after treatment. For the most part, this complication can be prevented with posttreatment compression over the entire leg (not just the treated area), which is adequate in terms of both duration and degree.

When prevention is not successful, the treatment of thrombophlebitis consists of maintaining adequate compression, NSAIDs, drainage, frequent ambulation, and, at times, low-molecular-weight heparin (LMWH).

Emboli and Deep Venous Thrombosis

Fortunately, pulmonary emboli and DVT are rare occurrences subsequent to sclerotherapy. Nonetheless, the incidence of DVT is probably grossly underestimated because it is often overlooked and not diagnosed as such. Although many cases are not properly or promptly diagnosed, there are clinical signs that should alert the practitioner. Among these signs are the cardinal signs of inflammation (redness, heat, swelling, pain, loss of function), dilated superficial veins, some laboratory markers, such as plasma D-dimers, as well as venous Doppler and impedance phlebography results. DVT usually presents 8 to 10 hours after treatment, particularly during times when vascular stasis is greatest. Pulmonary emboli typically occur from 5 to 7 days after thrombus formation. Because the mortality rate from a DVT and pulmonary emboli, without treatment, is alarmingly high, a thorough assessment of the patient and their risk factors, as well as careful posttreatment monitoring, are essential components of care. Patient education is also important. The patient and family members must be informed about the signs and symptoms of DVT and emboli and the importance of immediately reporting their observations to the physician.

Although the cause of DVT is largely unknown, it appears that both intrinsic patient-related factors (a hypercoagulability predisposition) and extrinsic treatment-related factors (vascular stasis and endothelial damage) have an impact on the occurrence of DVT. Limiting the volume of the sclerosing agent to only 0.5 to 1 mL per site, adequate compression with properly fitted graduated support hose (30 to 40 mm Hg pressure), and encouraging physical activity (muscular movement) immediately after the procedure will reduce thromboembolic complications. In addition, use extreme caution when the patient has a thrombophilia to prevent this serious postsclerotherapy complication.

The treatment of DVT must be immediate, decisive, and highly effective. A rapid reduction of clots can be accomplished with peripheral or direct infusions of a thrombolytic agent, such as urokinase or a tissue plasminogen activator (t-PA). Alternative treatment consists of the administration of anticoagulation therapy using intravenous (IV) heparin, which is then followed by warfarin, heparin subcutaneously, or a LMWH preparation, such as enoxaparin sodium (Lovenox).

Air Embolism

Small amounts of air entering the venous system do not pose a threat because these minimal amounts usually absorb into the blood, without ill effect, before the bloodstream reaches the pulmonary circulation. Larger amounts of air, however, such as may occur when using foams, can potentially lead to air emboli that manifest with migraines, nausea, and visual disturbances, all of which are usually self-limiting and without any long-term, adverse effects.

Distal necrosis may occur from an inadvertent injection into an artery. This complication is quite rare, but it perpetually plagues the thoughts of the physician because no sclerosing treatment is totally risk free of this complication, a complication that mandates intense immediate action. Arterial injection of a sclerosing agent can lead to emboli, occlusion, blood flow stasis, and necrosis. The most vulnerable areas include the groin, the medial or posterior malleolar area, and the back of the knee.

This complication requires instantaneous action. The sclerosing agent and blood should be aspirated immediately on the realization that this inadvertent injection has occurred. This action should be immediately followed by an injection of heparin (10,000 units) using the same needle kept in place with only the replacement of the syringe containing heparin, often a feat for only the ambidextrous, particularly when the patient is experiencing acute and severe pain. Ongoing treatment consists of the application of ice to the affected area, a heparin regimen for 6 or more days, IV dextran 10% for 3 days, and nifedipine, hydralazine, or prazosin orally for 30 days. At times, direct thrombolytic therapy is indicated.

An inadvertent injection into an artery is best prevented with arterial visualization using duplex imagery and having the patient in an upright position when the challenging malleolar area is injected (Fig. 23.28).

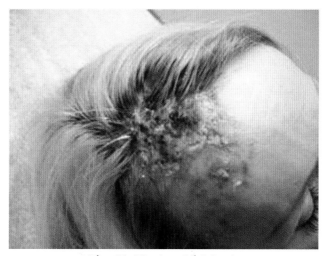

■ **Fig. 23.28** Arterial injection.

Allergic Reactions

Systemic allergic reactions are rare; nonetheless, they can occur. Some allergic reactions are minor and transient, whereas others can be severe and life threatening. Nonetheless, all patients with even minor allergic reactions must be assessed and monitored for any signs of a more serious reaction, including bronchospasm, angioedema, anaphylaxis, pulmonary toxicity, renal toxicity, and cardiac toxicity.

Minor allergic reactions, such as urticaria, are typically treated with an antihistamine, such as hydroxyzine (Atarax) or diphenhydramine (Benadryl). Prednisone may also be added for a brief course of therapy. Angioedema, with and without respiratory stridor, is treated with an oral antihistamine and intramuscular diphenhydramine in combination with IV corticosteroids, respectively. Aminophylline intravenously, an inhaled bronchodilator, corticosteroids, and antihistamines usually successfully treat bronchospasm without any further intervention; however, the practitioner must be aware that bronchospasm may signal the onset of anaphylaxis.

The earliest warning signs of impending anaphylaxis include urticaria, angioedema, itching, rising levels of anxiety, wheezing, coughing, and other, more-subtle warnings. The three classic signs of actual anaphylaxis, a severe life-threatening condition that requires immediate attention, are bronchospasm, respiratory airway edema, and vascular collapse (systemic vasodilation and cardiac failure). Emergency treatment and transport to an acute care facility in the community are most often necessary. This condition is treated with epinephrine to maintain blood pressure, intubation, theophylline, and oxygen to establish and maintain adequate oxygenation as well as other medications such as corticosteroids and diphenhydramine.

Some of the sclerosing agents that are most often associated with an allergic reaction include:

- Ethanolamine oleate
- Sodium morrhuate
- STS
- Chromated glycerin
- Plain glycerin
- POL
- Polyiodinated iodine
- HS
- Heparin
- Sodium salicylate
- Lidocaine (an additive to glycerin and HS)

Cutaneous Necrosis

This most often self-limiting complication can occur, albeit rarely, irrespective of sclerosing agent type. Several factors impact on the occurrence of cutaneous necrosis. These include extravasation, injection into an arteriole, reactive vasospasm, lymphatic injection, and excessive compression.

The extent and degree of extravasation are functions of both the type of the sclerosing agent and the concentration given. Despite good technique, a small amount of the sclerosing solution may leak into the surrounding tissue as the needle is withdrawn or when numerous punctures are necessary, thus leading to extravasation. More toxic solutions pose greater threats to subcutaneous damage than less toxic ones. For example, glycerin and CG are less toxic to tissue than STS.

Inadvertent arteriolar injection may occur as a result of a rapid, large volume injection of a sclerosing agent into telangiectasias with microshunts. Glycerin solutions are believed to be the least offensive in terms of arteriolar injection and subsequent tissue ulceration. Likewise, lymphatic vessel injection can also lead to cutaneous necrosis, particularly if the patient has lymphovenous anastomoses and the solution is caustic. Reactive arterial vasospasm also plays a role in terms of cutaneous necrosis. Some people, for unknown reasons, tend to have a predisposition to these vasospasms. Vigorous massage, in combination with a topical nitroglycerin ointment, may alleviate or eliminate this problem. Last, cutaneous ulceration, as a result of tissue ischemia and anoxia, may occur when there is excessive localized compression. It is therefore recommended that the patient wear a graduated compression stocking of no more than 40 mm Hg when in the supine position for long durations of time. Other preventive measures include the use of double stockings during nonbed rest times and the removal of the outer one during periods of bed rest so that the pressure can be lowered to an acceptable level.

Cutaneous necrosis can be prevented with the dilution of sclerosing solutions and the injection of hyaluronidase into multiple sites around the extravasation within 60 minutes of the episode, should extravasation occur (Fig. 23.29).

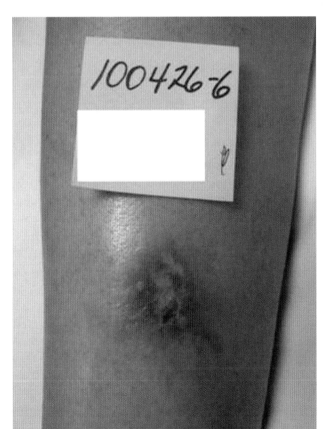

■ **Fig. 23.29** Ulcer.

Summary of Complications and Adverse Sequelae

The adverse sequelae and complications associated with sclerotherapy of telangiectatic veins and varicosities can often be prevented. However, these procedures can never be devoid of inherent risks, despite all preventive measures and superior technique. Some of these untoward events are minor, transient, and self-limiting, but some are life threatening and serious. Patients must be given complete information about the procedure, its benefits, risks, follow-up care, and alternatives for them to give informed consent before the procedure.

Comparative Effectiveness

Comparative research studies have been conducted to determine the relative effectiveness of the various sclerosants that are used for spider telangiectasias. Curlin and Ratz compared the effectiveness of STS 0.5%, POL 0.25%, and HS 20% with heparin. The results of this research indicated that POL was best tolerated, whereas HS and STS showed fastest clearing. In terms of effectiveness, there were no statistically significant differences among STS 0.5%, POL 0.25%, and HS 20% with heparin.[7]

Goldman[8] compared STS 0.25% with POL 0.5% and found little difference in terms of effectiveness. Another study, comparing 100% CG, POL 0.25% solution, and POL 0.25% foam, indicated that CG was associated with higher degrees of pain, better clearance, and no staining or matting, whereas foam POL caused the most staining and matting.[9] Another study, by Leach and Goldman, compared 72% glycerin diluted 2:1 with 1% lidocaine with epinephrine and STS 0.25%. This study showed significantly better and more rapid clearance with the glycerin and less staining than the STS.[10]

LASER TREATMENT OF SPIDER TELANGIECTASIAS

Historical Perspective

The laser is a relative newcomer to the treatment domain of lower extremity spider vein treatment; however, it is gaining increased popularity and refinement. This technologic newcomer's popularity is, interestingly, primarily driven by the consumer, not the practitioner, unlike most other new advances. Lasers are particularly useful for lower extremity spider veins that arise from matting or are refractory to sclerotherapy treatment. These treatments are also useful for people who have phobias, fears, and concerns relating to needles. Despite its advantages, however, laser use has some limitations, including the fact that they are an adjunctive and complementary therapy after sclerotherapy, rather than a substitute for it.

Basic Concepts and Terminology

Laser, an acronym for light amplification by stimulated emission of radiation, produces a beam of monochromic, coherent, collimated light of a specific wavelength. *Pumping* is a term used to describe the process of supplying the amount of energy necessary for the amplification of the laser beam. This energy can be delivered as light of varying wavelengths, or as an electrical current, which is measured in terms of joules (J). The amount of energy delivered to an area is referred to as *fluence,* and it can be represented as J per cm^2. The power with which the energy is delivered is referred to as *watts.* A watt (W) is equivalent to one joule per second. The number of watts that are delivered to a given unit area, typically indicated as W/cm^2, is called *irradiance.* Last, *pulse width* is the duration of laser exposure and it is documented in terms of milliseconds.

The therapeutic usefulness, as well as the possible untoward effects of laser treatments, are based on the fact that as a laser beam strikes the skin, it leads to four reactions: scattering, absorption, transmission, and reflection. Scattering is a function of wavelength and the presence of substances such as collagen, both of which can potentially have an impact on the occurrence of collateral, unintended tissue damage. For example, shorter wavelengths are associated with increased scattering compared with longer wavelengths. Laser photons are absorbed, and thus therapeutic, when they are not impeded by reflection, scattering, or transmission. The challenges to the practitioner arise from the fact that veins vary in terms of their ability to absorb the laser's energy, and each laser generator delivers only one wavelength without any built-in mechanisms to vary it, with one exception, the tunable dye laser. In other words, deeper veins require a longer wavelength than more superficial ones, but the wavelength of a specific generator is fixed; therefore no variation of wavelength is possible. Only power, spot size, and pulse width can be manipulated to attack the full thickness and circumference of the vein wall.

Lasers work by emitting the pulse of light that is absorbed by the hemoglobin in the blood vessel with just enough heat to the vein to cause irreparable, desired, damage to the vein but not enough to damage the skin as a result of the laser's absorption by melanin.

Ideally, the laser should deliver the precise amount of energy needed to damage the intended vein target but not cause any damage to the surrounding tissue, including the skin. It should also deliver this energy for precisely the correct duration to slowly coagulate the vessel's full thickness and entire circumference without rupturing it. In the real world, however, perfect techniques and equipment are not a reality, so the typical laser wavelength used is between 600 and 900 nm.

The shape of the beam and the wavelength of the emitted light for each type of laser give it its unique and specific characteristics. The use of lasers has some advantages in terms of telangiectasias treatment, and many of the complications associated with sclerotherapy are not likely to occur with noninvasive laser treatment. Furthermore, this diminished risk is not solely limited to the drug introduced into the body.

Shorter wavelength lasers have very good hemoglobin absorption, but they do not penetrate very deeply. They also have higher melanin absorption, something that competes with the hemoglobin. Longer wavelengths have both less hemoglobin absorption and less melanin absorption. They penetrate the skin more deeply. Deeper and larger spider telangiectasias respond better to longer, rather than shorter, wavelength lasers, and they are much better tolerated by darker skin tones, which are more tolerant and more forgiving than lighter skin tones.

Other factors are also important for the practitioner's consideration. For example, how much energy should be given, and how will that energy be delivered? Will it be given using a short burst or using a long pulse? Lasers also offer us a limited number of other variables that can be manipulated to optimize results. For example, stacking pulses allow cooling of the skin between pulses to take full advantage of the different heat specificities between skin and hemoglobin. In addition, there are methods to cool the skin to protect it from burns (cold air, ice packs, cold solutions through clear glass, and a cryogen spray).

Many different lasers have been used for the treatment of spider veins, but this section briefly addresses the most common lasers used today.

Types of Lasers

With rare exception, the primary lasers used today for leg veins are light sources and pulsed lasers. Included in these categories are the following types of lasers:

- Potassium titanyl phosphate (KTP 532 nm)
- Yellow-pulsed dye laser (585 nm to 605 nm)
- Alexandrite or infrared 755-nm laser
- Diode or infrared 810-nm, 940-nm, and 980-nm laser
- Neodymium:yttrium-aluminium-garnet (Nd:YAG) laser infrared to 1064 nm
- Intense pulsed light (IPL) broadband light source laser with 515 to 1200 nm

KTP and frequency-doubled Nd:YAG 532-nm lasers provide a very short pulse that works exceptionally well on the fine red spider veins. The shorter wavelength, however, does not penetrate very deeply, and it is absorbed by the melanin in the skin, making it not the treatment of choice among patients with darker skin types.

Diode lasers come in multiple wavelengths. The wavelengths used for the treatment of spider veins are 810 nm, 940 nm, and 980 nm. These spectrums have considerable hemoglobin absorption, lesser degrees of melanin absorption, and deeper penetration; thus they are suitable for the treatment of veins up to 1 mm in diameter.

The Nd:YAG 1064-nm laser has become the most widely used laser for the treatment of leg telangiectasias. It provides deeper penetration and less melanin absorption than the other wavelengths. It also has less hemoglobin absorption; however, it also increases water absorption. Higher energies are required with this laser, but these energies are well tolerated because they absorb low levels of melanin. Pain is a commonly occurring phenomenon, however, with this laser. A cooling intervention, such as cold air, cold water between glass, or cryogen spray, is frequently used to reduce any patient's discomfort. A topical anesthetic with lidocaine, for vasodilation, is also effective to combat the pain.

Regardless of the laser equipment used, however, there are some pitfalls and concerns that are common to all; therefore the physician should resist the temptation of overtreating the vessels by delivering unnecessary passes and/or greater than necessary fluences. These actions may lead to blanching, hypopigmentation, and/or necrosis with hyperpigmentation (Fig. 23.30).

Operative Steps

As previously discussed, the initial steps in laser treatment include a patient assessment, a thorough discussion of the benefits and potential risks of treatment, and photographic documentation. Next, the practitioner must decide which laser to use and what settings should be used for the particular patient.

As discussed previously, smaller red spider veins are typically very superficial veins, therefore shorter wavelength lasers are the treatment of choice. For example, the KTP 532-nm laser has been used successfully on these fine red spider veins. On the other hand, the Nd:YAG 1064-nm laser works better than the KTP 532-nm laser on larger veins up to, and including, the small reticular veins.

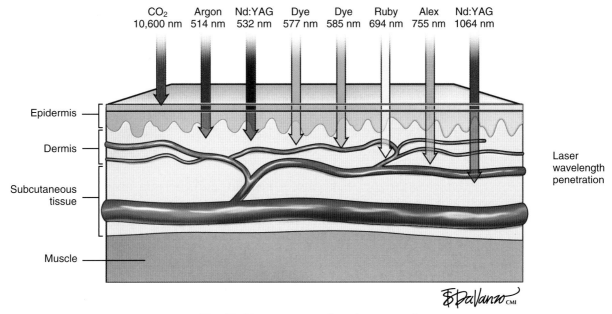

■ **Fig. 23.30** Laser wavelength penetration.

The next decision-making point is determining spot size or the diameter of the laser beam needed to treat the area. The smaller the spot diameter, the more concentrated is the energy, therefore less energy is needed. Smaller veins can be treated with small spot sizes as low as 1 mm. Larger spider veins, of about 1 mm, require a 2-mm to 4-mm spot size to effectively cover the vein. Larger veins, that is, those over 1 mm, are best treated with 6-mm spot size.

Following are determinations regarding the best pulse duration, the best duration between pulses, and the amount of energy to use. Pulse duration is another variable that can be manipulated to achieve optimal results based on the particular vein that will be treated. Smaller veins heat up more quickly than larger veins; therefore very short pulses are necessary to alleviate this potential hazard when treating the smaller veins. Larger veins take longer to heat up so longer pulses are needed to achieve desired outcomes.

Some lasers will stack pulses allowing for cooling intervals between pulses; therefore a delay time between pulses may be part of the settings, something that may have to be adjusted according to the unique needs of the patient. Darker skin tones have to cool longer between pulses then lighter skin tones. Energy settings can be by watts or by joules; joules take into account the pulse duration whereas watts do not. Most lasers are set by joules. Again, larger veins need more energy.

Finally, there are different cooling devices from which the practitioner must choose. Some of these choices include cooled air blown on the skin, ice packs, and cryogen air. Regardless of choice, however, each alternative must be carefully implemented either just before and/or just after the pulse of laser light. Pulsed cryogen air timing has to be scrupulously managed because too liberal use may lead to vasospasm and a decrease in the amount of hemoglobin necessary for light absorption. Because cooling prevents or alleviates patient discomfort and also provides protection against skin injury, it should be a routine aspect of laser treatment.

The most frequently encountered complication associated with cutaneous lasers is a skin burn that could result in a blister, pigmentary changes, and/or scarring. The extent of any burn is affected by several factors, including the wavelength used, the amount of energy delivered, the patient's skin type, and sun exposure before the treatment. Shorter wavelengths are more likely to injure the skin than longer ones because shorter wavelengths have a higher degree of melanin absorption. For this reason, short wavelength lasers should be used with caution in darker skin types.

The amount of energy delivered is also a factor that impacts on the occurrence and extent of any skin injury. Enough energy at virtually all wavelengths will cause skin injury. Joules, again, are calculated as watts per second; therefore 100 J given in over 100 ms is very different than 100 J given over 20 ms. More optimal results are sometimes achieved by treating darker skinned individuals with the long pulsed 1064-nm Nd:YAG laser, especially for larger spider veins.

Darker skin types have more melanin, and melanin absorbs energy from light as well as hemoglobin. People with darker skin tones are more likely to have an injury from laser treatment, and therefore should be approached with caution. Possibly even more important than skin type, however, is recent sun exposure. Sun exposure stimulates melanin production, so even people with light-colored skin may have increased melanin after sun exposure, thus increasing the risk of injury with laser treatment. The patient should be advised to avoid sun exposure for at least 2 weeks before the anticipated treatment and to continue sun avoidance for at least 2 weeks postprocedure.

Eye injury, for both the patient and the practitioner, is also a potential complication of laser treatment. It is essential therefore that adequate protective eyewear be worn to block the laser wavelength. Lead shields are also used, especially if the laser is used near the eyes (Figs. 23.31A–C–23.33).

Comparative Effectiveness

To date, there have been only a few studies comparing cutaneous laser treatment of spider telangiectasia and sclerotherapy. In 2002 research supported the fact that lasers were more effective for sclerotherapy than for spider telangiectasia.[11] A second study led to similar results, but a greater degree of patient satisfaction was observed with sclerotherapy.[12] In 2004 a sequential study comparing Nd:YAG 1064-nm laser treatment followed by sclerotherapy and sclerotherapy followed by laser treatment. The results of this research suggested that the best results were achieved with sclerotherapy followed by laser treatment.[13]

The current consensus is that sclerotherapy remains the primary treatment of choice for leg telangiectasias, but some are convinced that a combination of sclerotherapy and laser may have synergistic effects. This belief was challenged, however, in 1990 by Goldman and Fitzpatrick.[14] Their research indicated there were no statistically significant improvements in terms of outcome with this combination. Furthermore, increased complications were observed when compared with the complications encountered with sclerotherapy alone.

In summary, current data do not support laser treatment as the preferred modality for the treatment of leg telangiectasias when compared with sclerotherapy. It can and should be used as an adjunct to it or with needle-phobic patients and those with allergies to the commonly used sclerosants.

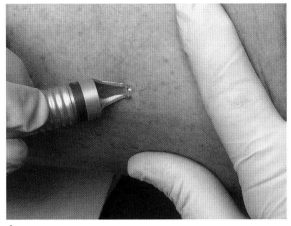
A

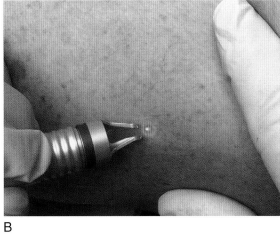
B

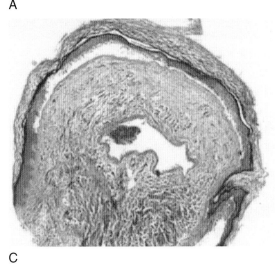
C

■ **Fig. 23.31** (A) Treating telangiectasia with 940-nm laser. (B) Posttreatment of telangiectasia with 940-nm laser. (C) Histologic slide of telangiectasia treated with 940-nm laser.

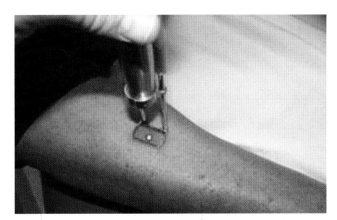

■ **Fig. 23.32** Sciton Nd:YAG laser.

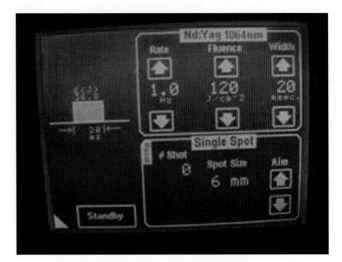

■ **Fig. 23.33** Sciton screen settings.

REFERENCES

1. Biegeleisen HI. Telangiectasia associated with varicose veins: treatment by microinjection technique. *JAMA.* 1934;102:2092.
2. Foley WT. The eradication of venous blemishes. *Cutis.* 1975;15:665.
3. Nootheti PK, Cadag KM, Magpantay A, et al. Efficacy of graduated compression stockings for an additional 3 weeks after sclerotherapy treatment for reticular and telangiectatic leg veins. *Dermatol Surg.* 2009;35:53–57.
4. Rao J, Wildemore JK, Goldman MP. Double-blind prospective comparative trial between foamed and liquid polidocanol and sodium tetradecyl sulfate in the treatment of varicose and telangiectatic leg veins. *Dermatol Surg.* 2005;31:631–635.
5. Morrison N, Neuhardt DL, Rogers CR, et al. Comparison of side effects using air and carbon dioxide foam for endovenous chemical ablation. *J Vasc Surg.* 2008;47:830–836.
6. Sarvananthan T, Shepherd AC, Willenberg T, et al. Neurological complications of sclerotherapy for varicose veins. *J Vasc Surg.* 2012;55(1):243–251.
7. Curlin MC, Ratz JL. Treatment of telangiectasia: comparison of sclerosing agents. *J Dermatologic Surg Oncol.* 1987;13:1181.
8. Goldman MP. Treatment of varicose and telangiectatic leg veins: double-blind prospective trial between aethoxysclerol and sotradecol. *Derm Surg.* 2002;28:52.
9. Kern P, Ramelet AA, Wutschert R, et al. Single-blind, randomized study comparing chromated glycerin, polidocanol solution and polidocanol foam for treatment of telangiectatic leg veins. *Dermatol Surg.* 2004;30:367–372.
10. Leach B, Goldman MP. Comparative trial between sodium tetradecyl sulfate and glycerin in the treatment of telangiectatic leg veins. *Dermatol Surg.* 2003;29:612.
11. Lupton JR, Alster TS, Romero P. Clinical comparison of sclerotherapy vs long pulsed Nd:YAG laser treatment of lower extremity telangiectasia. *Derm Surg.* 2002;28:694–697.
12. Coles MC, Werner RS, Zelickson BD. Comparative pilot study evaluating the treatment of leg veins with a long pulse Nd:YAG laser and sclerotherapy. *Lasers Surg Med.* 2002;30:154–159.
13. Levy J, Elbahr C, Jouve E, et al. Comparison and sequential study of long pulsed Nd:YAG 1064 nm laser and sclerotherapy in leg telangiectasia treatment. *Lasers Surg Med.* 2004;34:273.
14. Goldman MP, Fitzpatrick RE. Pulsed-dye laser treatment of leg telangiectasia with and without simultaneous sclerotherapy. *J Derm Surg Oncol.* 1990;16:338–344.

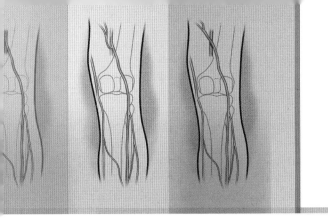

CHAPTER 24

Endovenous Management of Central and Upper Extremity Veins

Constantino S. Peña and Ashley Nicole Adamovich

Because of the increased use of central venous catheters and implantable pacemakers and defibrillators, upper extremity deep venous thrombosis (UEDVT) has become more frequent. Central vein stenosis and thrombosis, usually from neointimal hyperplasia, are commonly seen in dialysis-dependent patients or in patients who have had placement of an indwelling central venous catheter. Traditional risk factors also include thrombophilia and cancer. It is estimated that approximately 10% of all cases of deep venous thrombosis (DVT) occur in the upper extremity veins. Even though these cases are less likely to result in pulmonary embolism and postthrombotic syndrome than in lower extremity DVT, they are associated with a risk of pulmonary embolism (5.6%), venous gangrene, and disabling arm or neck swelling requiring proper recognition, diagnosis, and treatment.

PRIMARY UPPER EXTREMITY DEEP VENOUS THROMBOSIS: PAGET SCHROETTER SYNDROME

UEDVT can be classified as primary, when it occurs without an inciting cause, and secondary, when it is related to an underlying catheter or previous catheter. Primary UEDVT, also known as effort thrombosis, usually occurs in healthy young individuals (third decade of life) who present with sudden, severe swelling of the upper extremity that may be associated with cyanosis and arm paresthesia. The condition is usually seen in patients after a repetitive activity and is known by the eponym Paget-Schroetter syndrome after a British and a German physician who simultaneously reported it. These patients usually have a compressive phenomenon at the thoracic outlet. It is traditionally

659

seen at the level of the clavicular head and first rib. The scalenus anterior muscle and tendon, along with the bony structures, may compress the subclavian vein at this level, particularly at some stressed positions of the arm. The process can also be seen with the cervical ribs (Figs. 24.1 and 24.2). The combination of the compression of the costoclavicular portion of the axillosubclavian vein and repetitive stress leads to intimal damage and subsequent fibrotic reactions of the underlying vein. This intimal damage along with the diminished flow from the compression then promotes thrombosis. Patients with effort thrombosis must be identified because if this condition is not treated, it can progress, and patients may experience chronic disability (25%–74%).

Treatment

As opposed to patients with secondary UEDVT, in these patients there is an extrinsic venous compression responsible for the thrombosis. The goal of treatment is to restore venous patency and relieve the compression. When effort thrombosis is suspected in a patient, a catheter-directed chemical thrombolysis (if the patient is a candidate) is performed followed by a limited angioplasty, if needed, to restore flow. The results of the angioplasty are variable depending on the underlying injury to the vein. The hope is that the vein can be gently dilated to attempt to maintain patency; the patient can then undergo anticoagulation until decompression surgery can be performed. It is important to diagnose the compression during the thrombolysis procedures and understand that the long-term patency of angioplasty will be limited in the setting of external compression. Stents should never be placed in this compressive environment.

There is controversy about whether to operate immediately or several weeks after thrombolysis. Some surgeons will only operate in the setting of persistent symptoms. Typically, patients are treated with immediate surgery shortly after thrombolysis to relieve the compression. Several weeks after surgery, the status of the vein can be reassessed with ultrasound and angioplasty can be performed as needed to maintain or reestablish flow. There is also controversy whether it is worthwhile to resect the rib in patients who are asymptomatic with well-established collaterals; however, most institutions will proceed with first rib resection to attempt to reestablish patency of the axillosubclavian vein.

Before treatment, it is common for patients to have a venous duplex ultrasound demonstrating thrombosis. A computed tomography (CT) scan or magnetic resonance image highlighting the venous phase may be helpful in demonstrating the compression and excluding other sources of central occlusion (Fig. 24.3). Ultrasound-guided vascular access is achieved traditionally into the basilic or brachial vein to obtain direct access into the axillosubclavian vein. It is important to establish that the vein being punctured is patent. A 4-Fr or 5-Fr ministick microcatheter system is used to perform an initial venogram and document the extent of thrombosis (Fig. 24.4). Once the entry vein is found to be satisfactory, a 5-Fr or 6-Fr vascular sheath is placed. The axillosubclavian thrombosis is crossed with a soft tip guidewire (Bentson wire; Cook Medical, Bloomington, IN) and an angled catheter (Kumpe or multipurpose). The catheter is exchanged for a thrombolysis catheter that is placed across the area of thrombosis (Fig. 24.5). The catheter infusion length is matched to the length of thrombosis, and the patient is treated overnight with thrombolytics. The choice and dose are usually dependent on the operator's choice, amount of thrombus, and patient risk factors. We usually coadminister peripheral low-dose heparin during the infusion, typically 300 units of heparin per hour (Fig. 24.6). In the setting of an acute decompensation requiring rapid thrombectomy or a patient who may not be a candidate for chemical thrombolysis, mechanical thrombectomy may be performed.

Text continued on p. 665

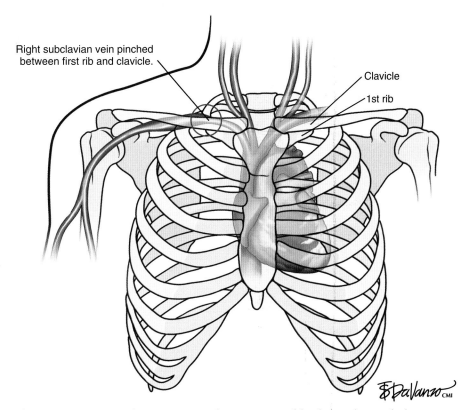

Right subclavian vein pinched
between first rib and clavicle.

Clavicle

1st rib

■ **Fig. 24.1** Diagram demonstrating the junction of both brachiocephalic veins into the superior vena cava.

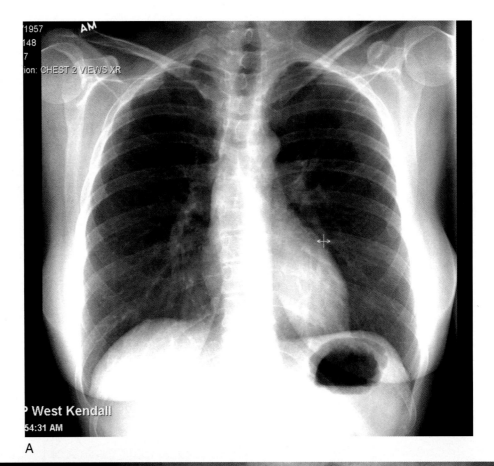

A

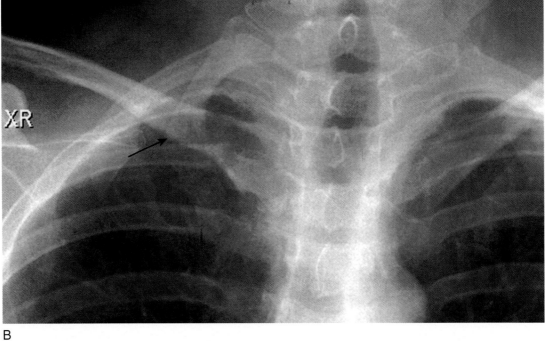

B

■ **Fig. 24.2** A frontal chest radiograph (A) and magnified view (B) depict the presence of a right-sided cervical rib *(arrow)*. This is just one of the possible causes of anatomic compression of the axillosubclavian vein.

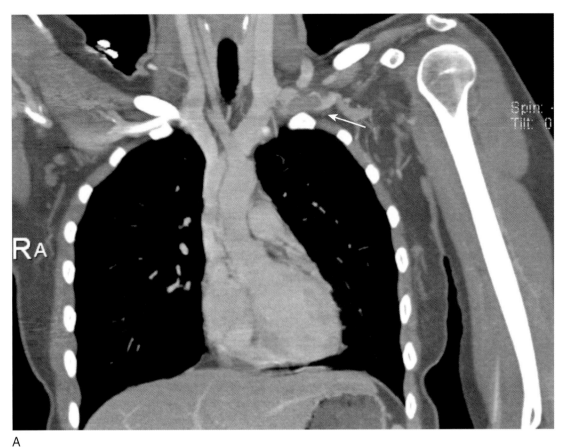

A

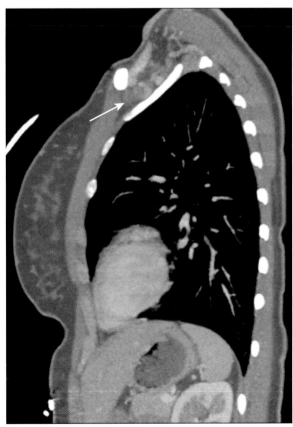

B

■ **Fig. 24.3** (A) A coronal reformation of a computed tomography (CT) scan during the venous phase demonstrating a focal thrombosis of the left axillosubclavian vein *(arrow)*. (B) A sagittal reformation of a CT scan during the venous phase demonstrating a focal thrombosis of the left axillosubclavian vein *(arrow)*. Note location of the vein between the clavicle and the first in both reformations.

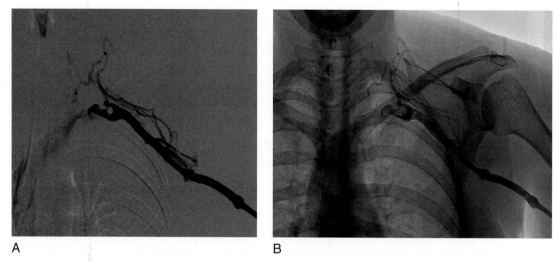

◼ **Fig. 24.4** A frontal left upper extremity venogram demonstrating occlusion with thrombosis of the left axillosubclavian vein in a subtracted (A) and unsubtracted (B) image.

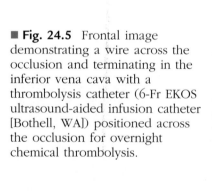

◼ **Fig. 24.5** Frontal image demonstrating a wire across the occlusion and terminating in the inferior vena cava with a thrombolysis catheter (6-Fr EKOS ultrasound-aided infusion catheter [Bothell, WA]) positioned across the occlusion for overnight chemical thrombolysis.

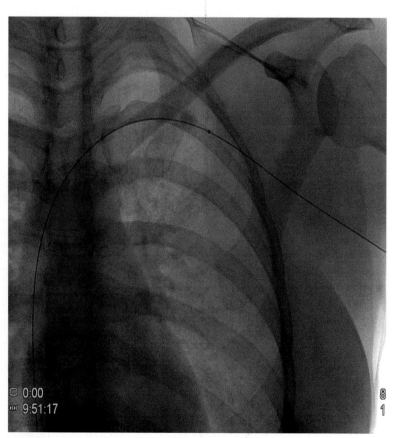

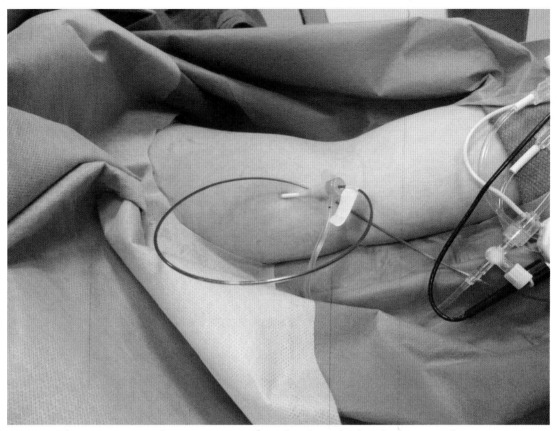

■ **Fig. 24.6** Image demonstrating a 6-Fr sheath in the brachial vein with an EKOS infusion catheter through the sheath. This patient received 0.5 mg per hour of r-tPA (alteplase; Genentech, San Francisco, CA) infused via the EKOS catheter and 300 units per hour of heparin via the sheath.

After overnight catheter directed thrombolysis, a venogram is performed to assess the patency of the axillosubclavian vein (Fig. 24.7). Usually, overnight thrombolysis is sufficient to clear the associated thrombus, but in certain patients, a second day of thrombolysis may be necessary. As with any thrombolysis procedure, the patient is informed of the potential risk of bleeding and monitored carefully, as well as with fibrinogen levels. A venogram is then performed in a provocative position to assess the amount of compression and secure the diagnosis. We usually abduct and externally rotate the arm over the patient's head. The area of compression on the vein is usually still present after thrombolysis (Figs. 24.8 and 24.9). Angioplasty can then be performed if there is a persistent high-grade stenosis (Fig. 24.10). A low-pressure balloon is used, not solely to treat the venous obstruction but also to assess the amount of fibrosis and neointimal damage because a severely damaged vein may require a venous patch at the time of surgical decompression. The surgical decompression may be performed from a transaxillary or supraclavicular approach. A portion of the first rib along with the tendinous attachment of the transected anterior scalene muscle is usually removed (Fig. 24.11).

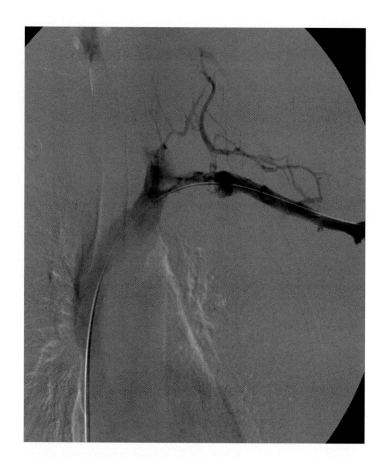

■ **Fig. 24.7** Venogram after overnight thrombolysis demonstrating clearing of thrombus with minimal irregularity at the level of compression.

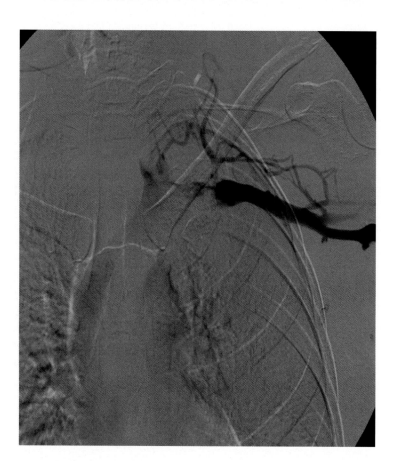

■ **Fig. 24.8** Venogram performed with the patient in a stressed position.

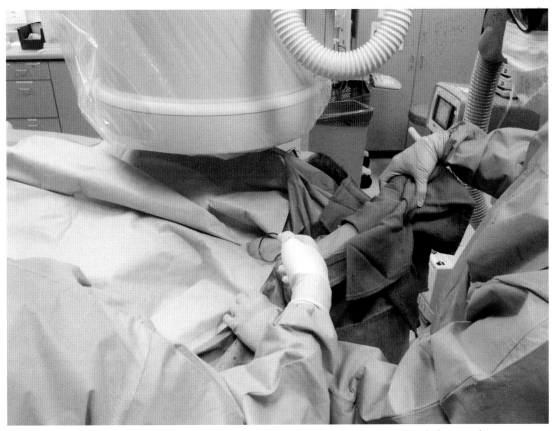

■ **Fig. 24.9** Positioning of patient for stressed views. We usually abduct and externally rotate the arm.

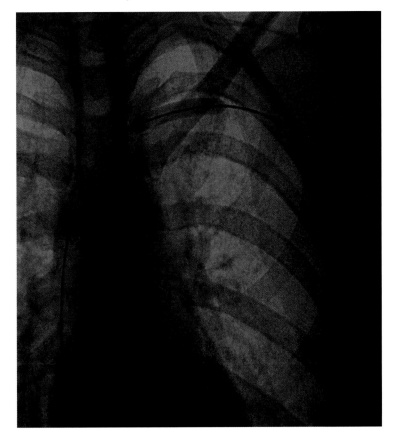

■ **Fig. 24.10** Dilating the residual narrowing or venous thickening after lysis.

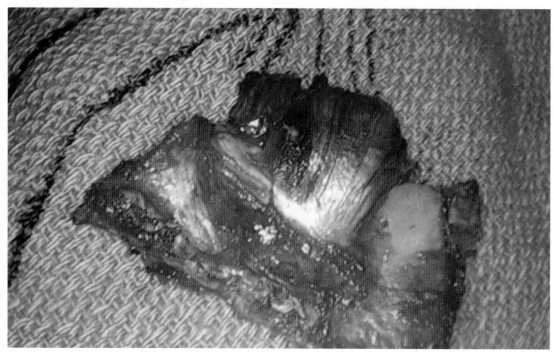

■ **Fig. 24.11** Surgical specimen of the first rib with associated anterior scalene tendinous attachment. *(From Abilio Coello, MD, FACS, Miami Vascular Specialists.)*

SECONDARY UPPER EXTREMITY DEEP VENOUS THROMBOSIS

Provoked or secondary upper extremity DVT is usually related to catheters and devices and has increased the incidence of upper extremity venous stenosis and DVT accounting for nearly 75% of these cases. These patients usually present with pain and/or arm swelling. Patient symptoms and extent of thrombosis determine if anticoagulation should be initiated for peripheral upper extremity venous thrombosis. Axillary, subclavian, and jugular thrombosis is usually treated with anticoagulation to improve symptoms and prevent pulmonary embolism. CHEST guidelines favor anticoagulation while maintaining a functional catheter in place if the catheter is necessary. The placement of superior vena cava (SVC) filters in patients who are intolerant of anticoagulation is controversial, and usually only patients who have a suspected upper extremity thrombus pulmonary embolism or are at high risk of a life-threatening pulmonary embolism are treated with SVC filters. SVC filter placement is a higher risk procedure that should be carefully considered, especially because the incidence of life-threatening pulmonary embolism from an upper extremity source is unknown.

Patients with a central-catheter–associated thrombosis are at slightly higher risk of pulmonary embolism. Pulmonary embolism has also been associated with the removal of these catheters in the acute setting of thrombosis. Treatment with anticoagulation in these patients and removal of the central catheters, only if the patient's symptoms persist or worsen on anticoagulation, is recommended. Prevention of unnecessary subclavian punctures and catheter placement may limit the amount and extent of subclavian venous stenosis and thrombosis.

DIALYSIS ACCESS–RELATED CENTRAL VENOUS STENOSIS

Central venous stenosis occurs in a significant number (11%–40%) of patients on hemodialysis. It is the leading cause of shunt dysfunction and is associated with venous hypertension and arm swelling. The cause of dialysis-associated central vein stenosis is unknown but is likely multifactorial. The neointimal fibrosis responsible for these central stenotic lesions may be associated with prior, centrally placed catheters. The damage caused by previous subclavian punctures has led the authors of the Kidney Disease Outcomes Quality Initiative (KDOQI) guidelines to strongly discourage unnecessary subclavian punctures, but the presence of a central catheter, even from the jugular approach, may cause sufficient endothelial damage from the trauma associated with its continual motion within the body. The turbulent and high flow associated with upper extremity hemodialysis access may explain central venous stenosis in patients who have never received a central catheter.

Central venous stenosis not only can be symptomatic with severe arm swelling but also may limit the function of a hemodialysis access. The treatment of central vein stenosis associated with hemodialysis is traditionally angioplasty. Unfortunately, the 1-year patency of these treatments has been reported to be between 10% and 30%, and the use of multiple, additional procedures to maintain secondary patency is the rule. The initial use of stents to treat central venous stenosis has been discouraged because of a similar patency rate to that of angioplasty and the possibility of stent compression in the thoracic outlet. In addition, there are no US Food and Drug Administration (FDA)–approved uncovered stents for the venous system. Even though the results from angioplasty are limited, endovascular dilatation of these stenoses is preferred over surgical options because of its availability, noninvasiveness, low risk of morbidity, and ability to repeat as needed. KDOQI guidelines recommend stent placement for central lesions that recur within 3 months after angioplasty and demonstrate immediate vessel recoil greater than 50% after angioplasty and vessel perforation. The patency of a stent in central venous stenosis is similar to that of angioplasty, but the ability of retreatment becomes limited (Figs. 24.12 and 24.13). The use of covered self-expandable stents has shown promise, particularly in the setting of peripheral dialysis graft anastomotic stenoses. Their use will likely increase in the central veins; however, the operator needs to be careful in not excluding other draining veins with a central covered stent.

Technically, angioplasty of central venous stenosis associated with hemodialysis is usually performed from the fistula and/or graft. In the setting of vessel occlusion, femoral access may also be needed. A sheath is placed in the access site, and a complete shunt study is performed with venography. The lesion is best treated over a working wire (Amplatz, Rosen, Torque). We usually begin with a low-pressure balloon (10-atm to 12-atm burst pressure). The sizing of the balloon is essential to prevent rupture. The dilatation of the stenosis is performed using a 3-minute inflation and an insufflator device to control the pressure administered. Care must be taken not to thrombose the access. If the stenosis cannot be dilated by the low-pressure balloon, a high-pressure balloon is used (Blue Max; Boston Scientific, Natick, MA, or Conquest; Bard, Tempe, AZ). If the stenosis was dilated by the low-pressure balloon inflation but demonstrated recoil, the decision can be made to stent the lesion, attempt a high-pressure balloon, or score the stenosis with a cutting balloon or similar product. It is important not to simply redilate with a larger-diameter balloon because this may risk rupturing the vein.

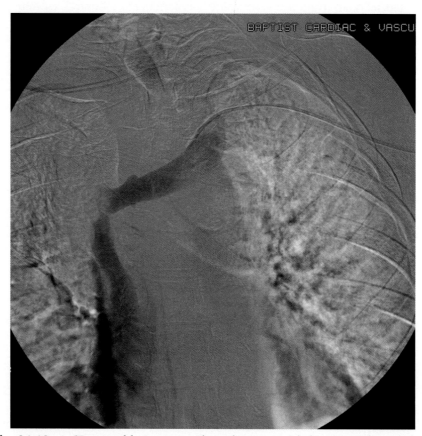

■ **Fig. 24.12** A 57-year-old woman with end-stage renal disease and central stenosis at the junction of the left brachiocephalic vein and superior vena cava. The patient has an occluded right upper extremity system.

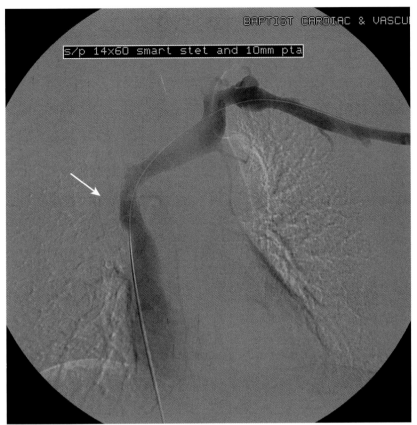

■ **Fig. 24.13** A 57-year-old woman with central stenosis resistant to venoplasty and treated with a 14-mm × 60-mm Smart stent (self-expanding nitinol; Cordis Johnson & Johnson [Bridgewater, NJ]) dilated to 10 mm *(arrow)*.

SUPERIOR VENA CAVA SYNDROME

Patients with SVC syndrome present with symptoms that include arm, neck, and facial swelling, as well as edema, erythema, orthopnea, and paresthesia. The symptoms may worsen with the patient in the recumbent position. SVC syndrome can develop progressively or acutely and is usually related to advanced oncologic disease, such as lung cancer or mediastinal disease. However, SVC stenosis and its associated syndrome can also occur as a consequence of benign fibrosing conditions of the mediastinum, such as sarcoidosis as well as previous radiation therapy and long-standing hemodialysis and the use of central venous catheters. The underlying condition consists of occlusion or severe stenosis of the central veins, preventing sufficient venous blood flow from returning into the right atrium. The jugular veins on each side of the neck join the subclavian vein to form the brachiocephalic vein in the chest. The right and left brachiocephalic veins then join to form the SVC. The lesions may occur in the SVC or in a number of central extremity veins, creating the equivalent to an SVC lesion. Treatment for SVC syndrome in the setting of cancer can include chemotherapy or radiation therapy, especially for chemosensitive and radiosensitive masses, but the response may take a few days, which may be unacceptable to patients with severe symptoms.

Even though there are no FDA-approved stents for the venous system, stents are used "off-label" in patients with SVC syndrome with improvement in 70% to 90% of patients' symptoms. Remember that the goal of treatment in patients with SVC syndrome from cancer is palliation. The long-term effects and patency of stents may not be relevant in patients with malignant obstruction or life-threatening symptoms. There is controversy surrounding stenting in the setting of SVC obstruction because a percentage of patients develop collateral pathways and may not become symptomatic. It is important to evaluate every patient individually, assessing symptoms and all available treatment options (Figs. 24.14–24.16). It is common for patients on hemodialysis to present with SVC syndrome caused by central occlusions and stenosis (Figs. 24.17–24.19).

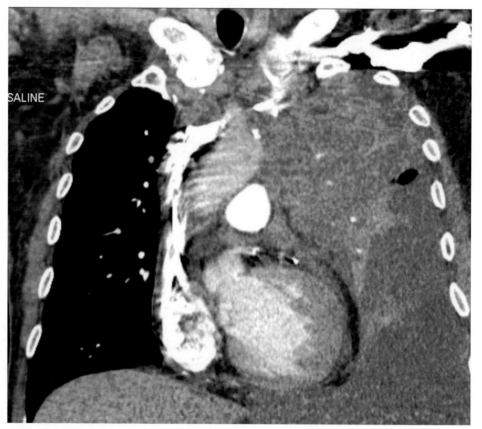

■ **Fig. 24.14** A 61-year-old patient with left upper lobe lung cancer presents with left arm and face swelling. Computed tomography scan suggests brachiocephalic compression.

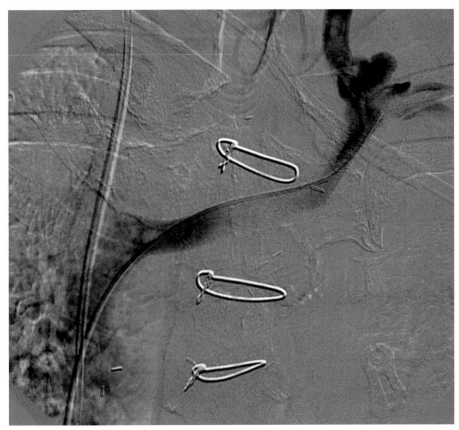

■ **Fig. 24.15** Venogram confirms compression and severe stenosis.

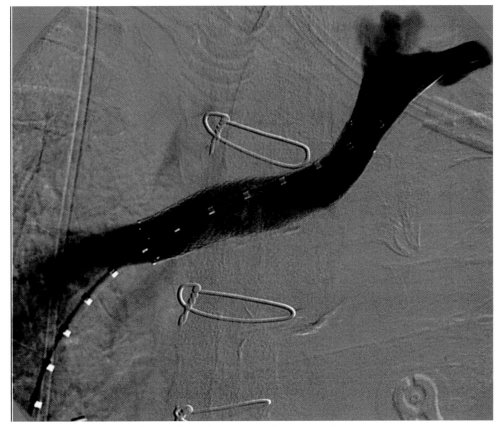

■ **Fig. 24.16** Venogram after stent placement.

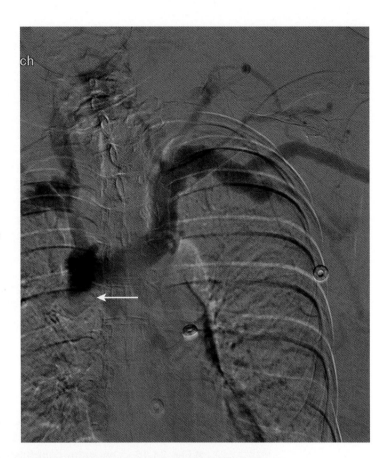

■ **Fig. 24.17** A 48-year-old woman with end-stage renal disease presented with a swollen head and face and was found to have obstruction of the proximal superior vena cava *(arrow)*.

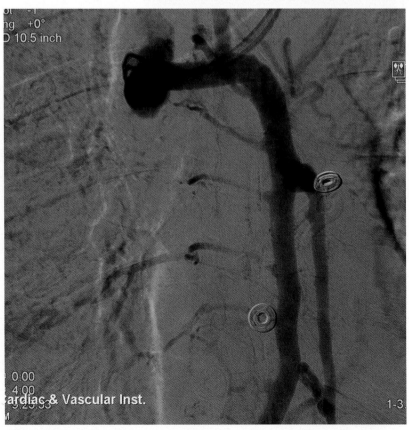

■ **Fig. 24.18** Venogram demonstrates central outflow via dilated hemiazygos system.

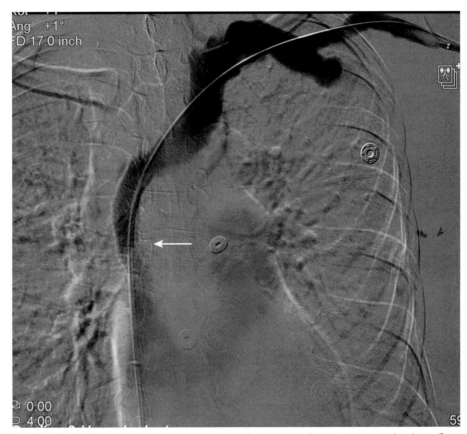

■ **Fig. 24.19** After angioplasty and stent placement, there is restored inline flow into the right atrium with prompt symptom improvement *(arrow)*.

Patients with SVC syndrome are initially studied using venography. A complete ultrasound examination including pulsed-wave Doppler and greyscale imaging may be helpful to establish the number and degree of stenoses or occlusions before the venogram. If possible, a cross-sectional study such as a CT angiogram or magnetic resonance angiogram with a venous phase may be obtained to confirm the level of stenosis and occlusion, as well as highlight the amount of underlying mass effect or malignancy (Fig. 24.20).

Although it may not be necessary to treat both innominate veins to achieve a clinical outcome, bilateral central venous stenting may be needed to reestablish optimal flow. The goal is to restore flow into the right atrium (Figs. 24.21–24.23). The patency of the jugular veins is important because its intact drainage centrally is usually sufficient to relieve face and head symptoms. At the time of venography, brachial vein access is complemented by femoral and possibly jugular access. In the setting of acute thrombosis, chemical or mechanical thrombolysis may be necessary to uncover the underlying stenosis and minimize embolization. At our institution, we usually attempt to place the central stents first and then extend additional stents peripherally to help anchor the stents in place as needed. Stent migration is a complication and may be limited by the use of proper oversizing of the stents. The SVC is a thin vessel, and aggressive dilatation of stents should be avoided because caval perforation may occur, especially in patients after radiation therapy (Figs. 24.24–24.26).

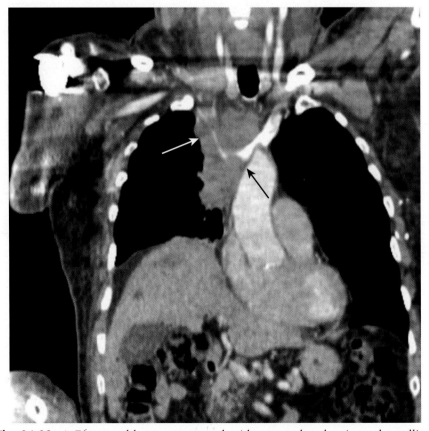

■ **Fig. 24.20** A 76-year-old man presented with severe head pain and swelling. Computed tomography scan demonstrates known lung cancer, which is causing narrowing of both brachiocephalic veins. The right brachiocephalic vein appears occluded (*arrows*).

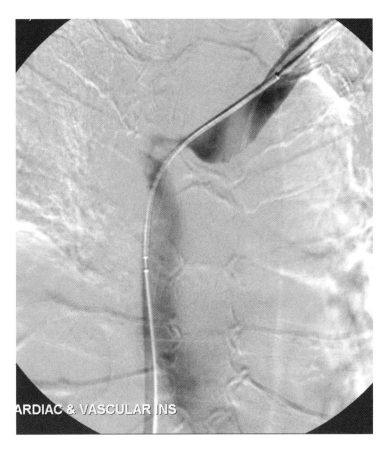

■ **Fig. 24.21** A 76-year-old man with lung cancer and superior vena cava syndrome. Left upper extremity venogram demonstrates severe stenosis of the distal left brachiocephalic vein with a self-expandable stent being positioned for treatment.

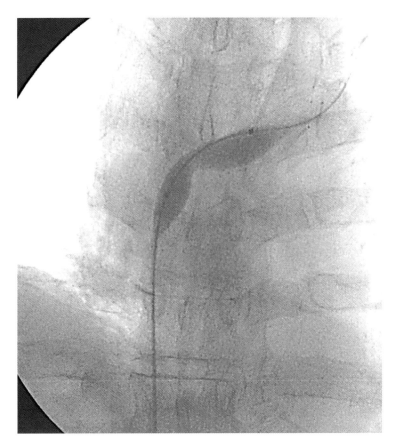

■ **Fig. 24.22** Dilatation of the stent with a 12-mm balloon.

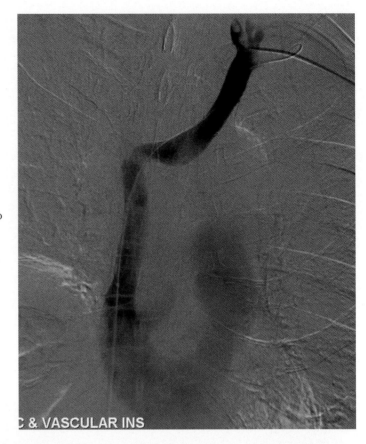

■ **Fig. 24.23** Venogram poststent placement demonstrates prompt flow into the superior vena cava with dramatic improvement in the patient's symptoms.

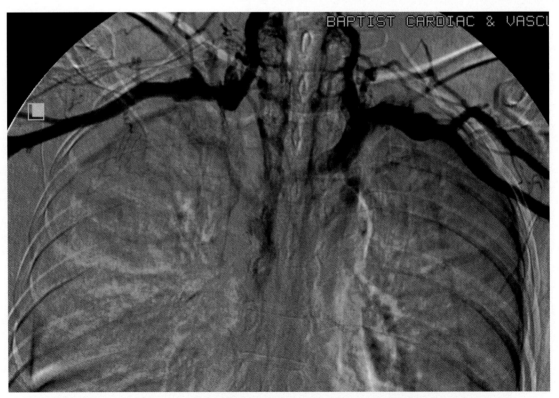

■ **Fig. 24.24** A 61-year-old woman with superior vena cava syndrome whose bilateral upper extremity venogram demonstrates bilateral brachiocephalic vein occlusion.

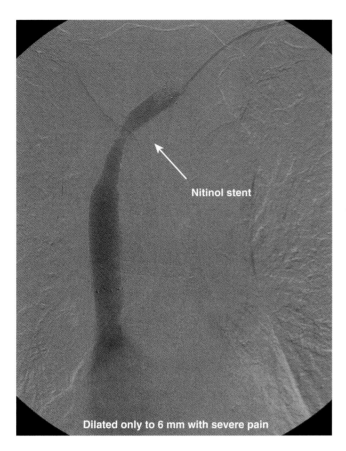

■ **Fig. 24.25** Postrecanalization of left brachiocephalic vein; a 14-mm × 80-mm nitinol stent (SMART) was placed *(arrow)*. Stent could be dilated only to 6 mm because of severe pain.

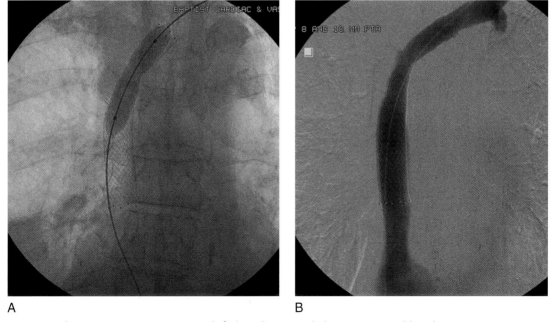

■ **Fig. 24.26** Patient returned 6 days later, and the stent was dilated to 8 mm and 10 mm. (A) With improved flow. (B) With further improvement in symptoms.

CROSSING UPPER EXTREMITY CENTRAL VENOUS OCCLUSIONS

Occlusion of the upper extremity central venous system may occasionally require endo-vascular revascularization. Traditional techniques used in the lower extremity central venous system may be used, but the risk of pericardial extravasation and potentially lethal pericardial hemorrhage should always be considered. In addition, the ability to cross a venous occlusion from both access points maybe helpful and increases the ability to successfully recanalize these occlusions. Initial attempts usually include a hydrophilic wire and catheter system that is escalated to a coaxial or triaxial support system with a sheath and support catheters. The need for sharp recanalization techniques is usually reserved for select lesions that have failed conservative techniques. These lesions are usually studied carefully with CT imaging to clearly establish the anatomy before attempting these approaches.

SUGGESTED READINGS

Bashit B, Parisi A, Frager DH, et al. Abdominal CT findings when the superior vena cava, bra-chiocephalic vein or subclavian vein is obstructed. *AJR Am J Roentgenol.* 1996;167:1457–1463.

Bleker SM, van Es N, Kleinjan A, et al. Current management strategies and long-term clinical outcomes of upper extremity venous thrombosis. *J Thromb Haemost.* 2016;14(5):973–981.

Carlon TA, Sudheendra D. Interventional Therapy for Upper Extremity Deep Vein Thrombosis. *Semin Intervent Radiol.* 2017;34(1):54–60.

Demondion X, Herbinet P, Van Sint Jan S, et al. Imaging assessment of thoracic outlet syndrome. *Radiographics.* 2006;26:1735–1750.

Fassiadis N, Roidl M, South M. Are we managing primary upper limb deep venous thrombosis aggressively enough in the district? *Int Angiol.* 2005;24:255–257.

Haskal Z, Trerotola S, Dolmatch A, et al. Stent graft versus balloon angioplasty for failing dialysis-access grafts. *N Engl J Med.* 2010;362:494–503.

Kapur S, Paik E, Rezaei A, et al. Where there is blood there is a way: unusual collateral vessels in superior and inferior vena cava obstruction. *Radiographics.* 2010;30:67–78.

Kearon C, Aki E, Ornelas J, et al. Antithrombotic Therapy for VTE Disease: CHEST Guideline and Expert Panel Report. *Chest.* 2016;149(2):315–352.

Kucher N. Deep-vein thrombosis of the upper extremities. *N Engl J Med.* 2011;364:861–869.

Lee WA, Hill BB, Harris EJ, et al. Surgical intervention is not required for all patients with sub-clavian vein thrombosis. *J Vasc Surg.* 2000;32:57–67.

Lindblad B, Bornmyr S, Kullendorff B, et al. Venous haemodynamics of the upper extremity after subclavian vein thrombosis. *Vasa.* 1990;19:218–222.

Lugo J, Tanious A, Armstrong P, et al. Acute Paget-Schroetter syndrome: does the first rib rou-tinely need to be removed after thrombolysis? *Ann Vasc Surg.* 2015;29(6):1073–1077.

Madan AK, Allmon JC, Harding M, et al. Dialysis access-induced superior vena cava syndrome. *Am Surg.* 2002;68:904–906.

Owens CA, Bui JT, Knuttinen MG, et al. Pulmonary embolism from upper extremity deep vein thrombosis and the role of superior vena cava filters: a review of the literature. *J Vasc Interv Radiol.* 2010;21:779–787.

Thomas IH, Zierler BK. An integrative review of outcomes in patients with acute primary upper extremity deep venous thrombosis following no treatment or treatment with anticoagulation, thrombolysis or surgical algorithms. *Vasc Endovasc Surg.* 2005;39:163–174.

Tilney ML, Griffiths HJ, Edwards EA. Natural history of major venous thrombosis of the upper extremity. *Arch Surg.* 1970;101:792–796.

Vemuri C, Salehi P, Benarroch-Gapei J, et al. Diagnosis and treatment of effort-induced thrombosis of the axillary Subclavian vein due to venous thoracic outlet syndrome. *J Vasc Surg Venous Lymphat Disord.* 2016;4(4):485–500.

CHAPTER 25

Venous Malformations

Constantino S. Peña and Guilherme Dabus

Vascular malformations are likely the single most misdiagnosed entity in the vascular system. Essentially, vascular malformations are errors in vasculogenesis with the particular characteristics of the lesion determined by the vessel in the vascular system that is involved. As a result, these malformations can include arteries, veins, lymphatic vessels, or capillaries. These lesions occur in about 1.5% of the population and over 90% are present at birth. Venous malformations are the most common vascular anomalies. Although these lesions can have mass effect on adjacent structures, they are not tumors.

An organized, histologically based classification system was initially presented by Mullikan, Glowacki, and colleagues in 1992, and a more recently modified classification system was adopted in 2014 by the International Society for the Study of Vascular Anomalies (ISSVA). The classification system clearly separates tumors (e.g., hemangiomas) from the vascular spaces that characterize a vascular malformation[1] (Table 25.1).

WHAT ARE HEMANGIOMAS? ARE THEY ARTERIOVENOUS MALFOMATIONS?

Hemangiomas are childhood masses characterized histologically by high endothelial cell turnover and by cell markers (GLUT-1, merosin, Lewis Y) that are traditionally found only in human placental tissue and that display phasicity characterized by a rapid proliferative phase, plateau phase, and slow involutional phase. The proper nomenclature for these lesions is *infantile hemangioma*. Infantile hemangiomas are benign vascular tumors that are not usually present at the time of birth but instead become evident

TABLE 25.1 Abbreviated International Society for the Study of Vascular Anomalies Classification for Vascular Anomalies

Vascular Anomalies				
Vascular Tumors			Vascular Malformations	
Benign	Locally Aggressive	Malignant	Simple	Combined
Infantile hemangioma	Kaposiform hemangioendothelioma	Angiosarcoma	Capillary malformation (CM)	CVM, CLM
Congenital hemangioma	Retiform hemangioendothelioma	Epithelioid hemangioendothelioma	Lymphatic malformation (LM)	LVM, CLVM
Tufted hemangioma	PILA, Dabska tumor		Venous malformation (VM)	CAVM
Spindle-cell hemangioma	Composite hemanigoendothioma		Arteriovenous malformation (AVM)	CLAVM
Epithelioid hemangioma	Kaposi sarcoma		Arteriovenous fistula	
Pyogenic granuloma				

CAVM, Capillary-arteriovenous malformation; *CLAVM,* cerebral-lymphatic-arteriovenous malformation; *CLM,* capillary-lymphatic-malformation; *CLVM,* capillary-lymphatic-venous malformation; *CVM,* capillary-venous-malformation; *LVM,* lymphatic-venous-malformation.
Abbreviated ISSVA classification for Vascular Anomalies by International Society for the Study of Vascular Anomalies is licensed under a Creative Commons Attribution 4.0 International License.

within the first 2 to 3 weeks of life. They are the most common, benign tumor of infancy. There is a subgroup of hemangiomas that present fully formed at birth known as congenital hemangiomas. These congenital hemangiomas (as opposed to infantile hemangiomas) do not exhibit the expected accelerated postnatal growth. Some congenital hemangiomas involute quickly over the first year of life and are called *rapidly involuting congenital hemangiomas* (RICHs), whereas some may persist indefinitely without treatment and are called *noninvoluting congenital hemangiomas* (NICHs).[2]

The majority of infantile hemangiomas are localized and, although disconcerting to parents and care providers, are nonthreatening.[3] For these lesions, observation and routine monitoring by the pediatrician or dermatologist are acceptable treatment options. A minority of infantile hemangiomas can, however, cause significant morbidity. These require early recognition, timely referral to a specialist, and prompt intervention to minimize complications. Worrisome presentations include multiple hemangiomas and sensitive locations such as beard distribution, periocular, perioral, nasal tip, large regions of the face and neck, and the lumbosacral spine region. In general, larger hemangiomas located on the face are more likely to require treatment. One of the strongest indications for the use of the laser is the presence of ulceration. Other symptoms necessitating therapeutic intervention include congestive heart failure, airway obstruction, dysphagia, infection, failure to thrive, external auditory canal occlusion, visual axis impairment, and severe facial deformity.

Hemangiomas in adults are not hemangiomas; a hemangioma is a childhood-only birthmark. If a vascular birthmark was not present in the childhood stage, then it is not a hemangioma. Hemangiomas are not arteriovenous malformations (AVMs), and vice versa. Although there is arterial inflow that identifies both these lesions, hemangiomas demonstrate typical tumor vascularity with a central arterial pedicle, and there is fairly minimal, if any, shunting identified in the outflow vessels. An AVM, on the other hand, may have significant venous shunting, with resultant low-resistance arterial inflow and arterialized pulsatility in the venous outflow vessels. Venous enlargement is also common in AVMs, resulting from the pressurized, shunted, arterial flow into the nidus.

Muscular skeletal hemangiomas are not hemangiomas. They are venous malformations that occur in the muscle. With the correct clinical history, a properly performed magnetic resonance imaging (MRI) examination should be almost pathognomonic. Vertebral body hemangiomas are also not hemangiomas; they are venous malformations that occur in bone. Review of the literature demonstrates numerous studies showing "increased vascularity" of these lesions. However, the increased vascularity is from the venous pooling in the lesion and not from arterial hypertrophy and neovascularity. Liver hemangiomas are not hemangiomas; they are venous malformations occurring in the liver.

VASCULAR MALFORMATIONS

Vascular malformations are malformed or dysplastic embryologic spaces that are characterized by normal endothelial cell turnover and abnormal vascular anatomy characterized by the dysplastic vessels involved. All vascular malformations can be placed into one of three groups: low flow, high flow, and combined.

Low-Flow Vascular Malformations—Venous Malformations

Low-flow venous malformations are the most common form of vascular malformation; simplified, they are a number of tortuous vascular channels. They will be evident at birth and will grow with the child. These are common birthmarks present at birth, although they can be clinically occult if deep in location and usually do not become symptomatic until late childhood/early adolescence. Deep subcutaneous or intramuscular venous malformations often manifest with only local swelling and pain. The diagnosis can be difficult because extremity varicosities may be the only visible sign, especially in deep venous malformations. Superficial venous malformations can be seen with bluish-purple skin discoloration. Venous malformations can be divided into truncal and extratruncal lesions. On physical examination, these lesions are soft and easily compressible and will often demonstrate engorgement, especially when the affected extremity is placed in a dependent position. Extratruncal lesions occur from remnants of primitive vessels early in development and are usually dysplastic and diffusely infiltrative. They commonly involve the deep soft tissue structures, but patients may have constant pain. Truncal venous malformations occur in differentiated and later-stage vascular structures and patients may have an impressive cutaneous manifestation with limb swelling and varicosities. Diffuse malformations involve multiple areas or regions and are usually part of a syndrome such as Klippel-Trenaunay syndrome. Diagnosis of venous malformations can usually be made by clinical examination. However, imaging studies, such as MRI, are performed to evaluate the extent and guide treatment. On MRI, venous malformations

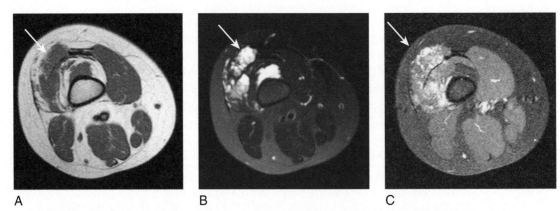

■ **Fig. 25.1** A 10-year-old boy with focal thigh swelling and pain. Axial T1-weighted (A), T2-weighted (B), and T1-weighted after gadolinium (C) images demonstrating a T1 isointense and T2 hyperintense signal and enhancement after gadolinium in a venous malformation *(arrow)* in the lateral aspect of left lower extremity.

are T1 isointense to muscle and T2 hyperintense and demonstrate late enhancement (Fig. 25.1).

Low-Flow Vascular Malformations—Lymphatic Malformations

These lesions are abnormalities of lymphatic etiology that often appear in infancy or early childhood, with more than 90% of patients presenting by age 2 years. More than 75% of these lesions are seen in the craniocervical region. Patients with these lesions usually present for treatment earlier than those with venous malformations, secondary to the cosmetic concerns of the localized mass effect or swelling caused by the lesions. Lymphatic malformations (LMs) will often fluctuate in size secondary to trauma, inflammation, or intralesional hemorrhage. Antibiotics are administered for fever or erythema. Unlike venous malformations, LMs are not usually painful. Larger LMs, however, can result in airway obstruction, speech abnormalities, and dysphagia. In the past, these lesions were called lymphangiomas or cystic hygromas. These outdated terms should no longer be used in clinical practice.

There are two subtypes of LMs: macrocystic LM and microcystic LM. Because the imaging characteristics and treatment options are different, it is important to recognize these subtypes. Macrocystic LMs appear similar to venous malformations on MRI except that they only demonstrate minimal, if any, peripheral enhancement. Macrocystic LMs are often easily accessible for sclerotherapy treatments. On the other hand, microcystic LMs are often only observed, with treatment options usually limited to surgical debulking and percutaneous management of cutaneous complications such as recurrent cellulitis or sclerotherapy treatment of bleeding superficial vesicles.

Low-Flow Vascular Malformations—Capillary Malformations

Capillary malformations (CMs) are capillary dilatations. They are characterized by ectatic papillary dermal capillaries and postcapillary venules in the upper reticular dermis and were commonly referred to as "port-wine" stains. CMs are present at birth and grow in size commensurate with the child because they have no tendency toward involution. At birth, CMs are usually pink or reddish and will usually darken with advancing age. They present as solitary lesions but can be associated with other vascular malformations. A typical worrisome location is the midline lower back region because CMs in this location may be associated with tethered spinal cord. Facial CMs may be associated with Sturge-Weber syndrome. Other conditions associated with CMs include Klippel-Trenaunay syndrome and Proteus syndrome.

High-Flow Vascular Malformations—Arteriovenous Fistulas

Arteriovenous fistulas (AVFs) are an abnormal connection between an artery and a vein. Although these high-flow lesions can be congenital, often they are acquired as the result of surgery, penetrating trauma, or erosion by adjacent disease processes. As blood follows the path of least resistance, flow in both the inflow artery and outflow vein increases. The resistance in the fistula can be low enough that the fistula tract causes a "steal phenomenon" to arterial supply distally and can actually cause a reversal of arterial flow in the distal arterial segment. This "parasitic circulation" can result in decreased arterial pressures in the distal capillary beds and cause tissue ischemia and pain. Treatment is usually from an endovascular approach, but this depends on the location of the AVF.

High-Flow Vascular Malformations—Arteriovenous Malformations

AVMs are abnormal connections between an artery and a vein that have a tortuous segment of dysplastic vessels (called the nidus) between the supplying artery or arteries and the draining vein or veins. Usually, these lesions are asymptomatic, but they can have varied symptoms, including heart failure, neuropathy, pain, or bleeding. Symptomatic, small, and superficial AVMs are occasionally treated with surgical resection; however, most AVMs are inoperable because they are large and diffuse in nature and involve important normal adjacent structures. With improvement of catheter technology, super-selective techniques, and the use of liquid embolic agents, embolotherapy has emerged as the primary mode of treatment for the management of peripheral AVMs.

YAKES ARTERIOVENOUS MALFORMATION CLASSIFICATION

The Yakes classification is a relatively new system that characterizes AVMs based on their angioarchitectures suggesting possible treatment strategies. A type I AVM is a direct arteriovenous fistula that can be occluded with mechanical devices such as coils or plugs. A type IIa AVM has multiple inflow arteries into a traditional central nidus with direct artery to arteriolar and vein to venule communication. A type IIb AVM similarly has multiple inflow arteries, which supplies a characteristic nidus that shunts into an enlarged draining vein. Type II AVM therapy should focus on sclerosing the nidus, either through the arterial inflow vessel or direct injection. A type IIIa AVM features multiple artery-to-arteriole communications into an enlarged central vein where the vein wall serves as the nidus. Its treatment includes transarterial embolization of the nidus along with possibly direct puncture and occlusion of the venous outflow vessel. A type IIIb AVM features multiple artery to arterioles communications into an enlarged central vein with multiple, usually dilated, outflow veins. Its treatment includes a strategy of transarterial embolization of the inflow as well as puncture and occlusion of the enlarged dominant venous outflow along with the occlusion of the other outflow veins with coils or plugs. A type IV AVM has multiple small arteriolar to venule communications that diffusely infiltrate tissues that should be addressed with superselective ethanol (50%) injection via direct injection or transcatheter approach.

TREATMENT OF VENOUS MALFORMATIONS

Treatment of venous malformations has improved over the past decade as a result of advances in percutaneous and transcatheter embolotherapy and sclerotherapy. Localized and diffuse venous malformations have been treated with sclerotherapy, whereas some localized lesions may be resected. Sclerotherapy can be performed with ethanol, liquid, and foam detergents. In our practice, we treat venous malformations with ethyl alcohol or sodium tetradecyl sulfate (STS) sclerotherapy. When dehydrated ethyl alcohol is used, however, the potential for serious complications is increased by an order of magnitude. Local ethanol complications are related to the transmural necrosis of the agent and spread to the surrounding tissues.

Preprocedure evaluation of a malformation with either ultrasound or MRI is helpful not only in defining the extent of the abnormality but also in aiding practitioners to determine possible direct access into the lesion (Figs. 25.2 and 25.3). Access into the malformation is usually performed with ultrasound and fluoroscopic guidance (Fig. 25.4). Biplane fluoroscopy can be used if the location of the lesion allows. Direct comparison with the magnetic resonance images can also be very helpful. Proper positioning on the angiographic table is critical to successfully access the malformation and to allow proper

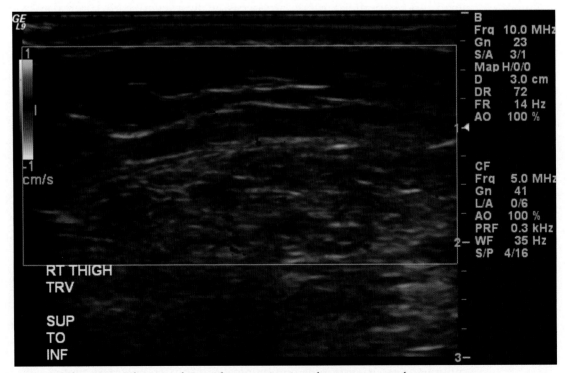

■ **Fig. 25.2** Ultrasound Doppler examination demonstrates a heterogeneous lesion with no increased flow consistent with a low-flow vascular venous malformation.

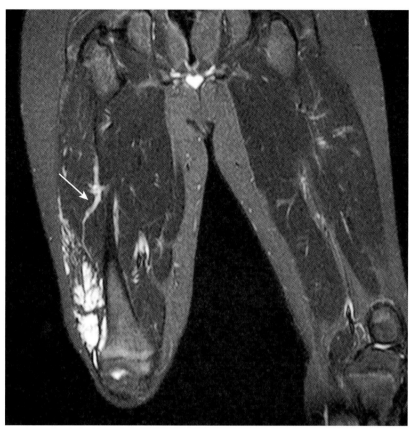

■ **Fig. 25.3** Coronal fat-saturated T1-weighted image. After the addition of gadolinium, enhancement of the dysplastic draining vein is demonstrated *(arrow)*.

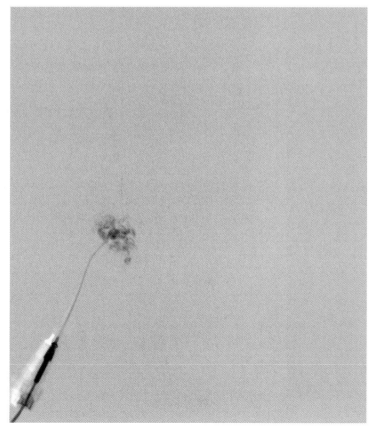

■ **Fig. 25.4** Initial venogram with dilute contrast.

anesthesia monitoring. All alcohol embolization procedures are performed with the patient under general anesthesia to allow for proper sedation and pain management, as well as to prepare should complications of treatment (such as cardiovascular collapse) occur. In addition, a tourniquet for control with a calibrated cuff can be used if the location of the lesions allows. When using a tourniquet, we do not exceed diastolic blood pressure and often only use minimal pressures in the 20 to 40 mm Hg range.

The technique for alcohol administration has evolved. Previously, dehydrated ethanol was opacified with a small amount of ethiodized oil (Ethiodol) to increase the visualization of the administered alcohol under fluoroscopic control. Currently, we use a negative contrast technique. This consists of opacification of the malformation with contrast, followed by administration of the ethyl alcohol that replaces the contrast on live fluoroscopic evaluation (Fig. 25.5). Once we have either treated the entire lesion or reached our sclerosant limits, the procedure is concluded (Fig. 25.6). The absolute maximum for ethyl alcohol is 1 mL per kg. In our practice, we rarely exceed 0.5 mL per kg in one procedure. A good working dose limit for ethyl alcohol is 0.25 mg per kg for the entire case. We also limit our total injected volume to 0.1 mL per kg per injection and allow at least 5 minutes between alcohol administrations. By adhering to these recommendations, we have completed safe treatment for many patients, without the use of pulmonary arterial catheter monitoring. Similarly, STS can be injected as a liquid or as a foam. (Fig. 25.7) The foam is more viscous and slightly easier to control. It can be applied via a transcatheter or direct puncture approach. A negative contrast technique is used during the injection (Figs. 25.8–25.10).

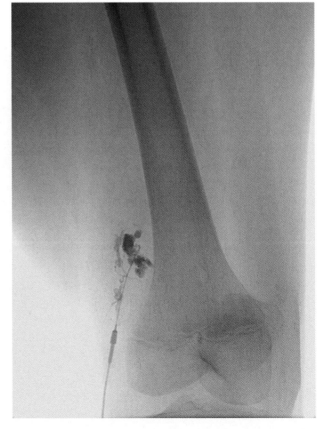

■ **Fig. 25.5** Direct puncture venography using a small angiocatheter.

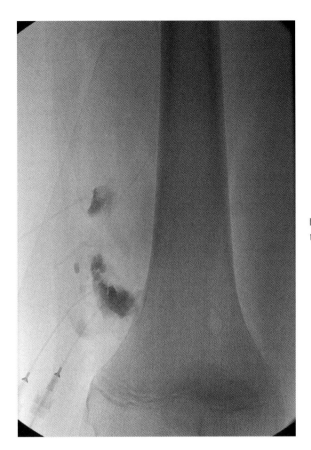

■ **Fig. 25.6** Posttreatment scout film demonstrating two separate treatment punctures.

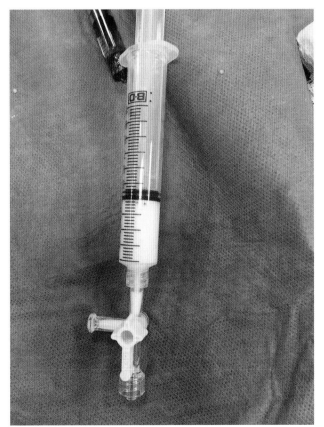

■ **Fig. 25.7** Syringe of 3 mL of 3% sodium tetradecyl sulfate used to create foam.

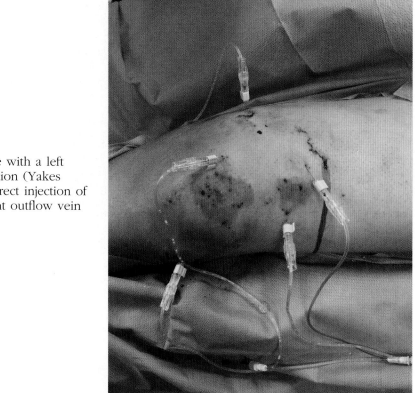

◾ **Fig. 25.8** A 22-year-old male with a left thigh painful venous malformation (Yakes IIIa). The patient underwent direct injection of the nidus vessels. The dominant outflow vein was later closed.

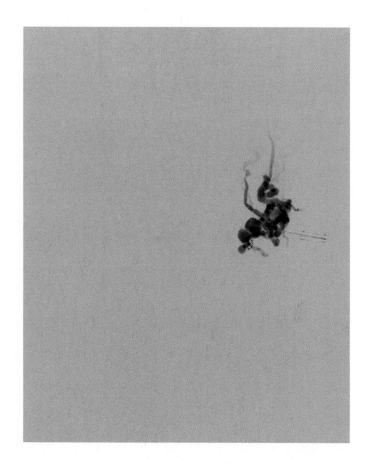

◾ **Fig. 25.9** Direct venogram demonstrating filling of the nidus vessels.

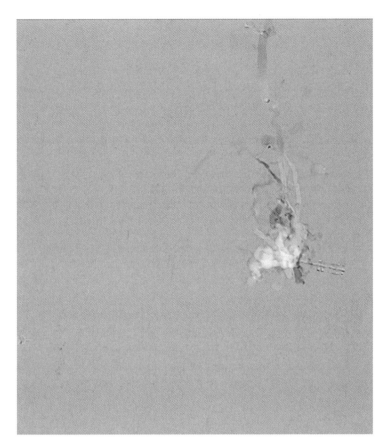

■ **Fig. 25.10** Images after the injection of sodium tetradecyl sulfate foam using negative-contrast technique.

Occasionally, a lesion can be treated in one session; however, most require several (two to four) treatments to reach our clinical endpoint of treating the pain associated with a symptomatic malformation. We do not treat asymptomatic lesions unless there is a significant cosmetic issue, which can occur with lesions on the face and neck. Treatments are usually spaced apart by 3 to 4 months to allow for postprocedural edema to resolve.

Our standard postprocedure orders include intravenous ketorolac, dexamethasone, and antibiotic coverage for the first 24 hours of treatment. Following overnight observation, patients are discharged home with an outpatient oral medication regimen of a methylprednisolone dose pack, ibuprofen therapy, and oral antibiotics.

Evaluation of the venous drainage of venous malformations is essential in their treatment. Malformations with no or limited venous drainage can be treated with embolic agents with higher effectiveness and less risk than malformations with normal draining vessels, whereas lesions with drainage into dysplastic veins or a venous ectasia can be most problematic to treat. Venous malformations may have a number of large-diameter connections to the deep venous system. It is important to control the injection to prevent the liquid embolics from entering these central veins. Burrows et al. have reported good result in 75% to 90% of their patient cohort treated with serial alcohol administration. However, many patients have chronic pain symptoms, and their clinical improvement may lag significantly behind a more technically successful treatment.

SELECTED READINGS

Al-Adnani M, Williams S, Rampling D, et al. Histopathological reporting of paediatric cutaneous vascular anomalies in relation to proposed multidisciplinary classification system. *J Clin Pathol.* 2006;59:1278–1282.

Bauman NM, Burke DK, Smith RJ. Treatment of massive or life-threatening hemangiomas with recombinant alpha (2a)-interferon. *Otolaryngol Head Neck Surg.* 1997;117:99–110.

Cho SK, Do YS, Kim DI, et al. Peripheral arteriovenous malformations with a dominant outflow vein: results of ethanol embolization. *Korean J Radiol.* 2008;9:258–267.

Merrow A, Gupta A, Patel M, et al. 2014 revised classification of vascular lesions from the international society for the study of vascular anomalies: radiologic-pathologic update. *Radiographics.* 2016;36:1494–1516.

Rosenblatt M. Endovascular management of venous malformations. *Phlebology.* 2007;22:264–275.

van der Linden E, Pattynama PMT, Heeres BC, et al. Long-term patient satisfaction after percutaneous treatment of peripheral vascular malformations. *Radiology.* 2009;251:926–932.

van Rijswijk CSP, van der Linden E, van der Woude H-J, et al. Value of dynamic contrast-enhanced MR imaging in diagnosing and classifying peripheral vascular malformations. *AJR Am J Roentgenol.* 2002;178:1181–1187.

Yakes WF. Yakes' AVM classification system. *J Vasc Interv Radiol.* 2015;26:S224.

REFERENCES

1. ISSVA Classification of Vascular Anomalies 2014 International Society for the Study of Vascular Anolamies at ISSVA.org/classification Accessed May 31, 2017.

2. Mulliken JB, Young AE. Vascular Birthmarks: Hemangiomas and Malformations. Philadelphia: WB Saunders; 1988.

3. Bittles MA, Sidhu MK, Sze RW, et al. Multidetector CT angiography of pediatric vascular malformations and hemangiomas: utility of 3-D reformatting in differential diagnosis. *Pediatr Radiol.* 2005;35:1100–1106.

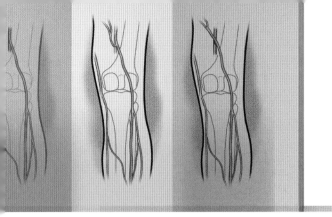

CHAPTER 26

Severity Scoring and Outcomes Measurement

Marc A. Passman

HISTORICAL BACKGROUND

The past few decades have marked a change of focus in reporting outcomes for venous disease and therapy. Although treatments were regularly being offered for many venous conditions, the outcomes were only sporadically evaluated, and reporting methods were not standardized, preventing comparison trials and confounding reported results. The realization that the language of diagnostic and treatment information needs to be universal has shifted the focus of physicians to organize information to provide a framework for clinical practice and research.[1] Reporting standards to address important elements of assessment, including clinical classification of disease, a grading system for risk factors, categorization of operations and interventions, complications encountered with grades for severity or outcomes, and criteria for improvement, deterioration, and failure has become a priority.[2] Results should be evaluated alongside other options, such as the natural course of the disease itself, nonsurgical therapies, additional surgical interventions, or alternative ways of performing an intervention.[3]

Developing and using proper venous severity and outcomes assessment tools should be paramount to those treating venous disease. The assessment of outcomes in chronic venous disease is multifactorial and is more complicated than in other vascular conditions. The end points of comparison must be objective usable measures that reflect signs, symptoms, and patient quality of life.[4] This chapter will review current venous assessment tools to determine severity of venous disease for both thrombotic and chronic venous insufficiency, which forms the core of outcome measurements used to determine quality benchmarking and comparative analysis. A general algorithm for use of these venous severity scoring systems will be recommended, highlighting the pearls and pitfalls of these outcome measurement tools.

VENOUS SEVERITY ASSESSMENT TOOLS

Venous Thromboembolism Risk Assessment—Caprini Score

Prevention of deep venous thrombosis (DVT) and pulmonary embolism (PE) is important because initial diagnosis is challenging, treatment is not always successful, long-term sequelae can include postthrombotic syndrome (PTS), and PE can cause sudden death. Using a venous thromboembolism (VTE) risk assessment will allow for more precise risk stratification of surgical and nonsurgical patients at potential risk for VTE, compared with risk of bleeding before instituting pharmacologic thromboprophylaxis prevention strategies. The Caprini score was introduced in 2005 to evaluate patient risk of developing VTE if placed into a high-risk situation (such as surgical procedure, major injury or other hospitalizations, malignancy, or prolonged immobility).[5] The Caprini score (Table 26.1) weighs out VTE risk factors with 1 to 5 points for each. The total risk factor score then is used to group patients into one of four categories (low, moderate, high, and highest risk), each of which corresponds to a recommended prophylactic regimen.[6] Practitioners should weigh in prophylactic safety against increased risks of bleeding in prophylactic decision making.

TABLE 26.1 Venous Thromboembolism Risk Assessment—Caprini Score

1 Point	2 Points	3 Points	5 Points
Age 41–60 years	Age 61–74 years	Age ≥ 75 years	Stroke (<1 month)
Minor surgery	Arthroscopic surgery	History of VTE	Elective arthroplasty
BMI ≥ 25[a]	Major open surgery (≥45 minutes)	Family history of VTE	Hip, pelvis, or leg fracture
History of major surgery (<1 month)	Laparoscopic surgery (>45 minutes)	Positive factor V Leiden	Multiple trauma (<1 month)
Varicose veins	Cancer (past or present)	Positive prothrombin 20210A	Acute spinal cord injury (<1 month)
Swollen legs	Patient confined to bed (>72 hours)	Elevated serum homocysteine	
Acute myocardial infarction	Immobilizing plaster cast (<1 month)	Positive lupus anticoagulant	
Congestive heart failure (<1 month	Central venous access	Elevated anticardiolipin antibodies	
Sepsis (<1 month)		Heparin-induced thrombocytopenia	
Serious lung disease, such as pneumonia (<1 month)		Other congenital or acquired thrombophilia	
Chronic obstructive pulmonary disease			
Medical patient on bed rest			

Recommended Prophylactic Strategy Based on Caprini Thrombosis Risk Factor Assessment Score[b]

Number of Risk Factors	Risk Category	Recommended Regimen
1	Low	Early ambulation plus elastic compression stockings
2–4	Moderate	Early ambulation plus elastic compression stockings plus sequential compression device anticoagulant
>4	High	Early ambulation plus elastic compression stockings plus sequential compression device plus LMWH, heparin, or warfarin

BMI, Body mass index; *LMWH,* low-molecular-weight heparin; *VTE,* venous thromboembolism.
[a]From Caprini JA. Thrombosis risk assessment as a guide to quality patient care. *Dis Mon.* 2005;52:70–78.
[b]From Caprini JA. Risk assessment as a guide for the prevention of the many faces of venous thromboembolism. *Am J Surg* 2010;S3–10.

Postthrombotic Syndrome—Villalta Score

The Villalta scale (Table 26.2) was proposed in the 1990s as a clinical scale to diagnose and classify the severity of PTS.[7] Based on a cross-sectional study of patients with documented DVT, the scale consists of five patient-rated venous symptoms (pain, cramps, heaviness, paresthesia, pruritus) and six clinician-rated physical signs (pretibial edema, skin induration, hyperpigmentation, pain during calf compression, venous ectasia, redness), which are each rated on a 4-point scale (0 = none, 1 = mild, 2 = moderate, 3 = severe). Points are summed to produce a total score (range, 0–33). Subjects are classified as having PTS if the score is 5 or more, or if a venous ulcer is present in a leg with previous DVT. The severity of PTS is categorized as mild/moderate if the score is 5 to 14, and as severe if the score is 15 or greater, or if a venous ulcer was present, regardless of the total score. In recent studies, the mild/moderate category has been subcategorized as mild if the score is 5 to 9 and moderate if the score is 10 to 14. Although several PTS scoring systems have been described, the Villalta score has been validated and has been shown to be reliable and reproducible.[8]

TABLE 26.2 Villalta Scale for Postthrombotic Syndrome

Symptoms/Clinical Signs	None	Mild	Moderate	Severe
Symptoms				
Pain	0 points	1 point	2 points	3 points
Cramps	0 points	1 point	2 points	3 points
Heaviness	0 points	1 point	2 points	3 points
Paresthesia	0 points	1 point	2 points	3 points
Pruritus	0 points	1 point	2 points	3 points
Clinical Signs				
Pretibial edema	0 points	1 point	2 points	3 points
Skin induration	0 points	1 point	2 points	3 points
Hyperpigmentation	0 points	1 point	2 points	3 points
Redness	0 points	1 point	2 points	3 points
Venous ectasia	0 points	1 point	2 points	3 points
Pain on calf compression	0 points	1 point	2 points	3 points
Venous ulcer	Absent			Present

Mild: score 5–9
Moderate: score 10–14
Severe: score > 15
From Villalta S, Bagatella P, Piccioli A, et al. Assessment of validity and reproducibility of a clinical scale for the post-thrombotic syndrome (abstract). *Haemostasis.* 1994;24:158a.

Clinical, Etiologic, Anatomic, Pathophysiologic Classification

The clinical, etiologic, anatomic, pathophysiologic (CEAP) classification (Table 26.3), developed in 1994 and modified in 2004, is a widely used reporting standard as a common descriptive platform for the reporting of diagnostic information in chronic venous disease.[9] The clinical component is scored for active disease severity from 0 (none) to 6 (active ulcers). The etiology section categorizes the venous disease as congenital, primary, or secondary. The anatomic classification identifies affected veins as superficial, deep, or perforating. The pathophysiologic section details the presence or absence of reflux in the superficial, communicating, or deep veins and any incidence of outflow obstruction. The basic CEAP classification is a simplified version of the more comprehensive CEAP and is recommended for clinical practice, with the more comprehensive CEAP reserved for research purposes. Although an excellent descriptive tool, the revised CEAP classification is static and is limited in its ability to reflect response to treatment, especially in the C5 to C6 categories. This limitation is most evident if the CEAP classification is used as a standalone instrument. Despite this shortcoming, there has been general acceptance and wide dissemination of CEAP for both clinical and research purposes, making CEAP an essential component of venous disease classification.

TABLE 26.3 Clinical, Etiologic, Anatomic, Pathophysiologic Classification

Clinical Classification

C_0: no visible or palpable signs of venous disease

C_1: telangiectasic or reticular veins

C_2: varicose wins

C_3: edema

C_{4a}: pigmentation or eczema

C_{4b}: lipodermatosclerosis or atrophic blanche

C_5: healed venous ulcer

C_6: active venous ulcer

S: symptomatic, including ache, pain, tightness, skin irritation, heaviness, and muscle cramps, and other complaints attributable to venous dysfunction

A: asymptomatic

Etiologic Classification

Ec: congenital

Ep: primary

Es: secondary (postthrombotic)

En: no venous cause identified

Continued

TABLE 26.3 Clinical, Etiologic, Anatomic, Pathophysiologic Classification—cont'd

Anatomic Classification

    As: superficial veins

    Ap: perforator veins

    Ad: deep veins

    An: no venous location identified

Pathophysiologic Classification

Basic CEAP

    Pr: *reflux*

    Po: obstruction

    Pr,o: reflux and obstruction

    Pn: no venous pathophysiology identifiable

    Advanced CEAP: same as basic CEAP, with addition that any of *18* named venous segments can be used as locators for venous pathology

Superficial Veins

    Telangiectasic or reticular veins

    Great saphenous vein above knee

    Great saphenous vein below knee

    Small saphenous vein

    Nonsaphenous veins

Deep Veins

    Inferior vena cava

    Common iliac vein

    Internal iliac vein

    External iliac vein

    Pelvic: gonadal, broad ligament veins, other

    Common femoral vein

    Deep femoral vein

    Femoral vein

    Popliteal vein

    Crural: anterior tibial, posterior tibial, peroneal veins (all paired)

    Muscular: gastrocnemial, soleal veins, other

Perforating Veins

    Thigh

    Calf

CEAP, Clinical, etiologic, anatomic, pathophysiologic.
From Rutherford RB, Bergan JJ, Carpentier PH, et al. Revision of the CEAP classification for chronic venous disorders: consensus statement. *J Vasc Surg.* 2004;40:1248–1452.

Revised Venous Clinical Severity Scoring

The Venous Clinical Severity Scoring (VCSS) was designed in 2000 and revised in 2010 to include nine recognized features of venous disease with each scored from 0 to 3 based on severity[10] (Table 26.4). The revised VCSS included updated terminology, clarified application, and combined important language to reflect severity changes across the spectrum of symptomatic venous disease. The feature that sets the revised VCSS apart from other physician-assessed instruments is its ability to reflect status changes in response to therapy, owing to the nature of the categories, which are broken down into elemental aspects of venous disease. The clinical descriptors include vein size and location, the use of compression therapy, skin changes (including pigmentation, inflammation, induration, and ulcers), and edema and its distribution as noted by the patient at different points in the day; pain is identified as aching, heaviness, fatigue, soreness, and burning.

VCSS has proven to be a valuable measure of objective and subjective outcomes in treating chronic venous disease. Others have evaluated the VCSS in large populations, finding it generally useful. Some deficiencies have been noted, including the scope of the clinical descriptors used. Because a large part of the VCSS depends on patient responses to physician queries, the ability to interpret the description of symptoms and to match them to a category in the VCSS is crucial in generating accurate data. The VCSS is generated by the clinician based on straightforward questions asked of the patient during examination. Several categories, including inflammation, induration, pigmentation, ulcers, and veins, are objective and are scored by the physician based on clinical evidence. At the same time, other categories, including pain, edema, and the use of compression are scored based on the subjective responses of the patient. The range of categories covered by the VCSS is representative of chronic venous disease and compiles a more complete picture of quality of life than specialized instruments.

The revised VCSS has retained sensitivity, while better identifying issues of patients with milder venous disease. One of the advantages of the revised VCSS is its ability to provide visual scoring data in chronic venous insufficiency. With the use of revised clinical descriptors, patient-reported symptoms can be combined with physician assessment to more accurately translate the picture of venous disease. This has helped bridge the gap between physician-scored assessment instruments and patient-reported tools and to transport surveys further into the land of science with standardized language, reliability, and validity. A revised VCSS of 8 or higher indicates a patient with severe disease at risk for progression and may warrant additional diagnostics or treatment.

Patient-Reported Outcome Tools

Physician-generated assessment instruments provide another perspective on the management of venous disease and are valuable tools in determining the level of disease and the efficacy of treatment. A patient-reported outcome is any report of patient health condition made by the patient and reported, without physician interpretation. Such an instrument can be used during the diagnostic phase to measure symptoms or disease states and following therapy to evaluate changes and treatment effect. The US Food and Drug Administration recommends the use of a patient-reported outcome (PRO) instrument when the element being measured is best known and expressed by the patient.[11]

TABLE 26.4 Revised Venous Clinical Severity Score

	None: 0	Mild: 1	Moderate: 2	Severe: 3
Pain or other discomfort (i.e., aching, heaviness, fatigue, soreness, burning) presumes venous origin		Occasional pain or other discomfort (i.e., not restricting regular daily activity)	Daily pain or other discomfort (i.e., interfering with but not preventing regular daily activities)	Daily pain or discomfort (i.e., limits most regular daily activities)
Varicose veins must be ≥3 mm in diameter to qualify in the standing position		Few: scattered (i.e., isolated branch varicosities or clusters); also includes corona phlebectatica (ankle flare)	Confined to calf or thigh	Involves calf and thigh
Venous edema presumes venous origin		Limited to foot and ankle area	Extends above ankle but below knee	Extends to knee and above
Skin pigmentation presumes venous origin, but does not include focal pigmentation over varicose veins or pigmentation caused by other chronic diseases (e.g., vasculitis purpura)	None or focal	Limited to perimalleolar area	Diffuse over lower third of calf	Wider distribution above lower third of calf
Inflammation should be more than just recent pigmentation (e.g., erythema, cellulitis, venous eczema, dermatitis)		Limited to perimalleolar area	Diffuse over lower third of calf	Wider distribution above lower third of calf
Induration presumes venous origin of secondary skin and subcutaneous changes (i.e., chronic edema with fibrosis, hypodermitis) Includes white atrophy and lipodermatosclerosis		Limited to perimalleolar area	Diffuse over lower third of calf	Wider distribution above lower third of calf
Active ulcer number	0	1	2	≥3
Active ulcer duration (longest active)	N/A	<3 months	>3 months but <1 year	Not healed for >1 year
Active ulcer size (largest active)	N/A	Diameter < 2 cm	Diameter 2–6 cm	Diameter > 6 cm
Use of compression therapy	0 Not used	1 Intermittent use of stockings	2 Wears stockings most days	3 Full compliance: stockings

Instructions for Using the Revised Venous Clinical Severity Score

On a separate form, the clinician will be asked:

"For each leg, please check 1 box for each item (symptom and sign) that is listed below."

Pain or Other Discomfort (i.e., Aching, Heaviness, Fatigue, Soreness, Burning)

The clinician describes the four categories of leg pain or discomfort that are outlined later to the patient and asks the patient to choose, separately for each leg, the category that best describes the pain or discomfort the patient experiences.

TABLE 26.4 Revised Venous Clinical Severity Score—cont'd

None = 0: None

Mild = 1: Occasional pain or discomfort that does not restrict regular daily

Moderate = 2: Daily pain or discomfort that interferes with, but does not prevent, regular daily activities

Severe = 3: Daily pain or discomfort that limits most regular daily activities

Varicose Veins

The clinician examines the patient's legs and, separately for each leg, chooses the category that best describes the patient's superficial veins. The standing position is used for varicose vein assessment. Veins must be ≥3 mm in diameter to qualify as varicose veins.

None = 0: None

Mild = 1: Few, scattered varicosities that are confined to branch veins or clusters. Includes corona phlebectatica (ankle flare), defined as >5 blue telangiectases at the inner or sometimes the outer edge of the foot

Moderate = 2: Multiple varicosities that are confined to the calf or the thigh

Severe = 3: Multiple varicosities that involve both the calf and the thigh

Venous Edema

The clinician examines the patient's legs and, separately for each leg, chooses the category that best describes the patient's pattern of leg edema. The clinician's examination may be supplemented by asking the patient about the extent of leg edema that is experienced.

None = 0: None

Mild = 1: Edema that is limited to the foot and ankle

Moderate = 2: Edema that extends above the ankle but below the knee

Severe = 3: Edema that extends to the knee or above

Skin Pigmentation

The clinician examines the patient's legs and, separately for each leg, chooses the category that best describes the patient's skin pigmentation. Pigmentation refers to color changes of venous origin and not secondary to other chronic diseases (i.e., vasculitis purpura).

None = 0: None or focal pigmentation that is confined to the skin over varicose veins

Mild = 1: Pigmentation that is limited to the perimalleolar area

Moderate = 2: Diffuse pigmentation that involves the lower third of the calf

Severe = 3: Diffuse pigmentation that involves more than the lower third of the calf

Inflammation

The clinician examines the patient's legs and, separately for each leg, chooses the category that best describes the patient's skin inflammation. Inflammation refers to erythema, cellulitis, venous eczema, or dermatitis, rather than just recent pigmentation.

None = 0: None

Mild = 1: Inflammation that is limited to the perimalleolar area

Moderate = 2: Inflammation that involves the lower third of the calf

Severe = 3: Inflammation that involves more than the lower third of the calf

Induration

The clinician examines the patient's legs and, separately for each leg, chooses the category that best describes the patient's skin induration. Induration refers to skin and subcutaneous changes such as chronic edema with fibrosis, hypodermitis, white atrophy, and lipodermatosclerosis.

None = 0: None

Mild = 1: Induration that is limited to the perimalleolar area

Continued

TABLE 26.4 Revised Venous Clinical Severity Score—cont'd

Moderate = 2: Induration that involves the lower third of the calf

Severe = 3: Induration that involves more than the lower third of the calf

Active Ulcer Number

The clinician examines the patient's legs and, separately for each leg, chooses the category that best describes the number of active ulcers.

None = 0: None

Mild = 1: 1 ulcer

Moderate = 2: 2 ulcers

Severe = 3: ≥3 ulcers

Active Ulcer Duration

If there is at least one active ulcer, the clinician describes the four categories of ulcer duration that are outlined later to the patient and asks the patient to choose, separately for each leg, the category that best describes the duration of the longest unhealed ulcer.

None = 0: No active ulcers

Mild = 1: Ulceration present for <3 months

Moderate = 2: Ulceration present for 3–12 months

Severe = 3: Ulceration present for >12 months

Active Ulcer Size

If there is at least one active ulcer, the clinician examines the patient's legs, and separately for each leg, chooses the category that best describes the size of the largest active ulcer.

None = 0: No active ulcer

Mild = 1: Ulcer < 2 cm in diameter

Moderate = 2: Ulcer 2–6 cm in diameter

Severe = 3: Ulcer > 6 cm in diameter

Use of Compression Therapy

Choose the level of compliance with medical compression therapy.

None = 0: Not used

Mild = 1: Intermittent use

Moderate = 2: Wears stockings most days

Severe = 3: Full compliance: stockings

Patient-reported, disease-specific instruments have been used extensively in reporting chronic venous disease and therapy and have increased sensitivity to the element being measured because of their focus on particular disease processes and treatments. These patient-reported, venous disease-specific surveys provide valuable information on the individual effect of venous disease. Understanding the elements that compel patients to seek treatment is important in planning therapy that will address their main concerns.

The 36-Item Short Form Health Survey (SF-36) is a generic, patient-reported, quality-of-life survey designed to assess physical health (the patient's level of functioning) and mental health (an indication of well-being) by breaking these categories into eight domains: physical and social functioning, role limitations because of physical or emotional problems, mental health, pain, vitality, and perception of health.[12,13] This survey has been widely used and validated in large population based venous studies.

The Chronic Venous Insufficiency Questionnaire (CIVIQ) has had two versions. The first version, was developed originally in French in 1994 and was subsequently validated in English.[14,15] The survey evaluated physical, psychologic, social, and pain effects. Different numbers of questions were asked in each category, rendering the instrument difficult to score. A revised version, CIVIQ 20, equally distributed the effects across 20 questions ranked 1 to 5 in severity (1 = no pain/not bothered at all; 5 = intense pain/impossible to do) with responses then categorized for composite score. Both versions of the CIVIQ have been used and validated.

The Venous Insufficiency Epidemiological and Economic Study (VEINES) instrument consists of 35 items in two categories to generate two summary scores, one for quality of life and another for symptoms.[16] The quality-of-life survey has 25 items that estimate the effect of disease on quality of life, and the symptom survey has 10 items that measure symptoms. The focus is on physical manifestations rather than psychologic and social elements. Because the score is divided into categories of symptoms and disease effect, this makes the VEINES instrument useful for many clinical applications. The VEINES has been validated in multiple languages.

The Aberdeen Varicose Vein Questionnaire is a 13-question survey developed in the 1990s addressing all elements of varicose vein disease.[17] Examined are physical and social issues (including pain, ankle edema, ulcers, and the use of compression therapy) as well as the effect of varicose veins on daily life and as a result of cosmetic issues. It is scored from 0 (no effect) to 100 (maximum effect). Specifically addressing the effect of varicose veins on quality of life, including cosmetic impact, this questionnaire was designed to improve the sensitivity of response among all patients, even those with less severe physical symptoms. This survey has been validated and used for all types of venous disease.[18]

The Charing Cross Venous Ulceration Questionnaire was developed and validated in 2000 to provide a quality-of-life measure for patients with venous ulcers. Before the existence of this instrument, there was no standardized measure of the effects of treatment for venous ulcers. The survey contains 20 questions scored from 0 (no effect) to 5 (maximum effect). The instrument is scored from the sum of these individual question scores. It has been validated and used in patients with ulcers.[19]

The Specific Quality of Life and Outcome Response–Venous (SQOR-V) survey was initially validated in French in 2007 and subsequently translated to English in 2010. It differs from the other patient-reported surveys in its focus on the relationship between the patient's primary complaint and his or her venous disease. It groups questions regarding symptoms, cosmesis, effect on activities and habits, and concern about the health implications of venous disease. Most of its 15 questions are broken into specific subcategories to elucidate thorough information about each aspect of the patient's concerns.[20]

PEARLS AND PITFALLS

- Chronic venous disease is a complex condition with numerous possible presentations and manifestations. Diagnosis is not always straightforward, generally requiring the application of clinical experience and diagnostic testing. Recently, physician-based and patient-based survey instruments have been used to assess and quantify the disease. Although these surveys are not in themselves diagnostic, they may provide valuable information about the most beneficial therapeutic direction to take.
- Although physician-reported and patient-reported tools provide useful information on symptoms and sequelae, the primary difference between them is perspective. It has

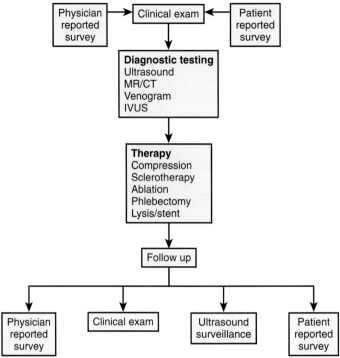

■ **Fig. 26.1** Algorithm for decision making and outcomes assessment in chronic venous disease. The initial clinical examination determines the appropriate diagnostic studies. Patient-generated and physician-generated assessment tools are administered as part of the decision-making process to help determine the therapy option that will address the most relevant concerns of physician and patient. In the follow-up period, routine ultrasound surveillance and clinical examination confirm the outcome of the procedure, whereas serial use of patient-generated and physician generated surveys follow clinical improvement and progress of patient concerns. *CT,* Computed tomography; *IVUS,* intravenous ultrasound; *MR,* magnetic resonance.

become evident that some combination of both types of instruments will provide the most comprehensive understanding of common elements. As shown in Fig. 26.1, this concept combines the more scientific, evidence-based approach of the physician instrument and the focus in the patient-reported assessment on disease elements that are of primary importance to the patient.[21–23]

- Although prevention strategies for VTE have been designed, the risk/benefit relationship of the instituting pharmacologic prevention varies when considered at the risk-profile level of the individual patient. Individualized VTE risk stratification, where patient-level factors are used to predict VTE risk, is a more precise approach especially given the large variation in VTE risk among the overall hospitalized patient population, targeted pharmacologic thromboprophylaxis strategies based on VTE risk assessment using the Caprini score can better optimize this risk/benefit relationship. A more precise approach to VTE risk stratification using Caprini scores may identify patients who will differentially benefit from pharmacologic thromboprophylaxis, compared with risk of bleeding when pharmacoprophylaxis is provided.

- For PTS, the Villalta score has been shown to have the highest degree of validation, excellent interobserver reliability, association with ambulatory venous pressures, correlation with severity of PTS, and ability to assess change in condition over time. The Villalta score should be used in all patients with prior documented DVT to determine diagnosis, severity, and treatment outcomes of PTS, with the consensus recommendation to combine Villalta with CEAP and VCSS for more accurate diagnosis of PTS.

● The course of outcomes assessment thus far has offered two choices for the type of assessment performed: physician assessed and patient reported. The data derived from physician-assessed instruments may not always be an indication of the effect of disease or the value to the patient of the changes following treatment, even seemingly slight improvements.[24] However, valuable data can be generated much more readily with little burden to the clinician. Input of these data into available online registries in the United States and in Europe is important to ensure that new therapies meet high standards of safety and reliability, and that they address the variables considered important to the physician and the patient.[25]

● A combination of clinical examination, duplex Doppler study, CEAP, and the revised VCSS is used to diagnose chronic venous disease and to plan therapeutic intervention. Any of these elements on its own would most likely provide insufficient information to plan a treatment strategy. By integrating these components, a more complete picture is obtained of the clinical severity of the venous disease and the elements most important to the patient. This multilevel strategy helps to guide therapy to achieve a successful outcome for the patient.

● Regardless of the instrument or approach chosen, the way the data are interpreted and reported is important in evaluating the effect of treatment. It is a long and exacting process for a survey tool to become a valid standardized reporting practice and eventually to evolve into a comprehensive measure of results that is widely accepted in clinical practice and research. Such surveys must be carefully chosen to address specific elements of the disease state in question. A generic measure such as the SF-36 may not address the specific elements of venous disease that are important to the clinician and patient, whereas an ulcer-specific survey such as the Charing Cross Venous Ulceration Questionnaire may not reflect the severity of other elements of venous disease. It is more relevant to have assessment instruments that are based on the specific language of venous disease. A carefully designed and chosen survey can initially aid in diagnosis and treatment planning. If it is serially applied throughout the treatment process, it can add valuable data on outcomes. When analyzed for a significant relevant population, these outcomes data add to the combined body of knowledge and clinical experience, providing evidence for the best practice treatment of chronic venous disease.

● Holding assessment instruments to the standard of psychometric analysis ensures the value of tests and their results. Psychometric standards have been used for years to apply standard practices to the development of tests in education, personality analysis, and skill assessment. The benchmarks for a good test are feasibility (whether the test is practical to administer and score), reliability (whether a score can be replicated when the same tester readministers the test), and validity (whether the scores are responsive to change).[26] Several generic and disease-specific instruments have been validated psychometrically. The physical and mental health summary measures of the SF-36 are based on the use of psychometric tests, and the instrument itself has been validated in large populations.[27] The VEINES instrument has been psychometrically tested in the areas of diagnostic elements (exclusion of classification of anatomic and physiologic variables that might aid choice of treatment) and outcomes scores (whether they could be scaled and if they accurately delineate clinical significance and degree of change over time).[28] The CIVIQ evaluates physical, psychologic, social, and pain dimensions and has been validated in large investigations. The Aberdeen Varicose Vein Questionnaire also measures physical symptoms and social issues but is specific to varicose veins. It has been used with the SF-36 and the VCSS in large studies to assess quality of life at specific intervals following intervention. The Charing Cross Venous Ulceration Questionnaire is specific to ulcers and has been used with the SF-36 to measure quality of life in patients with ulcers.

● The selection of outcomes variables to study and report is crucial. Clinical outcomes measure improvement in survival, symptoms, or quality of life as a result of therapy. Surrogate outcomes include diagnostic test results, physical signs, or physiologic variables. Examples include vein occlusion rates following ablation or venous stent patency rates. These often provide quantifiable results during a limited follow-up period. However, it is important to note that surrogate outcomes should not be held to the same standards as clinical outcomes. Although the change in response to treatment should still be predictive of benefit to the patient, the relationship between the two outcomes should be clear and well defined. Surrogate outcomes should not simply be correlated with clinical outcomes but should be predictive.

COMPARATIVE EFFECTIVENESS OF EXISTING TREATMENTS

For prevention of VTE in hospitalized patients, use of routine pharmacologic thrombo-prophylaxis compared with strategies that use VTE risk stratification and selective prevention carry different risk/benefit profiles.[29] For surgical patients who carry an unfavorable risk/benefit relationship between VTE and bleeding, precise strategies may be more favorable. A meta-analysis showed that individualized risk stratification using a Caprini score can identify a 14-fold variation in VTE risk among a larger group of surgical patients. Patients with Caprini scores of 7 to 8 and 8 or more have a demonstrable and significant VTE risk reduction when pharmacologic thromboprophylaxis is provided, without significant increase in bleeding.[30] Patients with Caprini scores of 6 or less, which includes approximately 75% of surgical patients, have an unfavorable or unknown risk/benefit relationship. Routine provision of pharmacologic thromboprophylaxis may be unnecessary for these patients thereby avoiding additional bleeding risk.

In patients with DVT, the principal factor influencing long-term quality of life and functional status is whether or not a patient develops PTS. The Villalta scale is a clinical scale to diagnose and classify the severity of PTS. In published studies that have provided data on the measurement properties of the Villalta scale, data are consistent in supporting that the Villalta scale is a reliable, valid, acceptable, and responsive measure of PTS in patients with previous documented DVT. Aspects of the Villalta scale that merit further evaluation include test–retest reliability, more detailed assessment of ulcer severity, and assessment of responsiveness across the full range of PTS severity.[31]

For chronic venous disease assessment, the basic CEAP classification is a simplified version of the more comprehensive CEAP and is recommended for clinical practice, with the more comprehensive CEAP reserved for research purposes. Whereas the CEAP classification system is useful for classifying stages of venous disease, its components have been recognized to be relatively static and insufficient for determining changes in venous disease severity. For example, a patient presenting with an active venous leg ulcer will be clinical CEAP C6 but when the ulcer heals, can improve at best only to clinical CEAP C5. Despite this shortcoming, there has been general acceptance and wide dissemination of CEAP for both clinical and research purposes, making CEAP an essential component of venous disease classification and comparative effectiveness.

For chronic venous insufficiency, the advantage of severity assessment tools, such as the revised VCSS can be illustrated in several clinical scenarios. For example, refractory unilateral leg swelling can be the result of many factors, including compromise of the muscle pump, venous outflow obstruction, or reflux of the deep, superficial, or perforator systems.[32] In conjunction with clinical examination and appropriate testing, the revised VCSS can help to track changes associated with therapy. Unilateral leg swelling that remains after initial treatment can be further evaluated to rule out other causes and to guide future interventions. Another example is chronic venous insufficiency without varicose veins, which can be difficult to discern on initial examination. The use of a survey such as the revised VCSS can help to elucidate patient symptoms consistent with underlying venous insufficiency and to guide the rest of the diagnostic process (Fig. 26.2). Finally, venous ulcers resulting from complex venous insufficiency at multiple levels can be difficult to manage, even with a staged approach to treatment. The revised VCSS can track changes with each therapeutic intervention and provide specific information on the ulcers, including number, size, and duration. This helps to maintain a record of the progress of ulcer healing over time (Figs. 26.3 and 26.4).[33]

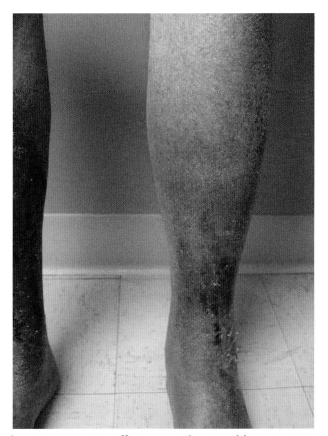

■ **Fig. 26.2** Chronic venous insufficiency without visible varicosities. Use of the Venous Clinical Severity Scoring system allowed patient symptoms to be followed and helped guide diagnostic decision making.

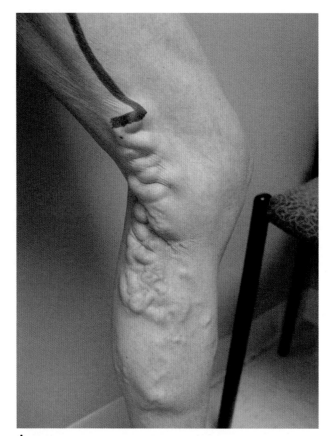

A

B

■ **Fig. 26.3** The language of revised Venous Clinical Severity Scoring (VCSS). Simplified clinician scoring and reporting allows for a common language of venous disease. (A) Pretreatment score, clinical, etiologic, anatomi, pathophysiologic (CEAP) 3—VCSS 8. (B) Posttreatment score, CEAP 3—VCSS 4.

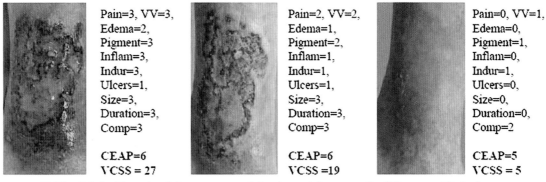

Pain=3, VV=3,
Edema=2,
Pigment=3
Inflam=3,
Indur=3,
Ulcers=1,
Size=3,
Duration=3,
Comp=3

CEAP=6
VCSS = 27

Pain=2, VV=2,
Edema=1,
Pigment=2,
Inflam=1,
Indur=1,
Ulcers=1,
Size=3,
Duration=3,
Comp=3

CEAP=6
VCSS =19

Pain=0, VV=1,
Edema=0,
Pigment=1,
Inflam=0,
Indur=1,
Ulcers=0,
Size=0,
Duration=0,
Comp=2

CEAP=5
VCSS = 5

■ **Fig. 26.4** The physician-generated "universal language" of Venous Clinical Severity Scoring and clinical, etiologic, anatomi, pathophysiologic scoring chronic venous disease. The same patient changes from C6–V27 to C6–V19 at last C5–V5.

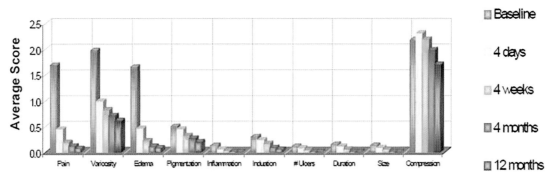

■ **Fig. 26.5** Average score for Venous Clinical Severity Scoring components over time. *(From Vasquez MA, Wang J, Mahathanaruk M, et al. The utility of the Venous Clinical Severity Score in 682 limbs treated by radiofrequency saphenous vein ablation.* J Vasc Surg. *2007;45:1008–1015.)*

Evidence-based medicine and outcomes assessment are critical tools for vascular surgery. The results of high-volume procedures should be followed up with a validated instrument. VCSS and each of its components is useful, significant, and easily applicable for the assessment of outcomes after endovenous ablation in limbs with symptomatic venous insufficiency[34] (Fig. 26.5). Modern surgical methods for treatment of chronic venous disease include superficial endovenous ablation, deep venous reconstruction, injection of sclerosing foam, percutaneous ablation of perforator veins, and iliac venous stenting. The use of physician-reported and patient-reported outcomes assessment instruments has been used effectively to determine long-term efficacy. Current clinical practice guidelines recommend that all patients with chronic venous disease be classified based on venous disease classification assessment that includes Caprini score for VTE risk assessment, Villalta score to assess PTS, CEAP, VCSS, and venous disease specific, patient-reported quality of life tools for all patients.[35,36]

ACKNOWLEDGMENT

The author gratefully acknowledges the contributions of the previous edition authors, Michael A. Vasquez and Carolyn E. Munschauer.

REFERENCES

1. Vasquez MA, Munschauer CE. The importance of uniform venous terminology in reports on varicose veins. *Semin Vasc Surg.* 2010;23:70–77.
2. Dayal R, Kent KC. Standardized reporting practices. In: Rutherford RB, ed. Vascular Surgery. 6th ed. Philadelphia: WB Saunders; 2005:41–52.
3. Rutherford RB. Presidential address: vascular surgery: comparing outcomes. *J Vasc Surg.* 1996;23:5–17.
4. Rutherford RB, Moneta GL, Padberg FT, et al. Outcome assessment in chronic venous disease. In: Gloviczki P, ed. Handbook of Venous Disorders. London: Hodder Arnold; 2009:684–693.
5. Caprini JA. Thrombosis risk assessment as a guide to quality patient care. *Dis Mon.* 2005;52:70–78.
6. Caprini JA. Risk assessment as a guide for the prevention of the many faces of venous thromboembolism. *Am J Surg.* 2010;199:S3–S10.
7. Villalta S, Bagatella P, Piccioli A, et al. Assessment of validity and reproducibility of a clinical scale for the post-thrombotic syndrome (abstract). *Haemostasis.* 1994;24:158a.
8. Kahn SR. Measurement properties of the Villalta scale to define and classify the severity of the post-thrombotic syndrome. *J Thromb Haemost.* 2009;7:884–888.
9. Rutherford RB, Bergan JJ, Carpentier PH, et al. Revision of the CEAP classification for chronic venous disorders: consensus statement. *J Vasc Surg.* 2004;40:1248–1252.
10. Vasquez MA, Rabe E, McLafferty RB, et al. Revision of the Venous Clinical Severity Score: venous outcomes consensus statement: special communication of the American Venous Forum Ad Hoc Outcomes Working Group. *J Vasc Surg.* 2010;52:1387–1396.
11. US Department of Health and Human Services. Guidance for Industry: Patient-Reported Outcome Measures: Use in Medical Product Development to Support Labeling Claims. Rockville, MD: Food and Drug Administration; December 2009.
12. Baker DM, Turnbull NB, Pearson JC, et al. How successful is varicose vein surgery? A patient outcome study following varicose vein surgery using the SF-36 Health Assessment Questionnaire. *Eur J Vasc Endovasc Surg.* 1995;9:299–304.
13. Garratt AM, Ruta DA, Abdalla MI, et al. SF 36 health survey questionnaire: II. Responsiveness to changes in health status in four common clinical conditions. *Qual Health Care.* 1994;3: 186–192.
14. Launois R, Reboul-Marty J, Henry B. Construction and validation of a quality of life questionnaire in chronic lower limb venous insufficiency (CIVIQ). *Qual Life Res.* 1996;5:539–554.
15. Jantet G. Chronic venous insufficiency: worldwide results of the RELIEF study: reflux assessment and quality of life improvement with micronized flavonoids. *Angiology.* 2002;53: 245–256.
16. Lamping DL, Schroter S, Kurz X, et al. Evaluation of outcomes in chronic venous disorders of the leg: development of a scientifically rigorous, patient-reported measure of symptoms and quality of life. *J Vasc Surg.* 2003;37(2):410–419.
17. Smith JJ, Garatt AM, Guest M, et al. Evaluating and improving health-related quality of life in pateints with varicose veins. *J Vas Surg.* 1999;30(4):710–719.
18. Garratt AM, Macdonald LM, Ruta DA, et al. Towards measurement of outcome for patients with varicose veins. *Qual Health Care.* 1993;2:5–10.
19. Smith JJ, Guest MG, Greenhalgh RM, et al. Measuring the quality of life in patients with venous ulcers. *J Vasc Surg.* 2000;31:642–649.
20. Guex JJ, Zimmet SE, Boussetta S, et al. Construction and validation of a patient-reported outcome dedicated to chronic venous disorders: SQOR-V (Specific Quality of Life and Outcome Response–Venous). *J Mal Vas.* 2007;32:135–147.
21. Meissner MH, Natiello C, Nicholls SC. Performance characteristics of the Venous Clinical Severity Score. *J Vasc Surg.* 2002;36:889–895.
22. Kundu S, Lurie F, Millward SF, et al. Recommended reporting standards for endovenous ablation for the treatment of venous insufficiency: joint statement of the American Venous Forum and the Society of Interventional Radiology. *J Vasc Surg.* 2007;46:582–589.

23. White JV. Proper outcomes assessment: patient based and economic evaluations of vascular interventions. In: Rutherford RB, ed. *Vascular Surgery*. 6th ed. Philadelphia: WB Saunders; 2005:35–41.

24. Lamping DL, Schroter S, Kurz X, et al. Evaluation of outcomes in chronic venous disorders of the leg: development of a scientifically rigorous, patient-reported measure of symptoms and quality of life. *J Vasc Surg*. 2003;37:410–419.

25. Smith JJ, Garratt AM, Guest M, et al. Evaluating and improving health-related quality of life in patients with varicose veins. *J Vasc Surg*. 1999;30:710–719.

26. Revicki DA, Cella D, Hays RD, et al. Responsiveness and minimal important differences for patient reported outcomes. *Health Qual Life Outcomes*. 2006;4:e70–e74.

27. Maurins U, Hoffmann BH, Lösch C, et al. Distribution and prevalence of reflux in the superficial and deep venous system in the general population—results from the Bonn Vein Study, Germany. *J Vasc Surg*. 2008;48:680–687.

28. Padberg F. Regarding "Evaluating outcomes in chronic venous disorders of the leg: development of a scientifically rigorous, patient-reported measure of symptoms and quality of life." *J Vasc Surg*. 2003;37:911–912.

29. Kearon C, Akl E, Ornealas J, et al. Antithrombotic therapy for VTE disease. CHEST Guideline and Expert Panel Report. *Chest*. 2016;149(2):315–352.

30. Pannucci CJ, Swistun L, MacDonald JK, et al. Individualized venous thromboembolism risk stratification using the 2005 Caprini score to identify the benefits and harms of chemoprophylaxis in surgical patients. A meta-analysis. *Ann Surg*. 2017;265:1094–1103.

31. Kahn SR, Shbaklo H, Lamping DL, et al. Determinants of health-related quality of life during the 2 years following deep vein thrombosis. *J Thromb Haemost*. 2008;6:1105–1112.

32. Eberhardt RT, Raffetto JD. Chronic venous insufficiency. *Circulation*. 2005;111:2398–2409.

33. Vasquez MA, Munschauer CE. Venous Clinical Severity Score and quality-of-life assessment tools: application to vein practice. *Phlebology*. 2008;23:259–275.

34. Vasquez MA, Wang J, Mahathanaruk M, et al. The utility of the Venous Clinical Severity Score in 682 limbs treated by radiofrequency saphenous vein ablation. *J Vasc Surg*. 2007;45:1008–1015.

35. Gloviczki P, Comerota AJ, Dalsing MC, et al. The care of patients with varicose veins and associated chronic venous diseases: clinical practice guidelines of the Society for Vascular Surgery and the American Venous Forum. *J Vasc Surg*. 2011l;53:2S–48S.

36. O'Donnell TF Jr, Passman MA, Marston WA, et al. Management of venous leg ulcers: clinical practice guidelines of the Society for Vascular Surgery and the American Venous Forum. *J Vasc Surg*. 2014;60:3S–59S.

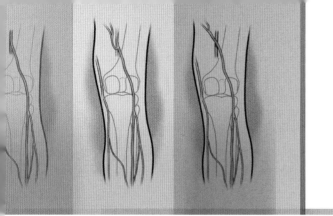

CHAPTER 27

Evidence-Based Summary of Guidelines From the Society for Vascular Surgery and the American Venous Forum

Peter Gloviczki, Monika Lecomte Gloviczki, and
Mark H. Meissner

Evidence-based medicine is best defined as "the conscientious, explicit, and judicious use of the current best evidence in making decisions about the care of individual patients."[1] Clinical practice guidelines evaluate the evidence in the scientific literature, assess the likely benefits and harms of a particular treatment, and aid the physicians to select the best care for the patient. The physician's clinical experience is important in this decision making and so are the patient's values and preferences. Cost of care and cost effectiveness have been playing an increasing role in deciding optimal and affordable medical care (Fig. 27.1). Assessment of rapidly increasing new technology is difficult because clinical studies with long-term efficacy are not available. It is important, however, that guidelines discuss approved emerging technologies and that patients are aware of any data on safety and early efficacy before they make a conscious decision.

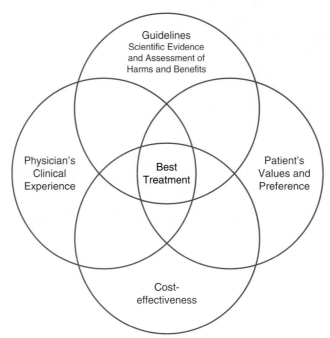

■ **Fig. 27.1** The optimal practice of evidence-based medicine.

THE EVIDENCE PYRAMID

The best evidence is usually provided by systematic reviews and meta-analyses of prospective randomized trials. Guidelines that adhere to accepted reporting standards and lack conflict of interest bring us the highest quality evidence on effectiveness of a therapy. Single prospective randomized trials, registry data, retrospective cohort studies, and case control studies are additional sources of evidence, although retrospective studies have limitations, and they provide a lower level of evidence. Case reports, editorials, and expert opinions as well as animal and in vitro research studies are at the bottom of the evidence pyramid, but even with very low level of evidence, they can support a treatment modality (Fig. 27.2). For high-quality evidence, the effects of therapy are precise, and further research is unlikely to change our confidence in the effect. In contrast, the estimated benefit provided by low-quality evidence may be unclear and subject to change as better-quality evidence becomes available.

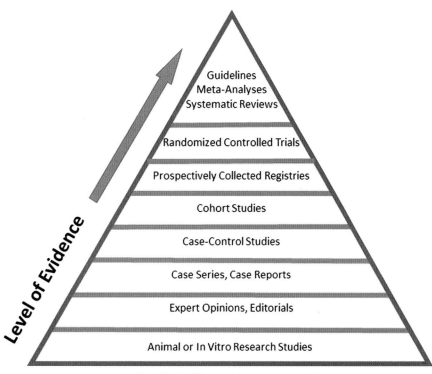

■ **Fig. 27.2** The evidence pyramid.

GRADING RECOMMENDATIONS AND EVIDENCE

Current approaches to the evaluation of clinical evidence are based largely on an assessment of the estimate of effect, beneficial or ill, associated with a treatment. The approach developed by the Grading of Recommendations, Assessment, Development, and Evaluation (GRADE) working group[2] has been adopted by the Society for Vascular Surgery (SVS) and the American Venous Forum in developing practice guidelines.[3] According to this system, there are two components to any treatment recommendation: the first a designation of the strength of the recommendation (1 = strong; 2 = weak) based upon the degree of confidence that the recommendation will do more good than harm; the second an evaluation of the strength of the evidence (A to D) based upon the confidence that the estimate of effect is correct (Table 27.1).

TABLE 27.1 GRADE Approach to Treatment Recommendations

Recommendation	Benefit Versus Risk	Quality of Evidence	Comment
1A	Clear	High: consistent results from RCTs or observational studies with large effects	Strong recommendation, generalizable
1B	Clear	Moderate: RCTs with limitations and very strong observational studies	Strong recommendation; may change with further research
1C	Clear	Low: observational studies Very low: case series, descriptive reports, expert opinion	Intermediate recommendation; likely to change with further research
2A	Balanced or unclear	High: consistent results from RCTs or observational studies with large effects	Intermediate recommendation: may vary with patient values
2B	Balanced or unclear	Moderate: RCTs with limitations and very strong observational studies	Weak recommendation; may vary with patient values
2C	Balanced or unclear	Low: observational studies Very low: case series, descriptive reports, expert opinion	Weak recommendation; alternative treatments may be equally valid

GRADE, Grading of recommendations, assessment, development, and evaluation; *RCTs,* randomized control trials.
Adapted from Guyatt G, Schunemann HJ, Cook D, et al. Applying the grades of recommendation for antithrombotic and thrombolytic therapy. *Chest.* 2004;126:179S–187S.

The strength of a recommendation (1 or 2) reflects the balance of benefits and risks, as well as cost to the health care system. Grade 1 recommendations are those in which the benefits of intervention clearly outweigh its risk and burdens. All well-informed patients would choose such a treatment, and the physician, often without a detailed knowledge of the underlying data, can securely recommend it. Grade 2 recommendations are weaker and reflect therapies in which the benefits and risks are either uncertain or more closely balanced. For such interventions, patients may choose different options based upon their underlying values. The SVS and the American Venous Forum have adopted the language of recommending the use of strong grade 1 guidelines and suggesting the use of weaker grade 2 guidelines.

The grade system is based on four levels (A to D) of methodologic quality (see Table 27.1), defined by the location of the evidence in the pyramid (see Fig. 27.2).[2] As mentioned earlier, studies on the top have high-quality, or grade A, evidence that usually comes from data of well-executed, randomized trials yielding consistent results and occasionally from large observational studies with significant effects. Moderate-quality evidence (grade B) frequently comes from randomized clinical trials with important limitations, registry data, and strong retrospective observational cohort studies. Low-quality to very low-quality evidence (grade C) includes most observational studies, cross-sectional or longitudinal, and experimental studies, located at the bottom of the pyramid (see Fig. 27.2). The term *best practice* has been adopted by expert panels to support treatments and procedures that have been used with success for years, but scientific evaluation has been sparse or not satisfactory to confirm significant benefit.

CLINICAL PRACTICE GUIDELINES ON VENOUS DISEASE

Evidence-based clinical practice guidelines of the SVS and the American Venous Forum (AVF) have been published in recent years on the care of patients with varicose veins and associated chronic venous diseases,[4] on the management of venous leg ulcers,[5] and on early thrombus removal strategies for the treatment of acute deep venous thrombosis (DVT).[6] Additional, major, national and international practice guidelines and reviews have also been published on prevention and treatment of acute venous thromboembolism[7] and chronic venous diseases,[8–12] and they all have been helpful to make decisions on how to evaluate and appropriately treat patients with venous diseases. These guidelines should be viewed as a summary of the best available clinical evidence to guide management of patients with chronic venous disease. However, consistent with the goals of evidence-based medicine, they are subject to the physician's clinical judgment, resources, and expertise and the patient's individual values and preferences. They should not be interpreted as a rigid standard of care.

This chapter summarizes the most important current guidelines on evaluation and management of patients with chronic venous disease adopted by our two major vascular societies, SVS and AVF. Details on evaluation and treatment are included in previous chapters of this book. For a list of the full venous guidelines of the SVS and the AVF, the readers should consult the original documents[4–6] and the recently published fourth edition of the Handbook of Venous and Lymphatic Disorders, which includes 300 of the latest evidence and consensus-based guidelines for the management of acute and chronic venous and lymphatic disorders.[13]

EVALUATION AND CLASSIFICATION

Evaluation of the patient with venous disease should include a thorough history, focusing on the underlying etiology (congenital, primary, or secondary), symptoms, and risk factors for venous disease. The degree of disability and effect on the patient's quality of life should also be assessed. Physical examination should focus on specific features of venous disease and exclusion of other etiologies of the patient's signs and symptoms. In clinical practice, every patient should be characterized using both the basic clinical, etiologic, anatomic pathophysiologic (CEAP) classification[14] (Table 27.2) and the Venous Clinical Severity Score (VCSS).[15]

Duplex ultrasonography, including an evaluation of reflux in the upright position, should be the initial diagnostic test in patients with suspected venous disease. Threshold values of greater than 500 ms are recommended for reflux in the saphenous, deep femoral, tibial, and perforating veins and greater than 1 second in the femoral and popliteal veins (see Table 27.2). Pathologic perforating veins should be differentiated from incompetent perforating veins. Pathologic perforating veins are those 3.5 mm or greater in diameter with outward flow of 500 ms or greater, located beneath an open or a healed venous ulcer defined by ultrasound (grade 1B).

Evaluation of patients with more advanced chronic venous insufficiency frequently includes additional physiologic and imaging studies, including computed tomography, magnetic resonance, or conventional contrast venography to delineate the underlying venous anatomy, pathology and plan therapy. For details of evaluation of these patients please consult Chapter 4.

TREATMENT

The treatment of varicose veins has rapidly evolved over the past several years, largely as a result of the advent of endovenous technologies. Current management options for symptomatic varicose veins include conservative management with compression hosiery and leg elevation, pharmacologic interventions, and superficial venous surgery. Substantial evidence has accumulated in recent years to support not only short-term or medium-term but also long-term effectiveness of many endovenous therapies.[16]

Treatment of more advanced, chronic venous insufficiency frequently includes additional drug therapies or interventions, such as local skin and ulcer care, and procedures to correct the underlying venous obstruction or valvular incompetence.

TABLE 27.2 Evaluation and Classification of Chronic Venous Disease

Guideline Number	Guideline	Grade of Recommendation (1: Strong; 2: Weak)	Grade of Evidence (A: High Quality; B: Moderate Quality; C: Low or Very Low Quality)
Classification			
1	We recommend using the CEAP (clinical, etiologic, anatomic, pathophysiologic) classification to describe chronic venous disorders	1	B
Evaluation with duplex ultrasound			
2	A cutoff value of 1 second is recommended to define reflux in the femoral and popliteal veins and of 500 ms for the great saphenous vein, the small saphenous vein, the tibial, deep femoral, and the perforating veins	1	B
3	We recommend that pathologic perforating veins include those with an outward flow of duration of ≥500 ms, with a diameter of ≥3.5 mm and a location beneath healed or open venous ulcers (CEAP class C5–C6).	1	B

Compression Therapy

Compression is considered first-line therapy for chronic venous disorders. For patients with simple varicose veins, the majority of comparative studies of compression stockings have evaluated surrogate hemodynamic parameters rather than patient-important outcomes, and it appears that stockings improve a variety of hemodynamic measurements.[17] However, the clinical benefits are less clear. Comparisons with placebo are very difficult but suggest some improvement in symptoms with the use of compression stockings. Definitive data regarding the optimal degree of compression are lacking. However, symptomatic improvement is clearly less than after surgical treatment of varicose veins,[18] and the authors of one systematic review concluded that the benefits of compression as a first-line treatment of varicose veins are limited.[17] Although 20 to 30 mm Hg compression stockings are suggested for patients with symptomatic varicose veins (grade 2C), all current guidelines recommend against their use as the primary treatment in patients who are candidates for superficial venous intervention (grade 1B, Table 27.3).[10,11,13]

For patients with open venous ulcers, compression stockings are recommended over surgery as the primary treatment.[19] A systematic review of 23 randomized and controlled clinical trials concluded that compression increases healing rates in comparison with no compression and that high compression is more efficacious than low compression.[20] However, it is not clear that there are substantial differences between the high compression alternatives. Compression therapy with superficial ablation was more effective to prevent ulcer recurrence than compression alone (see Table 27.3).[19]

Pharmacologic Therapy

Phlebotonic agents have been used to address many of the symptoms of chronic venous disorders, including leg pain, swelling, and pruritus. These include a heterogeneous group of plant extracts (rutosides, hidrosmine, diosmine, and others) as well as synthetic drugs with similar properties. A systematic review of 44 randomized, placebo-controlled trials evaluating oral phlebotonics suggested efficacy for some signs, such as edema, although the global evidence for their efficacy was insufficient to recommend routine use.[21] Although other preparations are available abroad, horse chestnut seed extract is the most studied preparation available in the United States. A systematic review of 17 randomized, controlled trials of horse chestnut seed extract suggests significant benefits with respect to leg pain, edema, and pruritus.[22] Two of these trials demonstrated similar improvements with horse chestnut seed extract and compression. Although the data are somewhat heterogeneous, and the consequences of long-term use are poorly documented, there is a suggestion that the venoactive drugs may have some benefit in patients with C2 to C3 disease (grade 2B, see Table 27.3).

There are few pharmacologic agents available for the treatment of C5–C6 disease, for those with healed or active venous ulcers. Pentoxifylline is available in the United States and it was found to be an effective adjunct to compression bandages for treating venous ulcers in a Cochrane review of 12 randomized trials involving 864 participants.[23] Randomized trials have similarly shown micronized purified flavonoid fraction, which is not available in the United States, to increase the odds of ulcer healing by 32% in comparison with compression and local wound care alone.[24] Despite the efficacy of theses pharmacologic adjuncts, they are probably indicated only for selected patients, with large or long-standing ulcers (grade 2B).

TABLE 27.3 Guidelines for Compression and Medical Therapy

Guideline Number	Guideline	Grade of Recommendation (1: Strong; 2: Weak)	Grade of Evidence (A: High Quality; B: Moderate Quality; C: Low or Very Low Quality)
Compression therapy			
4	We suggest compression therapy using moderate pressure (20–30 mm Hg) for patients with symptomatic varicose veins	2	C
5	We recommend against compression therapy as the primary treatment of symptomatic varicose veins in patients who are candidates for saphenous vein ablation	1	B
6	We recommend compression as the primary therapeutic modality for healing venous ulcers.	1	A
7	We recommend compression as an adjuvant treatment to superficial vein ablation for the prevention of ulcer recurrence.	1	A
Medical therapy			
8	We suggest venoactive drugs (diosmin, hesperidin, rutosides, sulodexide, micronized purified flavonoid fraction, or horse chestnut seed extract [aescin]) in addition to compression for patients with pain and swelling caused by chronic venous disease, in countries where these drugs are available	2	B
9	We suggest using pentoxifylline or micronized purified flavonoid fraction, if available, in combination with compression, to accelerate healing of venous ulcers	2	B

Surgical Management

The surgical management of varicose veins has evolved over the past century, with high ligation and stripping of the great saphenous vein being the standard approaches in past decades. High ligation alone fails to control reflux in a high proportion of patients. In comparison with high ligation alone, high ligation and stripping reduced the need for reoperation by two-thirds after 5 years of follow-up.[25] Surgical treatment of varicose veins has been shown to be more efficacious and cost effective than management with compression stockings. The randomized clinical trial, observational study, and assessment of cost-effectiveness of the treatment of varicose veins (REACTIV) trial[26] randomized 246 patients to conservative management (lifestyle advice and compression hosiery) versus surgery (saphenous ligation, stripping, and phlebectomy). There was significantly greater improvement in symptoms and quality of life in the surgical group and surgery was cost effective over a 10-year period. Notably 31% of patients did have some improvement in symptoms with compression hosiery alone, although 51.6% of patients assigned to conservative management crossed over to surgical treatment by the third year of follow-up. These data are supported by a Markov model demonstrating a variety of interventions for varicose veins, including surgical stripping, ultrasound-guided foam sclerotherapy, and endovenous thermal ablation (EVTA), to be more cost effective than conservative management.[27] Based upon this reasonably compelling evidence, interventions to ablate the incompetent superficial system, including surgery, EVTA, or foam sclerotherapy are recommended over compression stockings for symptomatic and fit patients with C2 to C3 disease (grade 1B, Table 27.4).

In patients with venous ulcers, the now classic randomized controlled ESCHAR (Effect of Surgery and Compression on Healing and Recurrence) trial confirmed the efficacy of surgery over compression therapy alone to prevent ulcer recurrence.[19] Some 500 patients with healed (C5) or open (C6) ulcers were randomized to compression, using a multilayer bandage for those with open ulcers, or surgery, which included great or small saphenous vein stripping and phlebectomy. Although there was no difference in 24-week healing rates, which were 65% in both arms, patients randomized to surgery had significantly lower 12-month recurrence rates (12% vs. 28%). These results were durable through 4 years of follow-up, at which point ulcer recurrence rates were significantly lower among patients randomized to compression plus surgery (31% vs. 56%).[19] After 3 years, patients randomized to surgery had 15 weeks more ulcer-free time than those receiving compression alone. Although superficial venous surgery did not improve ulcer healing rate compared with compression therapy alone (see Table 27.3), it can be considered a grade 1 recommendation for the prevention of ulcer recurrence, with moderate evidence B, considering the single, well-conducted, randomized control trial (RCT) that supports its benefit (see Table 27.4).

Endovenous Therapies

During the past 2 decades, an array of endovenous techniques have emerged and have largely replaced high ligation and stripping for the management of saphenous vein reflux.[16] These percutaneous, office-based procedures include radiofrequency ablation (RFA),[28,29] endovenous laser ablation (EVLA),[30] and ultrasound-guided foam sclerotherapy (UGFS).[31]

TABLE 27.4 Guidelines on Interventions

Guideline Number	Guideline	Grade of Recommendation (1: Strong; 2: Weak)	Grade of Evidence (A: High Quality; B: Moderate Quality; C: Low or Very Low Quality)
Surgical treatment of the incompetent saphenous vein			
10	For treatment of the incompetent saphenous vein in association with symptomatic varicose veins, we recommend saphenous vein ablation over compression therapy for appropriate candidates	1	B
11	For treatment of the incompetent great saphenous vein in association with symptomatic varicose veins, we suggest high ligation and inversion stripping of the saphenous vein to the level of the knee	2	B
12	For the treatment of the incompetent small saphenous vein associated with symptomatic various veins, we suggest high ligation at the knee-crease 3–5 cm distal to the saphenopopliteal junction and selective stripping of the vein	2	B
13	For prevention of venous ulcer recurrence, we recommend ablation of the incompetent superficial veins over compression therapy alone	1	B
Endovenous thermal ablation and ultrasound-guided foam sclerotherapy			
14	Endovenous thermal ablations (laser and radiofrequency ablations) and ultrasound-guided foam sclerotherapy are safe and effective, and we recommend them over surgery for treatment of saphenous incompetence	1	B
Emerging nonthermal nontumescent endovenous technologies (mechanical occlusion chemically assisted [MOCA], cyanoacrylate embolization [CAE], and V block assisted sclerotherapy [VBAS])			
15	We suggest MOCA for: • SSV incompetence with diameter < 10 mm • mildly tortuous GSV/SSV caused by steerable wire • BK GSV incompetence to the ankle for C2–C6 disease.	2	B
16	We suggest CAE for: • BK GSV incompetence • SSV incompetence	2	C
17	We suggest VBAS for AK GSV incompetence with diameter < 12 mm	2	C

AK, Above knee; *BK,* below knee; *GSV,* great saphenous vein; *SSV,* small saphenous vein.

Several RCTs showed early benefit of the percutaneous procedures over surgery causing less pain, less bruising, less wound complications, earlier return to work, and improvement in quality of life.[32–36] An RCT by Rasmussen et al. found that RFA and foam sclerotherapy were associated with the fastest recovery and had the least postoperative pain, although treatments with laser, radiofrequency, foam, and surgery were all efficacious.[35] Venous disease severity scores improved in all groups, supporting midterm benefit of all major vein ablation interventions.

Based largely on a systematic review of 12 RCTs,[36] two meta-analyses of a total of 30 RCTs,[37,38] and a Cochrane review,[39] all major guidelines recommend not only EVTA but also ultrasound-assisted foam sclerotherapy[40–44] over surgical ablation of the saphenous vein for the treatment of saphenous incompetence, a strong recommendation based on moderate quality of evidence.[4,11,45]

A recent report of the SVS/AVF coalition summarized evidence of both short-term and long-term effectiveness of EVTA.[16] Five-year data of RFA of the saphenous vein published by Proebstle et al.[29] confirmed sustained clinical and anatomic success for the vast majority of treated patients. Rasmussen et al. published 5-year follow-up of an RCT that compared EVLA (980 nm bare fiber) with high ligation and surgical stripping.[46] Data from this study demonstrated persistent and equivalent clinical and quality of life improvement at 5 years after both laser therapy and surgery and supported the fact that laser treatment is a valid alternative to open surgery.

Consensus-based recommendations of the AVF were recently published on cutting-edge, new technologies including the nonthermal nontumescent (NTNT) techniques. These include Mechanical Occlusion Chemically Assisted (MOCA) treatment, Cyanoacrylate Embolization (CAE) and V Block Assisted Sclerotherapy (VBAS). For the available literature and published efficacy of the NTNT techniques, the readers are referred to Chapter 8 of this atlas. Because long-term data on efficacy of NTNT treatments are not yet available, the recommendations are weak, and the evidence on efficacy is mostly at low or very low level (see Table 27.4). When choosing these treatments, patients must be made aware of the scant follow-up information that is available on these techniques.

Treatment of Varicose Vein Tributaries and Recurrent Varicose Veins

As discussed in detail in Chapter 10, for treatment of varicose vein tributaries our recommendation is to perform ambulatory mini phlebectomy as an outpatient procedure under local anesthesia, as an effective and definitive treatment for varicose veins. The procedure is performed after saphenous ablation, either during the same procedure or at a later stage (Table 27.5). Alternative, accepted treatments include power phlebectomy, thermal ablation, and foam and liquid sclerotherapy (see Chapter 10).

Treatment of recurrent varicose veins, after a thorough evaluation with duplex ultrasound, can be done with a combination of different techniques including ambulatory mini phlebectomy, foam or liquid sclerotherapy, or EVTA (see Table 27.5). We recommend against surgical reexploration of the saphenofemoral junction after previous high ligation and stripping and favor percutaneous techniques to minimize wound and lymphatic complications.

TABLE 27.5 Varicose Tributaries, Recurrent Varicose Veins and Perforating Veins

Guideline Number	Guideline	Grade of Recommendation (1: Strong; 2: Weak)	Grade of Evidence (A: High Quality; B: Moderate Quality; C: Low or Very Low Quality)
Varicose tributaries and recurrent varicose veins			
17	We recommend ambulatory mini phlebectomy, an outpatient procedure performed under local anesthesia, as an effective and definitive treatment for varicose veins; the procedure is performed after saphenous ablation, either during the same procedure or at a later stage	1	B
18	We suggest mini phlebectomy, foam sclerotherapy, or endovenous thermal ablation for recurrent varicose veins	2	B
Pathologic perforating veins (outward flow: >500 ms, diameter: >3.5 mm, located beneath healed or active ulcer)			
19	For open surgical treatment of incompetent pathologic perforating veins, we suggest against the modified open Linton procedure owing to associated morbidities	2	C
20	For those patients who would benefit from pathologic perforator vein ablation, we suggest treatment by percutaneous techniques over subfascial endoscopic perforator surgery (SEPS)	2	C
21	In a patient with advanced chronic venous insufficiency (C4b, C5, C6) and incompetent superficial veins in addition to pathologic perforating veins, we suggest ablation of both the incompetent superficial veins and perforator veins in addition to standard compressive therapy to aid ulcer healing and to prevent recurrence	2	C

Treatment of Pathologic Perforating Veins

Based on the currently available data, perforator interruption cannot be recommended in the treatment of C2 disease (grade 2B). However, the potential value of interruption of pathologic perforators (>3.5 mm, reflux ≥ 0.5 s, located near the ulcer bed) in C5–C6 disease cannot be excluded as detailed in Chapter 9, and it is suggested in appropriate patients with low level of evidence (grade 2C, see Table 27.5).

Treatment of Venous Obstruction

Symptomatic postthrombotic iliofemoral obstructions and nonthrombotic iliac vein lesions, such as a typical May-Thurner syndrome, caused by compression of the left common iliac vein by the overlying right common iliac artery, are frequently treated today with venous stents. A now classic study of Neglen et al. that included 982 patients confirmed primary and secondary 5-year stent patency rates of 57% and 86% for postthrombotic obstruction and 79% and 100% for symptomatic nonthrombotic iliac vein lesions.[47] A systematic review of iliac vein stenting analyzed data from 4959 patients and found lower patency rates with a wide range, but also noted that healing of venous ulcers occurred in 56% to 100% of the limbs in most patients after failure of conservative management. However, because of a lack of controlled prospective studies, the quality of evidence to support iliac vein stenting remains weak and a recent review by the Medicare Evidence Development and Coverage Advisory Committee (MEDCAC) panel scored the efficacy of venous stenting low.[16] Data of the completed and recently presented Acute Venous Thrombosis: Thrombus Removal With Adjunctive Catheter-Directed Thrombolysis (ATTRACT)[48] trial did not find significant difference in postthrombotic syndrome between those who were treated with conventional anticoagulation therapy versus those who had thrombolysis with or without iliac veins stenting. Thus results of additional prospective randomized studies, such as the Chronic Venous Thrombosis: Relief With Adjunctive Catheter-Directed Therapy (C-TRACT)[49] trial, are eagerly awaited. Based on overwhelmingly positive data of large cohort studies,[5,47,50] the guidelines of the SVS and the AVF suggest that stenting is safe, promising, and should be considered as an acceptable treatment for proximal venous obstruction, a strong recommendation with moderate level of evidence (grade 1B, Table 27.6). Open surgical bypass is rarely performed today, and it is reserved only for those symptomatic patients who are not candidates for or who failed endovascular treatment (grade 1B, see Table 27.6).[51]

CONCLUSION

Evidence-based clinical practice guidelines assist in recommending the best care to the patient, but they are not legal documents. Decisions on management should not be based on scientific data and cost of care alone but should incorporate the physician's personal experience and compassion and the well-informed patient's values and preferences.

TABLE 27.6 Treatment of Deep Vein Obstruction

Guideline Number	Guideline	Grade of Recommendation (1: Strong; 2: Weak)	Grade of Evidence (A: High Quality; B: Moderate Quality; C: Low or Very Low Quality)
Endovascular reconstruction for primary and postthrombotic iliac vein obstruction			
22	To alleviate pain and swelling and promote ulcer healing, we recommend venous stenting for treatment of primary iliac vein obstruction	1	B
23	To alleviate pain and swelling and promote ulcer healing, we recommend venous stenting for treatment of postthrombotic iliac vein obstruction	1	B
Open surgical treatment for iliac vein obstruction			
24	For patients who are not candidates for or have failed endovascular treatment, we suggest open surgical treatment using autologous vein as a suprapubic bypass (Palma procedure) or ePTFE for femorocaval or femorofemoral bypass in addition to standard compression therapy to aid severe venous claudication, venous leg ulcer healing, and to prevent ulcer recurrence	2	C

ePTFE, Expanded polytetrafluoroethylene.

REFERENCES

1. Sackett DL. Evidence-based medicine. *Spine.* 1998;23:1085–1086.
2. Guyatt G, Gutterman D, Baumann MH, et al. Grading strength of recommendations and quality of evidence in clinical guidelines: report from an American College of Chest Physicians task force. *Chest.* 2006;129:174–181.
3. Murad MH, Montori VM, Sidawy AN, et al. Guideline methodology of the Society for Vascular Surgery including the experience with the GRADE framework. *J Vasc Surg.* 2011;53:1375–1380.
4. Gloviczki P, Comerota AJ, Dalsing MC, et al. The care of patients with varicose veins and associated chronic venous diseases: clinical practice guidelines of the Society for Vascular Surgery and the American Venous Forum. *J Vasc Surg.* 2011;53:2S–48S.
5. O'Donnell TF Jr, Passman MA, Marston WA, et al. Management of venous leg ulcers: clinical practice guidelines of the Society for Vascular Surgery (R) and the American Venous Forum. *J Vasc Surg.* 2014;60:3S–59S.
6. Meissner MH, Gloviczki P, Comerota AJ, et al. Early thrombus removal strategies for acute deep venous thrombosis: clinical practice guidelines of the Society for Vascular Surgery and the American Venous Forum. *J Vasc Surg.* 2012;55:1449–1462.
7. Kearon C, Akl EA, Ornelas J, et al. Antithrombotic Therapy for VTE Disease: CHEST Guideline and Expert Panel Report. *Chest.* 2016;149:315–352.
8. Nicolaides AN, Allegra C, Bergan J, et al. Management of chronic venous disorders of the lower limbs: guidelines according to scientific evidence. *Int Angiol.* 2008;27:1–59.
9. Rabe E, Pannier F. Sclerotherapy of varicose veins with polidocanol based on the guidelines of the German Society of Phlebology. *Dermatol Surg.* 2010;36(suppl 2):968–975.
10. Varicose veins in the legs; 2013. The diagnosis and management of varicose veins. Clinical Guideline. Methods, evidence and recommendation. National Institute for Health and Care Excellence.
11. Wittens C, Davies AH, Baekgaard N, et al. Editor's choice—management of chronic venous disease: clinical practice guidelines of the European Society for Vascular Surgery (ESVS). *Eur J Vasc Endovasc Surg.* 2015;49:678–737.
12. Kahn SR, Galanaud JP, Vedantham S, et al. Guidance for the prevention and treatment of the post-thrombotic syndrome. *J Thromb Thrombolysis.* 2016;41:144–153.
13. Gloviczki P. Handbook of Venous and Lymphatic Disorders: Guidelines of the American Venous Forum. 4th ed. London: CRC Press, Taylor&Francis Group; 2017.
14. Eklof B, Rutherford RB, Bergan JJ, et al. Revision of the CEAP classification for chronic venous disorders: consensus statement. *J Vasc Surg.* 2004;40:1248–1252.
15. Vasquez Michael A, Eberhard R, Robert BM, et al. Revision of the venous clinical severity score: venous outcomes consensus statement: special communication of the American Venous Forum Ad Hoc Outcomes Working Group. *J Vasc Surg.* 2010;52:1387–1396.
16. Gloviczki P, Dalsing MC, Henke P, et al. Report of the Society for Vascular Surgery and the American Venous Forum on the July 20, 2016 meeting of the Medicare Evidence Development and Coverage Advisory Committee panel on lower extremity chronic venous disease. *J Vasc Surg Venous Lymphat Disord.* 2017;5:378–398.
17. Palfreyman SJ, Michaels JA. A systematic review of compression hosiery for uncomplicated varicose veins. *Phlebology.* 2009;24(suppl 1):13–33.
18. Michaels JA, Campbell WB, Brazier JE, et al. Randomised clinical trial, observational study and assessment of cost-effectiveness of the treatment of varicose veins (REACTIV trial). *Health Technol Assess.* 2006;10:1–196.
19. Gohel MS, Barwell JR, Taylor M, et al. Long term results of compression therapy alone versus compression plus surgery in chronic venous ulceration (ESCHAR): randomised controlled trial. *BMJ.* 2007;335:83.
20. Cullum N, Nelson EA, Fletcher AW, et al. Compression for venous leg ulcers. *Cochrane Database Syst Rev.* 2001;(2):CD000265.

21. Martinez MJ, Bonfill X, Moreno RM, et al. Phlebotonics for venous insufficiency. *Cochrane Database Syst Rev.* 2005;(3):CD003229.

22. Pittler MH, Ernst E. Horse chestnut seed extract for chronic venous insufficiency. *Cochrane Database Syst Rev.* 2006;(1):CD003230.

23. Jull AB, Arroll B, Parag V, et al. Pentoxifylline for treating venous leg ulcers. *Cochrane Database Syst Rev.* 2012;(12):CD001733.

24. Meissner MH, Eklof B, Smith PC, et al. Secondary chronic venous disorders. *J Vasc Surg.* 2007;46(supplS):68S–83S.

25. Dwerryhouse S, Davies B, Harradine K, et al. Stripping the long saphenous vein reduces the rate of reoperation for recurrent varicose veins: five-year results of a randomized trial. *J Vasc Surg.* 1999;29:589–592.

26. Michaels JA, Brazier JE, Campbell WB, et al. Randomized clinical trial comparing surgery with conservative treatment for uncomplicated varicose veins. *Br J Surg.* 2006;93:175–181.

27. Gohel MS, Epstein DM, Davies AH. Cost-effectiveness of traditional and endovenous treatments for varicose veins. *Br J Surg.* 2010;97:1815–1823.

28. Merchant RF, Pichot O. Long-term outcomes of endovenous radiofrequency obliteration of saphenous reflux as a treatment for superficial venous insufficiency. *J Vasc Surg.* 2005;42:502–509.

29. Proebstle TM, Alm BJ, Gockeritz O, et al. Five-year results from the prospective European multicentre cohort study on radiofrequency segmental thermal ablation for incompetent great saphenous veins. *Br J Surg.* 2015;102:212–218.

30. Min RJ, Khilnani N, Zimmet SE. Endovenous laser treatment of saphenous vein reflux: long-term results. *J Vasc Interv Radiol.* 2003;14:991–996.

31. Rabe E, Otto J, Schliephake D, et al. Efficacy and safety of great saphenous vein sclerotherapy using standardised polidocanol foam (ESAF): a randomised controlled multicentre clinical trial. *Eur J Vasc Endovasc Surg.* 2008;35:238–245.

32. Lurie F, Creton D, Eklof B, et al. Prospective randomized study of endovenous radiofrequency obliteration (closure procedure) versus ligation and stripping in a selected patient population (EVOLVeS Study). *J Vasc Surg.* 2003;38:207–214.

33. Rautio T, Ohinmaa A, Perala J, et al. Endovenous obliteration versus conventional stripping operation in the treatment of primary varicose veins: a randomized controlled trial with comparison of the costs. *J Vasc Surg.* 2002;35:958–965.

34. Hinchliffe RJ, Ubhi J, Beech A, et al. A prospective randomised controlled trial of VNUS closure versus surgery for the treatment of recurrent long saphenous varicose veins. *Eur J Vasc Endovasc Surg.* 2006;31:212–218.

35. Rasmussen LH, Lawaetz M, Bjoern L, et al. Randomized clinical trial comparing endovenous laser ablation, radiofrequency ablation, foam sclerotherapy and surgical stripping for great saphenous varicose veins. *Br J Surg.* 2011;98:1079–1087.

36. Eklof B, Perrin M. Review of randomized trials comparing endovenous thermal and chemical ablation. *Rev Vasc Med.* 2014;2:1–12.

37. Siribumrungwong B, Noorit P, Wilasrusmee C, et al. A systematic review and meta-analysis of randomised controlled trials comparing endovenous ablation and surgical intervention in patients with varicose vein. *Eur J Vasc Endovasc Surg.* 2012;44:214–223.

38. Murad MH, Coto-Yglesias F, Zumaeta-Garcia M, et al. A systematic review and meta-analysis of the treatments of varicose veins. *J Vasc Surg.* 2011;53:49S–65S.

39. Nesbitt C, Bedenis R, Bhattacharya V, et al. Endovenous ablation (radiofrequency and laser) and foam sclerotherapy versus open surgery for great saphenous vein varices. *Cochrane Database Syst Rev.* 2014;(7):CD005624.

40. Lattimer CR, Azzam M, Kalodiki E, et al. Cost and effectiveness of laser with phlebectomies compared with foam sclerotherapy in superficial venous insufficiency. Early results of a randomised controlled trial. *Eur J Vasc Endovasc Surg.* 2012;43:594–600.

41. Rasmussen L, Lawaetz M, Serup J, et al. Randomized clinical trial comparing endovenous laser ablation, radiofrequency ablation, foam sclerotherapy, and surgical stripping for great saphenous varicose veins with 3-year follow-up. *J Vasc Surg Venous Lymphat Disord.* 2013;1:349–356.

42. Biemans AA, Kockaert M, Akkersdijk GP, et al. Comparing endovenous laser ablation, foam sclerotherapy, and conventional surgery for great saphenous varicose veins. *J Vasc Surg.* 2013;58:727–734 e1.

43. Brittenden J, Cotton SC, Elders A, et al. A randomized trial comparing treatments for varicose veins. *N Engl J Med.* 2014;371:1218–1227.

44. Davies HO, Popplewell M, Darvall K, et al. A review of randomised controlled trials comparing ultrasound-guided foam sclerotherapy with endothermal ablation for the treatment of great saphenous varicose veins. *Phlebology.* 2016;31:234–240.

45. Varicose Veins in the Legs: The Diagnosis and Management of Varicose Veins; 2013. London: National Clinical Guideline Centre (July 2013).

46. Rasmussen L, Lawaetz M, Bjoern L, et al. Randomized clinical trial comparing endovenous laser ablation and stripping of the great saphenous vein with clinical and duplex outcome after 5 years. *J Vasc Surg.* 2013;58:421–426.

47. Neglen P, Hollis KC, Olivier J, et al. Stenting of the venous outflow in chronic venous disease: long-term stent-related outcome, clinical, and hemodynamic result. *J Vasc Surg.* 2007;46:979–990.

48. Vedantham S, Goldhaber SZ, Kahn SR, et al. Rationale and design of the ATTRACT Study: a multicenter randomized trial to evaluate pharmacomechanical catheter-directed thrombolysis for the prevention of postthrombotic syndrome in patients with proximal deep vein thrombosis. *Am Heart J.* 2013;165:523–530 e3.

49. Vedantham S. C-TRACT: what we've learned about DVT trial design. *Endovasc Today.* 2016;15:56–57.

50. Murphy E, Johns B, Varney E, et al. Deep venous thrombosis associated with caval extension of iliac stents. *J Vasc Surg Venous Lymphat Disord.* 2017;5.

51. Garg N, Gloviczki P, Karimi KM, et al. Factors affecting outcome of open and hybrid reconstructions for nonmalignant obstruction of iliofemoral veins and inferior vena cava. *J Vasc Surg.* 2011;53:383–393.

INDEX

Page numbers followed by *b* indicate boxes; *f*, figures; *t*, tables.